Diagnosis, Prevention and Treatment of Periodontitis

Diagnosis, Prevention and Treatment of Periodontitis

Editor: Joel Turner

FOSTER ACADEMICS
www.fosteracademics.com

www.fosteracademics.com

FOSTER ACADEMICS

Cataloging-in-Publication Data

Diagnosis, prevention and treatment of periodontitis / edited by Joel Turner.
p. cm.
Includes bibliographical references and index.
ISBN 978-1-63242-615-4
1. Periodontitis. 2. Periodontitis--Diagnosis. 3. Periodontitis--Treatment.
4. Periodontitis--Prevention. I. Turner, Joel.
RK450.P4 D53 2019
617.632--dc23

Foster Academics,
118-35 Queens Blvd., Suite 400,
Forest Hills, NY 11375, USA

ISBN 978-1-63242-615-4 (Hardback)

Printed and bound in China.

Contents

Preface

The main aim of this book is to educate learners and enhance their research focus by presenting diverse topics covering this vast field. This is an advanced book which compiles significant studies by distinguished experts in the area of analysis. This book addresses successive solutions to the challenges arising in the area of application, along with it; the book provides scope for future developments.

Periodontitis is a common medical condition. It is known as gingivitis in its early stage, which is characterized by swollen and bleeding gums. In its advanced stage, it leads to the inflammation of the periodontium. Ineffective oral hygiene may result in the accumulation of a bacterial and mycotic matrix on the gum line. This is known as dental plaque. It is the most common cause of periodontitis. Some ways to prevent periodontitis include following a healthy oral health regime including proper brushing and daily flossing, using an antiseptic mouthwash, regular dental check-ups, etc. The treatment methods of periodontitis include nonsurgical scaling and root planing, antibiotics and surgery in severe cases. This book elucidates the concepts and innovative models around prospective developments with respect to the diagnosis, prevention and treatment of periodontitis. It is a vital tool for all researching or studying dentistry.

It was a great honour to edit this book, though there were challenges, as it involved a lot of communication and networking between me and the editorial team. However, the end result was this all-inclusive book covering diverse themes in the field.

Finally, it is important to acknowledge the efforts of the contributors for their excellent chapters, through which a wide variety of issues have been addressed. I would also like to thank my colleagues for their valuable feedback during the making of this book.

Editor

The Novel Role of HtrA1 in Gingivitis, Chronic and Aggressive Periodontitis

Teresa Lorenzi[1*¶], Elena Annabel Niţulescu[2¶], Antonio Zizzi[3], Maria Lorenzi[1], Francesca Paolinelli[1], Simone Domenico Aspriello[4], Monica Baniţă[2], Ştefania Crăiţoiu[2], Gaia Goteri[3], Giorgio Barbatelli[1], Tommaso Lombardi[5], Roberto Di Felice[6], Daniela Marzioni[1*], Corrado Rubini[3], Mario Castellucci[1]

1 Department of Experimental and Clinical Medicine, Università Politecnica delle Marche, Ancona, Italy, **2** Department of Histology, University of Medicine and Pharmacy of Craiova, Craiova, Romania, **3** Pathological Anatomy, Department of Medical Sciences and Public Health, Università Politecnica delle Marche, United Hospitals, Ancona, Italy, **4** Department of Clinical Specialistic and Dental Sciences, Periodontology, Università Politecnica delle Marche, Ancona, Italy, **5** Laboratory of Oral and Maxillofacial Pathology, Division of Stomatology and Oral Surgery, University of Geneva, Geneva, Switzerland, **6** Private Dental Practice, San Benedetto del Tronto, Ascoli Piceno, Italy

Abstract

Proteolytic tissue degradation is a typical phenomenon in inflammatory periodontal diseases. HtrA1 (High temperature requirement A 1) has a serine protease activity and is able to degrade fibronectin whose fragments induce the expression and secretion of several matrix metalloproteinases (MMPs). The aim of this study was to investigate for the first time if HtrA1 has a role in gingivitis and in generalized forms of chronic and aggressive periodontitis. Expression of HtrA1 was investigated in 16 clinically healthy gingiva, 16 gingivitis, 14 generalized chronic periodontitis and 10 generalized aggressive periodontitis by immunohistochemistry and real-time PCR. Statistical comparisons were performed by the Kruskall-Wallis test. Significantly higher levels of HtrA1 mRNA and protein expression were observed in pathological respect to healthy tissues. In particular, we detected an increase of plasma cell HtrA1 immunostaining from gingivitis to chronic and aggressive periodontitis, with the higher intensity in aggressive disease. In addition, we observed the presence of HtrA1 in normal and pathological epithelium, with an increased expression, particularly in its superficial layer, associated with increasingly severe forms of periodontal disease. We can affirm that HtrA1 expression in plasma cells could be correlated with the destruction of pathological periodontal tissue, probably due to its ability to trigger the overproduction of MMPs and to increase the inflammatory mediators TNF-α and IL-1β by inhibition of TGF-β. Moreover, epithelial HtrA1 immunostaining suggests a participation of the molecule in the host inflammatory immune responses necessary for the control of periodontal infection.

Editor: Jens Kreth, University of Oklahoma Health Sciences Center, United States of America

Funding: This work was funded by Università Politecnica delle Marche with grants to G. G., G.B., D.M., C.R., M.C. EAN was supported by a fellowship from European Union - AM POS-DRU project with title "Supporting young people through PhD doctoral scholarships " ID –7603. The funders had no role in study design, data collection and analysis, decision to publish, or preparation of the manuscript.

Competing Interests: The authors have declared that no competing interests exist.

* Email: teresalorenzi@yahoo.it (TL); d.marzioni@univpm.it (DM)

¶ These authors contributed equally to this work.

Introduction

Periodontal diseases are characterized by an immune response to antigens in bacterial plaque as well as by alterations in connective tissue and morphological changes in the epithelium. This response is always clinically evidenced as gingivitis or periodontitis [1,2]. Gingivitis, a reversible inflammatory lesion, is the initial stage of gingival disease and the easiest to treat [3]. On the contrary, the periodontitis are characterized by the chronic activation of the immune system, alterations in connective tissue metabolism, production of cytokines and proteinases as well as the direct destruction of hard and soft tissue structures which support teeth by bacterial enzymes and virulence factors [3]. Among all the forms of periodontitis, chronic and aggressive periodontitis have received considerable attention due to their peculiar clinical presentation [4].

Interestingly, matrix metalloproteinases (MMPs) produced by immunoregulatory cells and fibroblasts play a destructive role in the inflammatory periodontal lesion progression [5]. It has been proposed that the expression and secretion of several MMPs are enhanced by fragments coming from the degradation of fibronectin [6,7]. This extracellular matrix glycoprotein is a natural substrate of HtrA1 (High temperature requirement A 1), a member of the family of HtrA proteins with serine protease activity [8]. HtrA1 is a secreted multidomain protein and it is characterized by the presence of a highly conserved trypsin-like serine protease domain and at least one protein interaction PDZ (PSD-95 (Postsynaptic density protein of Mr 95 kDa), Dlg (Drosophila Discs-Large protein) and ZO-1 (Zonula occludens protein 1)) domain [9] It also contains insulin-like growth factor-binding protein/follistatin/Mac25-like domain and a Kazal-type serine protease inhibitor motif at its N-terminus [9]. Serine protease HtrA1 is implicated in physiologic processes, such as the inhibition of TGF-β signalling [10], and in the pathogenesis of various diseases, including osteoarthritis, Alzheimer's disease and preeclampsia [7,8,11]. Since HtrA1 plays a role in extracellular matrix degradation acting directly by proteolytic cleavage of matrix protein components [12], or indirectly through HtrA1 ability to stimulate the overproduction of MMPs [7], we hypothesized an important role for HtrA1 in the onset of tissue destruction characterizing inflammatory periodontal diseases.

The aim of this study was to examine, for the first time, the profile of HtrA1 protein and mRNA expression by immunohistochemistry and real-time PCR, respectively, in gingivitis and in generalized forms of chronic and aggressive periodontitis, compared to clinically healthy gingiva. Our findings highlight a correlation of plasma cell HtrA1 expression with the occurrence of periodontal diseases and a possible contribution of epithelial HtrA1 to the control of periodontal infection.

Materials and Methods

Ethics statement

The experimental protocol was approved by the Ethics Committee of Università Politecnica delle Marche for human subjects and the study was conducted in accordance with the Helsinki Declaration of 1975, as revised in 2000. Written informed consent was granted from patients and parents on the behalf of the minors/children participants prior to inclusion in this study and recorded on file.

Individuals and Gingival Tissue Samples

The clinical and periodontal parameters of subjects were assessed by a single examiner (S.D.A.), as previously described [13]. A University of North Carolina (UNC)-15 calibrated periodontal probe (15 mm, probe tip diameter = 0.5 mm) (Hu Friedy, Chicago, IL, USA) was used for all the measurements.

Gingival tissue samples from 16 clinically healthy gingiva and 16 gingivitis (Table 1) were obtained from premolars of individuals not affected by periodontitis and showing no supporting tissue destruction, collected from sites requiring dental extraction for orthodontic treatment. Furthermore, 24 gingival specimens were collected from premolars of adults with periodontitis (14 generalized chronic periodontitis and 10 generalized aggressive periodontitis) (Table 1) during routine periodontal flap surgery after the initial phase of periodontal therapy, consisting of scaling and root planing. The clinical diagnosis of generalized chronic periodontitis was based on the presence of up to 30% of measured sites with clinical attachment loss (CAL) >5 mm [14]. The clinical diagnosis of generalized aggressive periodontitis was made in patients, aged between 18 and 40 years, showing an attachment loss greater than 6 mm affecting at least three permanent teeth other than the first molars and incisors [14]. In all the cases the histological framework was coherent with the clinical diagnosis.

The periodontal parameters (gingival index, probing depth and sulcus bleeding index) [13], were assessed at six different sites around each tooth (mesio-buccal, mid-buccal, disto-buccal, mesio-lingual, mid-lingual and disto-lingual). All the teeth enrolled in the study had homogeneous clinical parameters on all the six sites analyzed. The clinical status related to gingival biopsy sites is shown in Table 1.

None of the study participants: (i) had systemic diseases (endocrine disorders, immunodepression, diabetes), (ii) had used antibiotics, corticosteroids or non-steroidal anti-inflammatory drugs within the preceding 6 months, (iii) smoked or (iv) had used calcium channel-blockers, cyclosporine A, phenytoin, or any other drugs associated with gingival hyperplasia. Moreover, subjects who have undergone periodontal treatment within the previous 2 years were discarded.

From each subject, we obtained gingival tissue biopsies (n = 2) containing oral epithelium and subepithelial soft tissues, with a cubic shape of approximately 3 mm in length. In addition, first trimester placental tissue was used as positive control for real-time PCR [15], and for immunohistochemistry techniques [16], because it expresses both HtrA1 mRNA and protein.

For immunohistochemical analysis, specimens were fixed for 24 hours in 4% neutral buffered formalin at 4°C, and then embedded in paraffin. For molecular (real time-PCR) analysis, tissues were immediately frozen in liquid nitrogen and stored at −80°C.

Immunohistochemistry

3-μm paraffin-embedded tissue sections were deparaffinised and incubated for 60 min with 3% hydrogen peroxide in deionised water to inhibit endogenous peroxidase activity. Sections were washed in 50 mM Tris/HCl, pH 7.6 and pre-treated for 10 min at 98°C in 10 mM sodium citrate, pH 6.0. After blocking non-specific background for 1 hr at room temperature (RT) with Tris/HCl-6% non fat dry milk (Bio-Rad Laboratories, Milan, Italy), sections were incubated overnight at 4°C with rabbit polyclonal anti-human HtrA1 antibody (Abcam, Cambridge, UK), diluted 1:100 in Tris/HCl-3% non-fat dry milk. After washing in Tris/HCl, the sections were incubated for 1 hr at RT with goat anti-rabbit biotinylated antibody (Vector Laboratories, Burlingame, CA), diluted 1:200 in Tris/HCl-3% non fat dry milk. The peroxidase ABC method (Vector Laboratories) was applied for 1 hr at RT using 3′, 3′ diaminobenzidine hydrochloride (Sigma Chemical Co, St Louis, MO, USA) as the chromogen. Sections were counterstained in Mayer's haematoxylin, dehydrated and mounted with Eukitt solution (Kindler GmbH and Co., Freiburg, Germany). Negative controls were performed for gingival and placental tissues by omitting the primary or the secondary

Table 1. Clinical profile of gingival biopsy sites.

Individuals	N	Age (years) mean ± SD* range	Male	Gingival Index (mean ± SD)	Probing depth (mm) (mean ± SD)	Sulcus Bleeding Index (mean ± SD)
Healthy	16	23.87±5.53 17–35	8	0	2.50±0.43	0
Gingivitis	16	37±9.39 23–51	8	1.87±0.33	3.05±0.60	2.65±0.48
Chronic Periodontitis	14	47.25±5.52 42–57	6	2±0.70	6.87±0.78	4.12±0.60
Aggressive Periodontitis	10	25±4.55 20–35	5	2.12±0.78	7.37±1.11	4.62±0.48

*SD: Standard Deviation.

Table 2. Characteristics of the primers used for SYBR green Q-PCR assays.

Target gene	Primer*	Primer sequence (5′-3′)	Tm (°C)†	%GC	Amplicon length (bp)	Accession no.
Human HtrA1	hHTRA1_F hHTRA1_R	GGAAGATGGACTGATCGTGA CATAGTTGATGATGGCGTCG	57.3 57.3	50 50	347	NM_002775
Human SDHA	hSDHA_F hSDHA_R	AGCATCGAAGAGTCATGCAG TCAATCCGCACCTTGTAGTC	57.3 57.3	50 50	398	NM_004168

*Letters F and R after the primer name indicate forward and reverse orientation, respectively.
†Theoretical melting temperature (*Tm*) calculated using the MWG Oligo Property Scan (MOPS).

antibody. An isotype control antibody (Rabbit IgG, cat. n° I-100, Vector Laboratories, diluted 1:150) was used as a further negative control. The negative controls confirmed the specificity of the immunolabelling obtained with the primary antibody.

Two investigators evaluated simultaneously the cytoplasmic HtrA1 immunoreactivity in the more representative fields using images of the histological sections captured with a digital system. For this purpose, each field with area of 0.22 mm^2 was captured with a camera coupled to the light microscope and to a computer for digitalization of the image (Nikon Spa, Firenze, Italy). HtrA1 protein staining was classified with a five-point scale and was assigned a number value to each point: negative (− = 0), slight (+/− = 1), faint (+ = 2), moderate (++ = 3) and strong (+++ = 4). The evaluation of HtrA1 immunoreactivity provided by the two examiners was similar.

Preparation of cDNA for Q-PCR

Total RNA was extracted from frozen tissues (10 mg) using the Total RNA purification kit (Norgen, Biotek Corp., Thorold, Ontario, Canada), and then cleaned up and concentrated using the CleanAll RNA/DNA Clean-Up and Concentration Kit (Norgen), according to the manufacturer's instructions. The quality (A_{260}/A_{280}) and quantity (A_{260}) of extracted RNA were tested by a NanoDrop ND-1000 UV-Vis Spectrophotometer (Celbio, Milan, Italy). The integrity of the isolated RNA was checked by 1.5% denaturating agarose gel. 1 µg of RNA was reverse transcribed by the high-capacity cDNA RT kit (Applied Biosystems, Foster City, CA) using random primers.

Real-time PCR (Q-PCR) analysis

The sequences of the Q-PCR primers targeting HtrA1 gene are reported in Table 2. The reference gene SDHA (Succinate Dehydrogenase Complex Subunit A) was used as housekeeping gene for data normalization in order to correct for variations in RNA quality and quantity.

Real-time PCR was performed in a reaction mixture containing 10 µl of 2X iQ SYBR Green Supermix (Bio-Rad Laboratories), 0.1 µM of each primer, 0, 3 ng of sample template and RNase-

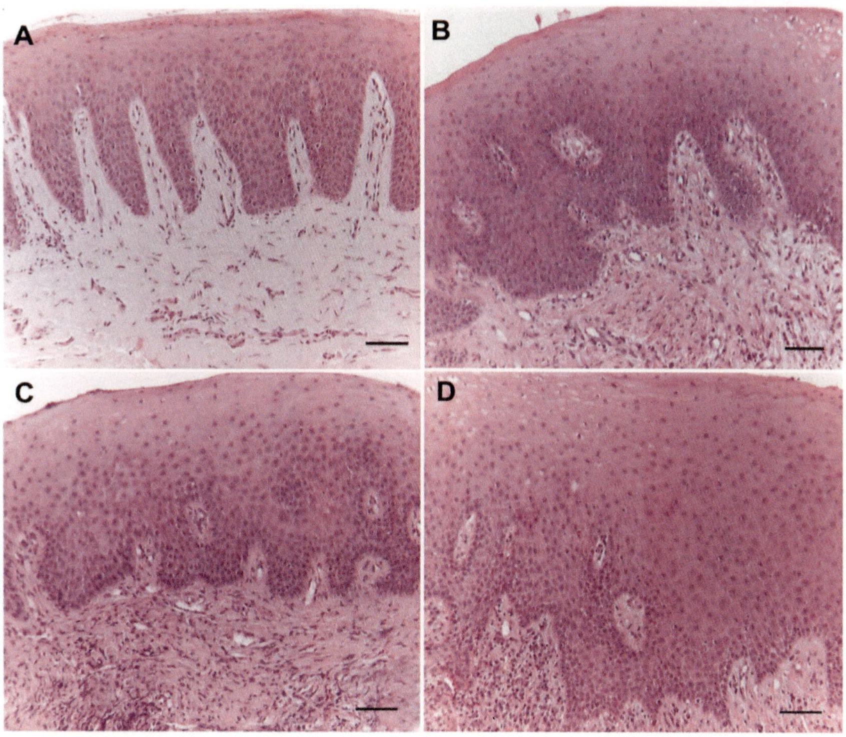

Figure 1. Haematoxylin and Eosin staining of periodontal tissues. A) healthy gingiva; **B)** gingivitis tissue; **C)** chronic periodontitis tissue; **D)** aggressive periodontitis tissue. Original magnification: 200x; scale bar: 50 µm.

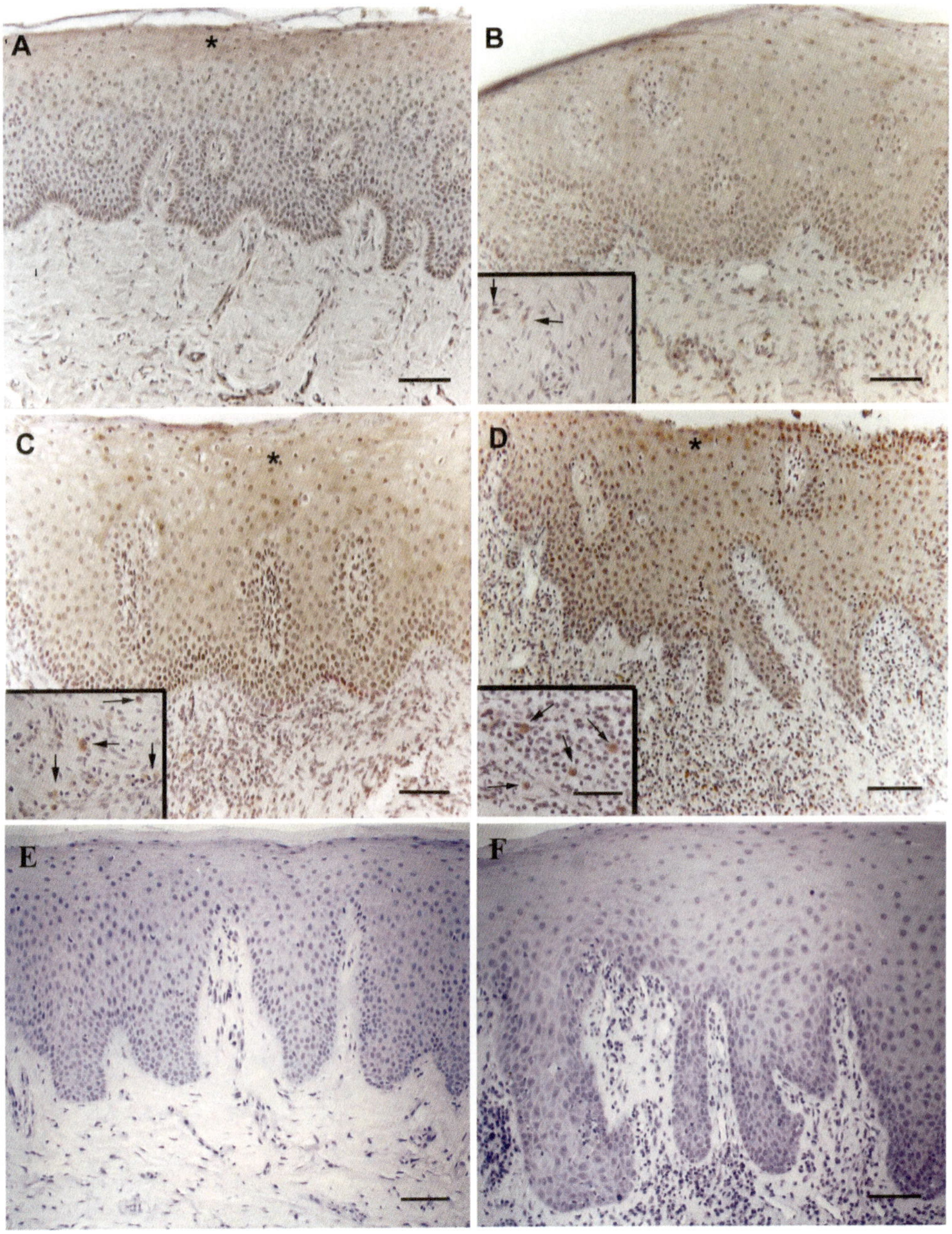

Figure 2. Expression of HtrA1, assessed by immunohistochemistry, in periodontal tissues. A) healthy gingiva; **B)** gingivitis tissue; **C)** chronic periodontitis tissue; **D)** aggressive periodontitis tissue. Negative control for healthy and aggressive periodontitis tissue is shown in panels **E)** and **F)**, respectively. Insets show the plasma cells positive to HtrA1 (arrows). The asterisk indicate the layer with the strongest HtrA1 immunostaining. Original magnification: 200x; scale bar: 50 μm. Original magnification of insets: 400x; scale bar: 25 μm.

free sterile water to a final volume of 20 μl. Amplification was performed using the iQ5 Multicolor Real-Time PCR Detection System (Bio-Rad Laboratories) using the following program: (i) an initial denaturing step at 95°C for 15 min.; (ii) 45 cycles, with 1 cycle consisting of denaturation at 95°C for 10 s, annealing at 60°C for 30 s and extension at 72°C for 30 s. Q-PCR assays with CT values over 40 were considered negative. For each PCR run, a negative (no-template) control and a minus-reverse transcriptase ("-RT") control were used to test for false-positive results or DNA contamination, respectively. The absence of non-specific products or primer dimers was confirmed by observation of a single melting peak in a melting curve analysis. For each Q-PCR, the genes were run in duplicate and all samples were tested in three separate experiments. In addition, the standard curve for each gene was constructed using serial dilutions of the cDNA obtained from the first trimester placenta (positive control).

Since PCR efficiencies were found to be close to 100%, the $2^{-\Delta\Delta C_t}$ (Livak) method was applied to compare data from gingivitis and chronic/aggressive periodontitis to the healthy gingival tissues (reference group). The results were obtained as "fold changes" in relative gene expression of tissues affected by the periodontal diseases respect to the reference ones.

Table 3. Immunohistochemical staining for HtrA1 in studied groups.

	HEALTHY	GINGIVITIS	CHRONIC PERIODONTITIS	AGGRESSIVE PERIODONTITIS
EPITHELIUM				
Superficial	+	+	++	+++
Intermediate	+/−	+	+	++
Parabasal	−	+	+	++
Basal	+/−	+	+	++
DERMIS				
Collagen fibers	−	−	−	−
Fibroblasts	−	+	−	−
Plasma cells	/	+	++	+++
VESSELS	+	+	+	+

Statistical analysis

A Kruskall-Wallis test was performed for evaluating RT-PCR and immunohistochemical differences between groups. A level of probability of 0.05 was used to assess the statistical significance. Statistical analyses were performed using the SPSS 16 package (SPSS Inc., Chicago, IL, USA). Data were expressed as median and 1st–3rd quartiles.

Results

Histopathological features

Healthy gingival mucosa showed parakeratinized stratified squamous epithelium (Fig. 1A) and papillomatosis with rete pegs and connective tissue papillae. The connective tissue (or corium) was fibrous with some fibroblasts and low inflammatory cell infiltration, mainly in the marginal gingival zone (Fig. 1A).

Gingivitis specimens showed connective tissue with high vascularization and variable inflammatory cell infiltrates (Fig. 1B). At higher magnification we observed some plasma cells, indicating focal stimulation of the humoral immune system, but macrophages, neutrophils and lymphocytes were also present (data not shown). Epithelium was acanthotic and parakeratinized (Fig. 1B).

Chronic (Fig. 1C) or aggressive (Fig. 1D) periodontitis exhibited an epithelium lining the pockets that varies in thickness and sometimes was hyperplastic and acanthotic. In the underlying corium, a high vascularization and a high-grade inflammatory infiltrate were present, consisting mainly of lymphocytes, macrophages and plasma cells in varying proportions (data not shown).

HtrA1 immunohistochemistry

HtrA1 showed a *cytoplasmic* staining. First trimester placental tissue (positive control) was positive for HtrA1 (data not shown). Healthy gingival tissues (Fig. 2A) revealed a gradual increase in HtrA1 immunoreactivity from the basal to the superficial layer of epithelium (Table 3). In gingivitis sections (Fig. 2B), HtrA1 positivity resulted uniformly distributed in all layers (Table 3). In chronic (Fig. 2C) and aggressive (Fig. 2D) periodontitis we observed HtrA1 immunostaining in the whole thickness of the epithelium, but with a stronger intensity in the superficial layer (Table 3). In addition, aggressive periodontitis showed a more evident HtrA1 positivity in all layers than chronic periodontitis (Table 3). Our results demonstrated an increase of HtrA1 immunostaining in epithelium, particularly in its superficial layer, associated with increasingly severe forms of pathology (Table 3, Fig. 2). In addition, parakeratotic layer showed a negative HtrA1 reactivity in all studied groups (Fig. 2). Thus, the whole epithelium showed a significant increase of HtrA1 expression in chronic ($p = 0.037$) and aggressive ($p < 0.001$) periodontitis compared to healthy subjects (Fig. 3A). In the corium of inflamed gingival tissue, HtrA1 was mainly expressed in plasma cells (Table 3, Figs. 2-insets, 3B). Gingivitis samples contained a few faintly (Table 3, Figs. 2B, 3B) immunopositive plasma cells. In chronic and aggressive periodontitis plasma cells reactive to HtrA1 were more represented and strongly stained than in gingivitis (Fig. 2C, 2D), with an increasing intensity of the immunostaining from chronic (Table 3, Figs. 2C, 3B) to aggressive ($p < 0.001$) (Table 3, Figs. 2D, 3B) periodontitis.

Fibroblasts and collagen fibers resulted negative for HtrA1 in all cases, except in gingivitis where fibroblasts were faintly positive (Table 3, Fig. 2B). HtrA1 immunostaining intensity in dermal vessels was weakly positive in all groups (Table 3, Fig. 2).

Expression of HtrA1 mRNA in healthy and pathological gingival tissues

Results of quantitative real-time PCR indicate that HtrA1 transcript was present in first trimester placental tissue (positive control) (data not shown) and in gingivitis at levels that are ~2 fold higher than in healthy gingiva. This difference resulted statistically significant ($p < 0.001$) (Fig. 4). Real-time PCR analysis of HtrA1 in chronic and aggressive periodontitis showed higher levels of mRNA expression than healthy tissues. Also in these cases, significant differences were detected ($p = 0.004$ and $p = 0.009$ for chronic and aggressive periodontitis, respectively) (Fig. 4). The differences of mRNA expression among the analyzed pathologies were not significant.

Discussion

Periodontal diseases are infectious inflammatory pathologies characterized by the destruction of the tooth-supporting structures [17]. Besides the innate immune response, the mobilization of adaptive immunity mechanisms induced by periodontal bacteria are the leading causes of inflammation [18]. Indeed, we confirm an increase in the number of immunoglobulin-producing plasma cells in chronic and aggressive periodontitis compared to gingivitis specimens [19]. Interestingly, we found a greater amount of plasma cells positive to HtrA1 in the periodontitis lesions respect to gingivitis. In addition, we detected an increase of plasma cell HtrA1 immunostaining from gingivitis to chronic and aggressive periodontitis, with the higher intensity in aggressive disease.

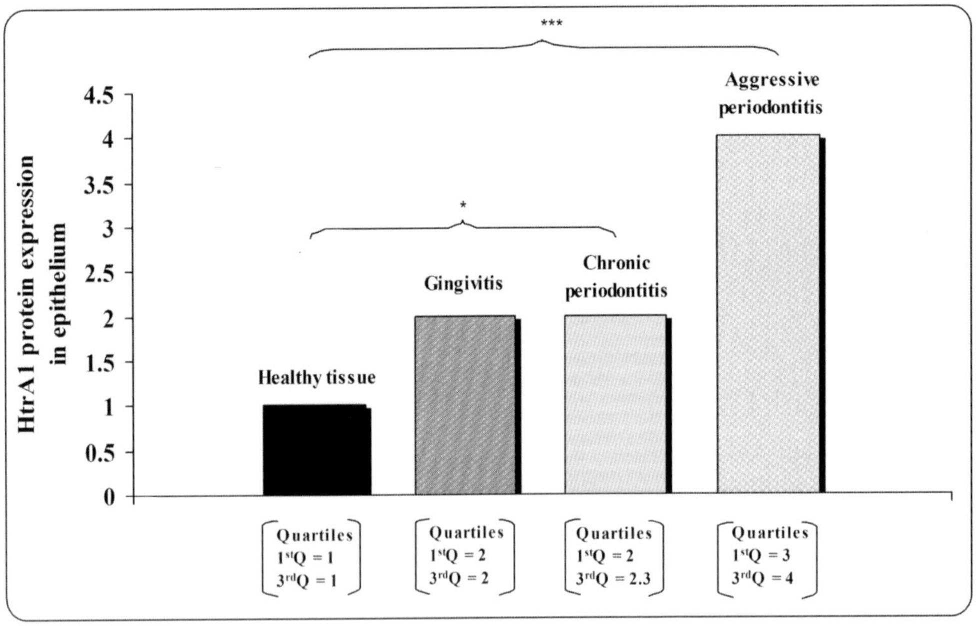

A

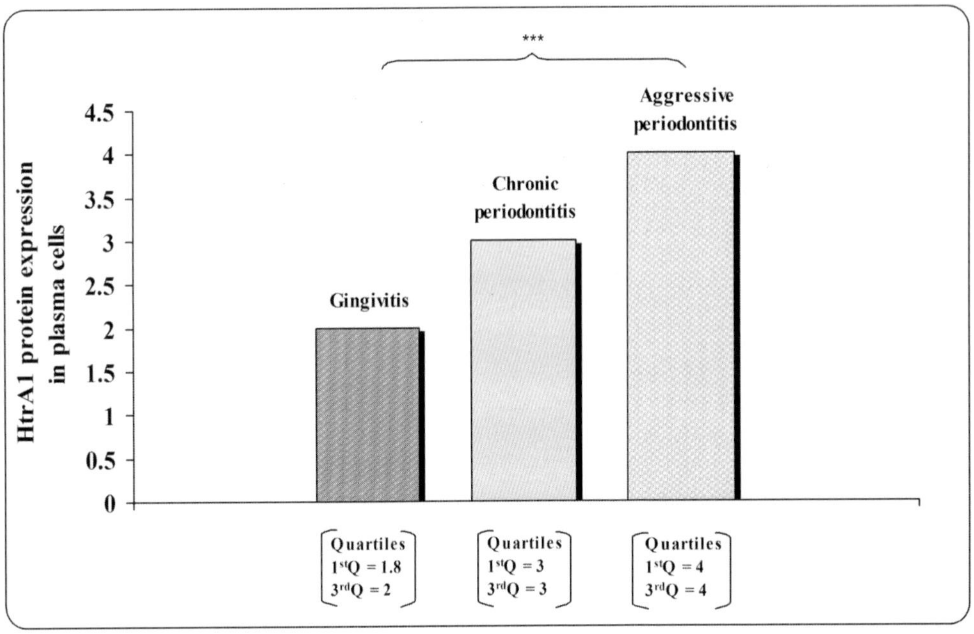

B

Figure 3. HtrA1 protein expression in A) epithelium and in B) plasma cells of studied groups. HtrA1 expression was classified with a five-point scale and was assigned a number value to each point: negative (neg = 0), slight (+/− = 1), faint (+ = 2), moderate (++ = 3) and strong (+++ = 4). $p<0.05$ (*); $p<0.001$ (***).

It is known that HtrA1 is able to digest fibronectin [8], and that the accumulation of fibronectin fragments instigates the expression and secretion of several MMPs [7]. MMPs, a family of zinc- and calcium-dependent proteases, have been often associated with the remodelling of periodontal tissues [20], because, together with tissue inhibitors of metalloproteinases (TIMPs), are supposed to control the extracellular matrix physiological turnover [21]. The *plasma cell expression* of HtrA1 *protein* in periodontal diseases, high in chronic but stronger in aggressive periodontitis, could trigger the overproduction of matrix metalloproteinases, causing an increase in the *MMP/TIMP-ratio* in periodontal tissues with the resulting tissue destruction. Moreover, it is known that HtrA1 functions as

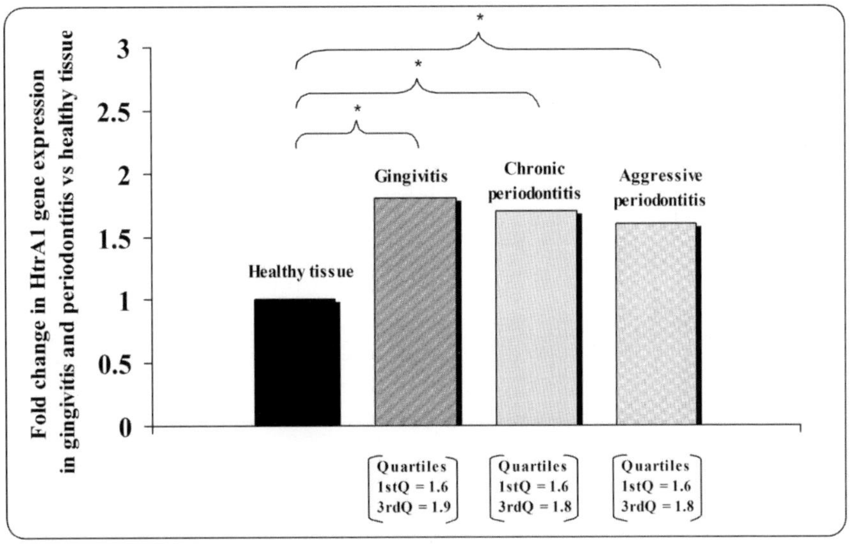

Figure 4. Quantitative real-time PCR of HtrA1 in periodontal tissues. Data are expressed as "fold changes" in relative gene expression of HtrA1 in periodontal diseases respect to the normal tissue. HtrA1 mRNA expression profile shows a statistically significant upregulation of its transcript in the analyzed periodontal diseases respect to healthy tissue. $p<0.05$ (*); $p<0.01$ (**).

an inhibitor of transforming growth factor (TGF)-β signalling [10], and seems to be able to bind and inhibit signalling of a wide range of TGF-β family proteins [10]. TGF-β is a pleiotropic cytokine that down-regulates the transcription of pro-inflammatory molecules, such as *Tumor Necrosis Factor*-α (TNF-α), and MMPs [22,23]. TNF-α plays a central role in inflammatory reaction in periodontal tissues. In particular, TNF-α up-regulates other classic pro-inflammatory innate immunity cytokines production, such as Interleukin-1β (IL-1β) [24]. We suggest that the strong HtrA1 positivity observed in plasma cells of tissues from patients affected by chronic and aggressive periodontitis could reduce the inhibitory effects of TGF-β, allowing the increase of inflammatory mediators (TNF-α; IL-1β) promoting disease progression. The lack of HtrA1 immunoreactivity in the pathological connective tissue rules out the involvement of the serine protease in the direct tissue destruction by proteolytic cleavage of matrix protein components. Therefore, the present study supports the hypothesis that HtrA1 protein expressed in plasma cells can indirectly take part in periodontal lesions, contributing to pathological tissue remodelling in periodontal diseases.

An essential feature found in chronic and aggressive periodontitis is the strong HtrA1 positivity in the epithelium, higher than in the epithelial layers of healthy and gingivitis specimens. Recent studies have demonstrated that TNF-α may also play important functions in the control of bacterial levels in the periodontal environment [25]. In addition, mouse models point to relevant role for TNF-α in the control of periodontal infection [26]. The epithelial immunolocalization of HtrA1 and its strong positivity, particularly in the upper part of the epithelium, suggest us that HtrA1 may have a role in controlling the environment outside the tissue. In particular, HtrA1 probably increases the transcription of TNF-α by inhibition of TGF-β signalling, thus acting as one factor of the immune protection necessary to counteract the growth, the invasion and the toxin production of bacteria organized as a dental biofilm in the deepened periodontal pockets [27]. The increase of HtrA1 immunostaining in the epithelial superficial layer associated with increasingly severe forms of periodontitis appears to confirm the correlation between HtrA1 expression and the altered periodontal environment.

Gingivitis, chronic and aggressive periodontitis showed significantly higher levels of HtrA1 mRNA and protein expression respect to healthy tissues. This behaviour provides the demonstration that HtrA1 expression in periodontal pathologies is genetically determined. HtrA1 protein expression in aggressive periodontitis was higher than gingivitis and chronic periodontitis, while no differences were found in HtrA1 mRNA levels between the three pathologies. This may show that HtrA1 gene expression is not a marker for a particular type of periodontitis but more probably for periodontal inflammation in general. The discrepancy between HtrA1 protein and gene expression is probably due to a possible regulation of HtrA1 mRNA translation by G-quadruplexes, structural elements formed in the 5′-UTRs of many genes recognized to influence the translation [28]. Another explanation could be provided by the 26S proteasome-mediated proteolysis degradation of proteins, such as HtrA1, involved in biological processes as control of cell proliferation and differentiation and programmed cell death (apoptosis) [29,30]. Since deregulation of proteasome function is known to occur in various human diseases [30], HtrA1 proteolysis could be different among the analyzed periodontal pathologies.

Acknowledgments

We are grateful to Prof. Rosaria Gesuita (Center of Epidemiology, Biostatistics, and Medical Information Technology, School of Medicine, Università Politecnica delle Marche, Ancona, Italy) for her valuable assistance in the statistical analysis of the data.

Author Contributions

Conceived and designed the experiments: T. Lorenzi ML MC. Performed the experiments: T. Lorenzi EAN ML FP. Analyzed the data: T. Lorenzi EAN AZ ML FP CR. Contributed reagents/materials/analysis tools: SDA GG GB DM CR MC. Wrote the paper: T. Lorenzi AZ. Critically revised the manuscript for important intellectual content: MB SC T. Lombardi RDF DM MC.

References

1. Berglundh T, Donati M (2005) Aspects of adaptive host response in periodontitis. J Clin Periodontol 32: 87–107.
2. Sanz M, Quirynen M (2005) Advances in the aetiology of periodontitis. Group A consensus report of the 5th European Workshop in Periodontology. J Clin Periodontol 32: 54–56.
3. Offenbacher S (1996) Periodontal diseases: Pathogenesis. Ann Periodontol 1: 821–878.
4. Ford PJ, Gamonal J, Seymour GJ (2010) Immunological differences and similarities between chronic periodontitis and aggressive periodontitis. Periodontol 2000 53: 111–123.
5. Beklen A, Ainola M, Hukkanen M, Gürgan C, Sorsa T, et al. (2007) MMPs, IL-1, and TNF are Regulated by IL-17 in Periodontitis. J Dent Res 86: 347–351.
6. Stanton H, Ung L, Fosang AJ (2002) The 45 kDa collagen-binding fragment of fibronectin induces matrix metalloproteinase-13 synthesis by chondrocytes and aggrecan degradation by aggrecanases. Biochem J 364: 181–190.
7. Grau S, Richards PJ, Kerr B, Hughes C, Caterson B, et al. (2006) The role of human HtrA1 in arthritic disease. J Biol Chem 281: 6124–6129.
8. Grau S, Baldi A, Bussani R, Tian X, Stefanescu R, et al. (2005) Implications of the serine protease HtrA1 in amyloid precursor protein processing. Proc Natl Acad Sci U S A 102: 6021–6026.
9. Clausen T, Southan C, Ehrmann M (2002) The HtrA family of proteases: implications for protein composition and cell fate. Mol Cell 10: 443–455.
10. Oka C, Tsujimoto R, Kajikawa M, Koshiba-Takeuchi K, Ina J, et al. (2004) HtrA1 serine protease inhibits signaling mediated by TGF-β family proteins. Development 131: 1041–1053.
11. Lorenzi T, Marzioni D, Giannubilo S, Quaranta A, Crescimanno C, et al. (2009) Expression patterns of two serine protease HtrA1 forms in human placentas complicated by preeclampsia with and without intrauterine growth restriction. Placenta 30: 35–40.
12. Tocharus J, Tsuchiya A, Kajikawa M, Ueta Y, Oka C, et al. (2004) Developmentally regulated expression of mouse HtrA3 and its role as an inhibitor of TGF-beta signaling. Dev Growth Differ 46: 257–274.
13. Aspriello SD, Zizzi A, Tirabassi G, Buldreghini E, Biscotti T, et al. (2011) Diabetes mellitus-associated periodontitis: differences between type 1 and type 2 diabetes mellitus. J Periodontal Res 46: 164–169.
14. Armitage GC (1999) Development of a classification system for periodontal diseases and conditions. Ann Periodontol 4: 1–6.
15. Nie G, Hale K, Li Y, Manuelpillai U, Wallace EM, et al. (2006) Distinct expression and localization of serine protease HtrA1 in human endometrium and first-trimester placenta. Dev Dyn 235: 3448–3455.
16. Marzioni D, Quaranta A, Lorenzi T, Morroni M, Crescimanno C, et al. (2009) Expression pattern alterations of the serine protease HtrA1 in normal human placental tissues and in gestational trophoblastic diseases. Histol Histopathol 24: 1213–1222.
17. Tonetti MS, Claffey N, European Workshop in Periodontology group C (2005) Advances in the progression of periodontitis and proposal of definitions of a periodontitis case and disease progression for use in risk factor research. Group C consensus report of the 5th European Workshop in Periodontology. J Clin Periodontol 32: 210–213.
18. Cutler CW, Jotwani R (2004) Antigen-presentation and the role of dendritic cells in periodontitis. Periodontol 2000 35: 135–157.
19. Artese L, Simon MJ, Piattelli A, Ferrari DS, Cardoso LA, et al. (2011) Immunohistochemical analysis of inflammatory infiltrate in aggressive and chronic periodontitis: a comparative study. Clin Oral Investig 15: 233–240.
20. Hannas AR, Pereira JC, Granjeiro JM, Tjäderhane L (2007) The role of matrix metalloproteinases in the oral environment. Acta Odontol Scand 65: 1–13.
21. Gonçalves LD, Oliveira G, Hurtado PA, Feitosa A, Takiya CM, et al. (2008) Expression of metalloproteinases and their tissue inhibitors in inflamed gingival biopsies. J Periodontal Res 43: 570–577.
22. Okada H, Murakami S (1998) Cytokine expression in periodontal health and disease. Crit Rev Oral Biol Med 9: 248–266.
23. Steinsvoll S, Halstensen TS, Schenck K (1999) Extensive expression of TGF-beta1 in chronically-inflamed periodontal tissue. J Clin Periodontol 26: 366–373.
24. Graves DT, Cochran D (2003) The contribution of interleukin-1 and tumor necrosis factor to periodontal tissue destruction. J Periodontol 74: 391–401.
25. Garlet GP (2010) Destructive and protective roles of cytokines in periodontitis: a re-appraisal from host defense and tissue destruction viewpoints. J Dent Res 89: 1349–1363.
26. Garlet GP, Cardoso CR, Campanelli AP, Ferreira BR, Avila-Campos MJ, et al. (2007) The dual role of p55 tumour necrosis factor-alpha receptor in Actinobacillus actinomycetemcomitans-induced experimental periodontitis: host protection and tissue destruction. Clin Exp Immunol 147: 128–138.
27. Haffajee AD, Socransky SS (2005) Microbiology of periodontal diseases: introduction. Periodontol 2000 38: 9–12.
28. Bugaut A, Balasubramanian S (2012) 5′-UTR RNA G-quadruplexes: translation regulation and targeting. Nucleic Acids Res 40: 4727–4741.
29. Chien J, Staub J, Hu SI, Erickson-Johnson MR, Couch FJ, et al. (2004) A candidate tumour suppressor HtrA1 is downregulated in ovarian cancer. Oncogene 23: 1636–1644.
30. Bedford L, Paine S, Sheppard PW, Mayer RJ, Roelofs J (2010) Assembly, structure, and function of the 26S proteasome. Trends Cell Biol 20: 391–401.

2

High-Fat Diet Induces Periodontitis in Mice through Lipopolysaccharides (LPS) Receptor Signaling: Protective Action of Estrogens

Vincent Blasco-Baque[1,2,3], Matteo Serino[1,2], Jean-Noël Vergnes[3], Elodie Riant[1,2], Pascale Loubieres[1,2,3], Jean-François Arnal[1,2], Pierre Gourdy[1,2], Michel Sixou[3], Rémy Burcelin[1,2]*, Philippe Kemoun[3]*

1 Institut National de la Santé et de la Recherche Médicale (INSERM), Toulouse, France, **2** Université Paul Sabatier, Unité Mixte de Recherche (UMR) 1048, Institut de Maladies Métaboliques et Cardiovasculaires (I2MC), Toulouse, France, **3** L.U. 51, Parodontites et Maladies Générales, Université Paul Sabatier, Faculté de Chirurgie Dentaire, 3, Chemin des Maraîchers, Toulouse, France

Abstract

Background: A fat-enriched diet favors the development of gram negative bacteria in the intestine which is linked to the occurrence of type 2 diabetes (T2D). Interestingly, some pathogenic gram negative bacteria are commonly associated with the development of periodontitis which, like T2D, is characterized by a chronic low-grade inflammation. Moreover, estrogens have been shown to regulate glucose homeostasis *via* an LPS receptor dependent immune-modulation. In this study, we evaluated whether diet-induced metabolic disease would favor the development of periodontitis in mice. In addition, the regulatory role of estrogens in this process was assessed.

Methods: Four-week-old C57BL6/J WT and CD14 (part of the TLR-4 machinery for LPS-recognition) knock-out female mice were ovariectomised and subcutaneously implanted with pellets releasing either placebo or 17β-estradiol (E2). Mice were then fed with either a normal chow or a high-fat diet for four weeks. The development of diabetes was monitored by an intraperitoneal glucose-tolerance test and plasma insulin concentration while periodontitis was assessed by identification of pathogens, quantification of periodontal soft tissue inflammation and alveolar bone loss.

Results: The fat-enriched diet increased the prevalence of periodontal pathogenic microbiota like *Fusobacterium nucleatum* and *Prevotella intermedia*, gingival inflammation and alveolar bone loss. E2 treatment prevented this effect and CD14 knock-out mice resisted high-fat diet-induced periodontal defects.

Conclusions/Significance: Our data show that mice fed with a diabetogenic diet developed defects and microflora of tooth supporting-tissues typically associated with periodontitis. Moreover, our results suggest a causal link between the activation of the LPS pathway on innate immunity by periodontal microbiota and HFD-induced periodontitis, a pathophysiological mechanism that could be targeted by estrogens.

Editor: Massimo Federici, University of Tor Vergata, Italy

Funding: This work was supported by grants from Société Française d'Hypertension Artérielle and from the Société Francophone de Diabète. Part of this work is supported by a European grant from the Framework program 7 (FlorinashNo 241913) to RB. The funders had no role in study design, data collection and analysis, decision to publish, or preparation of the manuscript.

Competing Interests: The authors have declared that no competing interests exist.

* E-mail: remy.burcelin@inserm.fr (RB); philippe.kemoun@wanadoo.fr (PK)

Introduction

The prevalence of Type 2 diabetes (T2D) has dramatically increased over the past decade both in developed and developing countries. Furthermore, the complications of this metabolic disease are nowadays major causes of morbidity and mortality [1]. The pathophysiology of T2D is characterized by a low-grade chronic inflammation [2], with the release of inflammatory cytokines by innate immune cells, mainly macrophages and dendritic cells, that impair insulin action [3]. It was recently suggested that the intestinal microbiota contributes to the development of obesity and insulin-resistance [4,5]. A switch from a normal diet towards a fat-enriched diet, where the daily amount of dietary fibers is reduced, was associated with a change in the ecology of the intestinal microbiota [6,7] with an increase in gram-negative bacteria. The activation of the immune system by gram-negative bacteria depends on specific pattern recognition receptors (PRRs) such as Cluster of differentiation 14/Toll-like receptor-4 (CD14/TLR4) [8]. CD14/TLR4 knockout mice are protected against the metabolic impact of a high-fat diet (HFD) [4]. Hence, the interaction among gram-negative pathogens and the immune system is a key factor for the development of metabolic diseases [4,9]. Interestingly, periodontitis, a chronic infection of the soft and hard tissues supporting the tooth, is caused by gram-negative capnophilic bacteria [10]. This disease is characterised by an inflammation and a loss of both soft and hard tissues of the periodontium (e.g. the periodontal tissues) that protect the roots of the tooth and anchor them to the jaws. Most pathogens involved in periodontitis have been identified, and many of them are also known to be involved in metabolic diseases [5] and many systemic diseases [11,12]. *Prevotella intermedia* (Pi) is a key periodontal pathogen inducing innate immune responses partly involved in deep periodontal tissues destruction [13] The frequency of *Pi* detection in the periodontal pocket is higher in diabetic than in healthy subjects [14]. Another periopathogen, *Fusobacterium nucleatum* (Fn), was detected in human carotid endarteriectomy specimens and is thought to exert atherogenic effects [15]. Apolipoprotein E knockout mice (ApoE$^{-/-}$) infected by *Fn* display increased lipid depots in the arterial wall compared with controls [16]. Indeed, *Fn* systemic infection increases plasma levels of total cholesterol and LDL [17]. Thus, it can be postulated that diet-induced metabolic diseases may favor the development of periodontitis.

We recently showed that estrogens are key players in the control of metabolic diseases involving immune regulation [18]. Furthermore, numerous epidemiological studies strongly suggest that estrogen deficiency is linked to the appearance of periodontal diseases (PD) [19]. As previously reported, a significant increase in the incidence of PD is associated with the menopause, which is considered as the main physiological cause of estrogen depletion [20,21,22]. Moreover, it has been suggested that hormonal replacement therapy can protect menopausal women against periodontitis [23]. However, the influence of these sexual steroid hormones on the occurrence of PD in a dysmetabolic and inflammatory context has not been addressed to date.

In this study, we investigated whether a high-fat diet, known to induce inflammation-mediated insulin-resistance and glucose-intolerance, as previously described [18], would promote the development of PD in ovariectomised mice, and whether estrogen administration would regulate this process. Our data reported herein demonstrate that HFD-induced metabolic disturbances were associated with the occurrence of periodontitis, and that chronic estrogen administration, as well as the deletion of CD14, strongly prevents the HFD-induced defects of periodontal tissue in mice.

Materials and Methods

Ethical Statement

All animal experimental procedures were approved by the local ethical committee of Rangueil University Hospital, INSERM BP 84225, 31432 Toulouse under the authorization number "C 31 555 07", and the Ethical committee of Purpan Hospital (Toulouse).

Animals and Experimental Procedures

C57BL6/J wild-type (WT) (Charles River, L'Arbres, France) and *CD14*-deficient (*CD14*KO) female mice born in our animal facilities were group-housed (five mice per cage) in a specific pathogen-free controlled environment (inverted 12-hr daylight cycle, light off at 10:00 a.m.). Four week-old mice were ovariectomised (OVX) and then subcutaneously implanted with pellets releasing either placebo or 17β-estradiol (e.g. E2, 0.1 mg for 60 days, 80 µg/kg per day; Innovative Research of America, Sarasota, FL) [18] under general anesthesia. Mice have then been fed with a normal chow diet (i.e. NCD; energy content: 12% fat, 28% protein, and 60% carbohydrate; A04, Villemoisson sur Orge, France) or a diabetogenic, high-fat carbohydrate-free diet (i.e. HFD; energy content: 72% fat (corn oil and lard), 28% protein and less than 1% carbohydrate; SAFE, Augy, France) for four weeks. This particular diet has been developed to induce a diabetic state after 4 weeks, as previously described [9]. Animals were divided into eight groups: WT OVX+NCD with placebo (n = 27), WT OVX+NCD+E2 (n = 16), WT OVX+HFD with placebo (n = 25), WT OVX+HFD+E2 (n = 25), *CD14KO* OVX+NCD with placebo (n = 6), *CD14KO* OVX+NCD+E2 (n = 6), *CD14*KO OVX+HFD with placebo (n = 12) and *CD14*KO OVX+ HFD+E2 (n = 12). At the end of experiment, mice were sacrificed by cervical dislocation; tissues were collected and snap-frozen in liquid nitrogen.

Intraperitoneal Glucose-tolerance Test (IPGTT)

Six-hour-fasted mice were injected with glucose into the peritoneal cavity (1 g/kg) after 4 weeks of HFD diet. Blood glucose was measured with a glucometer (Roche Diagnostics, Meylan, France) on 3.5 µl of blood collected from the tip of the tail vein at −30, 0, 30, 60, and 90 min after the glucose injection [9].

Plasma Insulin Concentration

To assess plasma insulin concentration, 20 µl blood were sampled from the tip of the tail vein of 6-hr-fasted mice. The plasma was separated and frozen at −80°C. 5 µl plasma were used to determine the insulin concentration with an Elisa kit (Mercodia, Uppsala, Sweden) and following the manufacturer's instructions.

Real-Time Quantitative PCR (qPCR) Analysis

Total RNA from white adipose tissue, liver and gingival tissue was extracted using the TriPure reagent (Roche, Basel, Switzerland). cDNA was synthesized using a reverse transcriptase (Applied Biosystems, Fost City, USA) from 1 µg of total RNA. The primers (Eurogentec, San Diego, USA) used were (5′ to 3′): tumor necrosis factor-α (*TNF-α*), forward TGGGACAGTGACCTGGACTGT; reverse TCGGAAAGCCCATTTGAGT; Interleukin 1β(*IL-1β*) forward TCGCTCAGGGTCACAAGAAA; reverse CATCAGAGGCAAGGAGGAAAAC; plasminogen activator inhibitor-1(*PAI-1*) forward ACAGCCTTTGTCATCTCAGCC; reverse CCGAACCACAAAGAGAAAGGA and interleukin-6 (*IL-6*) forward ACAAGTCGGAGGCTTAATTACACAT; reverse TTGCCATTGCACAACTCTTTTC. The concentration of each mRNA was normalized for RNA loading for each sample using ribosomal protein L19 (*RPL19*) forward GAAGGTCAAAGGGAATGTGTTCA; reverse CCTTGTCTGCCTTCAGCTTGT, as an internal standard and the data were analysed according to the $2^{-\Delta\Delta CT}$ method [24].

Culture and Identification of Periopathogens

The composition of the sub-gingival microbiota was determined as previously described [10]. The selected site was cleaned with 75% ethanol to remove the supragingival bacterial biofilm. Cervicular fluid was sampled with three endodontic sterile paper points held in sterile pliers: paper points were inserted into the sub-gingival space and then placed in a 2-ml bottle of reduced transport medium VGMA-III of Moëller. After mixing for 30 sec at maximal speed on a Vortex mixer, the 2-ml bottles containing glass beads were opened in an anaerobic chamber and samples were serially diluted ten-fold in Wilkins–Chalgren broth (WC, Oxoid, Basingstoke, Hampshire, UK). Bacteria were cultured on non-selective or selective medium agar plates [10]. Identification of putative anaerobic bacteria was carried out according to Bergey's manual criteria [25]. Genomic bacterial DNA was extracted using a classical phenol/chloroform method followed by alcohol precipitation (ice-cold 70% alcohol vol/vol). Semi-quantitative PCR was carried out using 2 µl of the extracted DNA with specific primers [4]. The primers (Eurogentec, San

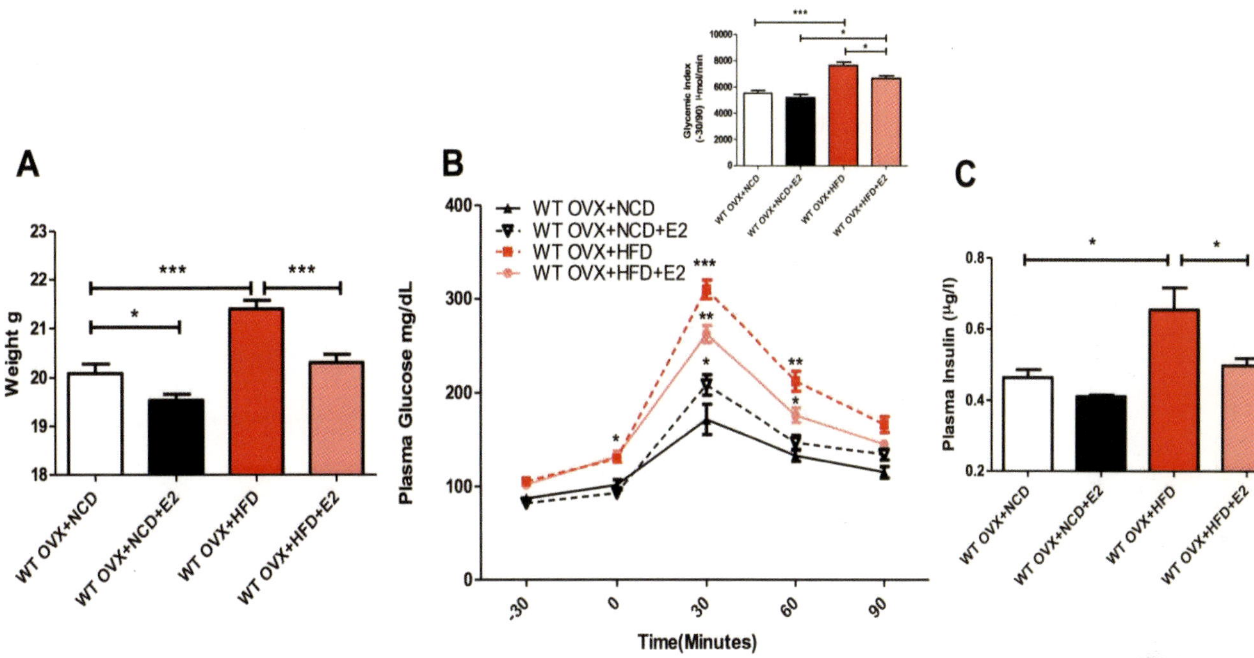

Figure 1. E2 administration prevents HFD-induced diabetic disorders. A) Body weight was assessed in 8-wk-old mice 4 weeks of diet: WT OVX+NCD (n = 27), WT OVX+NCD+E2 (n = 16), WT OVX+HFD (n = 15) and WT OVX+HFD+E2 (n = 15). **B**) Time course of glycemia (mg/dl) during an IPGTT. The inset represents the glycemic index for each group. **C**) Fasted plasma insulin concentration (µg/l) after 4 weeks of diet: WT OVX+NCD (n = 6), WT OVX+NCD+E2 (n = 6), WT OVX+HFD (n = 6) and WT OVX+HFD+E2 (n = 6). *P<0.05, **P<0.01, ***P<0.001 (one-way ANOVA followed by Tukey test for **A** and **C**; and Two-Way ANOVA with Bonferroni's post-test for **B**). Results are presented as means ± SEM.

Diego, USA) used were (5′ to 3′): *Fusobacterium nucleatum* forward AAGCGCGTCTAGGTGGTTATGT and reverse TGTAGTTCCGCTTACCTCTCCAG and *Prevotella intermedia* forward TCCACCGAT GAATCTTTGGTC and reverse ATCCAACCTTCCCTCCACTC.

Histological Examination

Gingival tissue surrounding the lower molars were excised, fixed in 4% paraformaldehyde for 48 hours and embedded in paraffin. Sections (4 µm thick), were then stained with hematoxylin/eosin. To quantify the infiltration of inflammatory cells, immune cells were counted in ten microscopic fields randomly selected from each group.

Quantification of Mandibular Alveolar Bone Resorption

To evaluate mandibular alveolar bone loss, hemi-mandibles were scanned using a high-resolution µCT (Viva CT40; Scanco Medical, Bassersdorf, Switzerland) [26]. Data were acquired at 45 keV, with a 10 µm isotropic voxel size. Six linear measurements were obtained from each molar by using a stereomicroscope with an on-screen computer-aided measurement package. The alveolar bone loss (in mm) was measured from the cemento-enamel junction (CEJ) to the alveolar bone crest (ABC) for each

Table 1. Positive bacterial cultures : intergroup comparisons among ovariectomised mice.

Bacterial cultures	Effect of diet			Effect of E2 supplementation			Effect of CD14 deletion		
	WT OVX NCD	WT OVX HFD	p[1]	WT OVX HFD	WT OVX HFD E2	p[1]	WT OVX HFD	*CD14*KO OVX HFD	p[1]
	n = 27 (%)	n = 25 (%)		n = 25 (%)	n = 25 (%)		n = 25 (%)	n = 12 (%)	
Fusobacterium nucleatum **(Fn)**	0 (0)	1 (4.0)	0.48	1 (4.0)	7 (28.0)	*** 0.04**	1 (4.0)	0 (0)	1.00
Prevotella intermedia **(Pi)**	1 (3.7)	4 (16.0)	0.18	4 (16.0)	0 (0)	0.11	4 (16.0)	1 (8.3)	1.00
Both Fn + Pi	1 (3.7)	6 (24.0)	*** 0.04**	6 (24.0)	0 (0)	**** 0.02**	6 (24.0)	3 (25.0)	1.00
Fn and/or Pi	2 (7.4)	11 (44.0)	**** <0.01**	11 (44.0)	7 (28.0)	0.37	11 (44.0)	4 (33.3)	0.72

[1]Fischer exact tests p-values, significant at p<0.05.
The table shows the qualitative analysis of periodontal microbiota in each group: WT OVX+NCD (n = 27), WT OVX+HFD (n = 25), WT OVX+HFD+E2 (n = 25) and *CD14*KO OVX+HFD (n = 12).
*P<0.05,
**P<0.01 (Fischer exact tests).

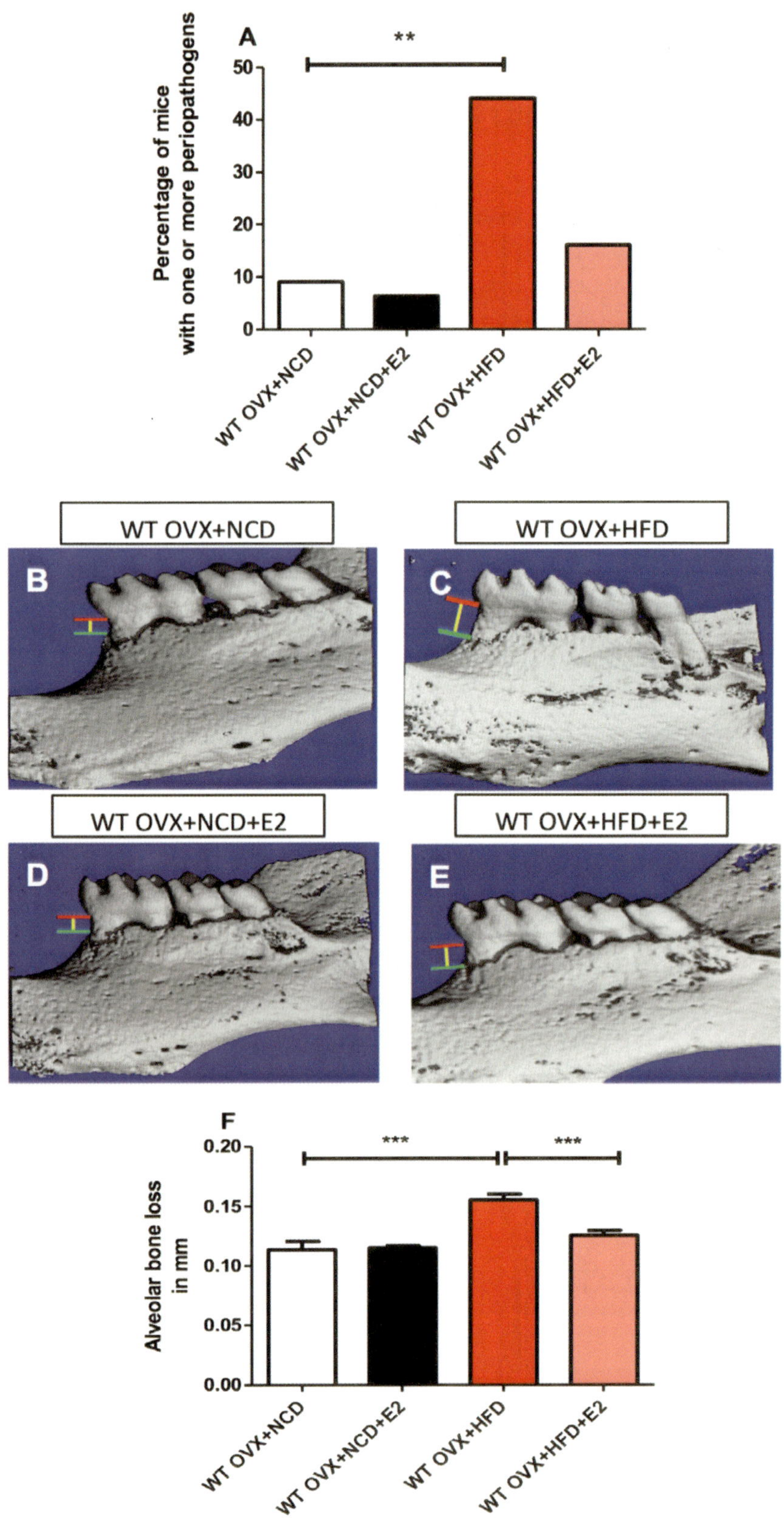

Figure 2. HFD induced periodontal disease in WT mice: reversal effect of E2-treatment. A) The occurrence of periodontal pathogens was analysed in 8-wk-old mice after 4 weeks of diet : WT OVX+NCD (n = 27), WT OVX+NCD+E2 (n = 16), WT OVX+HFD (n = 15) and WT OVX+HFD+E2 (n = 15). **B–G**) Hemi-mandible from each group, as reconstructed by the micro-CT. **F**) CEJ (red line: cemento-enamel junction)-ABC (green line: alveolar bone crest) distance to represent alveolar bone loss (yellow line) (n = 8 for each group). *P<0.05, **P<0.01, ***P<0.001 (one-way ANOVA followed by Tukey test). Results are presented as means ± SEM.

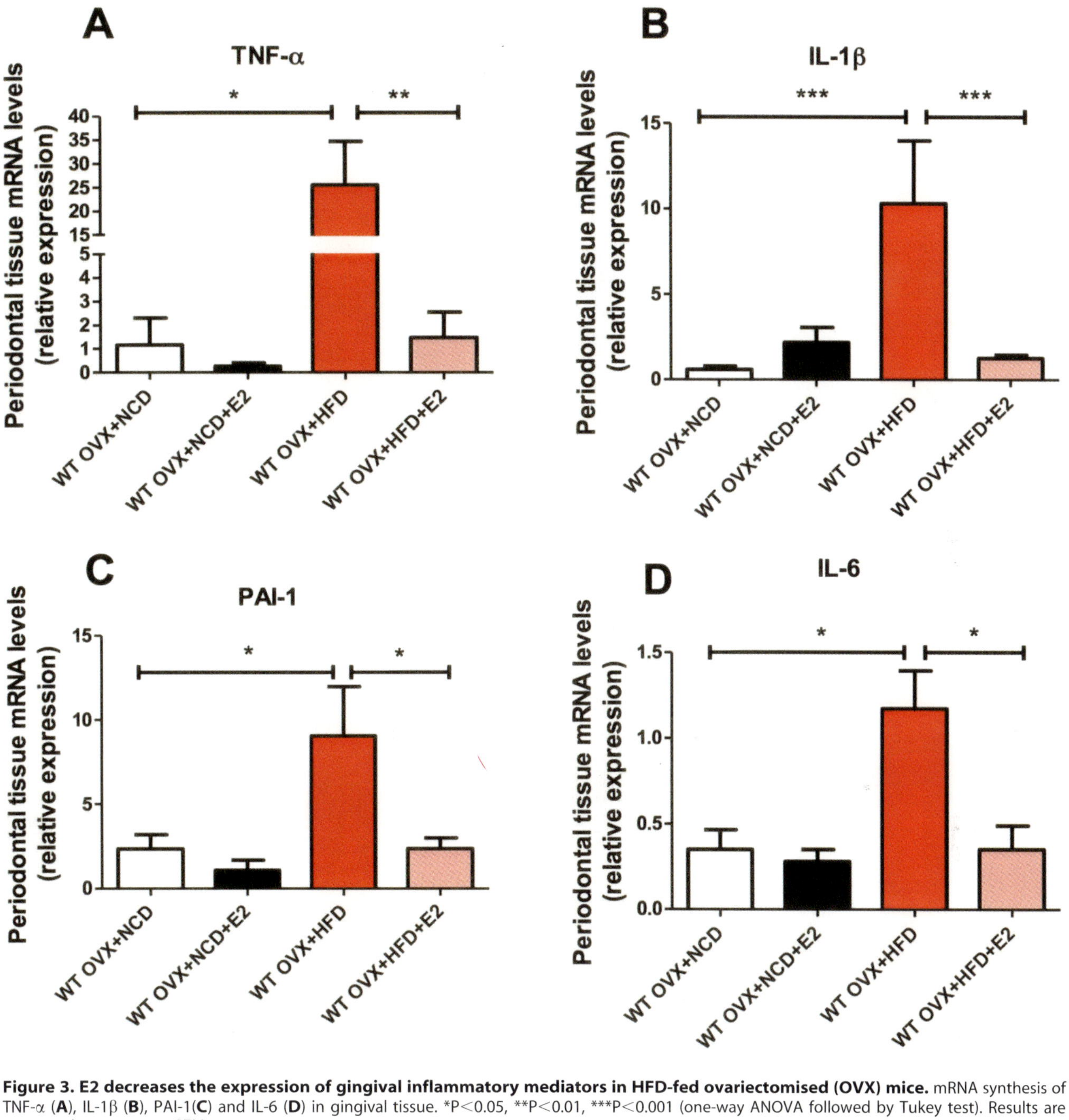

Figure 3. E2 decreases the expression of gingival inflammatory mediators in HFD-fed ovariectomised (OVX) mice. mRNA synthesis of TNF-α (**A**), IL-1β (**B**), PAI-1(**C**) and IL-6 (**D**) in gingival tissue. *$P<0.05$, **$P<0.01$, ***$P<0.001$ (one-way ANOVA followed by Tukey test). Results are presented as means ± SEM.

molar [27]. Three-dimensional reconstructions were generated from a set of 400 slices. After micro-CT analysis, the hemi-mandibles were cleaned with 0.1% hypochlorite over 20 min and then stained with 10% methylene blue.

Statistical Analysis

Results are presented as means ± SEM. One-way ANOVA followed by Tukey's post-test was used to assess the statistical significance between groups, except for the IPGTT analysis, where two-way ANOVA followed by Bonferroni's post-test was applied. The effects of diet, estrogen supplementation and *CD14* deletion on periodontal microbiota composition were tested using Fisher's exact test. A two-sided p-value <0.05 was considered statistically significant. Statistical analyses were performed using GraphPad Prism version 5.00 for Windows Vista (GraphPad Software, San Diego, CA), and R (version 2.12.1).

Results

Estradiol Prevents HFD-induced Metabolic Disorders in WT Ovariectomised Mice

Four-week-old wild-type C57Bl6/J female mice were ovariectomised then randomised according to both diet and E2-treatment, as reported in **Figure 1**. As expected, in comparison to NCD-fed mice, mice fed with a HFD for four weeks developed

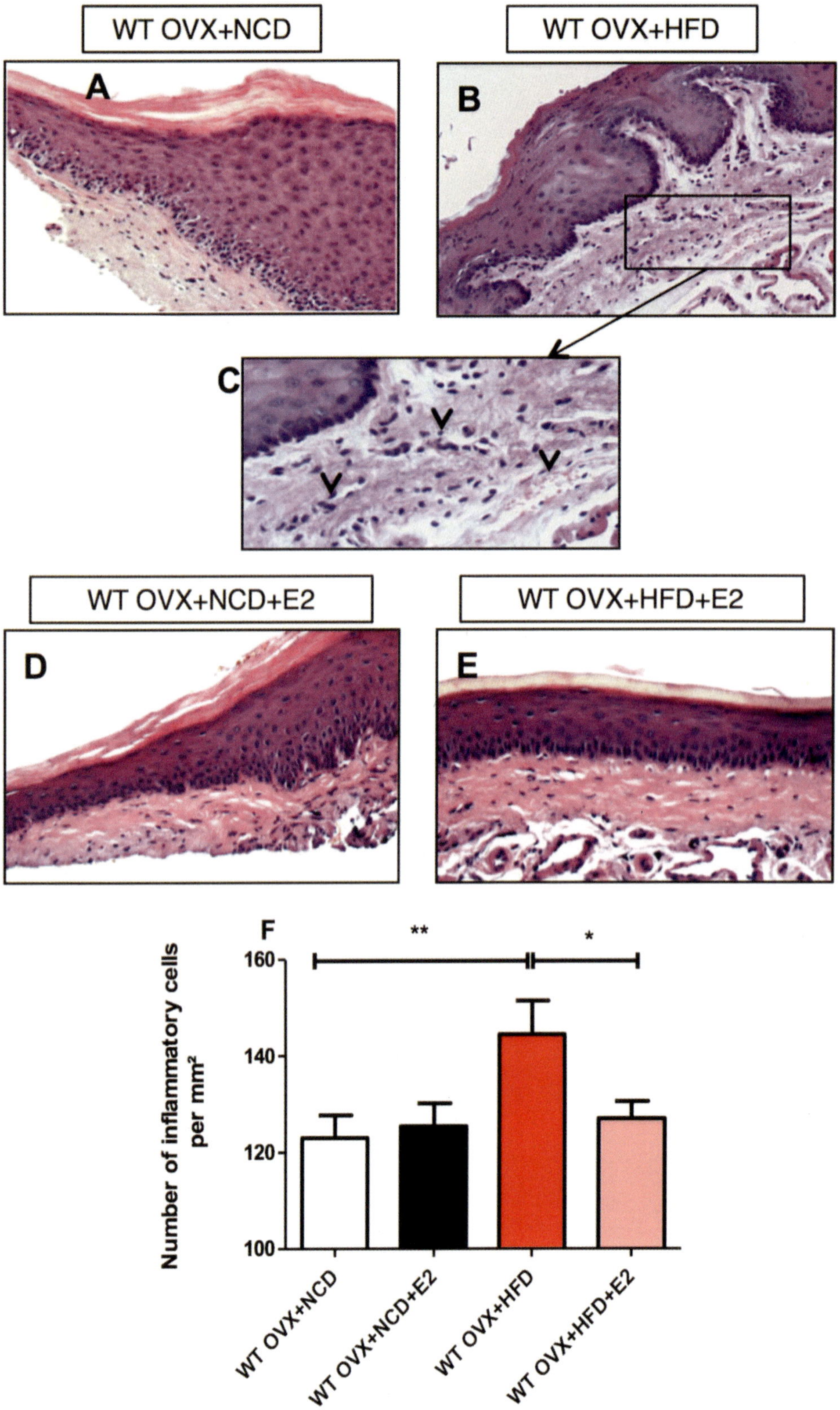

Figure 4. HFD-induced inflammatory cell infiltrate in gingival connective tissue is modulated by E2 in wild-type mice. Histological appearance of the gingival tissues with H/E coloration from WT OVX+NCD (**A**; n = 10),WT OVX+HFD (**B**; n = 10), WT OVX+NCD+E2 (**D**; n = 10), and WT OVX+HFD+E2 (**E**; n = 10). **C** Magnification of the inflammatory gingival tissue from HFD-fed mice. **F**. Number of inflammatory cells for each group. *P<0.05, **P<0.01, ***P<0.001 (one-way ANOVA followed by Tukey test). Results are presented as means ± SEM.

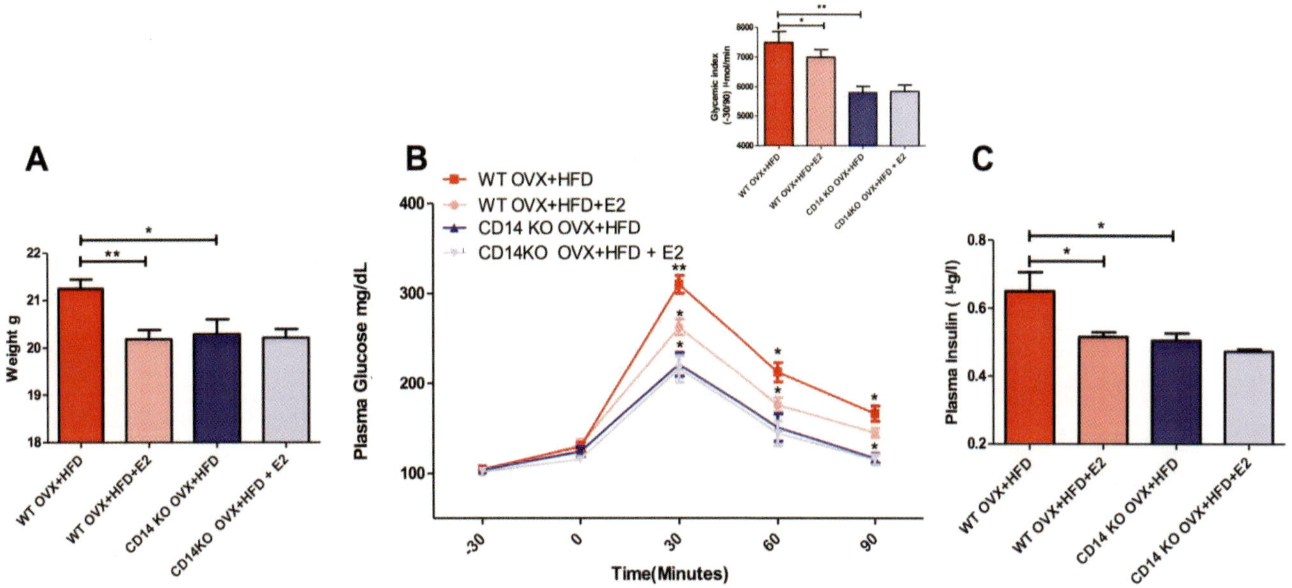

Figure 5. HFD-fed *CD14*KO mice did not exhibit metabolic disorders compared with WT. A) Body weight was assessed in 8-wk-old mice after 4 weeks of diet : WT OVX+HFD (n = 10), WT OVX+HFD+E2 (n = 10), CD14KO OVX+HFD (n = 12) and CD14KO OVX+HFD+E2 (n = 12). **B)** Time course of glycemia (mg/dl) during an IPGTT. The inset represents the glycemic index for each group. **C)** Fasted plasma insulin concentration (µg/l) after 4 weeks of diet : WT OVX+HFD (n = 6), WT OVX+HFD+E2 (n = 6), CD14KO OVX+HFD (n = 6) and CD14KO OVX+HFD+E2 (n = 6). *P<0.05, **P<0.01 (One-way ANOVA followed by Tukey's post-test for **A** and **C**; and Two-Way ANOVA with Bonferroni's post-test for **B**). Results are presented as means ± SEM.

a dysmetabolic phenotype characterised by increased body weight gain, impaired fasting glycemia, hyperinsulinemia and glucose-intolerance. It was noteworthy that the harmful effects of HFD on body weight, fasted plasma insulin and glucose homeostasis were largely prevented by E2-supplementation **(Fig. 1A–C)**.

HFD Promotes Periodontitis in the Absence of Estrogens

We then examined the respective influence of a HFD and estrogens on periodontal health. Without estrogen supplementation, the HFD significantly increased the percentage of animals with at least one and up to two periopathogen species, *Pi* and *Fn*, compared with control mice maintained on the NCD (**Fig. 2A; Table 1**). Furthermore, the HFD instigated the presence of *Pi/Fn* association in the periodontal microbiota of OVX-mice (**Table 1**), and induced alveolar bone resorption (a common feature of periodontitis) (**Fig. 2B–F**). Interestingly, E2-administration to OVX mice blunted the deleterious effects of the HFD on alveolar bone (**Fig. 2B–F)** and modified the periodontal microbiota by reducing the percentage of mice with *Pi* and *Fn* association (**Table 1**).

E2-treatment Prevents HFD-induced Inflammation of Periodontal Tissues

To determine whether E2 prevents HFD-induced periodontal disease by controlling inflammatory processes, we assayed the mRNA concentrations of several inflammatory mediators in the gingiva. TNF-α, IL-1β, PAI-1 and IL-6 expression significantly increased in the gingival connective tissue of OVX mice fed a fat-enriched diet when compared with their NCD-fed counterparts. Conversely, the proinflammatory effect of the HFD was abolished by E2-supplementation (**Fig. 3A–D**).

Microscopic examination of gingival connective tissue of HFD-fed mice highlighted an inflammatory cell infiltration (**Fig. 4A–F**), and red cells extravasation, compared with the NCD-fed OVX control mice (**Fig. 4A–F**). Interestingly, E2-supplementation reversed the HFD-induced periodontal soft tissue inflammation (**Fig. 4F**).

*CD14*KO Mice are Protected from HFD-induced Periodontitis

CD14 is an important modulator of the inflammatory responses induced by gram-negative bacteria. We therefore assessed the impact of *CD14* deletion on HFD-associated disorders including metabolic and periodontal alterations. According to our previous data [4] and in contrast to WT mice, *CD14*KO mice did not show increased body weight, fasted glycemia and plasma insulin concentration or glucose-intolerance, when fed a HFD (**Fig. 5A–C**) or a NCD (**Fig. S1A**) for four weeks.

Interestingly, the deletion of *CD14* also prevented the HFD-induced alveolar bone loss (**Fig. 6B–F**), although the association of *Pi/Fn* was unaffected in *CD14*KO HFD-fed mice (WT OVX+HFD 25% vs *CD14*KO OVX+HFD 24% **Table 1**). Like WT NCD-fed mice, *CD14*KO NCD-fed mice did not show a modified periodontal microbiota (**Table S1**). Furthermore, in contrast to the protective effect observed in WT mice, estrogen supplementation had no effect on the alveolar bone level in *CD14*KO mice (**Fig. 6A–F**).

The TNF-α, IL-1β, PAI-1 and IL-6 expression in the periodontal soft tissue of HFD-fed *CD14*KO mice was comparable to the controls (**Fig. 7A–D**). Moreover, in contrast to HFD-fed WT mice (**Fig. 8A–E**), the immune cell infiltration in gingival tissue was dramatically reduced in HFD-fed *CD14* mutant mice. In addition, E2 did not affect alveolar bone loss and overall inflammatory tone in *CD14*KO OVX+NCD (**Fig. S2A–F**).

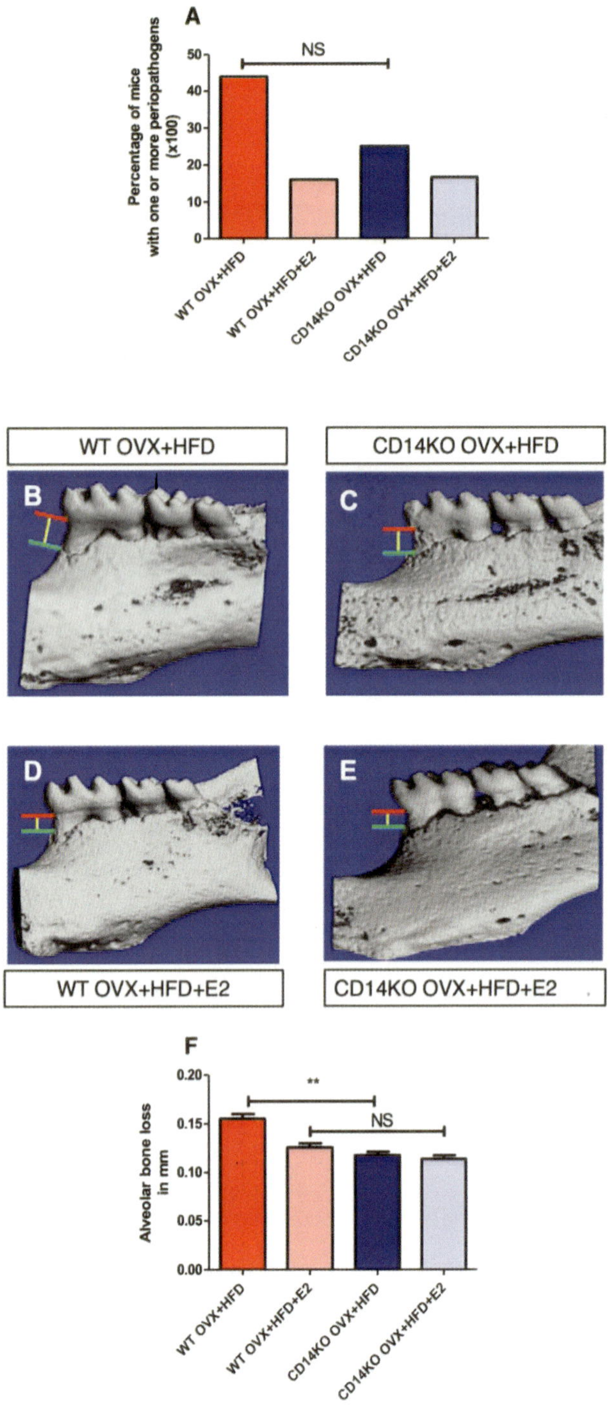

Figure 6. HFD-fed *CD14*KO mice are protected from periodontal disease compared with WT. A) The occurrence of periodontal pathogens was analyzed in 8-wk-old mice after 4 weeks of diet: WT OVX+HFD (n = 10), WT OVX+HFD+E2 (n = 10), CD14KO OVX+HFD (n = 12) and CD14KO OVX+HFD+E2 (n = 12). **B–G**) Hemi-mandible from each group, as reconstructed by the micro-CT. **F** CEJ (red line: cemento-enamel junction)-ABC (green line: alveolar bone crest) distance to represent alveolar bone loss (yellow line). $^*P<0.05$, $^{**}P<0.01$, $^{***}P<0.001$ (one-way ANOVA followed by Tukey test). Results are presented as means ± SEM.

Discussion

The data presented in this study showed that a fat-enriched diet combined with estrogen deficiency induced a periodontal disease in mice. Furthermore, our data strongly suggest that estradiol replacement may prevent HFD-induced metabolic and periodontal disorders.

Medium- or long-term diabetic patients with degenerative multi-organ complications [28], are also prone to frequent and severe periodontitis. To date, the mechanisms linking diabetes to periodontal diseases remain poorly understood. Our data showed that HFD increases the proportion of mice harbouring periodontal pathogens such as *Fusobacterium nucleatum* and *Prevotella intermedia*, known to be part of the subgingival plaque in periodontal pockets [29,30]. Indeed, it has been suggested that a fat-enriched diet may enhance the occurrence of oral pathogens in diabetic patients [31]. The reasons for this fundamental modification are still unclear. However, a switch to a high-fat diet induces a new intestinal ecology and, hence, a new periodontal ecology [32]. This modification increased the proportion of gram-negative bacteria producing inflammatory LPS, at least in the intestine [4]. Furthermore, the microbial diversity could explain the different metabolic phenotypes [33]. Therefore, an inappropriate immune function in reaction to the many bacterial antigens would generate a metabolic inflammation and the corresponding immune messengers may impair and maintain the metabolic disorders [2]. On the other hand, a microbiota composed of gram-negative bacteria produces LPS that directly move into the blood in human [34] or animal models to aggravate inflammation and systemic diseases [12,35]. Indeed, HFD-induced metabolic endotoxemia (an increase in plasma levels of LPS) was shown to be an initiator of metabolic diseases [35] *via* enhanced systemic inflammation [2]. Hence, the elevated systemic inflammation in diabetic patients could be linked to PD [36], demonstrating a two-sided relationship between these pathologies. Thus, inflammation could be a key feature of periodontitis to be targeted [5] and we can postulate that a fat-enriched diet may be a regulator of the relationship between microbiota and human host [36].

Although the mechanism through which periopathogens contribute to periodontal diseases is still not fully understood, studies have suggested that the pathogenic microbiota induces local and systemic inflammation [37,38], a common feature of metabolic disease [2]. As reported above, periodontitis is characterized by a complex biofilm composed of LPS-harboring gram-negative bacteria [32]. CD14, a cell-surface molecule involved in innate immunity [39], is a systemic modulator of LPS-induced metabolic disorders. In this context, we have demonstrated in the current study that *CD14*-ablation protects against HFD-induced inflammation-triggered diabetes and periodontitis. Indeed, HFD-fed *CD14*KO ovariectomised mice did not show any features of periodontitis such as alveolar bone loss or immune cell infiltration into the gingival connective tissue. Nevertheless, the number of mice exhibiting a periopathogenic microbiota was found to be increased. This result may suggest that a HFD induces metabolic disorders and periodontal damage through activation of innate immunity via LPS production by periodontal microbiota, rather than direct adverse effects on tissues by periopathogenic derivatives as previously suggested [40]. In agreement with our findings, previous studies have reported relationships between CD14, inflammation and PD in humans [41]. Therefore, the use of antibiotic treatment restricted to the periodontal pocket could be thought.

Homeostasis in periodontium involves multiple factors including variation in sex hormone production [42]. Many studies recently

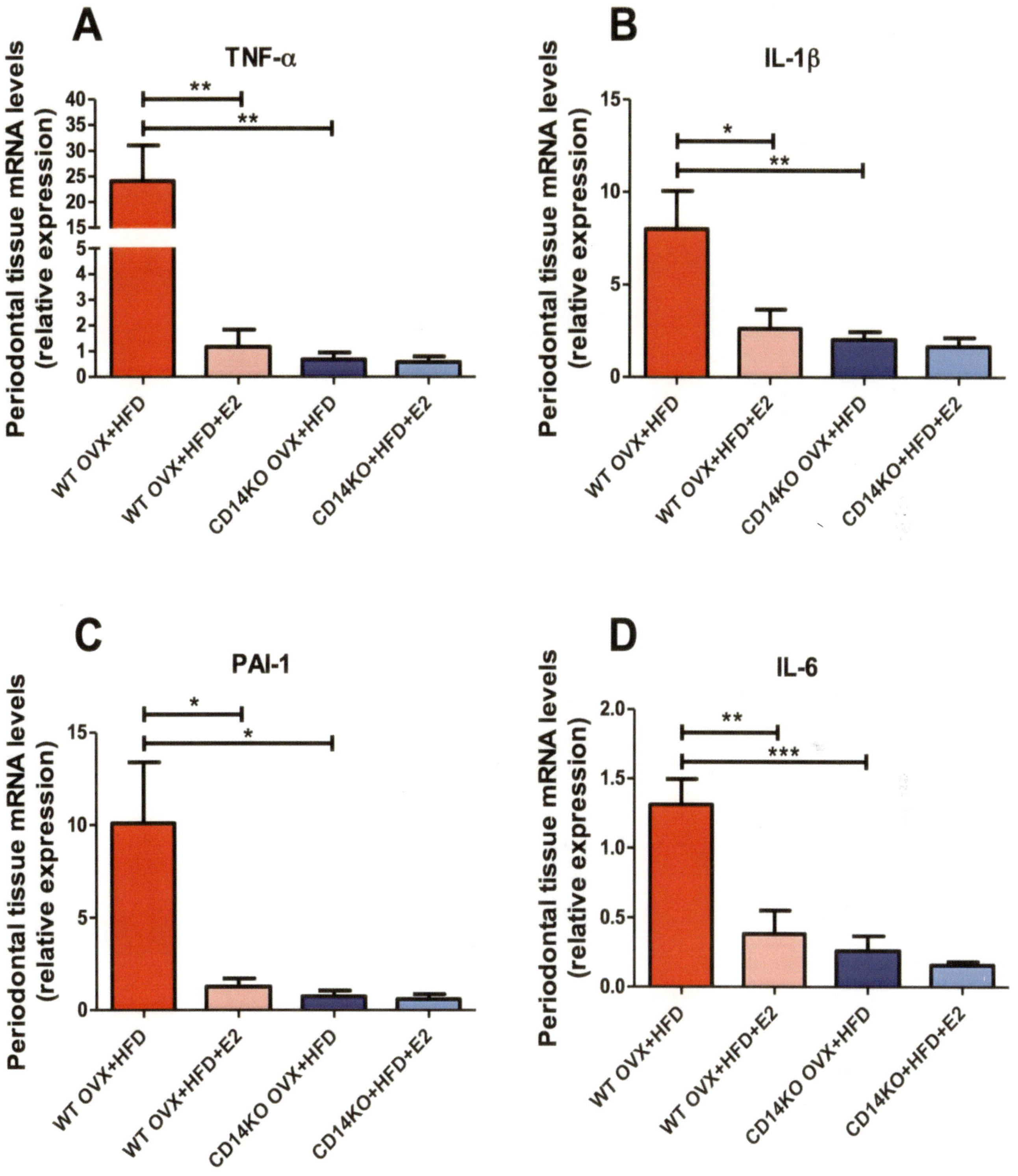

Figure 7. *CD14*KO mice did not display HFD-induced periodontal inflammation. mRNA expression of TNF-α (**A**), IL-1β (**B**), PAI-1(**C**) and IL-6 (**D**) in gingival tissue. *P<0.05, **P<0.01,***P<0.001 (one-way ANOVA followed by Tukey test). Results are presented as means ± SEM.

showed that modification of estrogenic status during menstrual cycles [43], puberty [44] and pregnancy [42], could be linked to the occurrence of gingivitis, an inflammation of soft periodontal tissue without loss of attachment [42]. Some studies hypothesized that estrogen therapy may be used in these periodontal pathologies [45]. However, this therapeutic strategy would be not applicable in gingivitis because it is spontaneously reversed after gingival plaque removing and/or menstrual cycle normalization [46]. Conversely, estrogen deficiency is considered a risk factor for periodontitis [19]. Importantly, we recently demonstrated that estrogen replacement reversed HFD-induced metabolic diseases [18,20]. Here, we report the reversal of the proportion of WT OVX mice

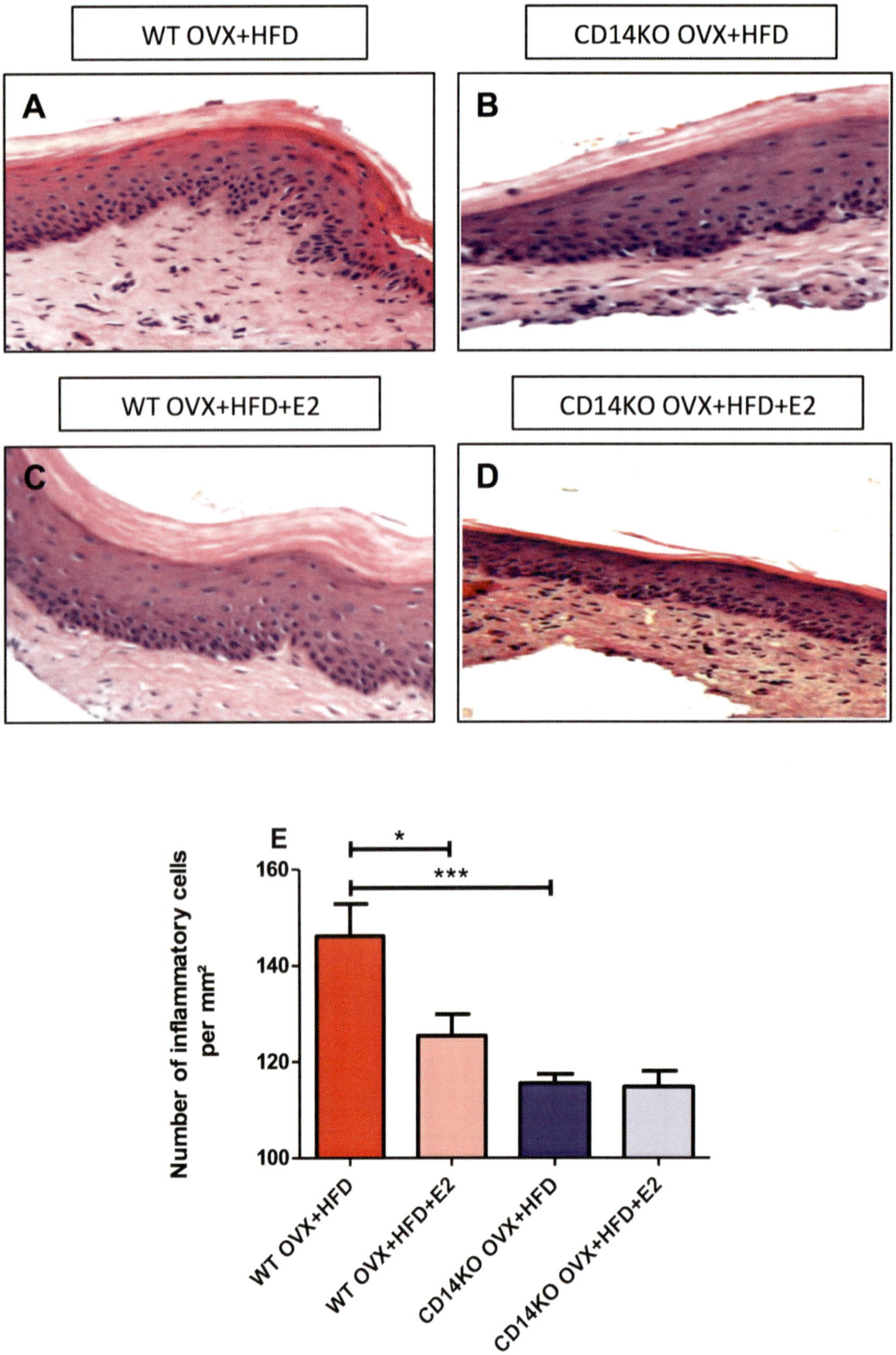

Figure 8. The depletion of *CD14* reduced HFD-induced inflammatory cell infiltration into gingival connective tissue. Histological appearance of the gingival tissues with H/E coloration from WT OVX+HFD (**A,** n = 6), *CD14*KO OVX+HFD (**B,** n = 6) WT OVX+HFD+E2 (**C,** n = 6), and *CD14*KO OVX+HFD+E2 (**D,** n = 6) **E**. Number of inflammatory cells for each group. *P<0.05,**P<0.01, ***P<0.001 (one-way ANOVA followed by Tukey test). Results are presented as means ± SEM.

with periodontal pathogenic microbiota by E2-treatment, as already reported in post-menopausal women using hormone replacement therapy [23]. While *in vivo* E2-administration enhanced systemic inflammation in mice [47], our results suggest that estrogen supplementation may have a specific protective effect on periodontal tissue by regulating the inflammation induced by a HFD [48]. Since E2 increases the thickness and keratinization of epithelia [49] we suggest that this hormone could reinforce the gingival epithelium against the colonization by specific periopathogens [48]. Moreover, E2 stimulates the innate immune response [50,51], increasing macrophage reactivity against aggressive bacteria [52]. As already suggested [53], our results support the hypothesis that E2-supplementation may have anti-inflammatory effects on periodontal tissue. Thus, we can propose that our present results could be the basis of further experimental trials dedicated to show the importance of hormone replacement therapy as well as that of a tight glycemic control to maintain periodontal health.

In conclusion, the data reported herein suggest a causal link between the activation of the LPS pathway on innate immunity by periodontal microbiota and the occurrence of HFD-induced periodontal defects. This pathophysiological mechanism could be targeted by estrogens, which may thus represent a new therapeutic perspective to prevent HFD-induced periodontal inflammation and reduce the occurrence of PD.

Supporting Information

Figure S1 NCD-fed CD14KO mice did not exhibit metabolic disorders. A) Body weight was assessed in 8-wk-old mice after 4 weeks of diet: CD14KO OVX+NCD (n = 12) and CD14KO OVX+NCD+E2 (n = 12). **B)** Time course of glycemia (mg/dl) during IPGTT. The inset represents the Glycemic index for each group. *P<0,05 (one-way ANOVA followed by Tukey test for A and Two-Way ANOVA with Bonferroni's post-test for B). Results are presented as means ± SEM.

Figure S2 NCD-fed CD14KO mice did not display periodontal disease. A) Alveolar bone loss of Hemi-mandibule from each group : CD14KO OVX+NCD (n = 5) and CD14KO OVX+NCD+E2 (n = 5), was explored B.C.D.E mRNA expression of TNF-α **(B)**, IL-1β **(C)**, PAI-1**(D)** and IL-6 **(E)** in gingival tissue. D. Number of inflammatory cells for each group *P<0,05 **P<0,01 ***P<0,001 (one-way ANOVA followed by Tukey test). Results are presented as means ± SEM.

Table S1 Rates of positive bacterial cultures in NCD-fed mice. The table shows the qualitative analysis of periodontal microbiota in each group : WT OVX NCD E2 (n = 16), CD14KO OVX+NCD (n = 5) and CD14KO OVX+NCD+E2 (n = 5). *P<0.05,**P<0.01 (Fischer exact tests).

Author Contributions

Conceived and designed the experiments: VBB MS JFA PG RB PK. Performed the experiments: VBB MS ER PL RB. Analyzed the data: VBB MS JNV. Wrote the paper: VBB MSJFA PG MS RB PK.

References

1. Preshaw PM, Alba AL, Herrera D, Jepsen S, Konstantinidis A, et al. (2012) Periodontitis and diabetes: a two-way relationship. Diabetologia 55: 21–31.
2. Hotamisligil GS (2006) Inflammation and metabolic disorders. Nature 444: 860–867.
3. Shoelson SE, Lee J, Goldfine AB (2006) Inflammation and insulin resistance. J Clin Invest 116: 1793–1801.
4. Cani PD, Amar J, Iglesias MA, Poggi M, Knauf C, et al. (2007) Metabolic endotoxemia initiates obesity and insulin resistance. Diabetes 56: 1761–1772.
5. Saito T, Shimazaki Y (2007) Metabolic disorders related to obesity and periodontal disease. Periodontol 2000 43: 254–266.
6. Turnbaugh PJ, Backhed F, Fulton L, Gordon JI (2008) Diet-induced obesity is linked to marked but reversible alterations in the mouse distal gut microbiome. Cell Host Microbe 3: 213–223.
7. Turnbaugh PJ, Ridaura VK, Faith JJ, Rey FE, Knight R, et al. (2009) The effect of diet on the human gut microbiome: a metagenomic analysis in humanized gnotobiotic mice. Sci Transl Med 1: 6ra14.
8. Neish AS (2009) Microbes in gastrointestinal health and disease. Gastroenterology 136: 65–80.
9. Cani PD, Delzenne NM, Amar J, Burcelin R (2008) Role of gut microflora in the development of obesity and insulin resistance following high-fat diet feeding. Pathol Biol (Paris) 56: 305–309.
10. Lakhssassi N, Elhajoui N, Lodter JP, Pineill JL, Sixou M (2005) Antimicrobial susceptibility variation of 50 anaerobic periopathogens in aggressive periodontitis: an interindividual variability study. Oral Microbiol Immunol 20: 244–252.
11. Blaizot A, Vergnes JN, Nuwwareh S, Amar J, Sixou M (2009) Periodontal diseases and cardiovascular events: meta-analysis of observational studies. Int Dent J 59: 197–209.
12. Blasco-Baque V, Kemoun P, Loubieres P, Roumieux M, Heymes C, et al. [Impact of periodontal disease on arterial pressure in diabetic mice.]. Ann Cardiol Angeiol (Paris).
13. Guan SM, He JJ, Zhang M, Shu L (2011) Prevotella intermedia stimulates tissue-type plasminogen activator and plasminogen activator inhibitor-2 expression via multiple signaling pathways in human periodontal ligament cells. FEMS Immunol Med Microbiol 62: 91–100.
14. Robert AA, Rass MD, Al-Zoman KH, Al-Sohail AM, Alsuwyed AS, et al. (2010) Determinants of periodontopathogens in microbiological monitoring of diabetic patients with periodontitis. Saudi Med J 31: 1044–1048.
15. Ford PJ, Gemmell E, Chan A, Carter CL, Walker PJ, et al. (2006) Inflammation, heat shock proteins and periodontal pathogens in atherosclerosis: an immunohistologic study. Oral Microbiol Immunol 21: 206–211.
16. Lee HR, Jun HK, Kim HD, Lee SH, Choi BK Fusobacterium nucleatum GroEL induces risk factors of atherosclerosis in human microvascular endothelial cells and ApoE(−/−) mice. Mol Oral Microbiol 27: 109–123.
17. Koren O, Spor A, Felin J, Fak F, Stombaugh J, et al. (2011) Human oral, gut, and plaque microbiota in patients with atherosclerosis. Proc Natl Acad Sci U S A 108 Suppl 1: 4592–4598.
18. Riant E, Waget A, Cogo H, Arnal JF, Burcelin R, et al. (2009) Estrogens protect against high-fat diet-induced insulin resistance and glucose intolerance in mice. Endocrinology 150: 2109–2117.
19. Haas AN, Rosing CK, Oppermann RV, Albandar JM, Susin C (2009) Association among menopause, hormone replacement therapy, and periodontal attachment loss in southern Brazilian women. J Periodontol 80: 1380–1387.
20. Bonds DE, Lasser N, Qi L, Brzyski R, Caan B, et al. (2006) The effect of conjugated equine oestrogen on diabetes incidence: the Women's Health Initiative randomised trial. Diabetologia 49: 459–468.
21. Donahue RP, Bean JA, Donahue RA, Goldberg RB, Prineas RJ (1997) Insulin response in a triethnic population: effects of sex, ethnic origin, and body fat. Miami Community Health Study. Diabetes Care 20: 1670–1676.
22. Lenfant F, Tremollieres F, Gourdy P, Arnal JF (2011) Timing of the vascular actions of estrogens in experimental and human studies: why protective early, and not when delayed? Maturitas 68: 165–173.
23. Tarkkila L, Kari K, Furuholm J, Tiitinen A, Meurman JH (2010) Periodontal disease-associated micro-organisms in peri-menopausal and post-menopausal women using or not using hormone replacement therapy. A two-year follow-up study. BMC Oral Health 10: 10.
24. Serino M, Waget A, Marsollier N, Masseboeuf M, Payros G, et al. (2011) Lipid-induced peroxidation in the intestine is involved in glucose homeostasis imbalance in mice. PLoS One 6: e21184.
25. Chan EC, McLaughlin R (2000) Taxonomy and virulence of oral spirochetes. Oral Microbiol Immunol 15: 1–9.
26. Wade-Gueye NM, Boudiffa M, Laroche N, Vanden-Bossche A, Fournier C, et al. (2010) Mice lacking bone sialoprotein (BSP) lose bone after ovariectomy and display skeletal site-specific response to intermittent PTH treatment. Endocrinology 151: 5103–5113.
27. Wilensky A, Gabet Y, Yumoto H, Houri-Haddad Y, Shapira L (2005) Three-dimensional quantification of alveolar bone loss in Porphyromonas gingivalis-infected mice using micro-computed tomography. J Periodontol 76: 1282–1286.
28. Munch IC, Larsen M, Borch-Johnsen K, Glumer C, Lund-Andersen H, et al. (2011) Cumulative glycaemia as measured by lens fluorometry: association with retinopathy in type 2 diabetes. Diabetologia 54: 757–761.
29. Takahashi K, Nishimura F, Kurihara M, Iwamoto Y, Takashiba S, et al. (2001) Subgingival microflora and antibody responses against periodontal bacteria of

young Japanese patients with type 1 diabetes mellitus. J Int Acad Periodontol 3: 104–111.
30. Field CA, Gidley MD, Preshaw PM, Jakubovics N (2012) Investigation and quantification of key periodontal pathogens in patients with type 2 diabetes. J Periodontal Res 47: 470–478.
31. Willershausen B, Haas G, Krummenauer F, Hohenfellner K (2004) Relationship between high weight and caries frequency in German elementary school children. Eur J Med Res 9: 400–404.
32. Burcelin R, Serino M, Chabo C, Blasco-Baque V, Amar J (2011) Gut microbiota and diabetes: from pathogenesis to therapeutic perspective. Acta Diabetol 48: 257–273.
33. Serino M, Luche E, Gres S, Baylac A, Berge M, et al. (2012) Metabolic adaptation to a high-fat diet is associated with a change in the gut microbiota. Gut 61: 543–553.
34. Amar J, Burcelin R, Ruidavets JB, Cani PD, Fauvel J, et al. (2008) Energy intake is associated with endotoxemia in apparently healthy men. Am J Clin Nutr 87: 1219–1223.
35. Cani PD, Bibiloni R, Knauf C, Waget A, Neyrinck AM, et al. (2008) Changes in gut microbiota control metabolic endotoxemia-induced inflammation in high-fat diet-induced obesity and diabetes in mice. Diabetes 57: 1470–1481.
36. Salvi GE, Yalda B, Collins JG, Jones BH, Smith FW, et al. (1997) Inflammatory mediator response as a potential risk marker for periodontal diseases in insulin-dependent diabetes mellitus patients. J Periodontol 68: 127–135.
37. Sahingur SE, Xia XJ, Schifferle RE (2012) Oral bacterial DNA differ in their ability to induce inflammatory responses in human monocytic cell lines. J Periodontol 83: 1069–1077.
38. Tew JG, El Shikh ME, El Sayed RM, Schenkein HA (2012) Dendritic cells, antibodies reactive with oxLDL, and inflammation. J Dent Res 91: 8–16.
39. Goyert SM, Ferrero E, Rettig WJ, Yenamandra AK, Obata F, et al. (1988) The CD14 monocyte differentiation antigen maps to a region encoding growth factors and receptors. Science 239: 497–500.
40. Feghali K, Tanabe S, Grenier D (2011) Soluble CD14 induces cytokine release by human oral epithelial cells. J Periodontal Res 46: 147–152.
41. Ren L, Jiang ZQ, Fu Y, Leung WK, Jin L (2009) The interplay of lipopolysaccharide-binding protein and cytokines in periodontal health and disease. J Clin Periodontol 36: 619–626.
42. Carrillo-de-Albornoz A, Figuero E, Herrera D, Cuesta P, Bascones-Martinez A (2012) Gingival changes during pregnancy: III. Impact of clinical, microbiological, immunological and socio-demographic factors on gingival inflammation. J Clin Periodontol 39: 272–283.
43. Krejci CB, Bissada NF (2002) Women's health issues and their relationship to periodontitis. J Am Dent Assoc 133: 323–329.
44. Oh TJ, Eber R, Wang HL (2002) Periodontal diseases in the child and adolescent. J Clin Periodontol 29: 400–410.
45. Giuca MR, Carli E, Pasini M, Bonfigli D, Cappe MR (2009) Evaluation of efficacy of estrogen and phytotherapy in oral cavity alterations of women in menopause. Minerva Ginecol 61: 13–22.
46. Baser U, Cekici A, Tanrikulu-Kucuk S, Kantarci A, Ademoglu E, et al. (2009) Gingival inflammation and interleukin-1 beta and tumor necrosis factor-alpha levels in gingival crevicular fluid during the menstrual cycle. J Periodontol 80: 1983–1990.
47. Calippe B, Douin-Echinard V, Laffargue M, Laurell H, Rana-Poussine V, et al. (2008) Chronic estradiol administration in vivo promotes the proinflammatory response of macrophages to TLR4 activation: involvement of the phosphatidylinositol 3-kinase pathway. J Immunol 180: 7980–7988.
48. Mascarenhas P, Gapski R, Al-Shammari K, Wang HL (2003) Influence of sex hormones on the periodontium. J Clin Periodontol 30: 671–681.
49. Arnal JF, Laurell H, Lenfant F, Douin-Echinard V, Brouchet L, et al. (2006) Estradiol action in atherosclerosis and reendothelialization. Ernst Schering Found Symp Proc: 69–86.
50. Corcoran MP, Meydani M, Lichtenstein AH, Schaefer EJ, Dillard A, et al. (2010) Sex hormone modulation of proinflammatory cytokine and C-reactive protein expression in macrophages from older men and postmenopausal women. J Endocrinol 206: 217–224.
51. Gillgrass A, Chege D, Bhavanam S, Kaushic C (2010) Estradiol limits viral replication following intravaginal immunization leading to diminished mucosal IgG response and non-sterile protection against genital herpes challenge. Am J Reprod Immunol 63: 299–309.
52. Maekawa T, Takahashi N, Tabeta K, Aoki Y, Miyashita H, et al. (2011) Chronic oral infection with Porphyromonas gingivalis accelerates atheroma formation by shifting the lipid profile. PLoS One 6: e20240.
53. Mirza BA, Syed A, Izhar F, Ali Khan A (2010) Bidirectional relationship between diabetes and periodontal disease: review of evidence. J Pak Med Assoc 60: 766–768.

3

Tobacco Smoke Augments *Porphyromonas gingivalis* - *Streptococcus gordonii* Biofilm Formation

Juhi Bagaitkar[1], Carlo A. Daep[1], Carol K. Patel[2], Diane E. Renaud[2], Donald R. Demuth[1,2], David A. Scott[1,2]*

1 Department of Microbiology and Immunology, University of Louisville, Louisville, Kentucky, United States of America, 2 Center of Oral Health and Systemic Disease, University of Louisville, Louisville, Kentucky, United States of America

Abstract

Smoking is responsible for the majority of periodontitis cases in the US and smokers are more susceptible than non-smokers to infection by the periodontal pathogen *Porphyromonas gingivalis*. *P. gingivalis* colonization of the oral cavity is dependent upon its interaction with other plaque bacteria, including *Streptococcus gordonii*. Microarray analysis suggested that exposure of *P. gingivalis* to cigarette smoke extract (CSE) increased the expression of the major fimbrial antigen (FimA), but not the minor fimbrial antigen (Mfa1). Therefore, we hypothesized that CSE promotes *P. gingivalis-S. gordonii* biofilm formation in a FimA-dependent manner. FimA total protein and cell surface expression were increased upon exposure to CSE whereas Mfa1 was unaffected. CSE exposure did not induce *P. gingivalis* auto-aggregation but did promote dual species biofilm formation, monitored by microcolony numbers and depth (both, $p<0.05$). Interestingly, *P. gingivalis* biofilms grown in the presence of CSE exhibited a lower pro-inflammatory capacity (TNF-α, IL-6) than control biofilms (both, $p<0.01$). CSE-exposed *P. gingivalis* bound more strongly to immobilized rGAPDH, the cognate FimA ligand on *S. gordonii*, than control biofilms ($p<0.001$) and did so in a dose-dependent manner. Nevertheless, a peptide representing the Mfa1 binding site on *S. gordonii*, SspB, completely inhibited dual species biofilm formation. Thus, CSE likely augments *P. gingivalis* biofilm formation by increasing FimA avidity which, in turn, supports initial interspecies interactions and promotes subsequent high affinity Mfa1-SspB interactions driving biofilm growth. CSE induction of *P. gingivalis* biofilms of limited pro-inflammatory potential may explain the increased persistence of this pathogen in smokers. These findings may also be relevant to other biofilm-induced infectious diseases and conditions.

Editor: Roy Martin Roop II, East Carolina University School of Medicine, United States of America

Funding: This study was funded by a National Institutes of Health award to DAS (R01DE019826). The funders had no role in study design, data collection and analysis, decision to publish, or preparation of the manuscript.

Competing Interests: The authors have declared that no competing interests exist.

* E-mail: dascot07@louisville.edu

Introduction

Periodontitis is an infectious, chronic inflammatory disease of the supportive structures of the teeth. Smokers often exhibit periodontal disease that is more severe than in non-smokers, with increased alveolar bone loss [1], attachment loss [2], tooth mobility, and tooth loss [3] all apparent and odds ratios of 3 to 7 commonly reported [4]. Moreover, smokers are more likely to be refractory to treatment than non-smokers [5]. Indeed, smoking has been reported to be responsible for more than half of the 15 million periodontitis cases in the US, with 42% and 11% attributable to current and former smoking, respectively [6]. The resultant health burden consumes > $14 billion per annum [7].

Dental plaque in healthy individuals is predominantly comprised of Gram positive commensals, with oral streptococci such as *Streptococcus gordonii* estimated to represent up to 70% of the total bacterial population [8,9,10]. However, in periodontitis there is a bacterial succession to a microflora rich in Gram negative, obligate anaerobes that is responsible for the onset and progression of disease [8,9]. Multiple studies have shown that smokers are more likely to be infected with the key etiological agent of periodontitis, *P. gingivalis*, to harbor higher numbers of *P. gingivalis*, and to exhibit more persistent infection by this pathogen [11,12,13,14], relative to non-smokers.

P. gingivalis persistence in the oral cavity of smokers can be attributed to a compromised immune response and/or increased bacterial virulence. We have recently shown, for example, that *P. gingivalis* adapts to the environmental stress presented by cigarette smoke extract (CSE) by altering the expression of several genes and outer membrane proteins that are key in lowering its inflammatory potential. Interestingly, specific genes (PG2133 and PG2134) in the operon coding for the synthesis and assembly of the major fimbrial antigen of *P. gingivalis* (*fimA*) were induced on exposure to CSE, while several genes in the capsular biosynthesis locus (*capK*, PG0117, PG0118 and *wecC*) were suppressed [15].

During the development of dental plaque, primary colonizers first bind to the salivary pellicle on the tooth surface and provide an attachment stratum that facilitates bacterial succession through multimodal, receptor-ligand mediated, co-adhesive interactions. In order for *P. gingivalis* to establish an oral infection, interactions with primary or early colonizers, such as *S. gordonii*, are critical [16,17]. For example, the long fimbriae (FimA) of *P. gingivalis* bind to *S. gordonii* glyceraldehyde-3 phosphate dehydrogenase (GAPDH) [17,18] while the shorter fimbriae (Mfa1) bind to streptococcal surface protein B (SspB) protein [19]. We have previously shown that an 80 amino acid sequence on SspB is critical for Mfa1 adhesion, with a synthetic peptide of this SspB region, named BAR

(SspB Adherence Region), a potent inhibitor of Mfa1-dependent *P. gingivalis - S. gordonii* biofilms formation [20]. On the other hand, *P. gingivalis* capsule production has been shown to be inversely related to biofilm growth [21].

As CSE-exposure down-regulates capsular genes and upregulates *fimA*-related gene activity, but not Mfa1 activity, we hypothesized that CSE exposure would augment *P. gingivalis - S. gordonii* biofilms formation via a FimA-dependent mechanism. We set out to test this hypothesis in a dual species, open flow biofilm model.

Materials and Methods

Materials

P. gingivalis 33277 and *Streptococcus gordonii* DL1 were purchased from the American Type Culture Collection (Manassas, VA). *Escherichia coli* TOP10, pBAD gIIIA expression plasmid and Platinum PCR Supermix High Fidelity were from Invitrogen (Carlsbad, CA). Gifu Anaerobe Medium [GAM] came from Nissui Pharmaceutical (Tokyo), while brain heart infusion (BHI) media and yeast extract were purchased from Beckton Dickinson (Sparks, MD). HRP-linked anti-Rabbit IgG was from Cell Signaling Technology (Beverly, MA), while anti-FimA and anti-Mfa1 specific antibodies were custom generated by Cocalico Biologicals (Reamstown, PA). Alexa Fluor 488 protein labeling kit to tag anti-*P. gingivalis* antibodies as well as hexidium iodide were purchased from Invitrogen. Tetramethylbenzidine, Manostat Carter 4/8 cassette peristaltic pump, 15 mm×40 mm cover glass, 0.89 mm diameter, platinum-cured silicone tubing and Falcon PVC plates were all purchased from Fisher Scientific (Suwanee, GA). HiTrap Chelating HP affinity columns came from Amersham Biosciences Corp. (Piscataway, NJ). FC71 flow cells were obtained from Biosurface Technologies Corp. (Bozeman, MT). Cloning primers were bought from Biosynthesis (Lewisville, TX) with initial TA-cloning performed using pGEM-T Easy from Promega (Madison, WI) followed by cloning into the pBAD gIIIA expression plasmid from Invitrogen. BAR peptide was synthesized by Biosynthesis Inc. (Lewisville, TX). Standard 3R4F reference cigarettes were obtained from Kentucky Tobacco Research and Development Center (Lexington, KY). West Pico chemiluminescent substrate kits and bacterial protein extraction reagent (B-PER) were purchased from Thermo Scientific (Rockford, IL). α-Bungarotoxin, BSA and 3,3′-Diaminobenzidine (DAB) substrate were purchased from Sigma Aldrich (St. Louis MO). Nitrocellulose membranes came from BioRad (Hercules, CA). TNF-α and IL-6 ELISA kits were purchased from eBioscience (San Diego, CA). Hydroxyapatite discs were purchased from Clarkson Chromatography Products (South Williamsport, PA).

Bacterial culture and *in vitro* modeling of tobacco exposure

S. gordonii DL-1 was cultured in BHI supplemented with 0.5% yeast extract under aerobic conditions, without shaking, at 37°C. *P. gingivalis* 33277 was grown in GAM or GAM conditioned with CSE (GAM-CSE) under anaerobic conditions (86% N_2, 4% H_2, 10% CO_2) at 37°C in a Coy Laboratories (Grass Lake, MI) anaerobic chamber. Bacteria were harvested at mid- to late-exponential phase (O.D. of 1 corresponds to 10^9 cells ml^{-1}). To prepare CSE, cigarette smoke was drawn through 50 ml GAM by using a three-way stopcock and a syringe, with 40 ml 'drags' performed over a period of 2 sec, one drag every 2 sec. Cigarette smoke extract (CSE)-conditioned medium was filtered (0.22 μm) and adjusted to pH 7.2. The nicotine [(S)-3-(1-methyl-2-pyrrolidinyl)pyridine] content of GAM-CSE was determined by gas–liquid chromatography, as previously described [22] and adjusted to physiologically relevant doses [22,23,24,25]. Unless otherwise noted, GAM-CSE was employed at a concentration of 4000 ng nicotine equivalents/ml. We have previously shown that *P. gingivalis* is tolerant, with respect to growth and viability, to such CSE doses [26]. In all experiments, *P. gingivalis* was either cultured in GAM or GAM-CSE for two passages. For specific experiments, CSE-exposed *P. gingivalis* was reconditioned by culturing back into GAM for two passages.

Expression and purification of rGAPDH and truncated SspB

Recombinant GAPDH was produced by PCR amplification of the coding gene from *S. gordonii* DL-1 using primers designed using the previously published sequence for the *GAPDH* gene in *S. gordonii* [27]. To facilitate directional cloning into the expression vector system, the restriction enzyme sites SacI and XbaI (underlined) were added at the beginning of each primer for GADPH, respectively:

5′-GCGGAGCTCGTAGTTAAAGTTGGTATTAACG-3′ (forward) and

5′-GCGTCTAGACCTTTAGCGATTTTTGCG-3′ (reverse).

The PCR product obtained was initially TA-cloned into pGEM-T Easy and subsequently directionally ligated into the pBAD gIIIA expression plasmid with a C-terminal 6X-histidine tag and transformed into expression strain *E. coli* Top10. rGAPDH was induced using 2 mM arabinose and purified using HiTrap chelating HP affinity columns, according to the manufacturer's protocol. Purity was confirmed by SDS-PAGE.

Synthesis of BAR and control peptides

BAR peptide (NH2-LEAAPKKVQDLLKKANITVKGAFQLFS-OH) and a control peptide in which BAR lysine residues were substituted with the D-enantiomers were synthesized commercially to ≥85% purity.

Total FimA and Mfa1 expression by *P. gingivalis*

P. gingivalis lysates (1×10^6 mid-late log cells) were obtained from cells grown in GAM, GAM-CSE or from reconditioned bacteria. Due to the large number of genes and proteins dysregulated by CSE [15,28], it was necessary to normalize western blots to *P. gingivalis* cell numbers, as previously described [20,28,29]. Western blots were probed with either rabbit anti-FimA or anti-Mfa1 IgG and HRP-linked anti-rabbit IgG. Immunoreactive bands were visualized by chemiluminescence. Imaging and densitometry were performed using a Kodak 4000 MM image station.

FimA and Mfa1 surface availability

FimA availability to antibody on mid- to late log phase CSE-exposed and control (GAM) *P. gingivalis* cells bound to PVC plates was determined by ELISA. Anti-FimA or anti-*P. gingivalis* IgG binding was quantified using an HRP-linked secondary antibody with tetramethylbenzidine as the chromogenic substrate, essentially as previously described by Pierce et al. [30]. Mfa1 availability to antibody was assessed identically. The FimA and Mfa1 signal was normalized to the total *P. gingivalis*. CSE-induced FimA and Mfa1 availability to antibody was expressed as percentage of the control (GAM).

P. gingivalis- S. gordonii dual species biofilms

P. gingivalis and *S. gordonii* biofilms were formed on saliva coated cover slips in FC 71 flow cells, as we have previously described [31,32]. Briefly, *S. gordonii* cells (25 ml cultures) were suspended in sterile PBS and labeled with hexidium iodide (1.6 mg/ml;) at room temperature for 15 min. Glass coverslips were coated with 0.22 μm filter-sterilized saliva and fixed in the flow cells. Labeled *S. gordonii* cells were then introduced into the flow cells using a Manostat Carter 4/8 cassette peristaltic pump at 6 ml per hour for approximately 2 hr. The flow cells were then washed with sterile PBS for 30 min to remove non-adherent *S. gordonii* cells. *P. gingivalis* cells, grown in GAM or GAM-CSE, were harvested by centrifugation, and re-suspended in PBS before being introduced into the flow system (flow rate of 6 ml per hour for 1 h). After washing in PBS, 30 min, bound *P. gingivalis* was detected using Alexa-488 labeled rabbit anti-*P. gingivalis* IgG. *P. gingivalis-S. gordonii* biofilms were visualized using an Olympus Fluoview confocal laser scanning microscope (Olympus, Pittsburgh, PA) under 60x magnification using the argon laser for visualization of Alexa488 labeling and the HeNe-G laser to visualize hexidium iodide-labeled streptococci. The number and height of *P. gingivalis* microcolonies were determined from 6 randomly chosen frames using the FluoView software. Microcolony depth was determined by performing *z*-plane scans from 0 μm to 50 μm above the cover glass surface.

Induction of TNF-α and IL-6 in human innate cells by *P. gingivalis* biofilms

P. gingivalis biofilms were grown on pellicle coated hydroxyapatite discs (10.6 mm Ø), essentially as described previously [33]. Briefly, hydroxyapatite discs were coated for 24 hours with growth medium (60% saliva pooled from 3 different donors, 10% FBS) for 24 hrs, 37°C to allow for pellicle formation. After 24 hrs, pellicle-coated hydroxyapatite discs were immersed in GAM or CSE in 6-well polystyrene cell culture plates and seeded with 10^9 *P. gingivalis* cells grown for two sequential passages in either GAM or CSE to initiate biofilm formation. Discs were incubated for 48 hr under anaerobic conditions (86% N_2, 4% H_2, 10% CO_2) at 37°C in a Coy Laboratories anaerobic chamber. To determine the inflammatory potential of *P. gingivalis* biofilms, hydroxyapatite discs were removed from GAM/CSE, washed once in PBS before placing them in 24-well polystyrene plates containing human PBMCs (10^6 per well). PBMCs were also simultaneously challenged with planktonic cultures of *P. gingivalis* grown in GAM or CSE for two passages (MOI 10:1).

Adherence of *P. gingivalis* to rGAPDH

Binding of *P. gingivalis* cells to immobilized protein was studied using a protocol adapted from Demuth et al [20]. 1, 5 and 10 μg of rGAPDH were immobilized on nitrocellulose membranes using a vacuum dot blot apparatus. Membranes were then blocked with 3% BSA for an hour followed by overnight incubation with *P. gingivalis* at 10^9 cfu/mL from GAM/CSE cultures at RT. Bound *P. gingivalis* was then quantified using rabbit anti- *P. gingivalis* IgG followed by HRP-tagged anti-rabbit secondary antibody and DAB substrate. Mean dot intensity from three independent blots was calculated using ImageJ software (NIH) and background signals (no immobilized protein) subtracted.

P. gingivalis aggregation assays

Fimbriae directly increase *P. gingivalis* adhesiveness by promoting inter-bacterial aggregation [34] [35] As CSE increases fimbrial density, we determined whether CSE promotes bacterial auto-aggregation. *P. gingivalis*, grown in GAM or CSE, was harvested by centrifugation and suspended in sterile PBS at O.D. ~1. Aggregation of *P. gingivalis* was assessed spectrophotometerically ($Abs_{600\ nm}$) over 8 hrs using an Eppendorf Biophotometer Plus spectrophotometer.

Influence of exogenous *S. gordonii* ligands (GAPDH and BAR) on dual species CSE-induced biofilms

CSE and control (GAM) *P. gingivalis-S. gordonii* biofilms were formed and analyzed, as described above with a slight modification. *P. gingivalis* grown in GAM or GAM-CSE was pre-treated with 3.4 μM GAPDH or BAR peptide for 30 minutes before introduction into the flow chamber. The number and height of *P. gingivalis* microcolonies were determined as described in the dual species biofilm section.

Statistical Analysis

Data were evaluated by two-tailed *t* tests and analysis of variance (ANOVA), as appropriate, using the InStat program (Graphpad Software, La Jolla, CA). Statistical significance was set at $p<0.05$.

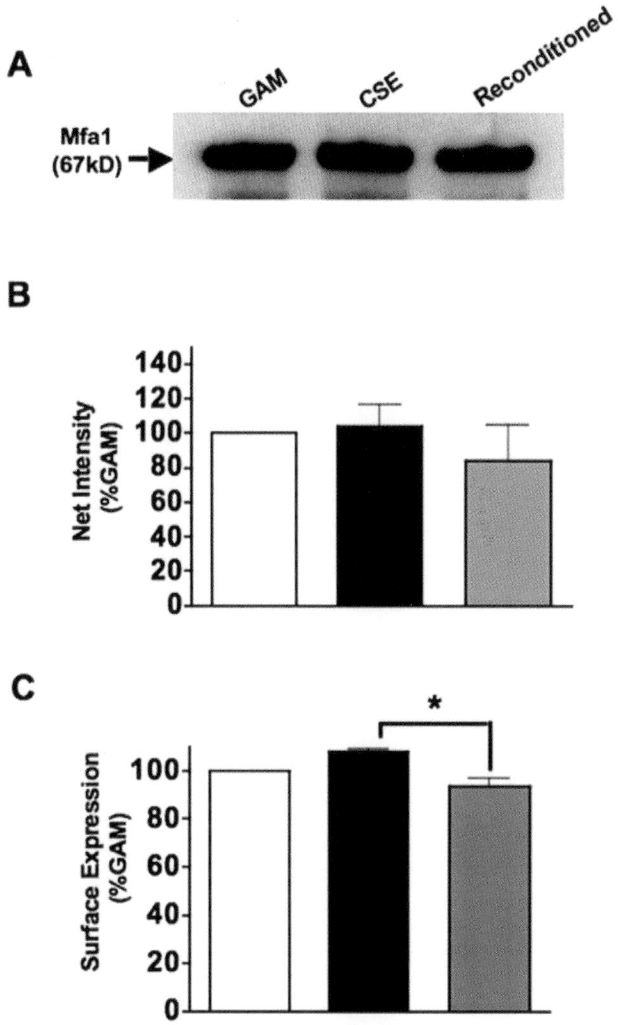

Figure 1. CSE exposure does not influence total protein levels or surface availability of Mfa1. (A) Western blots of 1 x 10^6 *P. gingivalis* cell lysates sequentially passaged in GAM, GAM-CSE, and then fresh GAM, respectively and re-probed with rabbit anti-Mfa1 antibody (blot was first probed for FimA, as shown in ***Supplemental Figure 1***). (B) Relative band intensities for Mfa1 expression (B) indicate Mfa1 protein levels remain unaltered by CSE exposure. Surface availability ELISAs for Mfa1 (C) confirm that Mfa1 availability on the *P. gingivalis* surface remains unchanged. *$p < 0.05$.

Results

CSE exposure upregulates surface expression of surface-available FimA but not Mfa1

Our previous studies suggested that exposure to CSE augments the expression of the major fimbrial antigen of *P. gingivalis* (FimA) at the transcriptional (microarray and RT-PCR) and protein levels, while simultaneously down-regulating capsular polysaccharides [15,28]. CSE-induced upregulation of FimA is confirmed in ***Figure S1***. However, CSE exposure has no effect on the absolute protein level of the minor fimbrial antigen of *P. gingivalis* (Mfa1; ***Figure 1A*** and ***B***) or on Mfa1 surface presentation, as assessed by availability to anti-Mfa1 antibodies (***Figure 1C***).

CSE exposure increases *P. gingivalis-S. gordonii* biofilm formation

Figures 2A and ***2B*** show representative z-stack images of microcolonies formed by *P. gingivalis* grown in GAM and GAM-CSE, respectively, on *S. gordonii*. As presented in ***Figure 2C and 2D***, CSE exposure resulted in an approximately 2-fold increase in the total number of *P. gingivalis-S. gordonii* microcolonies formed as well as an approximately 3-fold increase in microcolony height, relative to control biofilms ($p<0.05$ and $p<0.01$, respectively).

CSE exposure decreases the inflammatory activity of *P. gingivalis* biofilms

The pro-inflammatory activity of CSE-exposed *P. gingivalis* (Black bars) grown either in planktonic form or in monospecies biofilms was lower than that of unexposed bacteria (white bars), as determined by IL-6 and TNF-α release from primary human PBMCs, and- shown in ***Figure 3A and B*** respectively. Furthermore, this reduced immune potential was not influenced by á-bungarotoxin, an á7 nAChR and cholinergic anti-inflammatory pathway antagonist [36], (see ***Figure 3***). Therefore, it is unlikely that repressed cytokine production can be attributed to nicotine carry over from growth medium or bacterial sequestration and, rather, is a direct consequence of CSE-induced alteration to *P. gingivalis* itself.

CSE exposure does not induce *P. gingivalis* auto-aggregation

Aggregation of planktonic *P. gingivalis* did not occur in *P. gingivalis* grown in CSE or in GAM-CSE (see ***Figure S2***). Rather, the slow settling that is typical of this bacterium was apparent, suggesting that auto-aggregation does not contribute to CSE-induced *P. gingivalis-S. gordonii* biofilm formation.

CSE exposure increases *P. gingivalis* binding to immobilized FimA ligand (rGAPDH)

To determine whether CSE-induced FimA upregulation played a functional role in *P. gingivalis - S. gordonii* associations, adherence of *P. gingivalis* to immobilized rGAPDH was assessed. As shown in **Figure 4**, CSE-exposed *P. gingivalis* exhibited increased binding to rGAPDH ($p<0.01$ and $p<0.001$), compared to control bacteria (GAM), and did so in a dose-dependent manner.

CSE-induced *P. gingivalis-S. gordonii* biofilm formation is FimA-enhanced but Mfa1-dependent

The efficacy of rGAPDH protein to interfere with CSE-induced *P. gingivalis-S. gordonii* biofilms formation was subsequently assessed. CSE-exposed *P. gingivalis* associated strongly with *S. gordonii*, compared to controls (***Figures 5A*** and ***B***). While

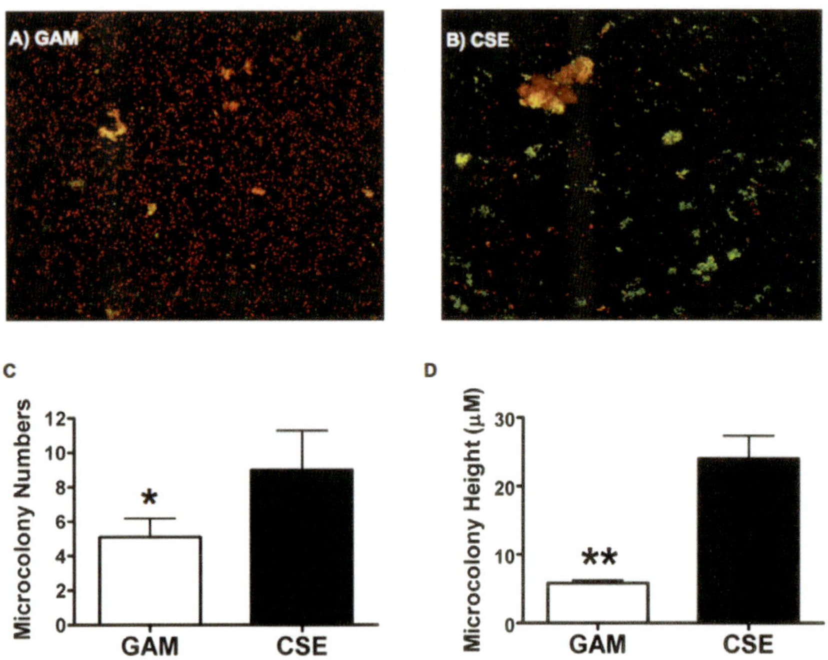

Figure 2. CSE exposure augments *P. gingivalis - S. gordonii* biofilm formation. Total number and height of microcolonies (yellow) formed by Hexidium iodide labeled *S. gordonii* (red) and Alexa-488 labeled *P. gingivalis* (green) biofilms, formed in an open flow system were quantified by taking optical section along the *x-y* and *z* axis at 1 μm intervals with a confocal microscope. CSE-exposed *P. gingivalis* associated strongly with *S. gordonii* as reflected by increased number of microcolonies formed (B) compared to control *P. gingivalis* grown in GAM (A). Total numbers (C) and average microcolony height (D) were quantified from 6 randomly chosen microscopic fields per biofilm using the FluoView software. *$p<0.05$; **$p<0.01$.

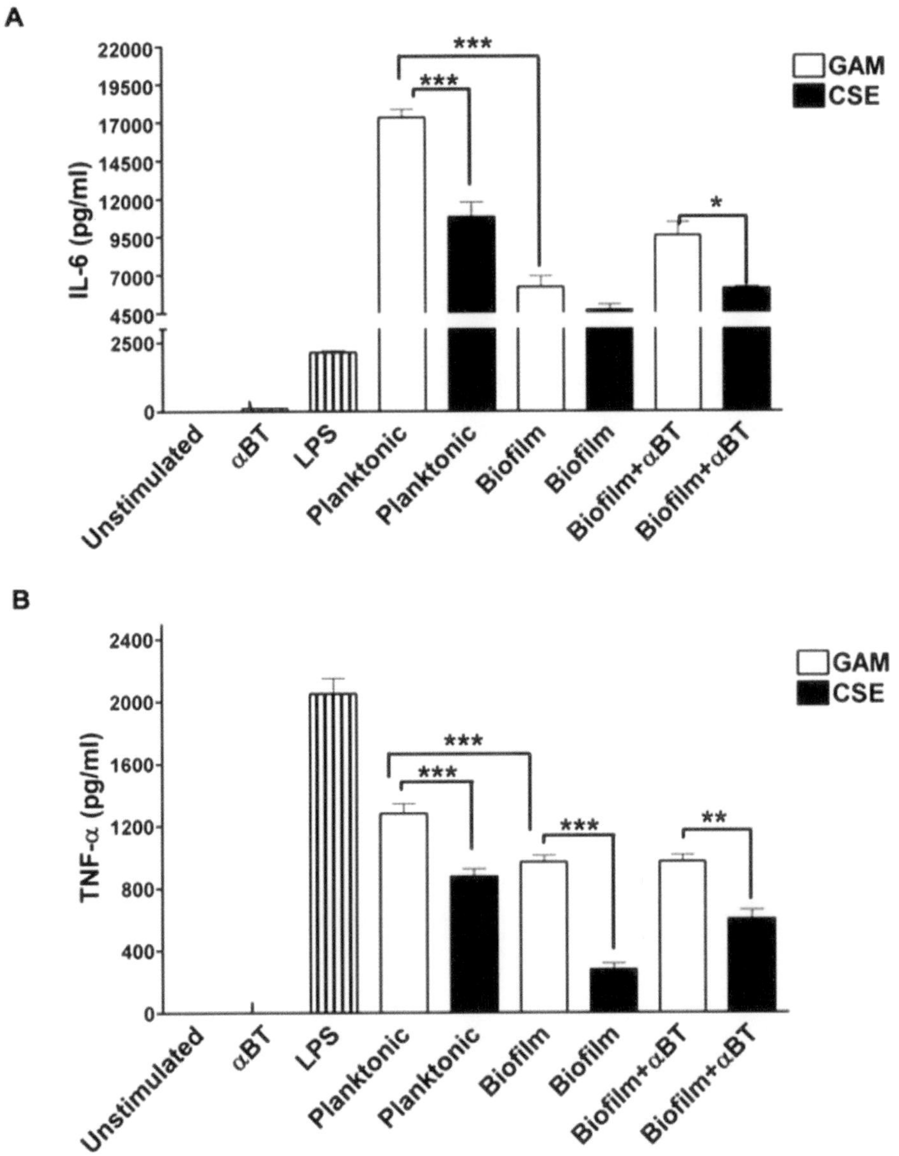

Figure 3. CSE exposure reduces inflammatory activity of *P. gingivalis* biofilms. Human PBMCs (1×10^{6}) were challenged with *P. gingivalis* grown in GAM or CSE as planktonic cultures (MOI 10:1) or with 48 hr *P. gingivalis* biofilms formed on HA discs in GAM or CSE and with 1 µg/ml *E. coli* LPS as positive control. Additionally, PBMCs were pre-treated with α–bungarotoxin (500 ng/ml for 30 min) before addition of biofilm discs. Cells were stimulated overnight and cell-free supernatants were analyzed for IL-6 (A) and TNF-α (B) levels by ELISA. **p*<0.05; ***p*<0.01; ****p*<0.001.

exogenous rGAPDH pretreatment did not have a significant influence on microcolony numbers, rGAPDH did decrease microcolony height by 65% relative to control biofilms ($p<0.05$ and $p<0.01$); (***Figures 5C and D***). We have previously shown that a synthetic BAR peptide, characterized by Daep et al, efficiently blocks the binding of Mfa1 to SspB [32,37]. Therefore, we used pre-incubation with BAR to ascertain the importance of Mfa1 in CSE-induced *P. gingivalis-S. gordonii* biofilm formation. As shown in ***Figure 5E*** and ***5F***, BAR peptide at 3.4 µM completely abrogated (100%) dual species biofilm formation under CSE-exposed and control conditions.

Discussion

Our prior work has established that CSE-exposure increases *P. gingivalis* monospecies biofilm formation. However, *in vivo* it is *P. gingivalis*-early colonizer (particularly streptococcal) interactions that are considered critical for *P. gingivalis* to establish itself and maintain a presence in dental plaque. Furthermore, microbes may interact with the immune response in different manners in biofilms than in planktonic form. Thus we have extended our prior studies to observe the influence of CSE on *P. gingivalis – S. gordonii*; mechanisms that promote CSE-induced *P. gingivalis – S. gordonii* interaction; and the pro-inflammatory potential of CSE-exposed biofilms.

We have previously reported, using microarrays representative of the *P. gingivalis* genome that CSE exposure resulted in the differential regulation of 6.8% of *P. gingivalis* genes in planktonic culture. Of particular relevance to biofilm formation were two major fimbriae synthesis genes that were induced by CSE (PG2133 and PG2134) as well as several genes in the capsular operon (*cap*K [PG0111], PG0117, PG0118 and *wec*C [PG0108])

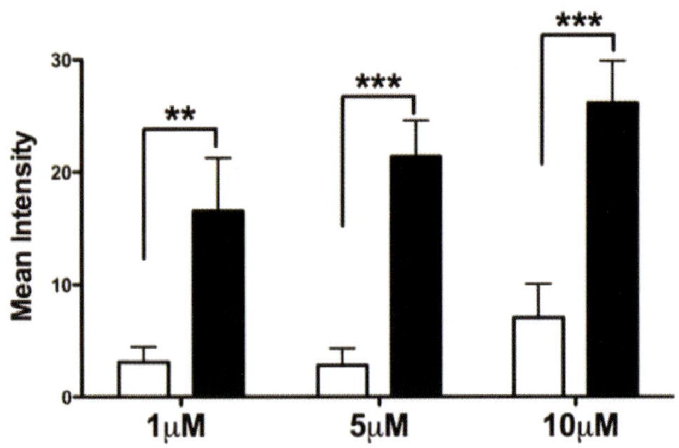

Figure 4. CSE exposure promotes adherence of intact *P. gingivalis* to rGAPDH. *P. gingivalis* adherence to immobilized rGAPDH was assessed by dot blot. 10^9 cfu/ml of *P. gingivalis*, grown either in GAM or CSE, were added to each blot and adherent bacteria detected using anti-*P. gingivalis* IgG. Averaged mean intensities from three independent blots indicate CSE exposure augments binding to GAPDH in a dose-dependent manner. $**p<0.01$; $***p<0.001$.

that were suppressed by CSE [15]. CSE dysregulation of capsular and fimbrial genes was reflected at the ultrastructural level, as confirmed by electron microcopy, and at the functional level, as shown by altered host-pathogen interactions [15,28].

We now show that CSE-exposure results in increased surface availability of FimA protein, but not Mfa1, and increases *P. gingivalis* biofilm formation in a dual species model. Thus, CSE-induced fimbrial gene dysregulation is functionally significant. FimA is known to play multiple roles in *P. gingivalis* virulence, but is best characterized as a fimbrial adhesin that is important in binding of *P. gingivalis* to the salivary pellicle [38].

Mfa1 is essential for *P. gingivalis-S. gordonii* biofilm formation, as illustrated by SspB-deficient mutants and competitive inhibition with BAR peptide [19,31,32,39]. We show herein that, nevertheless, FimA binds strongly to immobilized rGADPH; CSE-induced FimA surface upregulation significantly enhances dual species biofilm; and that the addition of an exogenous FimA ligand suppresses *P. gingivalis - S. gordonii* biofilms. FimA-GAPDH interactions are of much lower affinity than Mfa1-SSpB/BAR interactions, with IC_{50} values for inhibition of dual species biofilms reported to be in the region of 300-400 μg/ml and 4 μg/ml for GAPDH and SspB peptides respectively [31,32,40]. Thus, it would seem that a

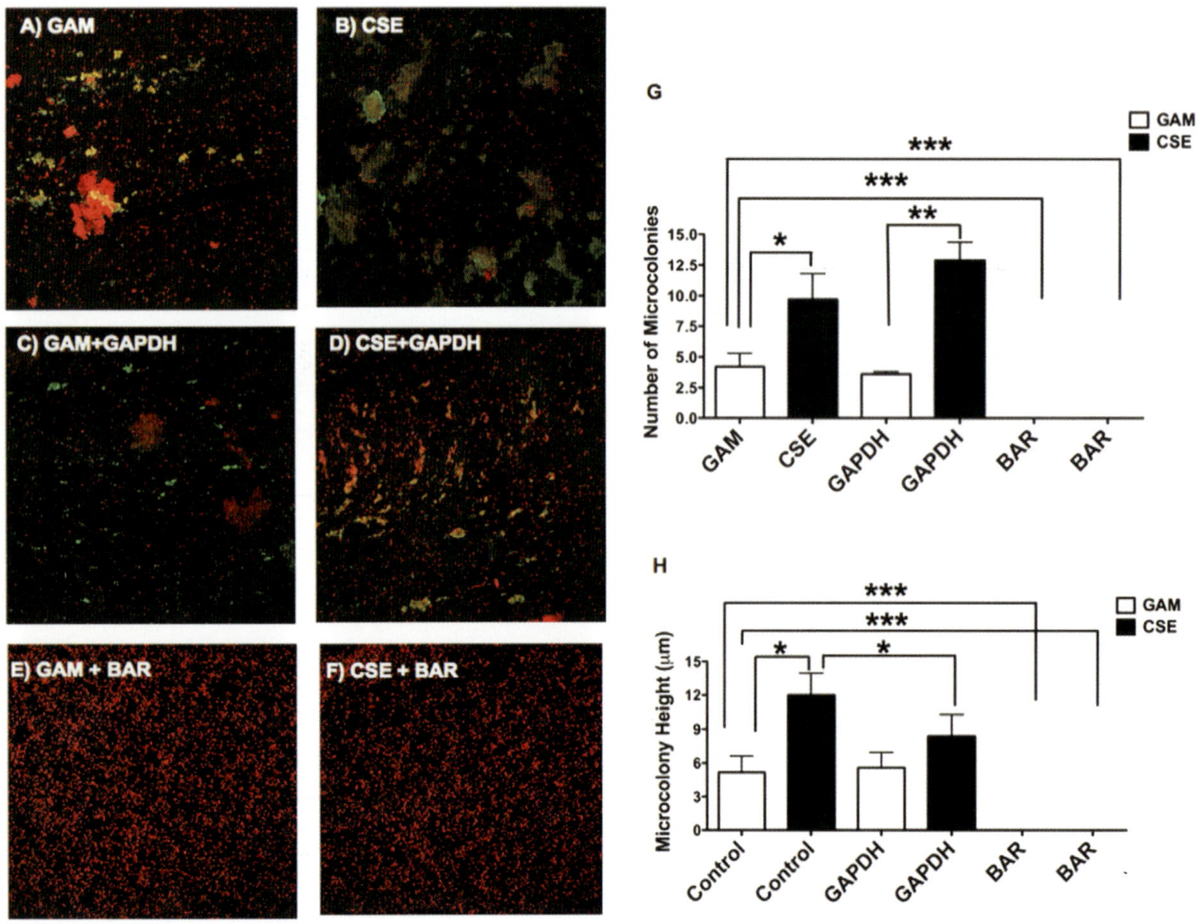

Figure 5. CSE augmentation of biofilm formation is FimA-enhanced and Mfa1-dependent. As shown previously CSE exposure significantly increased *P. gingivalis* association with *S. gordonii* (B) compared to control *P. gingivalis* grown in GAM (A) as reflected by total numbers of microcolonies (yellow) formed. Pre-treatment of *P. gingivalis* with rGAPDH (3.4 μM) reduced association (microcolony height and numbers) between CSE-exposed *P. gingivalis* and *S. gordonii* (D) but had no effect on control *P. gingivalis* grown in GAM (C). Pretreatment with BAR peptide (3.4 μM) completely abolished any association between *S. gordonii* and *P. gingivalis* grown either in GAM (E) or CSE (F). Total number and height of microcolonies (yellow) formed by Hexidium iodide labeled *S. gordonii* (red) and Alexa488 labeled *P. gingivalis* (green) biofilms formed in an open flow system were quantified by taking optical section along the *x-y* and *z* axis at 1 μm intervals under a confocal microscope and presented in figures (G) and (H) respectively. $*p<0.05$; $**p<0.01$; $***p<0.001$.

CSE-induced increase in FimA avidity enhances initial *P. gingivalis-S. gordonii* adhesive contacts. Subsequently, high affinity Mfa-SspB interactions are critical in stabilizing the biofilm and possibly promoting *P. gingivalis* persistence in the host.

While auto-aggregation in planktonic culture may not be directly related to biofilm formation *in vivo*, the lack of CSE-induced *P. gingivalis* auto-auggregation noted in vitro suggests that bacterial clumping did not contribute to increased biofilm formation in the flow cell system.

These data suggest that, in smokers and non-smokers alike, anti-biofilm strategies that target both FimA and Mfa1 may be more successful in inhibiting *P. gingivalis* colonization than the use of anti-Mfa1 agents alone. They also suggest that the considerable efforts currently underway to develop FimA-focused vaccination strategies [41,42] may be particularly relevant to tobacco users, the section of society who are most likely to harbor *P. gingivalis* and who share the largest periodontal disease burden. This hypothesis is supported by the discovery of a FimA binding domain (amino acid residues 166 to 183) on the GADPH protein produced by another oral streptococcus species, *S. oralis*, along with the realization that this peptide may represent another potent inhibitor of *P. gingivalis* colonization in the oral cavity [40].

It should also be remembered that enhancement of FimA surface expression may have other pathological consequences that are unrelated to streptococcal adhesion. Recently, for example, it has been shown that FimA binds several plasma factors, particularly prekallikrein, and may thus be involved in subversion of the kinin generating system to the benefit of *P. gingivalis* and disadvantage of the host [43]. FimA also appears to play important roles in the invasion and activation of host cells such as osteoblasts [44] and vascular endothelial cells [45] by *P. gingivalis*. Indeed, the invasion and activation of host cells is expected to be a critical step in many of the fatal and debilitating chronic systemic diseases associated with periodontal infections. Enhanced FimA expression may also promote *P. gingivalis* adherence to other periodontal pathogens like *Treponema denticola* [46] promoting establishment of a complex pathogenic plaque.

It is of interest that initial characterization of the host response to CSE-enhanced *P. gingivalis* mono-species biofilms suggests that they exhibit considerably reduced inflammatory potential than control biofilms, as assessed by stimulation of TNF-á and IL-6 from primary human innate cells. *P. gingivalis* does not express nicotinic receptors, does not internalize nicotine [47,48] and bacteria were washed prior to stimulating PBMCs with biofilms. Nevertheless, we thought it prudent to ensure that inflammatory suppression subsequent to engagement of the á7 nicotinic acetylcholine receptor by nicotine [36] did not occur. The reduced cytokine profile observed with CSE-exposed biofilms was not influenced by pre-incubation with the nAChR antagonist, á-bungarotoxin. Therefore, the possibility of nAChR-initiated activation of the cholinergic anti-inflammatory pathway by nicotine carry over is unlikely. These results are in keeping with our prior in vitro studies that have shown that intact *P. gingivalis* exposed to CSE elicit a reduced ability to induce cytokines under the transcriptional control of the NF-êB system [15,28]. While CSE promotes FimA expression, FimA itself is an inefficient TLR2-agonist and induces immune hyporesponsiveness in innate cells in a TLR2-IRAK-1-IκBα-dependent manner [28]. More recent data suggest that the TLR-engagement domain of FimA lies in the signal peptide with a cysteine residue at single amino acid position 19A essential [49]. Our findings are also consistent with established *in vivo* conditions. Patients who smoke exhibit increased susceptibility to periodontitis and are more likely to display severe disease and be refractory to treatment [5]. Paradoxically, smokers demonstrate reduced clinical inflammation, that is, diminished edema, bleeding on probing, and local cytokine production compared to non-smokers [5,50]. Thus, a reduced inflammatory capacity of CSE-exposed *P. gingivalis* biofilms is in keeping with the established clinical apparition of periodontitis in tobacco smokers.

In summary, the majority of periodontitis cases in the US have been directly attributed to tobacco smoking [6], yet the mechanisms underlying this smoking-induced and exacerbated infectious disease are poorly understood. CSE exposure results in increased dual species biofilm formation in a manner that is FimA-enhanced, Mfa1-dependent, and does not involve CSE-induced *P. gingivalis* aggregation. The dramatic CSE-induced promotion of biofilm formation is likely to contribute to the established clinical phenomenon of increased *P. gingivalis* infection and perseverance in the oral cavity of smokers. These findings are also relevant to ongoing efforts to develop effective anti-FimA vaccination strategies for the treatment of periodontal diseases and may have implications for other biofilm-associated diseases.

Supporting Information

Figure S1 CSE exposure increases total protein levels and surface availability of FimA. (A) Western blots of 1×10^6 *P. gingivalis* cell lysates sequentially passaged in GAM, GAM-CSE, and then fresh GAM, respectively and probed with rabbit anti-FimA antibody (A). (B) Relative band intensities for FimA expression indicate FimA is reversibly and significantly upregulated on CSE-exposure. Surface availability ELISA for FimA confirms that upregulated FimA is available on the *P. gingivalis* surface. *$p<0.05$; **$p<0.01$; ***$p<0.001$.

Figure S2 CSE does not induce *P. gingivalis* auto-aggregation. Aggregation of *P. gingivalis* (10^9 cells/ml) grown in either in GAM (grey line) or CSE (black line) and suspended in PBS was monitored by measuring optical density ($O.D._{600}$) of over time. CSE does not increase *P. gingivalis* aggregation.

Author Contributions

Conceived and designed the experiments: JB DRD DAS. Performed the experiments: JB CAD CKP DER. Analyzed the data: JB DAS. Contributed reagents/materials/analysis tools: CAD. Wrote the paper: JB DRD DAS.

References

1. Grossi SG, Genco RJ, Machtei EE, Ho AW, Koch G, et al. (1995) Assessment of risk for periodontal disease. II. Risk indicators for alveolar bone loss. Journal of Periodontology 66: 23–29.
2. Grossi SG, Zambon JJ, Ho AW, Koch G, Dunford RG, et al. (1994) Assessment of risk for periodontal disease. I. Risk indicators for attachment loss. J Periodontol 65: 260–267.
3. McGuire MK, Nunn ME (1996) Prognosis versus actual outcome. III. The effectiveness of clinical parameters in accurately predicting tooth survival. J Periodontol 67: 666–674.
4. Bagaitkar J, Demuth DR, Scott DA (2008) Increased susceptibility to bacterial infections in tobacco smokers. Tobacco Induced Diseases 4.
5. Palmer RM, Wilson RF, Hasan AS, Scott DA (2005) Mechanisms of action of environmental factors–tobacco smoking. J Clin Periodontol 32 Suppl 6: 180–195.
6. Tomar SL, Asma S (2000) Smoking-attributable periodontitis in the United States: findings from NHANES III. National Health and Nutrition Examination Survey. J Periodontol 71: 743–751.
7. Brown LJ, Johns BA, Wall TP (2002) The economics of periodontal diseases. Periodontol 2000 29: 223–234.

8. Rosan B, Lamont RJ (2000) Dental plaque formation. Microbes Infect 2: 1599–1607.
9. Marsh PD (1994) Microbial ecology of dental plaque and its significance in health and disease. Adv Dent Res 8: 263–271.
10. Christopher AB, Arndt A, Cugini C, Davey ME (2010) A streptococcal effector protein that inhibits Porphyromonas gingivalis biofilm development. Microbiology 156: 3469–3477.
11. Haffajee AD, Socransky SS (2001) Relationship of cigarette smoking to the subgingival microbiota. J Clin Periodontol 28: 377–388.
12. Zambon JJ, Grossi SG, Machtei EE, Ho AW, Dunford R, et al. (1996) Cigarette smoking increases the risk for subgingival infection with periodontal pathogens. J Periodontol 67: 1050–1054.
13. Eggert FM, McLeod MH, Flowerdew G (2001) Effects of smoking and treatment status on periodontal bacteria: evidence that smoking influences control of periodontal bacteria at the mucosal surface of the gingival crevice. Journal of Periodontology 72: 1210–1220.
14. Kamma JJ, Nakou M, Baehni PC (1999) Clinical and microbiological characteristics of smokers with early onset periodontitis. J Periodontal Res 34: 25–33.
15. Bagaitkar J, Scott DA, Williams LR, Renaud DE, Daep C, et al. (2009) Tobacco-induced alterations to Porphyromonas gingivalis-host interactions. Environmental Microbiology 11: 1242–1253.
16. Chung WO, Demuth DR, Lamont RJ (2000) Identification of a Porphyromonas gingivalis receptor for the Streptococcus gordonii SspB protein. Infect Immun 68: 6758–6762.
17. Maeda K, Nagata H, Yamamoto Y, Tanaka M, Tanaka J, et al. (2004) Glyceraldehyde-3-phosphate dehydrogenase of Streptococcus oralis functions as a coadhesin for Porphyromonas gingivalis major fimbriae. Infect Immun 72: 1341–1348.
18. Maeda K, Nagata H, Nonaka A, Kataoka K, Tanaka M, et al. (2004) Oral streptococcal glyceraldehyde-3-phosphate dehydrogenase mediates interaction with Porphyromonas gingivalis fimbriae. Microbes Infect 6: 1163–1170.
19. Park Y, Simionato MR, Sekiya K, Murakami Y, James D, et al. (2005) Short fimbriae of Porphyromonas gingivalis and their role in coadhesion with Streptococcus gordonii. Infect Immun 73: 3983–3989.
20. Demuth DR, Irvine DC, Costerton JW, Cook GS, Lamont RJ (2001) Discrete protein determinant directs the species-specific adherence of Porphyromonas gingivalis to oral streptococci. Infect Immun 69: 5736–5741.
21. Davey ME, Duncan MJ (2006) Enhanced biofilm formation and loss of capsule synthesis: deletion of a putative glycosyltransferase in Porphyromonas gingivalis. J Bacteriol 188: 5510–5523.
22. Fraser HS, Palmer RM, Wilson RF, Coward PY, Scott DA (2001) Elevated systemic concentrations of soluble ICAM-1 (sICAM) are not reflected in the gingival crevicular fluid of smokers with periodontitis. J Dent Res 80: 1643–1647.
23. McGuire JR, McQuade MJ, Rossmann JA, Garnick JJ, Sutherland DE, et al. (1989) Cotinine in saliva and gingival crevicular fluid of smokers with periodontal disease. J Periodontol 60: 176–181.
24. Chen X, Wolff L, Aeppli D, Guo Z, Luan W, et al. (2001) Cigarette smoking, salivary/gingival crevicular fluid cotinine and periodontal status. A 10-year longitudinal study. J Clin Periodontol 28: 331–339.
25. Scott DA, Palmer RM, Stapleton JA (2001) Validation of smoking status in clinical research into inflammatory periodontal disease. J Clin Periodontol 28: 715–722.
26. Bagaitkar J, Williams LR, Renaud DE, Bemakanakere MR, Martin M, et al. (2009) Tobacco-induced alterations to Porphyromonas gingivalis-host interactions. Environ Microbiol 11: 1242–1253.
27. Demuth DR, Davis CA, Corner AM, Lamont RJ, Leboy PS, et al. (1988) Cloning and expression of a Streptococcus sanguis surface antigen that interacts with a human salivary agglutinin. Infect Immun 56: 2484–2490.
28. Bagaitkar J, Demuth DR, Daep CA, Renaud DE, Pierce DL, et al. (2010) Tobacco upregulates P. gingivalis fimbrial proteins which induce TLR2 hyposensitivity. PLoS One 5: e9323.
29. Hritz M, Fisher E, Demuth DR (1996) Differential regulation of the leukotoxin operon in highly leukotoxic and minimally leukotoxic strains of Actinobacillus actinomycetemcomitans. Infect Immun 64: 2724–2729.
30. Pierce DL, Nishiyama S, Liang S, Wang M, Triantafilou M, et al. (2009) Host adhesive activities and virulence of novel fimbrial proteins of Porphyromonas gingivalis. Infect Immun 77: 3294–3301.
31. Lamont RJ, El-Sabaeny A, Park Y, Cook GS, Costerton JW, et al. (2002) Role of the Streptococcus gordonii SspB protein in the development of Porphyromonas gingivalis biofilms on streptococcal substrates. Microbiology 148: 1627–1636.
32. Daep CA, James DM, Lamont RJ, Demuth DR (2006) Structural characterization of peptide-mediated inhibition of Porphyromonas gingivalis biofilm formation. Infect Immun 74: 5756–5762.
33. Guggenheim B, Stathopolou P, Thurheer T, Kinane D (2009) In vitro modeling of host-parasite interactions: the 'subgingival' biofilm challenge of primary human epithelial cells. Nature Immunology - Technical Reports. In press.
34. Hongo H, Takano H, Morita M (2007) Dense fimbrial meshwork enhances Porphyromonas gingivalis adhesiveness: a scanning electron microscopic study. J Periodontal Res 42: 114–118.
35. Kuboniwa M, Amano A, Hashino E, Yamamoto Y, Inaba H, et al. (2009) Distinct roles of long/short fimbriae and gingipains in homotypic biofilm development by Porphyromonas gingivalis. BMC Microbiol 9: 105.
36. Rehani K, Scott DA, Renaud D, Hamza H, Williams LR, et al. (2008) Cotinine-induced convergence of the cholinergic and PI3 kinase-dependent anti-inflammatory pathways in innate immune cells. Biochim Biophys Acta 1783: 375–382.
37. Daep CA, Lamont RJ, Demuth DR (2008) Interaction of Porphyromonas gingivalis with oral streptococci requires a motif that resembles the eukaryotic nuclear receptor box protein-protein interaction domain. Infection and Immunity.
38. Koh EM, Kim J, Kim TG, Moon JH, Oh JH, et al. (2011) Cloning and characterization of heavy and light chain genes encoding the FimA-specific monoclonal antibodies that inhibit Porphyromonas gingivalis adhesion. Microbiol Immunol 55: 199–210.
39. Daep CA, Lamont RJ, Demuth DR (2008) Interaction of Porphyromonas gingivalis with oral streptococci requires a motif that resembles the eukaryotic nuclear receptor box protein-protein interaction domain. Infect Immun.
40. Nagata H, Iwasaki M, Maeda K, Kuboniwa M, Hashino E, et al. (2009) Identification of the binding domain of Streptococcus oralis glyceraldehyde-3-phosphate dehydrogenase for Porphyromonas gingivalis major fimbriae. Infect Immun 77: 5130–5138.
41. Shin EA, Park YK, Lee KO, Langridge WH, Lee JY (2009) Synthesis and assembly of Porphyromonas gingivalis fimbrial protein in potato tissues. Mol Biotechnol 43: 138–147.
42. Yu F, Xu QA, Chen W (2011) A targeted fimA DNA vaccine prevents alveolar bone loss in mice after intra-nasal administration. J Clin Periodontol 38: 334–340.
43. Rapala-Kozik M, Bras G, Chruscicka B, Karkowska-Kuleta J, Sroka A, et al. (2011) Adsorption of components of the plasma kinin-forming system on the surface of Porphyromonas gingivalis involves gingipains as the major docking platforms. Infect Immun 79: 797–805.
44. Zhang W, Ju J, Rigney T, Tribble GD (2011) Fimbriae of Porphyromonas gingivalis are Important for Initial Invasion of Osteoblasts, but Not for Inhibition of Their Differentiation and Mineralization. J Periodontol 82: 909–916.
45. Khlgatian M, Nassar H, Chou HH, Gibson FC, 3rd, Genco CA (2002) Fimbria-dependent activation of cell adhesion molecule expression in Porphyromonas gingivalis-infected endothelial cells. Infect Immun 70: 257–267.
46. Hashimoto M, Ogawa S, Asai Y, Takai Y, Ogawa T (2003) Binding of Porphyromonas gingivalis fimbriae to Treponema denticola dentilisin. FEMS Microbiol Lett 226: 267–271.
47. Cogo K, Calvi BM, Mariano FS, Franco GC, Goncalves RB, et al. (2009) The effects of nicotine and cotinine on Porphyromonas gingivalis colonisation of epithelial cells. Arch Oral Biol 54: 1061–1067.
48. Cogo K, Montan MF, Bergamaschi Cde C, E DA, Rosalen PL, et al. (2008) In vitro evaluation of the effect of nicotine, cotinine, and caffeine on oral microorganisms. Can J Microbiol 54: 501–508.
49. Shoji M, Yoshimura A, Yoshioka H, Takade A, Takuma Y, et al. (2010) Recombinant Porphyromonas gingivalis FimA preproprotein expressed in Escherichia coli is lipidated and the mature or processed recombinant FimA protein forms a short filament in vitro. Can J Microbiol 56: 959–967.
50. Johnson GK, Guthmiller JM (2007) The impact of cigarette smoking on periodontal disease and treatment. Periodontol 2000 44: 178–194.

4

Relationship between Periodontitis-Related Antibody and Frequent Exacerbations in Chronic Obstructive Pulmonary Disease

Tamaki Takahashi[1], Shigeo Muro[1]*, Naoya Tanabe[1], Kunihiko Terada[1], Hirofumi Kiyokawa[1], Susumu Sato[1], Yuma Hoshino[1], Emiko Ogawa[2], Kazuko Uno[3], Koji Naruishi[4], Shogo Takashiba[5], Michiaki Mishima[1]

1 Department of Respiratory Medicine, Kyoto University, Kyoto, Japan, **2** Health Administration Center, Shiga University of Medical Science, Shiga, Japan, **3** Louis Pasteur Center for Medical Research, Kyoto, Japan, **4** Division of Endodontology, Iwate Medical University, Department of Conservative Dentistry and Oral Rehabilitation, Iwate, Japan, **5** Department of Pathophysiology–Periodontal Science, Okayama University Graduate School of Medicine, Dentistry and Pharmaceutical Sciences, Okayama, Japan

Abstract

Background: To identify patients with chronic obstructive pulmonary disease (COPD) who are susceptible to frequent exacerbations is important. Although periodontitis aggravated by poor oral hygiene might increase the risk of lower respiratory tract infection, the relationship between periodontitis and COPD exacerbations remains unknown. This prospective cohort study investigates the relationship between periodontitis-related antibody and exacerbation frequency over a one-year period.

Methods: We assessed an IgG antibody titer against *Porphyromonas gingivalis,* which is a major pathogen of periodontitis, and then prospectively followed up 93 individuals over one year to detect exacerbations.

Results: The numbers of exacerbations and the rate of individuals with frequent exacerbations (at least two per year) were significantly lower in patients with higher IgG titer than those with normal IgG titer (0.8 vs. 1.2 per year, $p = 0.045$ and 14.3 vs. 38.6%, $p = 0.009$, respectively). Multivariate logistic regression analysis showed that being normal-IgG titer for periodontitis-related antibody significantly increased the risk of frequent exacerbations (relative risk, 5.27, 95% confidence interval, 1.30–25.7; $p = 0.019$) after adjusting for other possible confounders, such as a history of exacerbations in the past year, disease severity, COPD medication and smoking status.

Conclusions: Normal-IgG titer for periodontitis-related antibody can be an independent predictor of frequent exacerbations. Measuring periodontitis-related antibody titers might be useful to identify patients with susceptibility to frequent exacerbations so that an aggressive prevention strategy can be designed.

Editor: Clive M. Gray, University of Cape Town, South Africa

Funding: This study was supported by Grants-in-Aid for scientific research (B) (No. 16390234) and (C) (No. 21590964) and a grant to the Respiratory Failure Research Group from the Ministry of Health, Labour and Welfare, Japan. The funders had no role in study design, data collection and analysis, decision to publish, or preparation of the manuscript.

Competing Interests: The authors have declared that no competing interests exist.

* E-mail: smuro@kuhp.kyoto-u.ac.jp

Introduction

Chronic obstructive pulmonary disease (COPD) is the fourth leading cause of death worldwide, and it is associated with an increasing economic cost and social burden [1]. The natural history of COPD is punctuated by exacerbations, which consist of acute episodes of worsening symptoms that might warrant changes in regular medications. These exacerbations negatively impact lung function, health-related quality of life, prognosis and socioeconomic burden [1]. Thus, exploring predictors of exacerbations and identifying patients with susceptibility to frequent exacerbations are important to design an efficient preventive strategy.

Factors associated with exacerbation include disease severity [1], a history of exacerbations [2], smoking [3], chronic inflammation [4], bacterial colonization [5] and gastro-esophageal reflux disease [6]. In addition, we have reported an association between an impaired swallowing reflex and bacterial colonization, systemic inflammation and an increased risk of exacerbations [7]. Since an impaired swallowing reflex might cause the aspiration of oral bacteria leading to lower respiratory tract infection, and poor oral hygiene itself is involved in the risk of aspiration pneumonia [8–10], we speculated that poor oral hygiene would increase the frequency of exacerbations.

Periodontitis is a common oral infectious disease that is associated with poor oral hygiene among the general population. It is characterized by inflammation of the periodontium induced by subgingival plaque bacteria such as anaerobic gram-negative rods [11], that can also be associated with COPD exacerbation [12]. Chronic marginal periodontitis is more prevalent among patients with severe COPD than in other equally severe respiratory diseases [13] and the prevalence of periodontitis increases together with COPD severity [14]. In addition, serum antibody to *Porphyromonas gingivalis* (*P. gingivalis*), which is a frequently isolated pathogen, can be involved in systemic diseases such as cardiovascular disease [15–17]. However, the relationship between periodontitis and COPD exacerbation remains unclear.

We postulated that periodontitis is associated with COPD exacerbations. This prospective cohort study investigated the impact of baseline antibody titers for periodontal antigen (an index of periodontitis) on COPD exacerbation frequency for over one year. We also investigated the relationship between elevated-IgG titer for periodontitis-related antibody and inflammatory cytokines.

Methods

Ethics Statement

The study was approved by the ethics committee of Kyoto University (approval No. E182), and written informed consent was obtained from all participants.

Protocol and Study Participants

We recruited 109 patients with COPD from an outpatient clinic at Kyoto University Hospital, Japan, between September 2006 and August 2008 for this study. All patients provided written informed consent to participate. Blood and induced sputum samples were collected under stable conditions (as defined below) at entry for subsequent assay. We excluded 16 patients based on the following criteria: female, Brinkman index <10 pack-years, respiratory diseases other than COPD, daily intake of systemic corticosteroids and complicated with malignant diseases within 5 years. Thus, 93 patients were prospectively followed up for over one year to detect exacerbations.

Exacerbation Criteria

Exacerbations and stable periods were prospectively identified using diary cards as in our previous study [6,7]. We adopted a modified version of the East London cohort study criteria to define COPD exacerbations [6] based on an increase in any two "major" symptoms (dyspnea, sputum purulence and sputum quantity) or an increase in one "major" and one "minor" symptom (wheeze, sore throat, cough and nasal congestion/discharge) for at least two consecutive days [18]. Stable condition was defined as an exacerbation-free interval of >4 weeks [6].

Clinical Examinations

Pulmonary function tests (Chestac-65V; Chest MI Corp.; Tokyo, Japan) were performed after inhaling short-acting bronchodilators (salbutamol and ipratropium) at entry into the study. Lung volumes and diffusion capacity were measured using helium dilation and the single-breath method, respectively. The British Medical Research Council dyspnea scale (MRC) and Charlson Commorbidities index were also assessed.

Venous blood at entry was collected on the entry day during the stable period and stored at −80°C. Serum levels of immunoglobulin G (IgG) against *P. gingivalis* were measured using an enzyme-linked immunosorbent assay (ELISA) based on validated method [15,19,20]. Since the FDC381 and Su63 strains of *P. gingivalis* are serologically different, we separately measured antibody titers of *Pg*FDC381 and *Pg*Su63. We defined the cut-off point as the mean +2 SD of the controls based on the reported dataset of IgG titers to *Pg*FDC381 and *Pg*SU63 among 10 control individuals [20]. We divided COPD patients into two groups: one is patients whose antibody titers were higher than mean +2SD (High-IgG titer group), and the other includes those whose titers were lower than mean +2SD (Normal-IgG titer group).

Serum C-reactive protein (CRP) and γ-globulin were measured using the High Sensitivity CRP assay (Behring Diagnostics, Westwood, MA, USA), and cellulose acetate electrophoresis, respectively. We assayed 27 cytokines (PDGF, IL-1b, IL-1Ra, IL-2, IL-4, IL-5, IL-6, IL-7, IL-8, IL-9,IL-10, IL-12, IL-13, IL-15, IL-17, eotaxin, FGF, G-CSF, GM-CSF, IFN-γ, IP-10,MCP-1, MIP-1α, MIP-1β, RANTES, TNF-α and VEGF) in 62 patients using a multiplex bead-based immunoassay kit (Bioplex, Bio-Rad Laboratories, Life Science Research Group, Hercules, CA, USA).

Statistical Analysis

Data were statistically analyzed using the Mann-Whitney U-test and the χ^2 test with JMP 8.0 software (SAS Campus Drive, Cary, NC, USA) and all results are presented as medians and 25th-75th percentiles. Independent predictors of frequent exacerbations (defined as at least two exacerbations per year) were detected using multivariate logistic regression analysis. All *p*-values are two-sided and $p<0.05$ was considered significant.

Results

Baseline Characteristics of Study Patients

Table 1 shows the baseline characteristics of the 93 patients and the prevalence of elevated IgG antibody titer against *P. gingivalis*. The distribution of standardized IgG values were 1.29 (−0.05~3.75) for PgFDC 381 and 0.06 (−0.47~0.76) for Pg SU63. The rates of high IgG titer against *Pg*FDC381 and *Pg*Su63 were 52.7% and 23.7%, respectively. Table 2 shows that age, smoking status, smoking index, body mass index, forced expiratory volume in 1 second (FEV_1), Global Initiative for Chronic Obstructive Lung Disease (GOLD) stage, and MRC did not differ between High-IgG titer group and Normal-IgG titer group. Comorbidities assessed by Charlson Comrbidity index [21] were similar between these two groups. The frequency of using inhaled corticosteroid (ICS) was lower and serum γ-globulin levels were higher in High-IgG titer group than in Normal-IgG titer group, whereas the frequency of using tiotropium and long-acting β2 agonists (LABA), and of serum levels of CRP did not differ (Table 3). None of the patients received salmeterol/fluticasone propionate combination therapy.

Relationship between Elevated IgG Antibody Titer against *P. gingivalis* and Exacerbation Frequency

We hypothesized that more periodontitis lead to more exacerbations, but in contrast to our hypothesis, exacerbations were less frequent in High-IgG titer group than in Normal-IgG titer group (0.8 vs. 1.2 per year, $p = 0.045$, Figure 1 and Table 4). Moreover, the rate of patients who experienced frequent exacerbations (at least two per year) was also lower in High-IgG titer group than in Normal-IgG titer group (14.3% vs. 38.6%, $p = 0.009$, Table 4).

Multivariate Analysis to Detect Independent Predictors of Frequent Exacerbation

We performed multivariate logistic regression analysis to determine whether being normal IgG antibody titer against *P. gingivalis* could be an independent risk factor for frequent

Table 1. Patients' baseline characteristics (n = 93).

Age (y)	73 (45–88)
Body mass index (kg/m^2)	21.7 (14.3–30.5)
Smoking index (pack-years)	57 (20–220)
FEV_1 (% predicted)	55.0 (19.8–107.1)
GOLD stage, I/II/III/IV	12/46/30/5
High-IgG titer, n (%)	
*Pg*FDC381	49 (52.7)
*Pg*Su63	22 (23.7)

FEV_1, forced expiratory volume in one second;
GOLD, Global Initiative for Chronic Obstructive Lung Disease;
"High-IgG titer" includes subjects whose titers against *Porphyromonas gingivalis* (*Pg*FDC381 and *Pg*Su63) are above mean+2SD of healthy subsets [20].
Pg, *Porphyromonas gingivalis.* Data are expressed as median (25th–75th percentiles).

exacerbations (Table 5). This analysis included the occurrence of frequent exacerbations as a dependent categorical variable and higher IgG antibody titer against *P. gingivalis*, age, smoking status, body mass index, γ-globulin, CRP, use of ICS, tiotropium and LABA, FEV_1(%predicted) and a history of exacerbations in the year before entry as independent variables. We found that a history of exacerbation in the previous year and normal IgG antibody titer against *P. gingivalis* significantly increased the occurrence of exacerbations (Relative Risk [RR] 4.43, 95% confidence interval [95%CI] 1.20–19.6, p = 0.025; RR 5.27, 95%CI 1.30–25.7, p = 0.019, respectively).

Relationships between Elevated IgG Antibody Titer against *P. gingivalis* and Serum Inflammatory Cytokines: Subanalysis of Immune Status among 62 Patients

Tables S1 and S2 show the results of a comparison of 27 cytokines in 62 patients placed in groups that were higher-IgG titer or normal-IgG titer against *P. gingivalis* according to the multiplex bead-based immunoassay. Levels of serum IL-4 and IL-7 were significantly higher in Normal-IgG titer group than in High-IgG titer group, whereas the other cytokines did not significantly differ between them.

Discussion

We demonstrated that the frequency of exacerbations was higher among patients with COPD whose antibody titer against *P. gingivalis* was normal compared with those whose antibody titer against *P. gingivalis* was higher. Multivariate logistic regression analysis showed that being normal-IgG titer against *P. gingivalis* was independently associated with frequent exacerbations during the following year after adjustment for established exacerbation-related factors such as a history of exacerbation [2], FEV_1 [22,23] and the use of COPD medications [24,25]. These findings contradicted our hypothesis that periodontitis is a risk factor for COPD exacerbation. Nevertheless, the present findings are important because, to our knowledge, this is the first study to demonstrate a relationship between antibodies and COPD exacerbation, and to indicate the value of *P. gingivalis*-related antibodies as a predictor of exacerbation. There were no significant differences between High-IgG titer group and Normal-IgG titer group in age, FEV_1, GOLD stage, and exacerbation frequencies at the baseline characteristics.

It has been shown that a history of COPD exacerbations is a good predictor for the future exacerbation [2] and our result suggests that the possible mechanism for the frequent exacerbation, thus it seems apparently inconsistent that the frequencies of COPD exacerbation in the previous year are similar in the two groups in the baseline characteristics. However, it is also reported that considerable part of patients who experienced exacerbation in the previous year did not experience COPD exacerbation in the following year [2]. Moreover, we could not specify the timing that the antibody titers increased or decreased. It is possible that the severity of periodontitis, antibody titers or immune status might be different in the previous year and the actual prospective observational period. Further investigation is needed to verify these speculations.

Periodontitis is a disease that afflicts dentate people, so we checked only in cases with teeth. In the dentate patients group,

Table 2. Comparison of baseline characteristics between patients with normal and higher IgG titer against *Porphyromonas gingivalis.*

	Normal-IgG titer (n = 44)	**High-IgG titer (n = 49)**	***p* value**
Age (y)	74 (65–78)	73 (66–78)	0.83
Smoking status (Former : Current)	37:7	43:6	0.77
Smoking index (pack-years)	60 (47–102)	53 (40–80)	0.07
Body mass index (kg/m^2)	21.3 (19.5–23.3)	22.0 (20.1–23.5)	0.46
FEV_1 (% predicted)	54.4 (39.5–66.7)	56.5 (42.4–72.4)	0.39
GOLD stage (I/II/III/IV)	5/23/13/3	7/23/17/2	0.94
Numbers of patients with frequent exacerbations in the previous year, n (%)	22 (50.0)	24 (49.0)	1.00
MRC	1 (1–2)	1 (1–2)	0.86
Charlson comorbidity index	2 (1–3)	2 (1–3)	0.76

High-IgG titer group includes subjects whose titers against *Porphyromonas gingivalis* (*Pg*FDC381 and/or *Pg*Su63) are above mean+2SD of healthy subsets [20].
"Frequent exacerbations" are defined as ≥2 exacerbations per year.
FEV_1, forced expiratory volume in one second; GOLD, Global Initiative for Chronic Obstructive Lung Disease.; MRC, British Medical Research Council. Data are expressed as medians (25th–75th percentiles).

Table 3. Inflammatory markers in blood and use of COPD medication in patients between patients with normal and higher IgG titer against *Porphyromonas gingivalis.*

	Normal-IgG titer (n = 44)	High-IgG titer (n = 49)	*p* value
Blood			
γ-globulin, g/dL	1.04 (0.94–1.18)	1.20 (1.05–1.42)	0.0007
C-reactive protein, mg/L	0.82 (0.30–1.86)	0.94 0.36–1.71)	0.66
Use of COPD medications, n(%)			
Inhaled corticosteroid	23 (52.3)	15 (30.6)	0.038
Tiotropium	20 (45.5)	17 (34.7)	0.40
Long-acting β2 agonist	15 (34.1)	18 (36.7)	0.83
Salmeterol/fluticasone combination	0 (0)	0 (0)	1.00

High-IgG titer group includes subjects whose titers against *Porphyromonas gingivalis* (*Pg*FDC381 and/or *Pg*Su63) are above mean+2SD of healthy subsets [20]. Data area expressed as medians (25th–75th percentiles).

elevated serum IgG antibody titer didn't associated with exacerbation frequency directly, but frequent exacerbations (at least two per year) was lower in High-IgG titer group than in Normal-IgG titer group (15.6% vs. 44.0%, p = 0.018, Table S3).

Because periodontitis is often complicated with diabetic mellitus [26,27] or other systemic diseases [16,17,28–30], we also checked the comorbidities by using Charlson Comorbidities index. There was no difference between High-IgG titer group and Normal-IgG titer group. In this study population, comorbidities of COPD were not influenced on the periodontitis.

The importance of predictors of exacerbation is becoming recognized because identifying patients with susceptibility to frequent exacerbations allows the design of an aggressive prevention strategy [2]. We previously showed that an impaired swallowing reflex can predict frequent exacerbations [7]. Assuming that the aspiration of bacteria into the lungs especially among patients with an impaired swallowing reflex can cause lower respiratory tract infection, we postulated that the common oral infection, periodontitis, is associated with exacerbation.

Although a diagnosis of periodontitis requires a systematic approach including a comprehensive periodontal examination by a dentist, we used IgG antibody titers against periodontal pathogens as a surrogate marker. The validity of antibodies related to periodontitis in the management of periodontitis has been confirmed [15,20]. Serum pathogen-specific antibody levels reflect amounts of periodontal bacteria, and they are useful to assess the effects of periodontitis treatment [31,32].

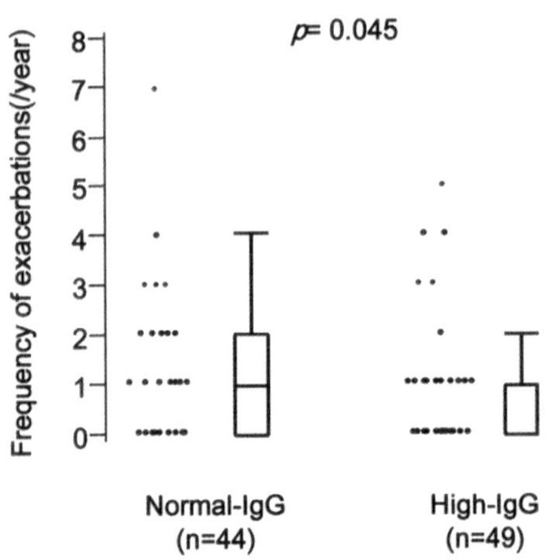

Figure 1. Frequency of exacerbations of patients with COPD and elevated serum IgG antibody titer against *Porphyromonas gingivalis.* Annual frequency of exacerbation is lower in patients with higher IgG titer than with normal IgG titer (1.2 vs. 0.8/year, p = 0.045).

Because periodontitis frequently occurs in patients with COPD [13], we assumed that such patients could be chronically exposed to periodontitis-related pathogens. Furthermore, *P. gingivalis* is the most frequently found pathogen in periodontitis [15]. Thus, serum levels of *P. gingivalis*-related antibody might reflect the ability to generate specific immune responses against infection with bacterial pathogens. This could be supported by the finding that serum γ-globulin levels were higher in High-IgG titer group than in Normal-IgG titer group. As bacterial infection is a major cause of COPD exacerbations [33], we speculated that an insufficient humoral immune response against bacteria in patients whose antibody titer against *P. gingivalis* was normal would be related to an increase in exacerbation frequency.

Our subanalysis of 27 cytokines using the multiplex bead-based immunoassay in 62 patients with COPD found higher serum levels of IL-4 and IL-7 in Normal-IgG titer group than High-IgG titer group (Table S1 and S2). Serum IL-4 level was measured by multiple testing in this study. The differences in the cytokine concentrations might be too small to attach a biological significance. However, some studies suggested that slight difference in the IL-4 concentration exerted biological difference [34,35]. We should be prudent to interpret these results.

The fact that higher serum levels of IL-4 and IL-7 in Normal-IgG titer group than High-IgG titer group seems to be contradictory to the fact that IL-4 functions as a B cell growth factor [36] and IL-7 simulates the proliferation of lymphoid progenitors [37]. However, we speculated that lower IgG could be a result from insufficient IgG production in spite of the intense producing stimuli such as IL-4 and IL-7 in some way that we could not identify in this research, and impaired negative feedback system on cytokine production might cause the higher level of IL-4 and IL-7. Another possible explanation is that Th2 cytokine suppression might influence our results. Papi A et al reported that airway eosinophil counts were increased during COPD exacerbations associated with virus detection [38] and some studies showed that virus infection lead to increase of IL-4 and made Th1/2 balance skew toward Th2 cytokines [39]. As a whole, it is possible that higher IgG titer and lower IL-4 might lead to systemic

Table 4. Frequency of exacerbations and elevated serum IgG antibody titer against *Porphyromonas gingivalis.*

	Normal-IgG titer (n = 44)	High-IgG titer (n = 49)	*p* value
Exacerbation frequency, per year			
Median (25th–75th percentiles)	1 (0–2)	0 (0–1)	0.045
Mean	1.2	0.8	
Rate of patients with frequent exacerbations, n (%)	17 (38.6)	7 (14.3)	0.009

High-IgG titer group includes subjects whose titers against *Porphyromonas gingivalis* (*Pg*FDC381 and/or *Pg*Su63) are above mean+2SD of healthy subsets [20].
Frequent exacerbations" are defined as ≥2 exacerbations per year.

suppression of Th2 immune programming resulting in the fewer exacerbation frequencies. However, the differences in these cytokines in this study were not so prominent and it is difficult to conclude definitely. Further studies are needed to clarify these speculations.

We previously showed that abnormal swallowing reflexes are associated with frequent exacerbations [7]. In the present study, we examined swallowing reflexes in 56 patients and separately evaluated the relationship between *P. gingivalis*-related antibody titers and exacerbation frequency in groups with normal and impaired swallowing reflexes. Table S4 shows that being normal-IgG titers for *P. gingivalis*-related antibody tended to increase exacerbation frequency in both groups. Although drawing a conclusive interpretation from the small sample cohort in the present study is difficult, we believe that the absence of *P. gingivalis*-related antibody contributes to exacerbation frequency regardless of the status of the swallowing reflex.

To evaluate the relationship between *P. gingivalis*-related antibody titers and airway inflammation, we induced sputum in 46 patients by having them inhale 3% hypertonic saline using an ultrasonic nebuliser (MU-32, Azwell Inc., Osaka, Japan). Table S5 shows that the total cell counts, profiles of inflammatory cells and inflammatory cytokines (IL-8 and TNF-α) in the supernatants did not differ between Normal-IgG titer group and High-IgG titer group. This finding supports the notion that antibody positivity

Table 5. Multivariable logistic regression analysis to identify risk factors for frequent exacerbation.

Variables	RR	95%CI	*p*-value
Age, per increase of 1 year	1.00	0.93–1.09	0.90
Smoking index, per increase of 1 pack-year	0.98	0.96–1.00	0.10
Body mass index, per increase of 1 kg/m^2	0.89	0.70–1.12	0.34
CRP, per increase of 1 µg/ml	0.99	0.99–1.00	0.70
γ-globulin, per increase of 1 g/dL	2.07	0.17–25.1	0.56
ICS, yes/no	2.01	0.57–7.55	0.28
Tiotropium, yes/no	1.53	0.41–5.80	0.52
LABA, yes/no	1.31	0.33–5.20	0.69
%FEV$_1$, per increase of 1%	0.99	0.94–1.02	0.49
Exacerbations in previous year, yes/no	4.43	1.20–19.6	0.025
Normal IgG antibody titer against *Porphyromonas gingivalis.*, yes/no	5.27	1.30–25.7	0.019

Frequent exacerbation is defined as ≥2 exacerbations per year.
RR, relative risk; CI, confidence interval; CRP, C-reactive protein; ICS, inhaled corticosteroid; LABA, long-acting β2 agonist.

reflects chronic low-level exposure to periodontitis-related pathogens rather than acute exaggerated airway inflammation induced by periodontitis-related pathogens.

This study has some limitations. Firstly, we could not find the significant correlation between periodontitis-related antibody titers and exacerbation frequency. (p = 0.1128, Figure S1). We speculated that the antibody titers might be determined by both the severity of the infection and the host reactivity, and COPD exacerbations were affected by various factors such as host defense mechanisms and the intensity of external insults, resulting in the difficulty for detecting the association between antibody titer and exacerbation frequency.

Secondly, since a dentist did not perform a comprehensive periodontal examination, we could not precisely diagnose periodontitis. However, the validity of the periodontitis-related antibody in the management of periodontitis has been confirmed [15,20]. We thus believe that patients with *Pg* FDC381 or *Pg* SU63 antibody had periodontitis, and that periodontitis itself might not be associated with exacerbation occurrence.

Thirdly, since oral pathogens were not quantitatively cultured, the extent of exposure to periodontal pathogens could not be determined. For example, *peptostreptococcus spp.* and *bacteroides spp.* colonized in the oral cavity and causes airway infection. In addition to that, other bacteria that can colonize in the oral cavity or nasopharynx except for periodontal pathogens such as *Haemophilus influenzae*, *Moraxella catarrhalis*, *Streptococcus pneumoniae*, *Staphylococcus aureus*, or *Pseudomonas aeruginosa* and Para *Haemophilus influenzae* were reported to be cultured from sputum at stable state COPD patients [40]. Also, Bafadhel et al. revealed that 55% of exacerbations were associated with bacterial infections and sputum cultures at exacerbations were associated with such bacteria [41,42]. But their association was still limited and periodontal pathogens were not investigated, so further investigations are needed.

Fourthly, we measured *P. gingivalis*-related antibody only once during an exacerbation-free state. Unlike paired examinations of the antibody titers, we could not discriminate bacterial colonization from new acquisition of pathogens. However, infection with *Pg* FDC381 and *Pg* SU63, both of which are common pathogens in periodontitis [15], mainly results in chronic inflammation of the periodontium. We thus speculated that levels of *P. gingivalis*-related antibody reflect the immune response to chronic infection with this pathogen.

Fifthly, we did not directly investigate the immunological status of the hosts, such as the ability to produce antibody, because a methodology has not yet been established.

Conclusion

In conclusion, normal-IgG titer for *P. gingivalis*-related antibody can be an independent predictor of exacerbation frequency. Measuring *P. gingivalis*-related antibody titers might be useful to identify patients with susceptibility to frequent exacerbations so that an aggressive strategy can be designed to prevent exacerbation.

Supporting Information

Figure S1 Frequency of exacerbations of patients with COPD and serum IgG antibody titer against *Porphyromonas gingivalis*. Annual frequency of exacerbation is not correlated with *Porphyromonas gingivalis*-related antibody titers (p = 0.1128).

Table S1 Patients' baseline characteristics (n = 62).

Table S2 Comparison of 27 cytokines between patients with normal and higher IgG titer against *Porphyromonas gingivalis*: subanalysis of 62 patients.

Table S3 Frequency of exacerbations and elevated serum IgG antibody titer against *Porphyromonas gingivalis* in dentate patients group.

Table S4 Frequency of exacerbations and elevated serum IgG antibody titer against *Porphyromonas gingivalis* in patients with normal and abnormal swallowing reflexes: subanalysis of 56 patients.

Table S5 Comparison of inflammatory markers in sputum from patients with normal and higher IgG titer against *Porphyromonas gingivalis*: subanalysis of 46 patients.

Acknowledgments

We thank Dr. Chieko Okuda for measuring the periodontitis antibody and Aya Inazumi and Yuko Maeda for excellent technical assistance.

Author Contributions

Conceived and designed the experiments: TT SM NT KT HK SS YH EO KU KN ST MM. Performed the experiments: TT SM NT KT HK SS KU KN. Analyzed the data: TT SM NT KT HK SS YH EO KU KN ST MM. Wrote the paper: TT SM NT.

References

1. Global strategy for diagnosis, management, and prevention of COPD updated 2010. Available from http://www.goldcopd.com.
2. Hurst JR, Vestbo J, Anzueto A, Locantore N, Mullerova H, et al. (2010) Susceptibility to exacerbation in chronic obstructive pulmonary disease. N Engl J Med 363: 1128–1138.
3. Stoller JK (2002) Clinical practice. Acute exacerbations of chronic obstructive pulmonary disease. N Engl J Med 346: 988–994.
4. Bhowmik A, Seemungal TA, Sapsford RJ, Wedzicha JA (2000) Relation of sputum inflammatory markers to symptoms and lung function changes in COPD exacerbations. Thorax 55: 114–120.
5. Patel IS, Seemungal TA, Wilks M, Lloyd-Owen SJ, Donaldson GC, et al. (2002) Relationship between bacterial colonisation and the frequency, character, and severity of COPD exacerbations. Thorax 57: 759–764.
6. Terada K, Muro S, Sato S, Ohara T, Haruna A, et al. (2008) Impact of gastro-oesophageal reflux disease symptoms on COPD exacerbation. Thorax 63: 951–955.
7. Terada K, Muro S, Ohara T, Kudo M, Ogawa E, et al. (2010) Abnormal swallowing reflex and COPD exacerbations. Chest 137: 326–332.
8. Kullberg E, Sjogren P, Forsell M, Hoogstraate J, Herbst B, et al. (2010) Dental hygiene education for nursing staff in a nursing home for older people. J Adv Nurs 66: 1273–1279.
9. Sjogren P, Kullberg E, Hoogstraate J, Johansson O, Herbst B, et al. (2010) Evaluation of dental hygiene education for nursing home staff. J Adv Nurs 66: 345–349.
10. Drinka P (2010) Preventing aspiration in the nursing home: the role of biofilm and data from the ICU. J Am Med Dir Assoc 11: 70–77.
11. Grossi SG, Zambon JJ, Ho AW, Koch G, Dunford RG, et al. (1994) Assessment of risk for periodontal disease. I. Risk indicators for attachment loss. J Periodontol 65: 260–267.
12. Brook I, Frazier EH (2003) Immune response to Fusobacterium nucleatum and Prevotella intermedia in the sputum of patients with acute exacerbation of chronic bronchitis. Chest 124: 832–833.
13. Leuckfeld I, Obregon-Whittle MV, Lund MB, Geiran O, Bjortuft O, et al. (2008) Severe chronic obstructive pulmonary disease: association with marginal bone loss in periodontitis. Respir Med 102: 488–494.
14. Deo V, Bhongade ML, Ansari S, Chavan RS (2009) Periodontitis as a potential risk factor for chronic obstructive pulmonary disease: a retrospective study. Indian J Dent Res 20: 466–470.
15. Yamazaki K, Honda T, Domon H, Okui T, Kajita K, et al. (2007) Relationship of periodontal infection to serum antibody levels to periodontopathic bacteria and inflammatory markers in periodontitis patients with coronary heart disease. Clin Exp Immunol 149: 445–452.
16. Pussinen PJ, Jousilahti P, Alfthan G, Palosuo T, Asikainen S, et al. (2003) Antibodies to periodontal pathogens are associated with coronary heart disease. Arterioscler Thromb Vasc Biol 23: 1250–1254.
17. Bohnstedt S, Cullinan MP, Ford PJ, Palmer JE, Leishman SJ, et al. (2010) High antibody levels to P. gingivalis in cardiovascular disease. J Dent Res 89: 938–942.
18. Anthonisen NR, Manfreda J, Warren CP, Hershfield ES, Harding GK, et al. (1987) Antibiotic therapy in exacerbations of chronic obstructive pulmonary disease. Ann Intern Med 106: 196–204.
19. Murayama Y, Nagai A, Okamura K, Kurihara H, Nomura Y, et al. (1988) Serum immunoglobulin G antibody to periodontal bacteria. Adv Dent Res 2: 339–345.
20. Sugi N, Naruishi K, Kudo C, Hisaeda-Kako A, Kono T, et al. (2011) Prognosis of periodontitis recurrence after intensive periodontal treatment using examination of serum IgG antibody titer against periodontal bacteria. J Clin Lab Anal 25: 25–32.
21. Charlson ME, Pompei P, Ales KL, MacKenzie CR (1987) A new method of classifying prognostic comorbidity in longitudinal studies: development and validation. J Chronic Dis 40: 373–383.
22. Miravitlles M, Guerrero T, Mayordomo C, Sanchez-Agudo L, Nicolau F, et al. (2000) Factors associated with increased risk of exacerbation and hospital admission in a cohort of ambulatory COPD patients: a multiple logistic regression analysis. The EOLO Study Group. Respiration 67: 495–501.
23. Garcia-Aymerich J, Farrero E, Felez MA, Izquierdo J, Marrades RM, et al. (2003) Risk factors of readmission to hospital for a COPD exacerbation: a prospective study. Thorax 58: 100–105.
24. Tashkin DP, Celli B, Senn S, Burkhart D, Kesten S, et al. (2008) A 4-year trial of tiotropium in chronic obstructive pulmonary disease. N Engl J Med 359: 1543–1554.
25. Calverley PM, Anderson JA, Celli B, Ferguson GT, Jenkins C, et al. (2007) Salmeterol and fluticasone propionate and survival in chronic obstructive pulmonary disease. N Engl J Med 356: 775–789.
26. Bascones-Martinez A, Matesanz-Perez P, Escribano-Bermejo M, Gonzalez-Moles MA, Bascones-Ilundain J, et al. (2011) Periodontal disease and diabetes-Review of the Literature. Med Oral Patol Oral Cir Bucal 16: e722–729.
27. Mealey BL, Oates TW (2006) Diabetes mellitus and periodontal diseases. J Periodontol 77: 1289–1303.
28. Pussinen PJ, Alfthan G, Tuomilehto J, Asikainen S, Jousilahti P (2004) High serum antibody levels to Porphyromonas gingivalis predict myocardial infarction. Eur J Cardiovasc Prev Rehabil 11: 408–411.
29. Renvert S (2003) Destructive periodontal disease in relation to diabetes mellitus, cardiovascular diseases, osteoporosis and respiratory diseases. Oral Health Prev Dent 1 Suppl 1: 341–357; discussion 358–349.
30. Pussinen PJ, Alfthan G, Rissanen H, Reunanen A, Asikainen S, et al. (2004) Antibodies to periodontal pathogens and stroke risk. Stroke 35: 2020–2023.
31. Sims TJ, Schifferle RE, Ali RW, Skaug N, Page RC (2001) Immunoglobulin G response of periodontitis patients to Porphyromonas gingivalis capsular carbohydrate and lipopolysaccharide antigens. Oral Microbiol Immunol 16: 193–201.
32. Lamster IB, Kaluszhner-Shapira I, Herrera-Abreu M, Sinha R, Grbic JT (1998) Serum IgG antibody response to Actinobacillus actinomycetemcomitans and Porphyromonas gingivalis: implications for periodontal diagnosis. J Clin Periodontol 25: 510–516.

33. Soler N, Torres A, Ewig S, Gonzalez J, Celis R, et al. (1998) Bronchial microbial patterns in severe exacerbations of chronic obstructive pulmonary disease (COPD) requiring mechanical ventilation. Am J Respir Crit Care Med 157: 1498–1505.
34. Surendar J, Mohan V, Rao MM, Babu S, Aravindhan V (2011) Increased Levels of Both Th1 and Th2 Cytokines in Subjects with Metabolic Syndrome (CURES-103). Diabetes Technology & Therapeutics 13: 477–482.
35. Baskar P, Silberstein DS, Pincus SH (1990) Inhibition of IgG-triggered human eosinophil function by IL-4. J Immunol 144: 2321–2326.
36. Paul WE, Ohara J (1987) B-cell stimulatory factor-1/interleukin 4. Annu Rev Immunol 5: 429–459.
37. Namen AE, Lupton S, Hjerrild K, Wignall J, Mochizuki DY, et al. (1988) Stimulation of B-cell progenitors by cloned murine interleukin-7. Nature 333: 571–573.
38. Papi A, Bellettato CM, Braccioni F, Romagnoli M, Casolari P, et al. (2006) Infections and airway inflammation in chronic obstructive pulmonary disease severe exacerbations. Am J Respir Crit Care Med 173: 1114–1121.
39. Becker Y (2006) Respiratory syncytial virus (RSV) evades the human adaptive immune system by skewing the Th1/Th2 cytokine balance toward increased levels of Th2 cytokines and IgE, markers of allergy–a review. Virus Genes 33: 235–252.
40. Zhang M, Li Q, Zhang XY, Ding X, Zhu D, et al. (2010) Relevance of lower airway bacterial colonization, airway inflammation, and pulmonary function in the stable stage of chronic obstructive pulmonary disease. Eur J Clin Microbiol Infect Dis 29: 1487–1493.
41. Bafadhel M, McKenna S, Terry S, Mistry V, Reid C, et al. (2011) Acute exacerbations of chronic obstructive pulmonary disease: identification of biologic clusters and their biomarkers. Am J Respir Crit Care Med 184: 662–671.
42. Rosell A, Monso E, Soler N, Torres F, Angrill J, et al. (2005) Microbiologic determinants of exacerbation in chronic obstructive pulmonary disease. Arch Intern Med 165: 891–897.

5

Macrophage Inflammatory Protein-1α Shows Predictive Value as a Risk Marker for Subjects and Sites Vulnerable to Bone Loss in a Longitudinal Model of Aggressive Periodontitis

Daniel H. Fine[1]*, Kenneth Markowitz[1], Karen Fairlie[1], Debbie Tischio-Bereski[1], Javier Ferrandiz[1], Dipti Godboley[1], David Furgang[1], John Gunsolley[2], Al Best[2]

1 Department of Oral Biology, School of Dental Medicine, Rutgers University, Newark, New Jersey, United States of America, **2** Department of Periodontics, School of Dentistry, Virginia Commonwealth of Virginia, Richmond, Virginia, United States of America

Abstract

Improved diagnostics remains a fundamental goal of biomedical research. This study was designed to assess cytokine biomarkers that could predict bone loss (BL) in localized aggressive periodontitis. 2,058 adolescents were screened. Two groups of 50 periodontally healthy adolescents were enrolled in the longitudinal study. One group had *Aggregatibacter actinomycetemcomitans* (*Aa*), the putative pathogen, while the matched cohort did not. Cytokine levels were assessed in saliva and gingival crevicular fluid (GCF). Participants were sampled, examined, and radiographed every 6 months for 2–3 years. Disease was defined as radiographic evidence of BL. Saliva and GCF was collected at each visit, frozen, and then tested retrospectively after detection of BL. Sixteen subjects with *Aa* developed BL. Saliva from *Aa*-positive and *Aa*-negative healthy subjects was compared to subjects who developed BL. GCF was collected from 16 subjects with BL and from another 38 subjects who remained healthy. GCF from BL sites in the 16 subjects was compared to healthy sites in these same subjects and to healthy sites in subjects who remained healthy. Results showed that cytokines in saliva associated with acute inflammation were elevated in subjects who developed BL (i.e., MIP-1α MIP-1β IL-α, IL-1β and IL-8; $p<0.01$). MIP-1α was elevated 13-fold, 6 months prior to BL. When MIP-1α levels were set at 40 pg/ml, 98% of healthy sites were below that level (Specificity); whereas, 93% of sites with BL were higher (Sensitivity), with comparable Predictive Values of 98%; $p<0.0001$; 95% C.I. = 42.5–52.7). MIP-1α consistently showed elevated levels as a biomarker for BL in both saliva and GCF, 6 months prior to BL. MIP-1α continues to demonstrate its strong candidacy as a diagnostic biomarker for both subject and site vulnerability to BL.

Editor: Paul J. Planet, Columbia University, United States of America

Funding: This study was funded in full by a grant from the National Institutes of Health DE 017968 to DHF. The funders had no role in study design, data collection and analysis, decision to publish, or preparation of the manuscript. The corresponding author accepts full responsibility for all aspects of the study and its resulting manuscript.

Competing Interests: DHF is the inventor of two patents pending titled "salivary bioassay for early detection of bone loss" (US08389015 B2) in which one of the biomarkers for detection is MIP-1alpha. DHF is the inventor of another patent pending titled "method for detection of active periodontal disease at the local tooth site" (Applic no. 13/183550) in which one of the biomarkers for detections is MIP-1 alpha. Both patents are owned by Rutgers University. DHF declares that the conduct of the study was not influenced by this conflict nor was the analysis or reporting of the data obtained from this study. There are no further patents, products in development or marketed products to declare.

* E-mail: finedh@sdm.rutgers.edu

Introduction

Improved diagnostics has been a major initiative in all phases of health care for the last 20 years with the anticipation that early diagnosis will lead to effective preventive treatment, reduced medical expenses, and improved overall health [1,2]. Periodontal research has been in the forefront of these efforts but the search for a biomarker for early prediction of disease has been elusive [3,4].

Periodontitis affects 47.2% of the adult American population and develops in response to a bacterial challenge; called plaque biofilm [5]. The disease initially affects the gingiva, a complex of tissue forming a collar around the base of the tooth enamel. The locus of infection is a "U" shaped crevice between the gingiva and its adjacent enamel. The gingival crevicular space is lined by epithelium separating the host from its external environment [6]. Periodontal disease is similar to other mucosal infections in that over time the provoking microbial challenge induces an aggressive inflammatory response in the underlying vascular connective tissue [7]. As inflammation progresses the boney structure supporting the tooth in the jawbone is undermined resulting in tooth loosening.

Periodontal researchers have an advantage over other mucosal scientists in that disease progression can be visualized and recorded over a span of time during which minimal irreversible damage occurs. Further, both bacterial initiators and host response elements can be collected from the crevice, the focus of disease activity, in a non-invasive manner [8]. Despite these advantages, progress in periodontal research has been hampered by; 1)

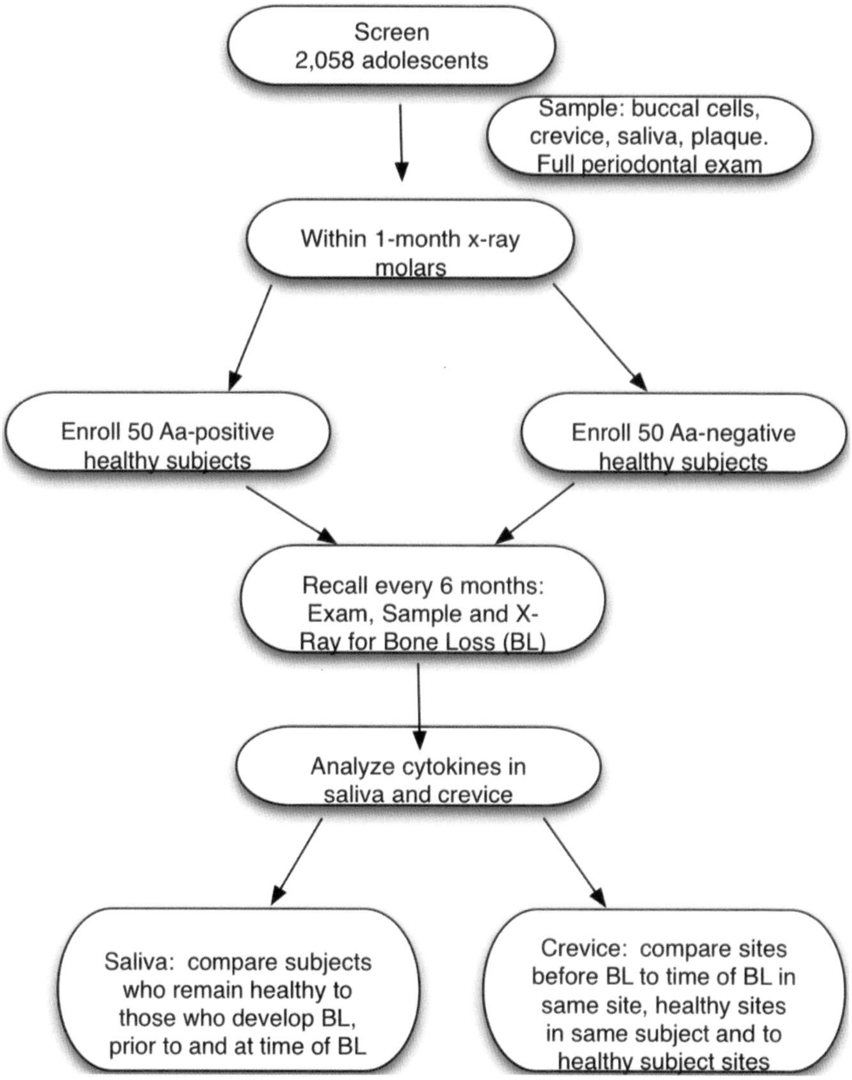

Figure 1. Flow Diagram of subjects participation in study. Fifty *Aa*-positive and 50 *Aa*-negative subjects were enrolled and followed every 6 months for up to 3 years. Cytokines from saliva and crevice fluid were collected every 6 months, stored, and then after bone loss was detected, salivary samples from 10 of those subjects (from a total of 16) and saliva from another 60 subjects who remained healthy was analyzed. In the case of crevice fluid, samples from 16 subjects who developed bone loss and another 38 who remained healthy was available for analysis.

difficulties tracking disease progression from beginning to end [9,10], and 2) difficulties identifying accurate and sensitive markers of disease [11,12].

Periodontal disease can be divided into two broad categories; a chronic form that occurs primarily in adults, named Chronic Adult Periodontitis (CAP), and an acute form that occurs in

Table 1. Demographic characteristics of subset of subjects for whom salivary cytokine analysis was performed.

Subject Ages (Mean ± Std Dev.)						
Race	**Healthy Aa + Subjects (N = 30)**		**Healthy Aa − Subjects (N = 30)**		**Bone Loss Subjects (N = 10)**	
	Age ± S.D. (Female)	**Age ± S.D. (Male)**	**Age ± S.D. (Female)**	**Age ± S.D. (Male)**	**Age ± S.D. (Female)**	**Age ± S.D. (Male)**
Hispanic (N = 17)	12.18±0.83 (6)	14.37±2.11 (5)	16.5±0.00 (3)	14.09±2.19 (5)	16.00±0.00 (1)	12.67±1.47 (2)
African-American (N = 31)	13.61±2.19 (10)	14.09±2.52 (6)	13.5±1.60 (10)	13.71±1.61 (12)	12.35±0.30 (3)	13.23±1.82 (4)
Asian (N = 3)	12.80±0.42 (2)	11.20±0.00 (1)	NA	NA	NA	NA
Total (N = 51)	**13.31±2.02 (30)**		**14.03±1.02 (30)**		**13.03±1.53 (10)**	

adolescents, named Localized Aggressive Periodontitis (LAP) [13]. CAP develops over a non-specified time-period, in an unspecified tooth location. CAP does not restrict itself to specific ethnic groups and is exacerbated by smoking [14]. These factors make CAP difficult to diagnose and follow. In contrast, LAP while less prevalent is relatively easy to diagnose and follow because it is localized to a few specific teeth, is found predominantly in adolescents of African and Hispanic descent, and is highly associated with *Aggregatibacter actinomycetemcomitans* (*Aa*), a Gram-negative microbe purported to be a specific pathogen associated with LAP [6].

The goal of our research has been to identify early markers of LAP, however, the current clinical pathway from health to periodontal disease presents several difficult roadblocks [15,16]. Standard measures of soft tissue loss, such as probing for pockets and clinical attachment level (CAL) loss, the current standards of diagnostic care, are relatively insensitive [17]. These measurements are particularly poor in LAP because these children are in their mixed dentition stage with teeth continuously erupting [18]. As a result, soft tissue measurements are relatively inaccurate because landmarks are constantly shifting. In contrast, bone measurements are related to specific physiological events that are well studied and occur in alveolar bone that is intimately related to stable tooth support [18]. While these soft-tissue landmarks vary, alveolar bone loss (BL) is irreversible to the greatest extent. However, both soft and hard tissue measurements are downstream relative to disease initiation and represent past historical data.

Notwithstanding these shortcomings identification of bone biomarkers in LAP could provide meaningful information for both forms of periodontal disease because the mechanisms for BL are host related, are common to both diseases (CAP and LAP), and should occur at least 6-months prior to detectable BL by radiograph [19]. Along these lines we have previously identified MIP-1α as a unique biomarker related to bone remodeling in LAP which has recently been confirmed by others in CAP [20–22]. However, longitudinal studies encompassing periodontal disease at both the subject and site level have not been done [20–22].

This report is part of an ongoing longitudinal cohort study of LAP in adolescents. The overall goals of the study are to identify host and microbial biomarkers of disease development. The purpose of this current study is to identify both subject and site-specific host-related biomarkers that could be predictive of BL in LAP subjects.

Materials and Methods

Ethics Statement

Approval for the conduct of this study was obtained from the Institutional Review Board of the University of Medicine and Dentistry of New Jersey (now Rutgers University).

The study was conducted in Newark, New Jersey because the majority of residents in Newark are African American and Hispanic, populations vulnerable to LAP. Both ascent and consent were received from each student's parent or guardian prior to screening.

Clinical Procedures

Screening. Screening was performed to select a group of healthy *Aa*-positive and *Aa*-negative subjects for enrollment into a longitudinal study designed to assess the association of *Aa*-carriage to host and microbial factors related to development of LAP. The examination consisted of a medical and dental history assessment, an oral examination, and collection of samples of saliva and buccal epithelial cells (BECs). Subjects were included if they were between the ages of 11–16, were medically healthy, and had a minimum of 4 first molars and 10 occluding teeth. Subjects were excluded if they had any medically related issues including but not limited to bleeding disorders, immune deficiencies, were taking either antibiotics or anti-inflammatories, or, if they had extensive dental caries [23]. A flow diagram illustrates the screened and enrolled population included in the study (Fig. 1).

Determination of Aa carriage. Buccal cells were used to determine whether the subject was *Aa*-positive or *Aa*-negative as described previously [23]. Briefly, BEC samples were obtained by scraping the cheek with a wooden tongue depressor using 5 strokes to obtain a sufficient amount of buccal material to analyze. The collection was suspended in 1 ml of phosphate buffered saline (PBS). A 100 µl aliquot of the re-suspended BEC sample was plated for determination of the presence or absence of *Aa*. Streaking, dilution and plating was done on AAGM agar for enumeration of *Aa* [23]. After plating on AAGM agar, culture dishes were placed in an incubator at 37°C with 10% CO_2 for 3–4 days [23]. Colonies seen on plates were identified as *Aa* based on their unique morphology and catalase activity. The polymerase chain reaction (PCR) was used for confirmation of cultural identification [23]. DNA obtained by the DNeasy tissue kit (Qiagen, Inc Valencia CA) for Gram-negative bacteria was used for this assessment [23]. Initially, categorization of subjects as *Aa*-positive was determined by the growth of *Aa* on agar. If no growth occurred on AAGM agar, DNA was extracted from the initial 1 ml BEC sample using the Gram-negative protocol described above for further proof that *Aa* was absent. As previously described DNA primers for the leukotoxin promoter region that is unique to *Aa* was used for these PCR determinations. This procedure was done a minimum of two times to confirm the presence or absence of *Aa* [23]. BECs were obtained from subjects at each visit to confirm their *Aa* status. To be considered to be *Aa*-negative no BEC or pocket sample could be *Aa*-positive. To be considered to be *Aa*-positive, subjects were required to show *Aa*-positivity for BECs or pocket samples at each visit.

Table 2. Demographic characteristics of subset of subjects studied for whom gingival crevicular fluid cytokine analysis on a site specific basis was performed.

Race	Subjects Remaining Healthy (N = 38)	Percent Aa Positive	Bone Loss Subjects (N = 15)	Percent Aa Positive
	Age ± S.D.		Age ± S.D.	
Hispanic	**13.47±1.95** (N = 15)	13%	**14.0±1.5** (N = 5)	**100%**
African-American	**13.3±1.52** (N = 20)	25%	**14.5±2.0** (N = 10)	100%
Not Reporting	**12.75±0.9** (N = 3)	33%		

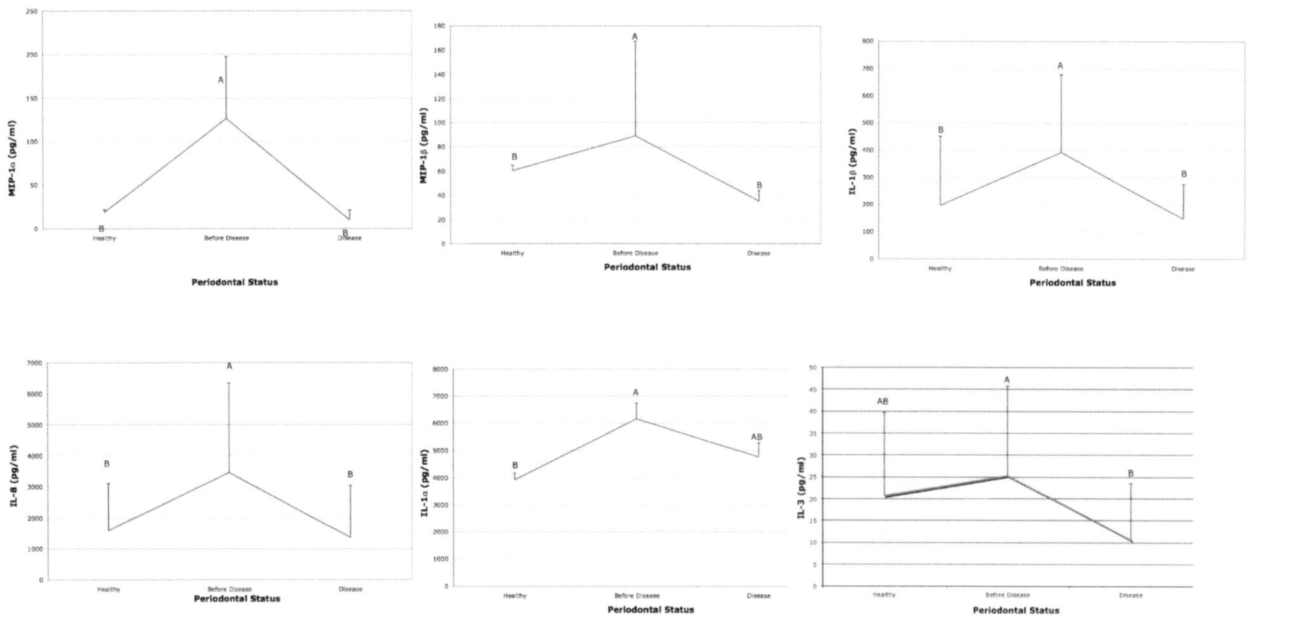

Figure 2. Salivary cytokines from healthy and bone loss subjects: Cytokines elevated prior to bone loss. Saliva from healthy subjects was compared to subjects who developed bone loss. The cytokines that showed significant differences are illustrated 6 months prior to bone loss and compared to levels at the time bone loss was detected (labeled disease) and to salivary levels found in subjects who started healthy and remained healthy. Letters that are different (A vs B) are significantly different at the $p<0.05$ level. Cytokines MIP-1α, MIP-1β, IL-1β, and IL-8 are all significantly elevated 6-mo. before BL when compared to saliva from healthy subjects and to saliva at the time disease was detected. IL-1α is significantly elevated prior to BL as compared to saliva from healthy subjects but is not significantly different than that seen at the time of disease detection.

Recall Visits

Periodontal examination. Our goal was to enroll at least 50 *Aa*-positive and 50 *Aa*-negative periodontally healthy adolescents and then to follow them and assess their periodontium for BL. Previous data indicated that 25% of *Aa*-positive adolescents develop BL over a 2–3 year period [23]. Probing was performed on six surfaces of all teeth with a Michigan 0 probe. Any pocket 5 mm or greater was examined for clinical attachment loss (CAL). The Loe-Brown definition of incipient disease was used to define subjects as "diseased" (pockets of ≥6 mm and CAL of ≥2 mm) for exclusion from the longitudinal study. Health was defined as pockets of 4 mm or less with no bleeding. A subject with one 5 mm pocket with no bleeding was also considered as healthy [23].

One month following the screening visit, all subjects were required to take four bite-wing radiographs. For purposes of the study, definitive diagnosis of disease was based on x-ray evidence of bone loss as opposed to soft tissue measurements. This decision was based on evidence that soft tissue measurement in this mixed dentition age group could produce shifting landmarks while radiographs provide a more stable diagnosis [23]. Bite-wing x-rays were taken for all subjects at 6-month intervals. BL was indicated by detection of loss of the lamina dura at the alveolar crest. Frequent calibration exercises were conducted for pocket probing, CAL, and radiographic interpretation. The two clinical examiners (KM and DTB) repeated the exercises to determine the accuracy of their readings. For soft tissue, examiners were considered to be in agreement if 80% of the sites they measured had identical readings and if 20% were within ±1 mm. The calibration exercise demonstrated 80% inter and 90% intra examiner repeatability. For x-ray calibration, 95% inter and intra examiner agreement was required.

Only periodontally healthy subjects were enrolled in the study and recalled at 6-month intervals. Samples of saliva, BECs, gingival crevicular fluid (GCF) and subgingival plaque were taken at each visit, given a coded number and stored for future analysis. To avoid disease progression, any subject who showed BL at any visit was exited from the study and provided with treatment at the dental school at no cost. A previous manuscript provides a more detailed description of the clinical procedures [23].

Sample Collection: Saliva

Students expectorated into a 50 ml wide mouthed polystyrene tube held over ice until approximately 5 ml of unstimulated whole saliva was collected. The salivary sample received a coded number and was subjected to centrifugation at 10,000-×g for clarification and then aliquoted prior to storage at −80°C [23]. After BL was detected samples from that visit and the previous visit were thawed for analysis and comparison [20]. Total protein content and cytokine analysis was performed. Saliva from a total of 16 subjects with BL was acquired; however, in 7 samples a limited amount of saliva was available due to prior analysis [20]. As a result we performed a sample size calculation to determine the number of subjects per group required for further analysis. For that calculation we used salivary IL-1β (as opposed to the MIP-1α data) since this data provided us with a more conservative estimate. Based on these calculations we determined that 9 subjects per group would be sufficient to find a statistically significant differential and to achieve a p value of 0.05. Using these calculations we randomly selected 30 *Aa*-positive subjects and 30 *Aa*-negative subjects who remained healthy to be compared to 10 of the 16 subjects who had LAP. As mentioned, duplicate testing with sufficient saliva was available for 10 subjects in the BL group. Saliva from the remaining 6 BL subjects was depleted and not available for these analyses. Saliva from another 60 healthy subjects who remained healthy was matched to the age and ethnicity of the 10 BL subjects (Table 1).

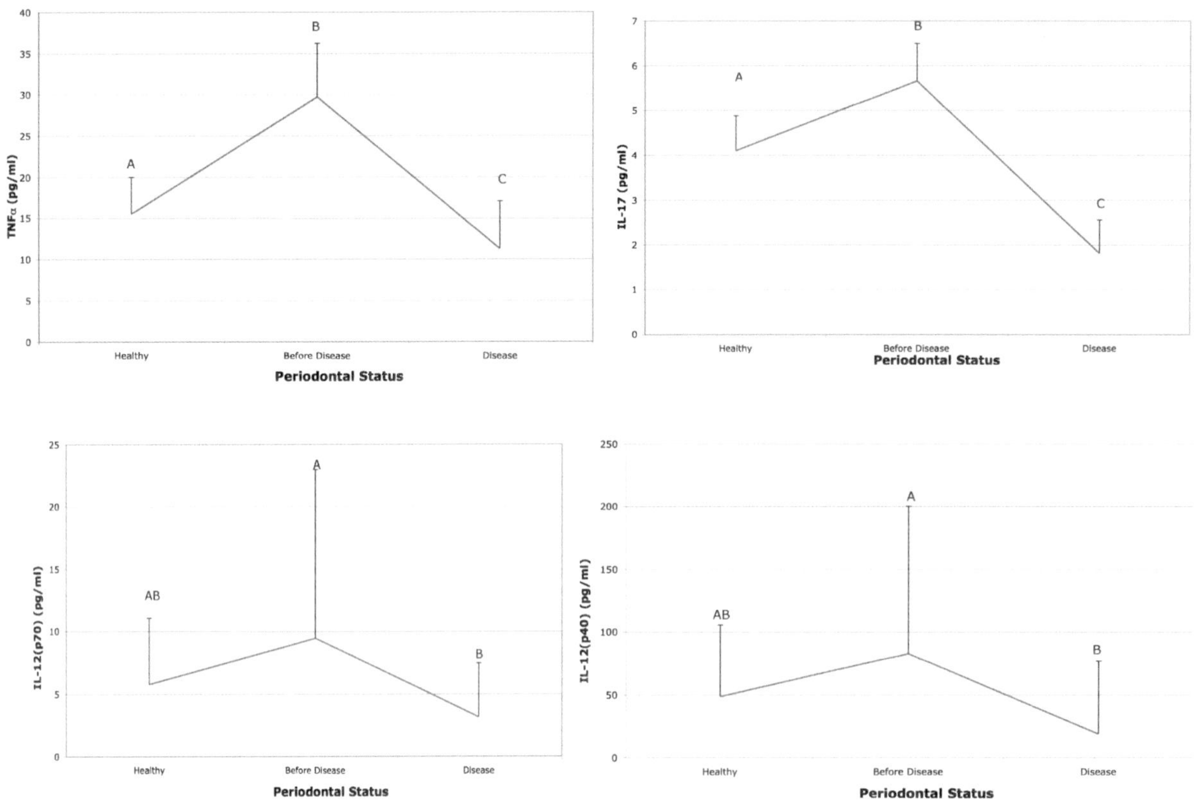

Figure 3. Salivary cytokines from healthy and bone loss subjects: Other salivary cytokines elevated prior to disease. Saliva from healthy subjects was compared to subjects who developed bone loss. The cytokines that showed significant differences are illustrated 6 months prior to bone loss and compared to levels at the time bone loss was detected (labeled disease) and to salivary levels found in subjects who started healthy and remained healthy. Letters that are different (A vs B) are significantly different at the $p<0.05$ level. Cytokines IL-17 and TNF-α are significantly elevated prior to disease as compared to health and at the time of BL detection; while IL-12 (p40) and IL-12 (p70) were significantly elevated prior to disease but were not significantly different from saliva obtained from healthy subjects $p<0.05$.

Sample Collection: Gingival Crevicular Fluid (GCF)

GCF collection was obtained from the mesial surface of each first molar at each visit. Each quadrant was isolated with cotton rolls and a saliva ejector. Teeth being sampled were gently debrided of supragingival plaque prior to placement of a periodontal paper crevicular collection strip (Oraflow Inc, Plainview NY USA). The collection strip was gently placed at the gingival margin of the molar collection site for 15 seconds. Individual strip samples were placed into coded eppendorf tubes for storage at −80°C [23]. After BL occurred, samples from the BL detection visit and the visit prior to BL were both thawed, eluted in phosphate buffered saline (PBS), and analyzed for protein content and cytokine levels.

For site-specific data we analyzed samples from 15 of the 16 subjects who developed BL. In two subjects, two sites showed BL. We recovered GCF from 17 sites in the 16 subjects who developed BL. For site related data three analyses were performed. First, we analyzed sites that developed BL. GCF was recovered from 15 sites (2 samples were unavailable prior to BL) and assessed those sites at the visit prior to BL (N = 15) as compared to these same sites at the visit BL was detected (N = 17). Second, we analyzed sites that remained healthy in these same 15 subjects (N = 45; the three healthy molars) and compared these sites to sites that developed BL (N = 15). In this case we examined all sites (three other first molar sites that remained healthy in these same subjects) at the visit prior to BL. The LAP samples from sites prior to BL were duplicate samples from the same sites in the previous analysis but were run in a blind manner and independently in a second Luminex analysis (see below). Third, we compared healthy sites in LAP subjects (N = 15) to healthy sites in subjects who did not develop BL (N = 26 for *Aa*-negative subjects and N = 12 for *Aa*-positive subjects). In this case, sample analysis was performed on samples obtained at the visit at the time BL was detected. Prior to selection of samples in this third assessment, we performed a sample size calculation using IL-6 data (as opposed to MIP-1α data). We assumed that IL-6 data would provide the most conservative estimate for sample size calculation. Our analysis indicated that 8 subjects per group would be sufficient to determine significance at the 0.05 level. These calculations indicated that we had sufficient material to proceed.

Subject samples were selected for analysis if there was a sufficient crevicular protein content for analysis and if the subjects were a match to the mean age and ethnicity of the BL subjects. As a result we randomly chose 26 *Aa*-negative subjects (N = 26 sites), 12 *Aa*-positive subjects (N = 12 sites) and 15 healthy sites from the 16 *Aa*-positive subjects who developed BL. All data was coded and analyzed in a blind manner.

For GCF analysis we selected a panel of seven cytokines. IL-1β, MIP-1α, and IL-8 were chosen as markers of acute inflammation. IL-2, IL-10 and IL-12 were chosen as markers of chronic inflammation [24]. We also selected IL-6, a cytokine that participates in both acute and chronic inflammation.

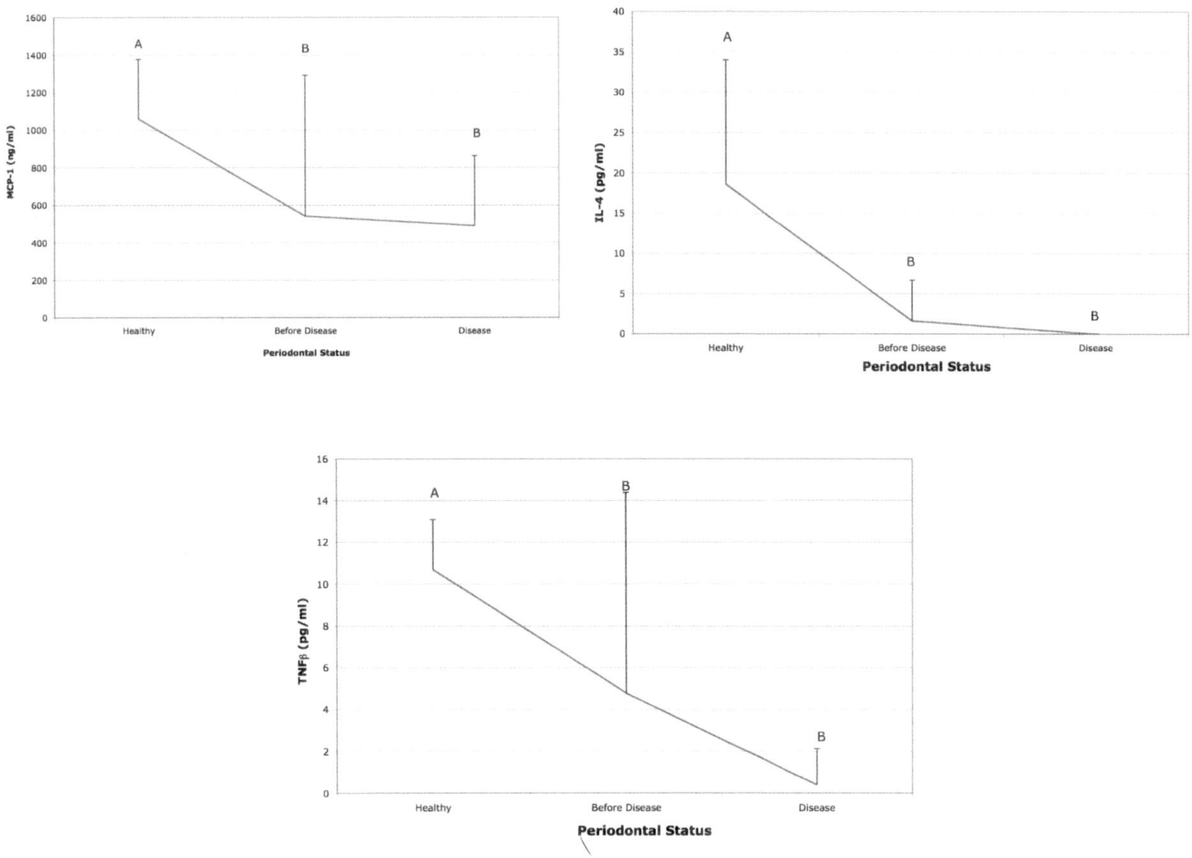

Figure 4. Salivary cytokines from healthy and bone loss subjects: Salivary cytokines elevated in health prior to disease detection. Saliva from healthy subjects was compared to subjects who developed bone loss. The cytokines that showed significant differences are illustrated 6 months prior to bone loss and compared to levels at the time bone loss was detected (labeled disease) and to salivary levels found in subjects who started healthy and remained healthy. Letters that are different (A vs B) are significantly different at the $p<0.05$ level. Cytokine MCP-1, IL-4 and TNF-β were significantly depressed before disease as compared to health but were not different when saliva prior to disease was compared to saliva at the visit disease was detected.

Cytokine Processing and Analysis

Saliva and GCF processing. For salivary analysis the presence and level of 21 chemo/cytokines were assessed using the Luminex/Millipore xMap system (Millipore, Billerica MA) [20]. A 100 μl sample was placed in the well of a 96-well plate containing its own internal controls for each of the chemo/cytokines to be analyzed. Excitation of each fluorochrome produced a signal that permitted detection of from 1–500 pg per chemo/cytokine [20]. All data was normalized to pg/ml based on a constant level of protein. For GCF analysis the presence and level of 7 chemo/cytokines were assessed as described. All test were done twice in duplicate.

Statistical Analysis

Chi-squared analysis was used to assess differences in race while a student's-t-test was used to analyze age to determine if the BL subjects differed from healthy controls with respect to age.

Salivary samples were assessed by analysis of variance (ANOVA) comparing 3 groups; samples from healthy subjects who remained healthy (N = 60), salivary samples at the visit prior to BL in healthy subjects who developed BL (N = 10), and samples from these same subjects at the visit BL was detected (N = 10). Tukey Kramer (HSD) analysis was performed to assess all means in pairwise comparisons within the ANOVA. Differences were significant if they achieved a p value of <0.05.

GCF data was subjected to three separate analyses. Initially, sites prior to BL (N = 15) were compared to that same site at the visit BL was detected (N = 17) using an ANOVA with Tukey Kramer analysis. In these same LAP subjects, BL sites in the visit prior to BL were compared to first molar sites that were diagnosed as healthy and remained healthy in these same subjects at that same visit. In this the second analysis, 45 healthy sites (three healthy first molar sites in 15 subjects) were compared to 15 BL sites prior to BL. The groups used for the third analysis were selected based on the sample size calculations derived from the second GCF analysis and were matched in age, race, and availability of GCF for analysis. This material was taken from healthy sites at the time of the BL detection visit from LAP subjects and compared to *Aa*-positive and *Aa*-negative subjects who started healthy and remained healthy. All data was analyzed by ANOVA with Tukey Kramer analysis coupled with a Bonferroni correction to protect against multiple testing (p value = 0.007 was set to achieve a level of significance of $p<0.05$). Sensitivity and specificity testing was performed using a cut point of >40 pg/ml for MIP-1α. We also calculated positive and negative predictive values using the same sample groups.

Specificity was calculated for another 26 subjects who were *Aa*-negative and remained healthy and another 12 subjects who were *Aa*-positive and remained healthy as compared to the 15 subjects who developed BL. In this analysis a cut point of MIP-1α levels of 40 pg/ml was used for GCF at the visit prior to BL. Specificity was

Table 3. Cytokine levels (pg/ml) in same molar sites prior to bone loss vs. same molar sites at visit bone loss detected.

Cytokine levels in pg/ml							
Site Status	**IL-1β**	**1L-2**	**IL-6**	**IL-8**	**IL-10**	**IL-12**	**MIP-1α***
Prior to Bone Loss N = 15	6.31±11.32	0.93±1.44	0.19±0.22	233±172	1.56±1.36	5.25±6.68	47.66±8.83
Time of Bone Loss N = 17	40.07±92.0	1.64±1.60	1.90±1.45	349±234	2.33±1.47	6.68±5.37	21.1±13.3

*MIP-1α levels are higher in crevice fluid obtained from sites prior to bone loss.

Table 4. Cytokine levels (pg/ml) in sites remaining healthy vs sites that develop bone loss in LAP subjects: visit prior to detection of BL.

Cytokine levels in pg/ml							
Site Status in LAP subjects (N = 15)	**IL-1β**	**1L-2**	**IL-6***	**IL-8**	**IL-10**	**IL-12**	**MIP-1α****
Sites Remain Healthy (N = 45)	25.9±60.3	1.10±1.48	1.05±1.47	386±445	2.55±1.46	4.72±3.83	14.79±11.04
Sites Develop Bone Loss (N = 15)	6.08±11.03	0.87±1.46	0.18±0.22	218±176.2	1.46±1.33	5.11±6.46	48.03±8.62

*IL-6 levels are higher in crevice fluid in sites that started healthy and remained healthy.
**MIP-1a levels are higher in crevice fluid obtained from sites piror to bone loss that developed bone loss.

Table 5. Cytokine levels (pg/ml) in healthy sites from LAP subjects vs Aa-negative and positive healthy subjects at visit BL was detected.

Cytokine levels in pg/ml							
Site Status	**IL-1β****	**IL-2***	**IL-6**	**IL-8*****	**IL-10**	**IL-12**	**MIP-1α***
Healthy Aa-neg (N = 26)	0.88±1.41	2.86±0.25	0.14±0.21	34.3±62.2	2.87±0.93	5.57±4.12	9.39±9.32
Healthy Aa-pos (N = 12)	**59.6±115.7**	**0.09±0.38**	1.47±4.91	138.8±10.5	1.04±0.65	3.28±2.90	11.04±8.22
LAP (Aa-pos) (N = 15)	26.85±69.8	***4.37±1.56***	0.94±1.84	**293±373**	2.55±3.90	15.5±4.60	15.5±11.38

*IL-2 higher in sites in LAP subjects vs. Aa-pos & Aa-neg healthy sites.
**IL-1β higher in Aa-pos healthy sites vs. Aa-negative healthy sites.
***IL-8 higher in LAP sites vs. Aa-negative healthy sites.

determined by calculating the number of healthy sites from these various subject groups showing MIP-1α levels >40 pg/ml. The rationale for determining the cut-off value for MIP-1α based on the fact that the range for MIP-1α was from 42.5 pg/ml to 52.7 pg/ml with a mean of 47.66 pg/ml and standard deviation of 8.82 pg/ml in sites that encountered BL at the visit prior to BL. A slightly lower level of 40 pg/ml was chosen for the cut point.

Finally, we constructed a statistical model analyzing both the sites (N = 15 BL sites from LAP subject +45 healthy sites from same LAP subject = 60) and the subjects (N = 15 BL subjects +12 healthy *Aa*-positive subjects +26 healthy *Aa*-negative subjects; N = 53) relative to levels of MIP-1α to determine whether the subject or the site was the most critical factor relative to levels of MIP-1α and its relationship to BL. In the analysis the subject was modeled as a random effect.

Results

Demographics

The demographic distribution of all students who participated in the study is shown in Tables 1 and 2. Salivary analysis compared 60 healthy subjects to 10 subjects who developed LAP. Fifty percent of the subjects were female with a mean age of 13.03+2 as compared to 13.7+2.3 for the male subjects (Table 1). The LAP group had a mean age of 13.03±1.5. Fifty percent of the healthy subjects were *Aa*-positive while 100% of the LAP subjects were *Aa*-positive. GCF analysis included 15 participants who developed BL in addition to another 26 healthy *Aa*-negative and 12 healthy *Aa*-positive participants. The age of the healthy subjects (13.38±1.9) was not significantly different from the LAP group (14.5±1.5) nor was the ethnic distribution of these participants (Table 2). However, while 20% of the healthy group was *Aa*-positive, 100% of the LAP group had *Aa* (Table 2).

Cytokine Analysis

Salivary cytokines. Cytokine levels associated with acute inflammation (IL-1β, IL-8, MIP-1α and MIP-1β) were elevated in subjects 6–9 months prior to detection of BL as compared to salivary levels at the time BL was detected and to saliva from subjects who remained healthy (Fig. 2). IL-3 and IL-1α were elevated prior to disease when compared to health but showed no difference when compared to the visit when BL was detected (Fig. 2). TNF-α and IL-17 were also elevated prior to BL and at the visit when BL was detected (Fig. 3). In addition, IL-12 was significantly elevated prior to BL in these same LAP subjects but was not elevated in comparison to subjects who remained healthy (Fig. 3). Moreover, IL-4, TNF-β, MCP-1 were all higher in saliva derived from healthy subjects as compared to LAP subjects (Fig. 4). Further, MIP-1α showed the greatest difference when compared to other cytokines and was elevated 13-fold in saliva prior to BL as compared to saliva from healthy subjects and to saliva at the visit BL was detected (Fig. 2). In addition, IL-2, IL-6, IL-7 IL-10 and INF-γ were similar in health and in the visit prior to detection of BL but where lower at the time of detection of BL (Fig. S1).

Crevice fluid cytokines. For GCF analysis, MIP-1α was significantly elevated prior to BL at the site of BL (N = 15) as compared to that same site (N = 17) at the time BL was detected (Table 3). In contrast, IL-6 was significantly reduced in sites that developed BL as compared to those sites that remained healthy (N = 45) in these same LAP subjects (N = 15) that developed BL. These assessments were performed on samples at the visit prior to detection of BL (Table 4). MIP-1α levels in GCF taken from these sites (N = 15) in the visit 6–9 months prior to BL showed elevated

Table 6. Predictive value of crevicular levels of MIP-1α of 40 pg/ml or above at sites that do or do not develop bone loss in same LAP subject at visit prior to bone loss.

MIP-1α levels	Bone Loss Positive Sites (N)	Bone Loss Negative Sites (N)	Sensitivity (%)	Specficity (%)	Postiive Predictive Value	Negative Predictive Value
MIP-1α >40 pg/ml	14	1				
MIP-1α <40 pg/ml	1	44				
			93.33	98.73	93.3	98.7
TOTAL SITES	15	45				

levels when compared to sites that remained healthy (N = 45) in these same subjects (Table 4; p<0.01).

In data taken from the third GCF analysis, IL-2 was lower in *Aa*-positive healthy sites as compared to *Aa*-negative healthy sites but was significantly higher in *Aa*-positive healthy sites from LAP subjects (p<0.01). IL-8 and IL-1β were significantly higher in *Aa*-positive healthy sites as compared to *Aa*-negative healthy sites (p< 0.01). IL-8 was also elevated in healthy *Aa*-positive sites from LAP subjects (p<0.01; see Table 5).

When a cut point was set at >40 pg/ml and healthy sites in LAP subjects (N = 45) were compared to sites prior to BL (N = 15) in LAP subjects, a specificity of 98.73% and a sensitivity of 93.33% was achieved as a predictive risk marker for MIP-1α in a site prior to BL that would develop BL (Table 6).

When 26 subjects who were *Aa*-negative and 12 subjects who were *Aa*-positive all of whom remained healthy were compared to 15 sites that remained healthy in LAP subjects, a specificity of 98% was obtained when the cut point was set at >40 pg/ml for MIP-1α (Table 7). Our statistical modeling indicated that the site status played the more dominant role than subject status relative to prediction of BL (p<0.0001).

Discussion/Conclusions

Our results indicate that elevated levels of MIP-1α in saliva can be used to identify subjects susceptible to BL, while MIP-1α in GCF can identify sites susceptible to BL. We followed adolescents vulnerable to LAP from health to disease over a 2–3 year period and found that elevated levels of MIP-1α were seen in advance of BL at both the site and subject level. These elevated levels were detected 6–9 months prior to radiographic visualization of BL. The relationship between MIP-1α and periodontal disease has been confirmed in two independent studies [21,22]. One study showed that MIP-1α was a superior salivary biomarker when compared to further downstream markers of BL that included osteoprotegrin (OPG), C-telopeptide pyrodiniline cross links of type 1 collagen, and a β-terminal C-type 1 collagen telopeptide [22]. MIP-1α showed a specificity of 92.7% and a sensitivity of 94% for periodontal disease and an 18-fold elevation in CAP subjects when their salivary biomarkers for bone remodeling were compared to healthy subjects. It was particularly revealing that MIP-1α (as an upstream mediator of bone loss) performed significantly better than mid (OPG) and downstream (telopeptides) markers of bone remodeling [22]. In a second study, statistically elevated levels of MIP-1α were found in GCF obtained from diseased pocket sites in LAP [21]. While both studies support the utility of MIP-1α as a biomarker, neither presented longitudinal data implicating MIP-1α as a predictor of BL and neither examined both salivary and crevicular biomarkers in the same subject.

Microbial profiles appear to be distinctly different when comparing acute (LAP) and chronic (CAP) forms of periodontitis [23]. This is reflected by evidence indicating that events related to Toll-like receptors expressed by the innate immune pattern recognition system are also distinctly different when it comes to differentiating between bacteria related to CAP and LAP [24]. However, as events move further and further downstream toward RANK and MIP-1α activation of osteoclasts, these events appear to flow into a common pathway [19,23]. Therefore, the data derived from this study is likely to be applicable to BL in CAP [22].

MIP-1α is chemotactic for polymorphonuclear leukocytes (PMNs) in acute inflammation and is stimulatory for monocytes in relation to osteoclastogenesis [25]. In vitro it has been shown that *Aa* lipopolysaccharide (LPS) can induce PMNs and epithelial cells to produce MIP-1α. MIP-1α can activate osteoclasts, which can also be synergized by IL-1β [25]. This relationship between *Aa*, MIP-1α, IL-1β and BL has been supported by clinical studies showing elevated MIP-1α and IL-1β in saliva of *Aa*-positive subjects prior to BL [20,22].

Ideally cytokines should be studied in a time and site dependent manner referencing levels found at that site and at that time in the

Table 7. Analysis of specificity of MIP-1a levels in healthy sites from Aa-negative and Aa-positive subjects who remained healthy as compared to healthy sites in LAP subjects where another site developed bone loss.

MIP-1α levels	Healthy site from Aa-negative subject (N = 26)	Healthy site from Aa-positive subject (N = 12)	Healthy site from LAP subject (N = 15)	Total Sites with MIP-1α levels > or < than 40 pg/ml
MIP-1α >40 pg/ml (N)	1	0	0	1
MIP-1α <40 pg/ml (N)	25	12	15	52
TOTALS ALL SITES	26	12	15	53

context of developing disease. Since cytokine networks are complex, interactive, continuously changing and have redundant functionality, interpretation of levels of cytokines at one point in time are fraught with errors [26]. Our assessments have taken these issues into account by evaluating a site-specific disease in the context of a subject in a longitudinal model. However, we recognize the vulnerability of our interpretation based on the fact that the time between our measurements was 6-months. We propose to use 3-month intervals in future studies; however, it seems reasonable to assume that calcium release from collagen in bone remodeling could take as long as 6–9 months to be seen radiographically [19]. Nevertheless, with these shortcomings in mind, this is the first report to implicate MIP-1α as a predictive risk biomarker with high specificity and sensitivity in both saliva and GCF at a specific site developing periodontal BL in a longitudinal cohort study.

In this study, cytokines such as IL-8, MIP-1α, and MIP-1β, were significantly elevated in whole saliva in LAP subjects prior to BL. These cytokines along with IL-1β are known to recruit and activate, PMNs, monocytes and macrophages and are consistent with an aggressive acute inflammatory response [24,27]. In addition, IL-17 and TNF-α were elevated in the saliva of the LAP subjects prior to BL. These cytokines as well as MIP-1α emerged from sites in LAP subjects and have also been associated with BL and thus could serve as diagnostic biomarkers for BL [21]. Saliva is known to collect GCF that emigrates from all sites in the dentition and thus saliva is a repository for both subject and site related material [8]. While saliva from the LAP subjects that were undergoing BL showed a significant overall shift toward markers of acute inflammation, healthy subjects who remained healthy, harbor a health related microflora [23] and showed elevated levels of chronic inflammatory markers in their saliva. Several other cytokines such as IL-4, TNF-β and MCP-3 as well as IL-10 and IL-13 were also elevated in saliva of healthy subjects (Fig. 4 and Fig. S1). These cytokines have been implicated in healing and response to injury [27]. In this case it is possible that the host cytokines controlled disease progression [28].

Of particular interest were the distinct differences seen when the four sites from the same LAP subject who developed BL were analyzed because only one of the four sites showed BL while the others remained healthy. In this case the one BL site prior to BL, unlike any of the other sites, showed elevated MIP-1α levels. It is noteworthy that sites that remained healthy showed IL-6 levels that were significantly elevated in these same LAP subjects that developed disease at another site. In a second analysis IL-8 showed elevated levels in LAP sites that remained healthy at the time disease was detected at another site. The relationship of IL-6 and IL-8 to MIP-1α needs to be better understood.

Previously we showed that subgingival sites harbored a microbial consortium consisting of *Aa*, *Filifator alocis* and *Streptococcus parasanguinis* 6–9 months prior to BL, while the other three sites that remained healthy in the same individual showed a health related flora [23]. These findings suggest that the consortium that colonized BL sites could be responsible for affecting the host response at that site (bacterial colonization precedes the host response). These LAP consortium microbes are known to be capable of suppressing immune responsiveness while *Aa*/LPS could activate epithelial cells or monocytes in the underlying connective tissue and thus could be responsible for elevated MIP-1α [29]. Therefore, as suggested by our statistical model and our microbiological data, the local site appears to be more relevant as a predictor of BL than subject derived data (see Tables 6 and 7) [23].

Several questions remain unanswered. Can we assume that the microbial shift causes the local cytokine response? Alternatively is it possible that the local cytokine reaction is responsible for the subsequent microbial shift? It seems likely that the leading edge of the massive subgingival bacterial front challenges the thinning pocket epithelial lining that lies in direct contact with the adjacent highly vascular connective tissue. Chemokines and cytokines secreted by the defending epithelial barrier produce innate response elements that are likely intended to induce a homeostatic balance [24]. While the presumed goal of this response is protection against disease, the specifics of these relationships still need to be proven in vivo [30]. Understanding these complex interactions could provide us with a better understanding of pathogenesis of periodontitis and other mucosally initiated infections.

With this data in hand a strategy should be considered to test MIP-1α as well as other potential inflammatory cytokines such as TNF-α and IL-17 as risk markers for BL on both a site and subject level in long term clinical studies. Using these tools, diagnosis of patients and sites at risk for disease can be improved which can lead to better more cost effective methods of prevention and treatment in this pandemic mucosal infectious disease.

Supporting Information

Figure S1 Salivary cytokines from healthy and bone loss subjects: Salivary cytokines depressed at the time bone loss was detected. Saliva from healthy subjects was compared to subjects who developed bone loss. The cytokines that showed significant differences are illustrated 6 months prior to bone loss and compared to levels at the time bone loss was detected (labeled disease) and to salivary levels found in subjects who started healthy and remained healthy. Letters that are different (A vs B) are significantly different at the $p<0.05$ level. IL-13, IL-6, IL-7 and IL-10 all show lower levels at time disease was detected.

Figure S2 Salivary cytokines from healthy and bone loss subjects: Other salivary cytokines depressed at the time bone loss was detected. Saliva from healthy subjects was compared to subjects who developed bone loss. The cytokines that showed significant differences are illustrated 6 months prior to bone loss and compared to levels at the time bone loss was detected (labeled disease) and to salivary levels found in subjects who started healthy and remained healthy. Letters that are different (A vs B) are significantly different at the $p<0.05$ level. IL-2 and IFN-γ are lower at time disease was detected as compared to health and prior to disease detection.

Acknowledgments

The authors would like to thank the administration of the School of Dental Medicine for their continuing support. We would also like to thank the Office of Health Services for the Newark Public Schools, the Superintendents Office for the Newark Public Schools. Finally we would like to thank all the principals, teachers, nurses, students, guardians and parents who assisted us and played a vital role in the success of this study.

Author Contributions

Conceived and designed the experiments: DHF. Analyzed the data: JG AB. Wrote the paper: DHF. Review and suggestions of manuscript: JG AB KM KF DTB JF DG DF. Contributed all reagents: DHF. Contributed all the analysis tools: JG AB. Responsible for laboratory work related to the samples: DF DG. Responsible for clinical assessments and for collection of samples: DTB KM. Responsible for contacting students and for all correspondence with subjects, parents, guardians and the Newark School System: KF. Responsible for data entry and monitoring: JF.

References

1. Schuetz P, Christ-Crane M, Muller B (2007) Biomarkers to improve diagnostic and prognostic accuracy in systemic infections. Curr Opin Crit Care 13: 578–585.
2. Yager P, Edwards T, Fu E, Helton K, Nelson K, et al. (2006) Multifluidic diagnostic technologies for global health. Nature 442: 412–418.
3. Golub LM, Kleinberg I (1976) Gingival crevicular fluid: a new diagnostic aid in managing the periodontal patient. Oral Sci Rev 8: 49–61.
4. Mandel ID (1993) Salivary diagnosis; promises, promises. Ann NY Acad Sci 694: 1–10.
5. Eke P, Dye BA, Wei L, Thornton-Evans GO, Genco RJ, et al. (2012) Prevalence of periodontitis in adults in the United States. J Dent Res 91: 914–920.
6. Fine DH, Kaplan JB, Kachlany SC, Schreiner HC (2006) How we got attached to *Actinobacillus actinomycetemcomitans*. Periodontol 2000 42: 114–157.
7. Pihlstrom BI, MIchalowicz BS, Johnson NW (2005) Periodontal diseases. Lancet 366: 1809–1820.
8. Giannobile WV, Beikler T, Kinney JS, Ramseler CA, Morelli T, et al. (2009) Saliva as a diagnostic tool for periodontal disease current state and future directions. Periodontol 2000 50: 52–64.
9. Goodson JM, Tanner ACR, Haffajee AD, Sornberger GC, Socransky SS (1982) Patterns of progression and regression of advanced destructive periodontal disease. J Clin Periodontol 9: 472–481.
10. Glavind L, Loe H (1967) Errors in clinical assessment of periodontal destruction. J Periodont Res 9: 180–184.
11. Listgarten MA (1980) Periodontal probing: what does it mean? J Clin Periodontol 7: 165–176.
12. Kinney JS, Ramseier CA, Giannobile WV (2007) Oral fluid-based biomarkers of alveolar bone loss in periodontitis. Ann NY Acad Sci 1098: 230–251.
13. Armitage GC (1999) Development of a classification system for periodontal diseases and conditions. Ann Periodontol 4: 1–6.
14. Albandar JM, Brunelle JA, Kingman A (1999) Destructive periodontal disease in adults 30 years of age and older in the United States. 1988–1994. J Periodontol 70: 13–29.
15. Brown LJ, Albandar JM, Brunelle JA, Loe H (1996) Early-onset periodontitis: progression of attachment loss during 6 years. J Periodontol 67: 968–975.
16. Haubek DL, Ennibi O-K, Poulsen, Vaeth M, Poulsen S, et al. (2008) Risk of aggressive periodontitis in adolescent carriers of the JP2 clone of Aggregatibacter (Actinobacillus) actinomycetemcomitans in Morocco: a prospective longitudinal cohort study. Lancet 371: 237–242.
17. Best A, Burmeister JA, Gunsolley JC, Brooks CN, Schenkein HA (1990) Reliability of attachment loss measurements in a longitudinal clinical trial. J Clin Periodontol 17: 564–569.
18. Clerehugh V, Lennon MA, Worthington HV (1990) 5-year result of a longitudinal study of early periodontitis in 14-to 19 year old adolescents. J Clin Periodontol 17: 702–08.
19. McCauley LK, Nohutcu RM (2002) Mediators of periodontal osseous destruction and remodeling: principles and implications for diagnosis and therapy. J Periodontol 73: 1377–1391.
20. Fine DH, Markowitz K, Furgang D, Fairlie K, Ferrandiz J, et al. (2009) Macrophage inflammatory protein 1-a: a salivary biomarker of bone loss in a longitudinal cohort study of children at risk for aggressive periodontal disease? J Periodontol 80: 106–113.
21. Shaddox L, Wiedey J, Bimstein E, Magnusson K, Clare-Salzler M, et al. (2010) Hyper-responsive phenotype in localized aggressive periodontitis. J Dent Res 89: 143–148.
22. Al-Sabbagh M, Alladah A, Lin Y, Kryscio RJ, Thomas MV, et al. (2012) Bone remodeling-associated salivary biomarker MIP-1a distinguishes periodontal disease from health. J Periodontal Res 47: 389–395.
23. Fine DH, Markowitz K, Fairlie K, Tischio-Bereski D, Ferrandiz J, et al. (2013) A consortium of *Aggregatibacter actinomycetemcomitans, Streptococcus parasanguinis* and *Filifactor alocis* is present in sites prior to bone loss in a longitudinal study of localized aggressive periodontitis. J Clin Microbiol 51: 2850–2860.
24. Preshaw P, Taylor JJ (2011) How has research into cytokine interactions and their role in driving immune responses impacted our understanding of periodontitis? Periodontol 2000 38: 60–84.
25. Ryu OH, Choi SJ, Linares AM, Song IS, Kim YJ, et al. (2007) Gingival epithelial cell expression of macrophage inflammatory protein-1-alpha induced by interleukin-1-beta and lipopolysaccharide. J Periodontol 78: 1627–1634.
26. Bettelli E, Korn T, Kuchroo VK (2007) Th17 the third member of the effector T cell trilogy. Curr Opin Immunol 19: 652–657.
27. Feghali CA, Wright TM. (1997) Cytokines in acute and chronic inflammation. Front Biosci 2: 12–26.
28. Harrington LE, Mangan PR, Weaver CT (2006) Expanding the effector CD4 T-cell repertoire: the Th17 lineage. Curr Opin Immunol 18: 349–356.
29. Aruni AW, Roy F, Fletcher HM (2011) *Filifactor alocis* has virulence factors that can enhance its persistence under oxidative stress conditions and mediate invasion of epithelial cells by *Porphyromonas gingivalis*. Infect Immun 79: 3872–3886.
30. Darveau RP (2010) Periodontitis: a polymicrobial disruption of host homeostasis. Nat Rev Microbiol 8: 481–490.

6

Antibody and T Cell Responses to *Fusobacterium nucleatum* and *Treponema denticola* in Health and Chronic Periodontitis

Jieun Shin[1], Sang-A Kho[2], Yun S. Choi[1], Yong C. Kim[1], In-Chul Rhyu[2], Youngnim Choi[1]*

1 Department of Immunology and Molecular Microbiology, BK21 CLS, School of Dentistry and Dental Research Institute, Seoul National University, Seoul, Korea,
2 Department of Periodontology, BK21 CLS, School of Dentistry and Dental Research Institute, Seoul National University, Seoul, Korea

Abstract

The characteristics of the T cell response to the members of oral flora are poorly understood. We characterized the antibody and T cell responses to FadA and Td92, adhesins from *Fusobacterium nucleatum*, an oral commensal, and *Treponema denticola*, a periodontal pathogen, respectively. Peripheral blood and saliva were obtained from healthy individuals and patients with untreated chronic periodontitis (CP, n = 11 paris) and after successful treatment of the disease (n = 9). The levels of antigen-specific antibody were measured by ELISA. In plasma, IgG1 was the most abundant isotype of Ab for both Ags, followed by IgA and then IgG4. The levels of FadA-specific salivary IgA (sIgA) were higher than Td92-specific sIgA and the FadA-specific IgA levels observed in plasma. However, the periodontal health status of the individuals did not affect the levels of FadA- or Td92-specific antibody. Even healthy individuals contained FadA- and Td92-specific $CD4^+$ T cells, as determined by the detection of intracytoplasmic CD154 after short-term *in vitro* stimulation of peripheral blood mononuclear cells (PBMCs) with the antigens. Patients with CP tended to possess increased numbers of FadA- and Td92-specific $CD4^+$ T cells but reduced numbers of Td92-specific $Foxp3^+CD4^+$ Tregs than the healthy subjects. Both FadA and Td92 induced the production of IFNγ and IL-10 but inhibited the secretion of IL-4 by PBMCs. In conclusion, *F. nucleatum* induced Th3 (sIgA)- and Th1 (IFNγ and IgG1)-dominant immune responses, whereas *T. denticola* induced a Th1 (IFNγ and IgG1)-dominant response. This IFNγ-dominant cytokine response was impaired in CP patients, and the Td92-induced IFNγ levels were negatively associated with periodontal destruction in patients. These findings may provide new insights into the homeostatic interaction between the immune system and oral bacteria and the pathogenesis of periodontitis.

Editor: Clive M. Gray, University of Cape Town, South Africa

Funding: This study was supported by the National Research Foundation of Korea Grant (2011-0028235) by the Korean Government funded through the Oromaxillofacial Dysfunction Research Center for the Elderly at Seoul National University. The funders had no role in study design, data collection and analysis, decision to publish, or preparation of the manuscript.

Competing Interests: The authors have declared that no competing interests exist.

* E-mail: youngnim@snu.ac.kr

Introduction

The surface of the human body is colonized by billions of commensal bacteria that live in harmony with their host. According to the current paradigm, the host immune system maintains tolerance to commensals but develops active immunity against harmful pathogens. Vaughan *et al.* reported that *Neisseria meningitidis*, an opportunistic pathogen colonizing the upper respiratory tract, induces mucosal T and B cell memory, but *N. lactamica*, a commensal bacterium, induces only a T cell-independent B cell response in humans [1]. Similarly in mice, a lack of classical immunological memory is observed in the intestinal IgA response against gut commensals [2]. However, the commensal *Lactobacillus*, which colonizes the nasal mucosa and crosses the nasal epithelial barrier, induces Th1, but not Treg or Th2, responses in mice [3].

The human oral cavity harbors a complex bacterial community composed of more than 700 species [4]. Most are commensals, and only a small number of species are known to be associated with oral diseases, such as dental caries and periodontitis. Periodontitis is a polymicrobial disease that arises from a microbial shift in the indigenous flora of the plaque biofilm rather than from the sudden introduction of a new pathogen [5]. To understand the immunopathogenesis of periodontitis, antibody (Ab) and T cell responses to periodontal pathogens have been widely studied. A number of studies have demonstrated the presence of IgG Abs against periodontal pathogens using whole bacteria or isolated proteins, such as fimbriae from *Porphyromonas gingivalis*, bacterial surface protein A from *Tannerella forsythia*, and leukotoxin from *Aggregatibacter actinomycetemcomitans* in human serum or gingival crevicular fluid [6–10]. Two decades ago, the presence of T cells specific to *P. gingivalis* in the peripheral blood of patients with periodontitis and of healthy subjects was shown by a limiting dilution assay without further characterization of the bacteria-specific T cells [11]. In the following decade, several groups established peripheral blood and gingival T cell clones specific to periodontal pathogens and characterized their cytokine production [12–14]. Kopitar *et al.* recently reported that the commensal oral bacteria *Streptococcus mitis* and *Propionibacterium acnes* prime human dendritic cells to induce *in vitro* differentiation of Th2 and Treg cells, respectively [15]. However, all previous studies have employed long-term *in vitro* stimulation with bacterial antigens (Ags) prepared from whole bacteria or outer membranes, which allows for the activation of naïve T cells by specific Ags or non-specific mitogens [16]. Thus, the nature of adaptive immunity to oral comensals and periodontal pathogens in humans are poorly understood.

The aims of the current study include i) to characterize the T-dependent Ab and T cell responses to *Fusobacterium nucleatum*, an oral commensal, and *Treponema denticola*, a periodontal pathogen, in healthy individuals, and ii) to determine difference in those Ab and T cell responses between healthy subjects and patients with chronic periodontitis (CP). Although the levels of *F. nucleatum* are significantly associated with increasing pocket depth [17], *F. nucleatum* is a prevalent member of plaque biofilm in healthy individuals and is considered a commensal or possibly beneficial bacterium due to its ability to induce antimicrobial peptides in gingival epithelial cells [18,19]. *T. denticola* is one of the major periodontal pathogens involved in CP [20]. To exclude components that are mitogenic or reactive to natural Abs produced in a T-independent manner, a single surface protein was chosen as a representative T-dependent Ag for each bacterium. FadA is an adhesin of *F. nucleatum* involved in adhesion and cellular invasion [21]. Td92 is an adhesin of *T. denticola* and an inducer of proinflammatory cytokines [22]. The vaccine protein tetanus toxoid (TT) was used as a control Ag to provide a comparison to a classical systemic immune response. Through the examination of Ab, Ag-specific $CD4^+$ T cells, and the cytokine response to these three Ags, here, we demonstrate that both *F. nucleatum* and *T. denticola* normally induce T cell memory in humans and that CP is associated with a reduced IFNγ/IL-4 cytokine ratio. These findings may provide new insights into the homeostasis of the immune system with oral bacteria and the pathogenesis of periodontitis.

Materials and Methods

Study Subjects and Periodontal Assessment

Individuals with CP (n = 11) were recruited from patients who visited the Department of Periodontology at the Seoul National University Dental Hospital. CP was diagnosed based on the classification system established at the International Workshop for a Classification of Periodontal Diseases and Conditions in 1999 [23]. Age- and gender-matched healthy control subjects (n = 11) were recruited through an advertisement. Control subjects were designated as healthy if they had both full-mouth probing pocket depth and full-mouth clinical attachment level not greater than 3 mm. All healthy subjects had no history of periodontal treatment or diagnosis with periodontitis. All subjects were in good general health and had no history of antimicrobial or periodontal treatment for 3 months before the start of the study. The study was performed according to the principles expressed in the Declaration of Helsinki, after receiving approval from the Institutional Review Board of the Seoul National University Dental Hospital. Written informed consent was obtained from all subjects. After collecting 20 ml peripheral blood and 5 ml saliva, the full-mouth pocket depth, clinical attachment level from the cementoenalmel junction, and bleeding on probing at six sites for each tooth were recorded by one calibrated examiner. All clinical parameters were measured with a manual probe (CP-12, Hu Friedy, Chicago, IL, USA). Four weeks after receiving quadrant scaling/curettage (four visits within four to six weeks), nine patients who were successfully treated and participated in a re-call check were re-sampled.

Human Materials

Plasma samples were obtained by centrifugation of 1 ml blood. The supernatant and solid pellet of saliva were separated. Plasma and the saliva supernatant were stored at −20°C until use. The solid pellet of saliva was subjected to DNA extraction. The remaining blood was layered on Ficoll-Hypaque (Amersham Bioscience, Uppsala, Sweden) after diluting in PBS at 1:1 and centrifuged at 400 g for 40 min. PBMCs in the buffy coat layer were separated and stored in a liquid nitrogen tank until use.

Recombinant FadA and Td92 Proteins

Escherichia coli M15 transformed with the Td92-containing pQE30 vector was kindly provided by Dr. Bong Kyu Choi at School of Dentistry, Seoul National University and the construction of Td92- containing pQE30 is previously reported [22]. The entire coding region for the FadA gene was amplified from the gDNA of *F. nucleatum* ATCC 25586 by PCR using the following primers: 5′-GGAATTCCATATGAAAAAATTTTTATTATTAGCAG-3′ and 5′-CCGCTCGAGGTTACCAGCTCTTAAAGCTTG-3′. The forward and reverse primers contained Nde I and Xho I sites (underlined), respectively. The amplified gene segments were cloned into the Nde I-Xho I sites of an expression vector pET-30(a) (QIAGEN, Valencia, CA, USA) and the plasmid was used to transform *E. coli* BL21. Expression of the recombinant proteins in *E. coli* was induced by treatment with 1 mM isopropyl-β-D-1-thiogalactopyranoside for 4 h. The recombinant FadA and Td92 were purified from the bacterial lysate using nickel-nitrilotriacetic acid agarose (Ni-NTA agarose; QIAGEN). The identities of the purified recombinant FadA and Td92 proteins were confirmed by SDS-PAGE gel electrophoresis and coomassie blue staining (Figure S1). The proteins were then dialyzed three times against 200 volumes of PBS for 24 h.

Measurement of Ag-specific IgA, IgG1, and IgG4 in the Plasma and Saliva

High binding 96-well EIA/RIA plates were coated with 200 ng/ml FadA, Td92 or TT (GreenCross, Yongin, Kyungki, Korea) at 4°C overnight. For the standard, two columns were coated with serially diluted (30 ng/ml to 0.04 ng/ml) human IgA, IgG1, or IgG4 mAb (Southern Biotech, Birmingham, AL, USA) instead of Ag. After blocking with 1% BSA in PBS at room temperature for 1 h 30 min, the plates were incubated with 100 µl plasma or saliva samples at room temperature for 1 h 30 min. For each sample, three serially diluted samples were prepared. All samples and standards were run in duplicate. After washing, the plates were incubated with 100 µl HRP-conjugated goat-anti-human-IgA, -IgG1, or -IgG4 polyclonal Ab (Sothern Biotech) in 1% BSA-PBS for 1 h. After washing, the bound detection Ab was developed with 100 µl 3, 3′, 5, 5′-tetramethylbenzidine substrate (Sigma, St. Louis, MO, USA) for 15 min. After stopping the reaction with 2 N H_2SO_4, the plates were immediately read at 450 nm. The levels of Ag-specific Abs were calculated using an equation generated from the standard curve.

Stimulation of PBMCs with Ag

PBMCs were thawed and stabilized in culture medium (RPMI 1640 medium with 10% heat-inactivated FBS, 2 mM L-glutamine, and 100 U/ml penicillin/streptomycin) at 37°C for 12 h. For flow cytometry analysis, PBMCs (2×10^6 cells/200 µl/well) were stimulated with 30 µg/ml Ag protein, 2 µg/ml anti-CD28 mAb (BD Bioscience, San Diego, CA, USA), and 2 µg/ml anti-CD49d mAb (BD Bioscience) in the presence of 20 µl of PE-conjugated anti-CD154 mAb (BD Bioscience) at 37°C for 16 h.

Monensin (2 μM, BD Bioscience) was added to the culture medium for the last 4 h prior to harvesting cells. To analyze effector cytokines produced in response to Ags, PBMCs (1×10^6 cells/200 μl/well) were stimulated with 30 μg/ml Ag protein, 2 μg/ml anti-CD28 mAb, and 2 μg/ml anti-CD49d mAb for 48 h. The concentration of the Ag and the stimulation time were determined by preliminary experiments to obtain the maximal difference in the number of $CD154^+CD4^+$ T cells and cytokine production compared to unstimulated cells. After thawing and stabilization, the PBMCs samples that did not have enough live cells for the experiment were excluded from the assay.

Cell Staining and Flow Cytometry Analysis

After stimulation, Ag-specific cells were identified by cytoplasmic staining of CD154. The harvested cells were blocked with 0.1% human serum and stained with APC-conjugated anti-CD4 mAb (BD Bioscience). Cells were then stained with FITC-conjugated anti-Foxp3 mAb (BD Bioscience) after permeabilization with Fix/Perm (BD Bioscience). Cells were analyzed with a FACSCalibur flow cytometer (BD Bioscience) using the CellQuest software (BD Bioscience). Lymphocytes gated based on forward and side scatters were plotted in the density plots of CD4 vs. CD154, and the percentage of $CD154^+$ $CD4^+$ T cells was determined. Then, the $CD154^+CD4^+$ T cells were gated and plotted against Foxp3 and CD4 to obtain the percentage of Ag-specific $Foxp3^+CD4^+$ T cells.

Measurement of Cytokines

The amount of IL-4, IL-10, IL-17, and IFNγ secreted into the culture medium was measured using ELISA kits (R&D Systems, Minneapolis, MN, USA) according to the manufacturer's instructions.

Quantification of F. nucleatum and T. denticola in Saliva

To estimate the level of *T. denticola* and *F. nucleatum* in the oral cavity, the relative proportion of each bacterium in saliva was determined by real-time PCR. Bacterial genomic DNA was extracted from the solid pellet of saliva using a G-spin^{TM} bacterial genomic extraction kit (iNtRON, Kyung-gi, Korea). One microgram of gDNA was subjected to real time-PCR amplification using universal primers that targeted a highly conserved region of 16s rRNA, and bacteria-specific primers that targeted a specific area in the 16s rRNA gene of *F. nucleatum* or *T. denticola*. A 20 μl reaction mix containing 1 μg gDNA, SYBR Premix Ex *Taq*, ROX Reference Dye (Takara Bio, Otsu, Japan), and each primer (0.2 μM) was prepared and subjected to amplification using a fluorescence thermocycler (Applied Biosystems 7500 Real-time PCR, Foster City, CA, USA) under the following conditions: initial denaturation at 94°C for 1 min, followed by 40 cycles of denaturation at 95°C for 15 s, annealing at 60°C for 15 s, and elongation at 72°C for 33 s. The specificity of the PCR product was verified by melting curve analysis. Relative copy numbers of *F. nucleatum* and *T. denticola* rRNA genes compared to the products of the universal rRNA primers were calculated using $2^{-\Delta Ct}$. Real-Time PCR was performed in triplicate for each gDNA sample. The primer sequences used are as follows: 5′-ACTCCTACGG-GAGGCAGC-3′ and 5′-CAATTCCTTTGAGTTTCACC-3′ for the universal primers; 5′-TGTAGTTCCGCTTACCTCTT-CAG-3′ and 5′-AAGCGCGTCTAGGTGGTTATGT-3′ for *F. nucleatum*; and 5′-TAATACCGAATGTGCTCATTTACAT-3′ and 5′-TCAAAGAAGCATTCCCTCTTCTTCTTA-3′ for *T. denticola*.

Statistics

The differences between the healthy subjects and CP patients were analyzed by Mann-Whitney U test. The differences in response to two different Ags or before and after treatment for the same subjects were analyzed by Wilcoxon signed-rank test. Pairwise correlation analysis was performed using Spearman's rank correlation test. All statistics were performed using the SPSS Statistics19 software (IBM, Seoul, Korea). Data were considered statistically significant at a p-value of <0.05.

Results

Clinical Parameters of Subjects

Compared to healthy subjects, patients with untreated CP had significantly increased levels of clinical attachment level, a parameter of periodontal destruction, and increased levels of bleeding on probing, a parameter of inflammation. Successful treatment of the disease improved both clinical parameters to the levels that are comparable to those of healthy subjects (Table 1).

Ab Responses in Plasma and Saliva

B cells specific to T-dependent Ags undergo class switching with the help of follicular B helper T cells that provide CD40L and multiple cytokines. The production of IgG1, IgG4, and IgA involves IFNγ, IL-4, and TGFβ, respectively [24–26]. Because the cytokine secretion patterns of follicular B helper T cells and peripheral effector helper T cells are similar, the production of IgG1, IgG4, and IgA reflect Th1, Th2, and Th3 responses, respectively [27]. Therefore, we determined the levels of IgG1, IgG4, and IgA in the plasma and the levels of IgA in the saliva by ELISA to characterize both the Ab and T cell responses to the Ags.

We first analyzed the Ab responses mounted against the three Ags in healthy subjects. In the plasma, IgG1 was the most abundant isotype of Ab for all three Ags, followed by IgA and then IgG4. However, lower levels of FadA- and Td92-specific IgG1 and IgG4 were present compared to those specific to TT. The levels of Td92-specific IgG1 were particularly low. The levels of FadA-specific salivary IgA (sIgA) were significantly higher than the levels of either Td92- or TT-specific sIgA (Figure S2). For FadA-specific IgA, the levels in saliva were higher than those observed in plasma ($P = 0.03$).

Next, the Ab responses of healthy subjects and CP patients were compared. Although slight increase in the levels of FadA- or Td92-specific sIgA, IgA, or IgG4 were observed in CP patients, the differences were not statistically significant. Similarly, the disease treatment did not significantly alter the levels of Abs compared with those before treatment of CP (Figure 1a, b, c, d).

These data show that different Ab responses were mounted against FadA, Td92, and TT, but the periodontal health status of the individuals had no significant effect on the levels of Abs against the three Ags.

The Presence of Ag-specific $CD4^+$ T cells and $Foxp3^+CD4^+$ Tregs

The presence of Ag-specific $CD4^+$ T cells was determined by the detection of intracytoplasmic CD154 (CD40L) following short-term *in vitro* stimulation of peripheral blood mononuclear cells (PBMCs) with Ags [28,29]. CD154 is transiently expressed on recently activated $CD4^+$ T cells and is regarded to be a reliable intracytoplasmic marker of Ag-specific $CD4^+$ T cells [30,31]. Because regulatory T (Treg) cells also upregulate CD154 upon activation [32], the proportion of Tregs among the Ag-specific

Table 1. Characteristics and clinical parameters of subjects.

	Healthy	Patients (Before)	*P* value†	Patients (After)	*P* value‡
Sex (female %)	36	36		33	
Smoker (%)	18	18		22	
Age	34.1±11.8§	34.5±11.7	P=0.867	32.3±3.2	P=0.301
Clinical attachment level (mm)	2.0±0.4‡	3.4±0.2	P<0.0001	2.3±0.2	P=0.078
Bleeding on probing (%)	5.2±4.4‡	66.6±32.1	P<0.0001	11.6±9.0	P=0.122

†Mann-Whitney U test between healthy and patients with CP before treatment.
‡Mann-Whitney U test between healthy and patients with CP after treatment.
§Mean ± standard deviation.

CD4+ T cells was simultaneously determined by intracellular Foxp3 staining (Figure 2a).

A small number of unstimulated CD4+ T cells were positive for CD154. These cells likely represent circulating effector cells that were activated *in vivo*. Stimulation with FadA, Td92, or TT significantly increased the number of CD154+CD4+ T cells in both healthy and CP groups (Figure 2b left panel), which suggests the presence of memory CD4+ T cells specific to these Ags. After subtracting the number of background stained cells, the mean percentages of FadA-, Td92-, and TT-specific cells out of the total CD4+ T cells in healthy subjects were 0.26±0.04, 0.42±0.14, and 0.21±0.05, respectively (Figure 2b right panel). There was no significant difference in the number of Ag-specific CD4+ T cells among the three Ags. Compared with healthy subjects, CP patients tended to contain increased numbers of CD154+CD4+ T cells for all three Ags and also for background (Figure 2a and b left

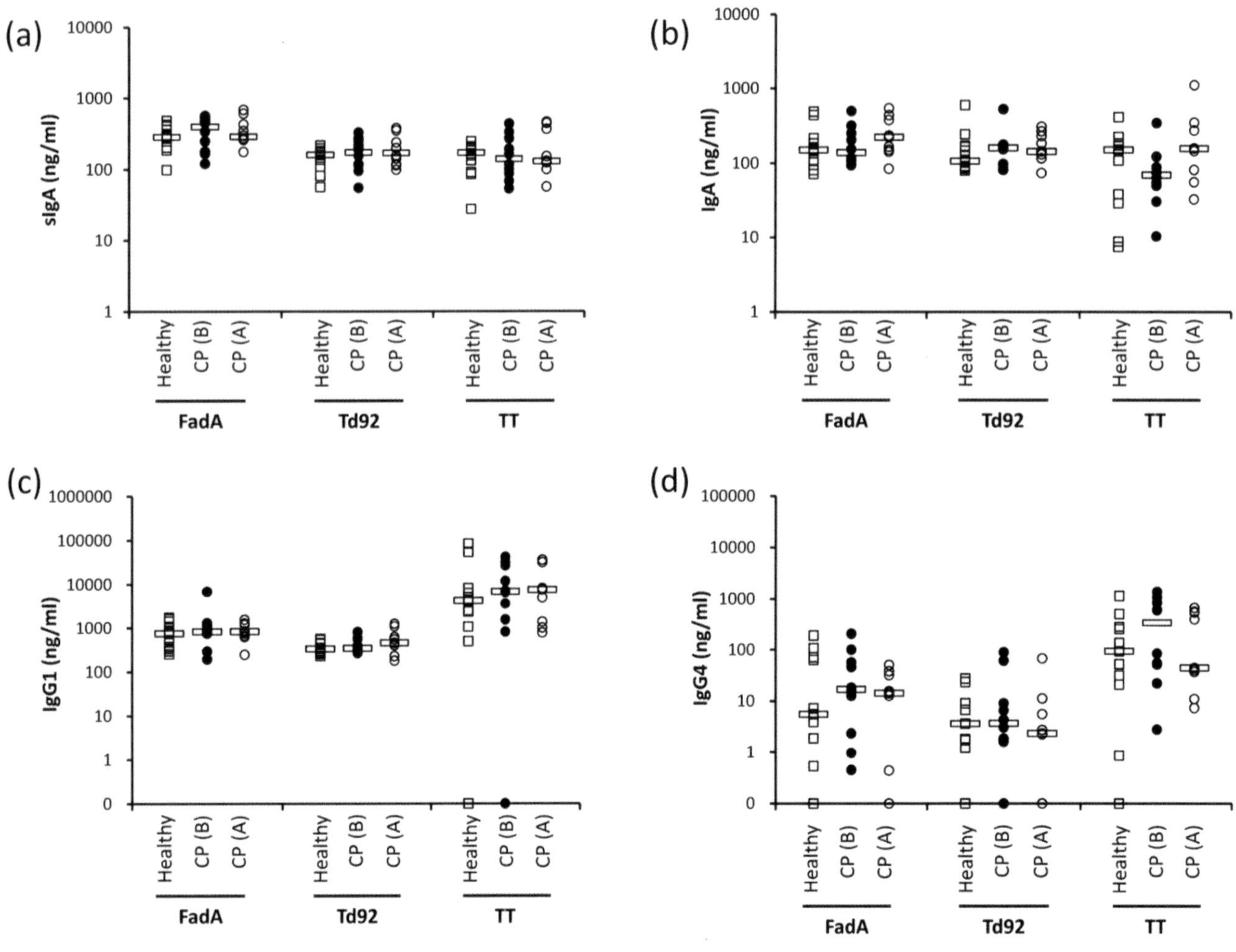

Figure 1. FadA-, Td92-, and TT-specific Abs in saliva and plasma. The levels of FadA-, Td92-, and TT-specific-IgA in saliva (a) and the Ag-specific-IgA (b), -IgG1 (c), and -IgG4 (d) in plasma were determined by ELISA. Bars indicate median values. CP (B): patients with chronic periodontitis before treatment. CP (A): patients with chronic periodontitis after treatment.

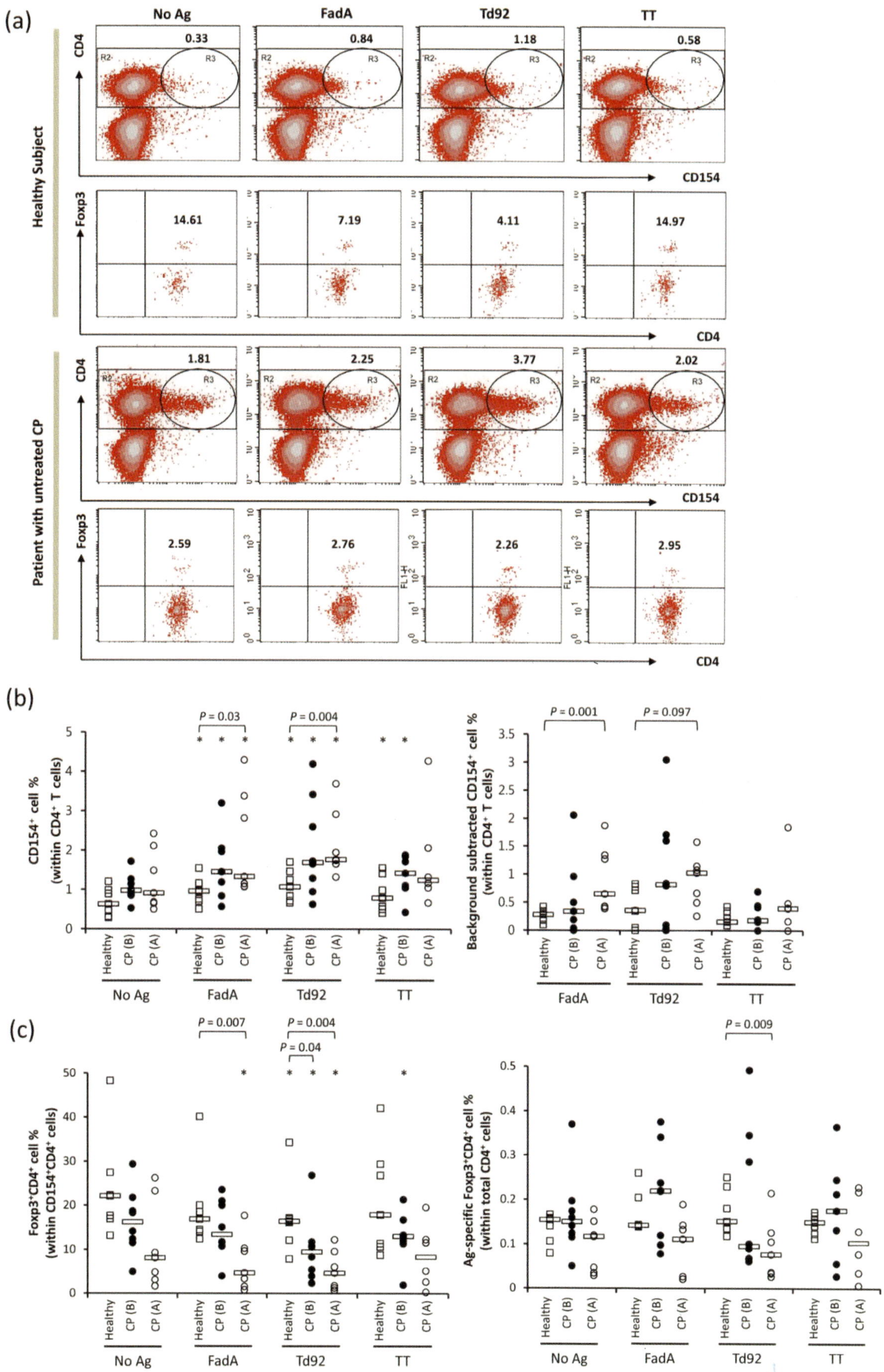
(a)
No Ag
FadA
Td92
TT
Healthy Subject
Patient with untreated CP
CD4
CD154
Foxp3
0.33
0.84
1.18
0.58
14.61
7.19
4.11
14.97
1.81
2.25
3.77
2.02
2.59
2.76
2.26
2.95
(b)
CD154⁺ cell % (within CD4⁺ T cells)
Background subtracted CD154⁺ cell % (within CD4⁺ T cells)
P = 0.03
P = 0.004
P = 0.001
P = 0.097
Healthy
CP (B)
CP (A)
(c)
Foxp3⁺CD4⁺ cell % (within CD154⁺CD4⁺ cells)
Ag-specific Foxp3⁺CD4⁺ cell % (within total CD4⁺ cells)
P = 0.007
P = 0.004
P = 0.04
P = 0.009

Figure 2. Presence of FadA-, Td92-, and TT-specific CD4$^+$ T cells and Ag-specific Foxp3$^+$CD4$^+$ Tregs in PBMCs PBMCs from healthy subjects (n = 7), patients with CP before (B) treatment (n = 8), and patients with CP after (A) treatment (n = 7) were stimulated with medium alone (No Ag), 30 μg/ml FadA, Td92, or TT for 16 hours in the presence of PE-conjugated anti-CD154 mAb, purified anti-CD28 mAb, and anti-CD49d mAb. Monensin was added during the last 4 h of culture. The stimulated cells were stained with an APC-conjugated anti-CD4 mAb and a FITC-conjugated anti-Foxp3 mAb. (a) Lymphocytes gated based on FSC vs. SSC were plotted by CD4 vs. CD154 in the density plots (Top and the third rows). The percentage of CD154$^+$ cells (R3) among the CD4$^+$ T cells (R2) is presented. CD154$^+$CD4$^+$ T cells were gated and plotted by Foxp3 vs. CD4 (the second and the fourth rows). Numbers indicate the percentage of Foxp3$^+$ cells among the gated CD154$^+$CD4$^+$ T cells. (b) The percentage of CD154$^+$ cells out of the total CD4$^+$ T cells was graphed (left panel). The percentage of Ag-specific cells out of the total CD4$^+$ T cells was graphed after subtracting the number of background stained cells (right panel). (c) The percentage of Foxp3$^+$CD4$^+$ Tregs among the CD154$^+$CD4$^+$ T cells was graphed (left panel). The percentage of CD154$^+$Foxp3$^+$CD4$^+$ T cells out of the total CD4$^+$ T cells was graphed (right panel). Bars indicate median values. *, $P<0.05$ compared to No Ag.

panel). After subtracting the number of background stained cells, the mean percentages of FadA-, Td92-, and TT-specific cells out of the total CD4$^+$ T cells in patients with untreated CP were 0.55±0.24, 1.02±0.38, and 0.14±0.17, respectively (Figure 2b right panel). CP treatment further increased the numbers of FadA- and Td92-specific CD4$^+$ T cells, resulting in significant differences from the levels observed in healthy subjects (Figure 2b).

In healthy subjects, the percentage of Foxp3$^+$CD4$^+$ Tregs out of the Ag-specific CD154$^+$CD4$^+$ T cells was decreased upon Ag stimulation (Figure 2c left panel). No significant differences were observed in the responses elicited by the various Ags. Interestingly, patients with CP presented with a reduced percentage of Foxp3$^+$CD4$^+$ Tregs out of the Ag-specific cells in both the unstimulated and Ag-stimulated conditions. This difference was increased upon clinical therapy, which resulted in a significant difference from healthy subjects upon stimulation with FadA or Td92 (Figure 2c left panel). Because the number of Ag-specific CD4$^+$ T cells was increased in CP patients, the percentage of Ag-specific Foxp3$^+$CD4$^+$ Tregs was adjusted to the total CD4$^+$ T cell population. The expansion of Ag-specific Foxp3$^+$CD4$^+$ Tregs was examined in several patients with untreated CP. However, after therapy, the patients presented lower levels of Td92-specific Foxp3$^+$CD4$^+$ Tregs than the healthy subjects (Figure 2c right panel).

In summary, the treated CP patients presented increased levels of FadA- and Td92-specific CD4$^+$ T cells but reduced levels of Td92-specific Tregs than the healthy subjects.

Cytokine Response

We examined Ag-induced production of IFNγ, IL-4, and IL-17 that are Th1, Th2, and Th17 effector cytokines, respectively, in addition to a regulatory cytokine IL-10. Although identification of Ag-specific CD4$^+$ T cells via flow cytometric detection of CD154 allows for the concurrent examination of cytokines, such as IL-2, TNFα, and IFNγ, the expression of IL-4 and IL-10 requires sorting and additional stimulation for 36 h [29], as confirmed in our preliminary study. Therefore, PBMCs were stimulated with Ags for 48 h, a time period that allows activation of memory T cells but limits that of naïve T cells, and the amounts of IFNγ, IL-4, IL-10, and IL-17 secreted into the supernatant were measured by ELISA. In healthy subjects, all three Ags increased the production of IFNγ and IL-10, and FadA and Td92 reduced IL-4 secretion compared to the basal levels (Figure S2). No significant change in the levels of IL-17 was observed upon Ag stimulation. TT induced the highest levels of IFNγ production among the three Ags, followed by Td92 and FadA. The levels of FadA-stimulated IL-17 production were lower than those induced by Td92 or TT (Figure S3).

Compared to healthy controls, PBMCs from CP patients failed to show a significant IFNγ response to either FadA or Td92 and tended to produce increased levels of IL-4 both at basal levels and following Ag stimulation. In addition, the patient PBMCs presented a tendency to produce consistently lower levels of IL-10 (Figure 3a, b, c, d). After clinical therapy, the differences in IFNγ and IL-4 levels were exaggerated, but the levels of IL-10 were restored (Figure 3a, b, c, d). Consequently, the patients with treated CP exhibited significantly reduced IFNγ/IL-4 ratios in response to all three Ags compared to the healthy subjects (Figure 3e).

These results indicate that different cytokine responses were induced by different Ags and by differences in the periodontal health status.

Relative Amounts of F. nucleatum and T. denticola in Saliva

To estimate the amounts of *F. nucleatum* and *T. denticola* colonizing the oral cavity, the relative proportion of each bacterium among total bacteria in saliva was determined by real-time PCR of 16S rRNA genes. With the exception of one individual, all healthy subjects carried detectable levels of *T. denticola*. Both healthy individuals and CP patients carried higher amounts of *F. nucleatum* than *T. denticola* ($P<0.0001$). Although statistical significance was not achieved, patients with CP contained a higher proportion of *T. denticola* than healthy subjects, which was restored by clinical therapy (Figure 4).

Correlations among Clinical, Immunological, and Microbial Parameters

Correlations among the examined periodontal, immunological, and microbial parameters were analyzed. We first asked if there were any parameters associated with periodontal destruction. The relative proportion of *T. denticola* had a positive correlation with CAL ($P=0.03$) in the combined population of healthy subjects and patients, but not in healthy group alone. In patients with untreated CP, the levels of Td92-induced IFNγ production and Td92-specific IgA in plasma had a negative and a positive correlation with CAL, respectively ($P=0.019$ and $P=0.02$, respectively). Meanwhile, the levels of Td92-specific sIgA were negatively associated with CAL in healthy subjects ($P=0.039$).

The increased proportion of Ag-specific CD4$^+$ T cells and the altered cytokine profile observed in CP patients may be a result of increased levels of bacteria. However, this correlation was not detected (data not shown). Interestingly, for almost all examined immunologic parameters, there were strong correlations between the Ags for each parameter. For example, high levels of FadA-specific sIgA correlated with high levels of Td92- and TT-specific sIgA (Table 2). This finding suggests that a certain intrinsic feature of each individual affects the individual's immune response to all Ags.

Discussion

Our results have revealed that humans normally develop T cell memory to both *F. nucleatum* and *T. denticola*, regardless of the

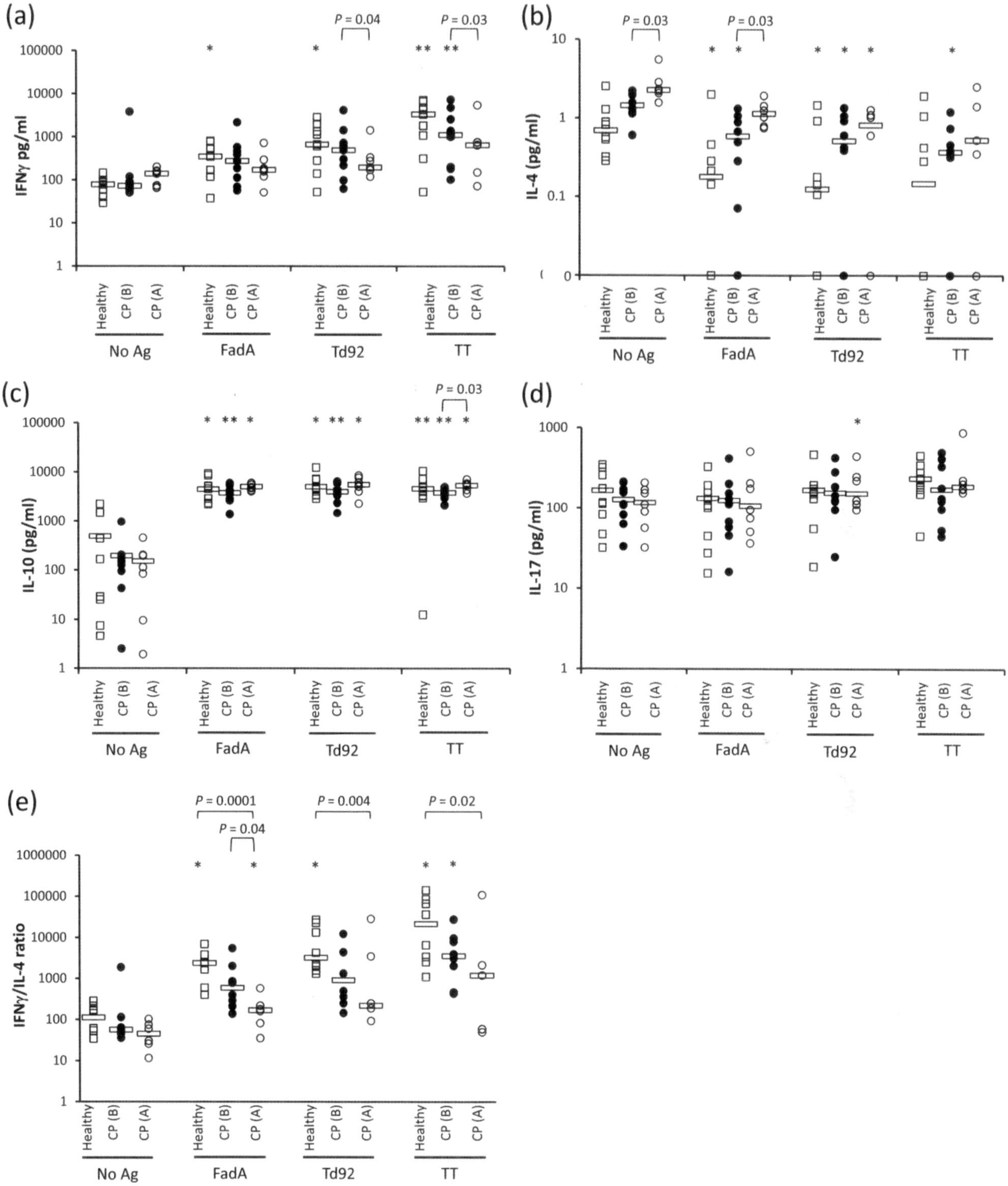

Figure 3. Cytokine production by PBMCs in response to FadA, Td92, or TT PBMCs from healthy subjects (n = 9), patients with CP before (B) treatment (n = 9), and patients with CP after (A) treatment (n = 7) were stimulated with medium alone (No Ag), 30 μg/ml FadA, Td92, or TT for 48 hours in the presence of purified anti-CD28 mAb and anti-CD49d mAb. (a–d) The amount of IFNγ, IL-4, IL-10, and IL-17 secreted into the supernatant was measured by ELISA. (e) The ratio of IFNγ/IL-4 was calculated and plotted. For the calculation of this ratio, half of the lowest detectable concentration (0.1 pg/ml) was arbitrarily assigned to IL-4 samples that had a zero value. Bars indicate median values. *, $P<0.05$; **, $P<0.01$ compared to No Ag.

periodontal health status, as evidenced by the presence of FadA- and Td92-specific CD4$^+$ T cells, IgG, and IgA as well as Ag-induced IFNγ production by PBMCs. The presence of FadA- and Td92-specific CD4$^+$ T cells was determined by detecting

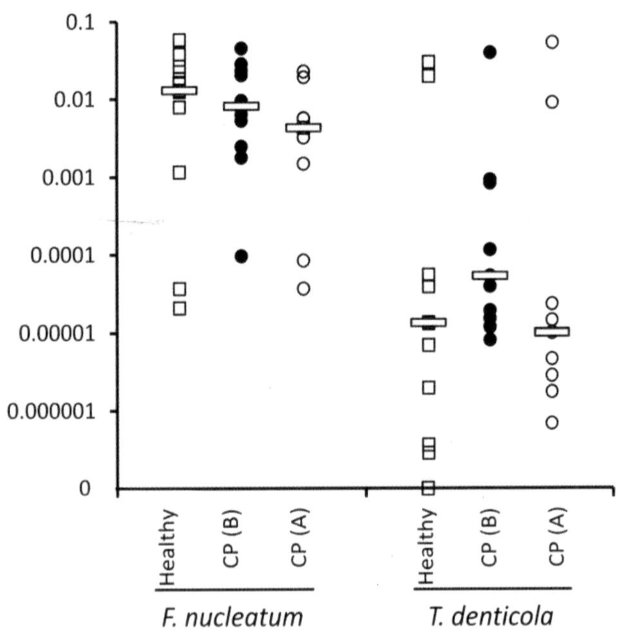

Figure 4. Relative amounts of F. nucleatum and T. denticola in saliva. The relative proportion of *F. nucleatum* or *T. denticola* among the total bacteria in saliva was determined by real-time PCR of 16S rRNA. Bars indicate median values.

intracytoplasmic CD154. The addition of anti-CD154 Ab to PBMC cultures during short-term *in vitro* stimulation with Ag stains only the specific T cells that have been previously activated with the Ag [30]. The CD154-stained Ag-specific T cells include $CCR7^+CD27^+$ central memory (T_{CM}) and $CCR7^-CD27^{+/-}$ effector memory T (T_{EM}) cells, and both populations contribute to cytokine production [30,31]. The presence of FadA- and Td92-specific $CD4^+$ T cells in PBMCs indicates that *F. nucleatum* and *T. denticola* can reach the systemic immune system to activate T cells, which may be attributable to the ability of these bacteria to invade gingival epithelial cells and/or gingival tissue [33,34]. Alternatively, transient bacteremia, which can be triggered by mastication, tooth brushing, and various dental procedures, might be the route by which oral bacteria encounter the systemic immune system [35]. The increased number of FadA- and Td92-specific $CD4^+$ T cells in patients, particularly after CP treatment, may reflect frequent bacteremia and the repeated activation of specific T cells. Compared to TT, FadA and Td92 induced lower levels of plasma IgG1 and IgG4 *in vivo*, and this coincides with the fact that both FadA and Td92 induced low levels of IFNγ production and down-regulated IL-4 production by PBMCs *in vitro*. When the FadA- and the Td92-induced responses were compared, significantly higher levels of FadA-specific sIgA and plasma IgG1 were observed, while Td92 induced higher levels of IFNγ and IL-17 production by PBMCs. Therefore, the immune evasive property of *T. denticola* reported in the innate immune compartment [19,36] was not observed in the adaptive immune compartment. These results also indicate that *T. denticola* preferentially induces a cell-mediated rather than a humoral response. *F. nucleatum* seems to be efficient in inducing mucosal immunity as evidenced by the high

Table 2. Correlations of the examined immunologic parameters between the Ags.

	Td92-specific/induced	TT-specific/induced
FadA-specific IgA in saliva	0.908[†] ($P<0.0001$)	0.845 ($P<0.0001$)
Td92-specific IgA in saliva	–	0.914 ($P<0.0001$)
FadA-specific IgA in plasma	0.858 ($P<0.0001$)	0.464 ($P=0.01$)
Td92-specific IgA in plasma	–	0.453 ($P=0.012$)
FadA-specific IgG1 in plasma	0.438 ($P=0.015$)	0.069 ($P=0.716$)
Td92-specific IgG1 in plasma	–	0.117 ($P=0.539$)
FadA-specific IgG4 in plasma	0.249 ($P=0.184$)	0.233 ($P=0.215$)
Td92-specific IgG4 in plasma	–	0.433 ($P=0.017$)
FadA-specific $CD154^+/CD4^+$ (%)	0.741 ($P<0.0001$)	0.944 ($P<0.0001$)
Td92-specific $CD154^+/CD4^+$ (%)	–	0.784 ($P<0.0001$)
FadA-specific $Foxp3^+/CD154^+CD4^+$ (%)	0.816 ($P<0.0001$)	0.833 ($P<0.0001$)
Td92-specific $Foxp3^+/CD154CD4^+$ (%)	–	0.818 ($P<0.0001$)
FadA-specific $Foxp3^+/CD4^+$ (%)	0.808 ($P<0.0001$)	0.814 ($P<0.0001$)
Td92-specific $Foxp3^+/CD4^+$ (%)	–	0.712 ($P<0.0001$)
FadA-induced IFNγ	0.929 ($P<0.0001$)	0.824 ($P<0.0001$)
Td92-induced IFNγ	–	0.870 ($P<0.0001$)
FadA-induced IL-4	0.691 ($P<0.0001$)	0.429 ($P=0.032$)
Td92-induced IL-4	–	0.427 ($P=0.033$)
FadA-induced IL-10	0.761 ($P<0.0001$)	0.908 ($P<0.0001$)
Td92-induced IL-10	–	0.754 ($P<0.0001$)
FadA-induced IL-17	0.859 ($P<0.0001$)	0.609 ($P=0.002$)
Td92-induced IL-17	–	0.778 ($P<0.0001$)

[†]Spearman's rho calculated using all values from healthy individuals and patients with CP before and after therapy.

levels of FadA-specific sIgA. Collectively, *F. nucleatum* induces Th3 (sIgA)- and Th1 (IFNγ and IgG1)-dominant immune responses, whereas *T. denticola* induces a Th1 (IFNγ and IgG1)-dominant immune response. One limitation of this study is that the presence of Ag-specific Th1 or Th3 cells was not directly shown. Because PBMC were used to examine cytokine profiles of Th subsets, $CD8^+$ T cells and NK cells could have contributed to the IFNγ production.

The Th1-response to FadA and Td92 observed in healthy individuals raises the question how our immune system maintains homeostasis with the *F. nucleatum* and *T. denticola* present in the oral cavity. The epithelial barrier and sIgA would normally prevent bacterial invasion and the constant activation of T cells by these bacteria. The negative correlation between Td92-specific sIgA and CAL observed in healthy subjects suggests a protective role of sIgA in disease onset. If the oral bacteria invade epithelia and underlying tissue, another potential mechanism to maintain homeostasis would be regulation via regulatory cells and cytokines. The numbers of FadA- and Td92-specific Tregs within the total $CD4^+$ T cells were comparable to the numbers of TT-specific Tregs. However, no significant difference observed in this study may be attributable to small sample size. Dendritic cells (DCs) conditioned by mucosal epithelial cells support the induction of several types of Tregs, including $CD4^+CD25^+Foxp3^+$ induced Treg (iTreg), $CD4^+CD25^-Foxp3^-LAP^+$ Th3, and $CD4^+CD25^-Foxp3^-IL\text{-}10^+$ Tr1 [37]. Thus, there is a possibility that the FadA- or Td92-specific $CD4^+$ T_{CM} cells may preferentially differentiate in the draining lymph nodes of the oral cavity *in vivo* into various types of Tregs. The low levels of FadA- and Td92-specific IgG1, IgG4, and IFNγ responses than TT-specific responses support this possibility. Ag stimulation of PBMCs induced high levels of the regulatory cytokine IL-10, but TT also elicited comparable levels of IL-10. Therefore, there is no sufficient evidence for or against the preferential regulation of immune response to FadA or Td92 through Tregs or IL-10. The best strategy to maintain the homeostatic relationship between the immune system and oral bacteria may be to keep bacteria outside tissue by competent epithelial barriers and sIgA.

Another important finding is the association of CP with a IFNγ/IL-4 cytokine imbalance. A number of conflicting results, including the dominance of Th1 cytokines [38,39], of Th2 cytokines [40,41], or no dominance [42,43] in the periodontal lesions, have been reported over the last 15 years. These reports have recently been reviewed, and it was suggested that a skewed balance toward Th2 is responsible for periodontitis expression [44]. Our study coincides with the Th2-skewed response to oral bacterial Ags. Considering that periodontitis is a polymicrobial disease, the responses to two recombinant proteins from two oral species may not reflect the whole picture of immune response associated with periodontitis. In our study, however, the IFNγ/IL4 imbalance was also observed in response to TT, an Ag irrelevant to periodontitis. Furthermore, the levels of FadA-induced IFNγ or IL-4 had strong correlations with those induced by Td92 and TT in the combined population of healthy subjects and patients. These findings suggest that the skewed response toward Th2-like type observed in the CP patients may be an intrinsic feature of each subject rather than an Ag-specific phenotype. Increased IL-5 production by PBMCs from patients with CP following stimulation with mitogen also supports the intrinsic nature of the Th2 bias in CP patients [45]. Importantly, the levels of Td92-induced IFNγ had a negative correlation with CAL in patients, suggesting a protective role of the Th1 response to *T. denticola* in disease progression. Similarly, the importance of the Th1-dependent immune clearance of *P. gingivalis* for protection against alveolar bone loss has been demonstrated in a mouse model of periodontitis [46]. The levels of IL-4 production did not correlate with any clinical parameters. Whether the IFNγ/IL-4 imbalance is the cause or the result of disease warrants further investigation in larger samples.

Another important question to be answered in the future is to what degree the T cell responses observed in PBMCs reflect those in gingival tissues. The T_{EM} cells from PBMCs maintain effector functions of heterogeneous Th subsets, such as Th1, Th2, and Th17 [47,48]. T_{CM} cells include committed pre-Th 1 and pre-Th 2 in addition to non-polarized cells [49]. Because the distinct cytokine profiles of Th or pre-Th subsets are maintained upon restimulation in the absence of polarizing factors [49], the IFNγ/IL-4 imbalance observed in the current study is likely to reflect that of the circulating memory T cell pool in each subject. Although the presence of Th17 cells in periodontal lesions has been reported [50], no IL-17 response to either FadA or Td92 was evident in our study using PBMCs. A study using gingival and peripheral blood T cells in parallel would clarify the relationship of Ag-specific T cells distributed in two compartments.

In conclusion, both *F. nucleatum* and *T. denticola* activate $CD4^+$ T cells and induce a Th1-type response in humans. CP is associated with an impaired IFNγ/IL-4cytokine balance. These findings may provide new insights into the homeostatic interaction between the immune system and oral bacteria and the pathogenesis of periodontitis.

Supporting Information

Figure S1 Recombinant Td92 and FadA proteins. The identities of the purified recombinant FadA and Td92 proteins were confirmed by SDS-PAGE gel electrophoresis and coomassie blue staining.

Figure S2 Comparison of Ab response to FadA, Td92, and TT in healthy individuals. From the results shown in Figure 1, the data of healthy subjects are graphed separately. *, $P<0.05$; **, $P<0.01$.

Figure S3 Comparison of cytokine response of PBMCs to FadA, Td92, and TT in healthy individuals. From the results shown in Figure 3, the data of healthy subjects are graphed separately. *, $P<0.05$; **, $P<0.01$ compared to No Ag. #, $P<0.05$; ##, $P<0.01$.

Author Contributions

Conceived and designed the experiments: JS IC-R YC. Performed the experiments: JS S-A K YSC YCK. Analyzed the data: JS S-AK YC. Wrote the paper: JS YC.

References

1. Vaughan AT, Brackenbury LS, Massari P, Davenport V, Gorringe A, et al. (2010) Neisseria lactamica selectively induces mitogenic proliferation of the naive B cell pool via cell surface Ig. J Immunol 185: 3652–3660.
2. Hapfelmeier S, Lawson MA, Slack E, Kirundi JK, Stoel M, et al. (2010) Reversible microbial colonization of germ-free mice reveals the dynamics of IgA immune responses. Science 328: 1705–1709.
3. Costalonga M, Cleary PP, Fischer LA, Zhao Z (2009) Intranasal bacteria induce Th1 but not Treg or Th2. Mucosal Immunol 2: 85–95.
4. Aas JA, Paster BJ, Stokes LN, Olsen I, Dewhirst FE (2005) Defining the normal bacterial flora of the oral cavity. J Clin Microbiol 43: 5721–5732.
5. Darveau RP (2010) Periodontitis: a polymicrobial disruption of host homeostasis. Nat Rev Microbiol 8: 481–490.

6. Tew JG, Smibert RM, Scott EA, Burmeister JA, Ranney RR (1985) Serum antibodies in young adult humans reactive with periodontitis associated treponemes. J Periodontal Res 20: 580–590.
7. Takeuchi Y, Aramaki M, Nagasawa T, Umeda M, Oda S, et al. (2006) Immunoglobulin G subclass antibody profiles in *Porphyromonas gingivalis*-associated aggressive and chronic periodontitis patients. Oral Microbiol Immunol 21: 314–318.
8. Hall LM, Dunford RG, Genco RJ, Sharma A (2012) Levels of serum immunoglobulin G specific to bacterial surface protein A of *Tannerella forsythia* are related to periodontal status. J Periodontol 83: 228–234.
9. Brage M, Holmlund A, Johansson A (2011) Humoral immune response to *Aggregatibacter actinomycetemcomitans* leukotoxin. J Periodontal Res 46: 170–175.
10. Pussinen PJ, Könönen E, Paju S, Hyvärinen K, Gursoy UK, et al. (2011) Periodontal pathogen carriage, rather than periodontitis, determines the serum antibody levels. J Clin Periodontol 38: 405–411.
11. Mahanonda R, Seymour GJ, Powell LW, Good MF, Halliday JW (1989) Limit dilution analysis of peripheral blood T lymphocytes specific to periodontopathic bacteria. Clin Exp Immunol 75: 245–251.
12. Wassenaar A, Reinhardus C, Thepen T, Abraham-Inpijn L, Kievits F (1995) Cloning, characterization, and antigen specificity of T-lymphocyte subsets extracted from gingival tissue of chronic adult periodontitis patients. Infect Immun 63: 2147–2153.
13. Nakajima T, Yamazaki K, Cullinan MP, Gemmell E, Seymour GJ (1999) T-cell antigen specificity in humans following stimulation with *Porphyromonas gingivalis*. Arch Oral Biol 44: 1045–1053.
14. Gemmell E, Carter CL, Grieco DA, Sugerman PB, Seymour GJ (2002) *P. gingivalis*-specific T-cell lines produce Th1 and Th2 cytokines. J Dent Res 81: 303–307.
15. Kopitar AN, Ihan Hren N, Ihan A (2006) Commensal oral bacteria antigens prime human dendritic cells to induce Th1, Th2 or Treg differentiation. Oral Microbiol Immunol 21: 1–5.
16. Geginat J, Sallusto F, Lanzavecchia A (2001) Cytokine-driven proliferation and differentiation of human naive, central memory, and effector memory CD4(+) T cells. J Exp Med 194: 1711–1719.
17. Socransky SS, Haffajee AD, Cugini MA, Smith C, Kent RL Jr (1998) Microbial complexes in subgingival plaque. J Clin Periodontol 25: 134–144.
18. Krisanaprakornkit S, Kimball JR, Weinberg A, Darveau RP, Bainbridge BW, et al. (2000) Inducible expression of human beta-defensin 2 by *Fusobacterium nucleatum* in oral epithelial cells: multiple signaling pathways and role of commensal bacteria in innate immunity and the epithelial barrier. Infect Immun 68: 2907–2915.
19. Ji S, Kim Y, Min BM, Han SH, Choi Y (2007) Innate immune responses of gingival epithelial cells to non-periodontopathic and periodontopathic bacteria. J Periodontal Res 42: 503–510.
20. Haffajee AD, Teles RP, Socransky SS. (2006) Association of *Eubacterium nodatum* and *Treponema denticola* with human periodontitis lesions. Oral Microbiol Immunol 21: 269–282.
21. Ikegami A, Chung P, Han YW (2009) Complementation of the fadA mutation in *Fusobacterium nucleatum* demonstrates that the surface-exposed adhesin promotes cellular invasion and placental colonization. Infect Immun 77: 3075–3079.
22. Jun HK, Kang YM, Lee HR, Lee SH, Choi BK (2008) Highly conserved surface proteins of oral spirochetes as adhesins and potent inducers of proinflammatory and osteoclastogenic factors. Infect Immun 76: 2428–2438.
23. Armitage GC (2000) Development of a classification system for periodontal diseases and conditions. Northwest Dent 79: 31–35.
24. Kawano Y, Noma T, Yata J. (1994) Regulation of human IgG subclass production by cytokines. IFN-gamma and IL-6 act antagonistically in the induction of human IgG1 but additively in the induction of IgG2. J Immunol 153: 4948–4958.
25. Gascan H, Gauchat JF, Aversa G, Van Vlasselaer P, de Vries JE (1991) Anti-CD40 monoclonal antibodies or CD4+ T cell clones and IL-4 induce IgG4 and IgE switching in purified human B cells via different signaling pathways. J Immunol 147: 8–13.
26. Stavnezer J (1995) Regulation of antibody production and class switching by TGF-beta. J Immunol 155: 1647–1651.
27. Reinhardt RL, Liang HE, Locksley RM (2009) Cytokine-secreting follicular T cells shape the antibody repertoire. Nat Immunol 10: 385–393.
28. Frentsch M, Arbach O, Kirchhoff D, Moewes B, Worm M, et al. (2005) Direct access to CD4+ T cells specific for defined antigens according to CD154 expression. Nat Med 11: 1118–1124.
29. Chattopadhyay PK, Yu J, Roederer M (2005) A live-cell assay to detect antigen-specific CD4+ T cells with diverse cytokine profiles. Nat Med 11: 1113–1117.
30. Stubbe M, Vanderheyde N, Goldman M, Marchant A (2006) Antigen-specific central memory CD4+ T lymphocytes produce multiple cytokines and proliferate *in vivo* in humans. J Immunol 177: 8185–8190.
31. Stubbe M, Vanderheyde N, Pircher H, Goldman M, Marchant A (2008) Characterization of a subset of antigen-specific human central memory CD4+ T lymphocytes producing effector cytokines. Eur J Immunol 38: 273–282.
32. Guiducci C, Valzasina B, Dislich H, Colombo MP (2005) CD40/CD40L interaction regulates CD4+CD25+ Treg homeostasis through dendritic cell-produced IL-2. Eur J Immunol 35: 557–567.
33. Ji S, Shin JE, Kim YC, Choi Y (2010) Intracellular degradation of *Fusobacterium nucleatum* in human gingival epithelial cells. Mol Cells 30: 519–526.
34. Lux R, Miller JN, Park NH, Shi W (2001) Motility and chemotaxis in tissue penetration of oral epithelial cell layers by *Treponema denticola*. Infect Immun 69: 6276–6283.
35. Forner L, Larsen T, Kilian M, Holmstrup P (2006) Incidence of bacteremia after chewing, tooth brushing and scaling in individuals with periodontal inflammation. J Clin Periodontol 33: 401–407.
36. Shin J, Ji S, Choi Y (2008) Ability of oral bacteria to induce tissue-destructive molecules from human neutrophils. Oral Dis 14: 327–334.
37. Weiner HL, da Cunha AP, Quintana F, Wu H (2011) Oral tolerance. Immunol Rev 241: 241–259.
38. Yamamoto M, Fujihashi K, Hiroi T, McGhee JR, Van Dyke TE, et al. (1997) Molecular and cellular mechanisms for periodontal diseases: role of Th1 and Th2 type cytokines in induction of mucosal inflammation. J Periodontal Res 32: 115–119.
39. Górska R, Gregorek H, Kowalski J, Laskus-Perendyk A, Syczewska M, et al. (2003) Relationship between clinical parameters and cytokine profiles in inflamed gingival tissue and serum samples from patients with chronic periodontitis. J Clin Periodontol 30: 1046–1052.
40. Tokoro Y, Matsuki Y, Yamamoto T, Suzuki T, Hara K (1997) Relevance of local Th2-type cytokine mRNA expression in immunocompetent infiltrates in inflamed gingival tissue to periodontal diseases. Clin Exp Immunol 107: 166–174.
41. Lappin DF, MacLeod CP, Kerr A, Mitchell T, Kinane DF (2001) Anti-inflammatory cytokine IL-10 and T cell cytokine profile in periodontitis granulation tissue. Clin Exp Immunol 123: 294–300.
42. Wassenaar A, Reinhardus C, Abraham-Inpijn L, Snijders A, Kievits F (1998) Characteristics of *Prevotella intermedia*-specific CD4+ T cell clones from peripheral blood of a chronic adult periodontitis patient. Clin Exp Immunol 113: 105–110.
43. Berglundh T, Liljenberg B, Lindhe J (2002) Some cytokine profiles of T-helper cells in lesions of advanced periodontitis. J Clin Periodontol 29: 705–709.
44. Berglundh T, Donati M (2005) Aspects of adaptive host response in periodontitis. J Clin Periodontol 32 Suppl 6: 87–107.
45. Sigusch B, Klinger G, Glockmann E, Simon HU (1998) Early-onset and adult periodontitis associated with abnormal cytokine production by activated T lymphocytes. J Periodontol 69: 1098–1104.
46. Liang S, Krauss JL, Domon H, McIntosh ML, Hosur KB, et al. (2011) The C5a receptor impairs IL-12-dependent clearance of *Porphyromonas gingivalis* and is required for induction of periodontal bone loss. J Immunol 186: 869–877.
47. Sallusto F, Lenig D, Forster R, Lipp M, Lanzavecchia A (1999) Two subsets of memory T lymphocytes with distinct homing potentials and effector functions. Nature 401: 708–712.
48. Acosta-Rodriguez EV, Rivino L, Geginat J, Jarrossay D, Gattorno M, et al. (2007) Surface phenotype and antigenic specificity of human interleukin 17-producing T helper memory cells. Nat Immunol 8: 639–646.
49. Rivino L, Messi M, Jarrossay D, Lanzavecchia A, Sallusto F, et al. (2004) Chemokine receptor expression identifies Pre-T helper (Th)1, Pre-Th2, and nonpolarized cells among human CD4+ central memory T cells. J Exp Med 200: 725–735.
50. Cardoso CR, Garlet GP, Crippa GE, Rosa AL, Júnior WM, et al. (2009) Evidence of the presence of T helper type 17 cells in chronic lesions of human periodontal disease. Oral Microbiol Immunol 24: 1–6.

Characterization of the Autocrine/Paracrine Function of Vitamin D in Human Gingival Fibroblasts and Periodontal Ligament Cells

Kaining Liu, Huanxin Meng*, Jianxia Hou

Department of Periodontology, Peking University School and Hospital of Stomatology, Beijing, China

Abstract

Background: We previously demonstrated that 25-hydroxyvitamin D_3, the precursor of 1α,25-dihydroxyvitamin D_3, is abundant around periodontal soft tissues. Here we investigate whether 25-hydroxyvitamin D_3 is converted to 1α,25-dihydroxyvitamin D_3 in periodontal soft tissue cells and explore the possibility of an autocrine/paracrine function of 1α,25-dihydroxyvitamin D_3 in periodontal soft tissue cells.

Methodology/Principal Findings: We established primary cultures of human gingival fibroblasts and human periodontal ligament cells from 5 individual donors. We demonstrated that 1α-hydroxylase was expressed in human gingival fibroblasts and periodontal ligament cells, as was cubilin. After incubation with the 1α-hydroxylase substrate 25-hydroxyvitamin D_3, human gingival fibroblasts and periodontal ligament cells generated detectable 1α,25-dihydroxyvitamin D_3 that resulted in an up-regulation of CYP24A1 and RANKL mRNA. A specific knockdown of 1α-hydroxylase in human gingival fibroblasts and periodontal ligament cells using siRNA resulted in a significant reduction in both 1α,25-dihydroxyvitamin D_3 production and mRNA expression of CYP24A1 and RANKL. The classical renal regulators of 1α-hydroxylase (parathyroid hormone, calcium and 1α,25-dihydroxyvitamin D_3) and *Porphyromonas gingivalis* lipopolysaccharide did not influence 1α-hydroxylase expression significantly, however, interleukin-1β and sodium butyrate strongly induced 1α-hydroxylase expression in human gingival fibroblasts and periodontal ligament cells.

Conclusions/Significance: In this study, the expression, activity and functionality of 1α-hydroxylase were detected in human gingival fibroblasts and periodontal ligament cells, raising the possibility that vitamin D acts in an autocrine/paracrine manner in these cells.

Editor: Christopher R. Weber, University of Chicago, United States of America

Funding: This research was funded by National Natural Science Foundations of China (http://www.nsfc.gov.cn/Portal0/default152.htm) (30772420, 81100749) and Beijing Natural Science Foundation (http://www.bjkw.gov.cn/n1143/n1240/n1465/n2276/index.html) (7102164). The funders had no role in study design, data collection and analysis, decision to publish, or preparation of the manuscript.

Competing Interests: The authors have declared that no competing interests exist.

* E-mail: kqhxmeng@bjmu.edu.cn

Introduction

Vitamin D_3 is a major component in the regulation of calcium and phosphorus metabolism. The function of vitamin D_3, via the active hormonal metabolite 1α,25-dihydroxyvitamin D_3 ($1,25OH_2D_3$), is to regulate the absorption of these essential minerals in the intestine, and their mobilization in bone tissues [1]. $1,25OH_2D_3$ also plays an important role in the regulation of T cell function and immunological reaction [2]. The biological function of $1,25OH_2D_3$ is orchestrated by vitamin D receptor (VDR). After binding with VDR, $1,25OH_2D_3$ acts on the vitamin D responsive element (VDRE) located upstream of its target genes (eg. CYP24A1, RANKL, et al.) and up-regulates their expression which results in the corresponding biological effects [3,4,5,6,7].

$1,25OH_2D_3$ is formed from vitamin D_3 in a two-step hydroxylation: 25-hydroxyvitamin D_3 ($25OHD_3$) hydroxylated in the liver is transported to the kidney by vitamin D binding protein (DBP) and is metabolized to $1,25OH_2D_3$ by the renal cytochrome P450 enzyme $25OHD_3$-1α-hydroxylase CYP27B1 [8].

Besides the kidney [9,10,11], there are extra-renal sites of $1,25OH_2D_3$ synthesis, including the skin [12], prostate [13], activated monocytes/macrophages [14], bone [15,16] and sebocytes [17]. Furthermore, local production of $1,25OH_2D_3$ in extra-renal tissues has been postulated to regulate parameters of cell growth and differentiation in an autocrine or paracrine fashion [15,18].

Periodontal tissues consist of two hard tissues, bone and cementum, and two soft tissues, gingiva and periodontal ligament. Although bone-derived cells, osteoblast-like cells and osteoblasts can synthesize $1,25OH_2D_3$ [15,16], it is unknown whether this also occurs in periodontal soft tissues. Human gingival fibroblasts (hGF) and human periodontal ligament cells (hPDLC) are two kinds of periodontal fibroblasts and are important components of gingiva and periodontal ligament, respectively. Whether $1,25OH_2D_3$ synthesis occurs in these cells warrants further investigation.

Our previous studies [19,20] demonstrated that levels of plasma $25OHD_3$ of patients with aggressive periodontitis were significantly higher than those of healthy controls; local $25OHD_3$ levels in gingival crevicular fluids were 300 times higher than plasma levels in these patients. It is not known why the precursor of $1,25OH_2D_3$ is abundant around periodontal soft tissues. Recently, McMahon et al. reported that $1,25OH_2D_3$ could enhance the antibacterial defense of human gingival epithelial cells [21]. Thus, if $25OHD_3$ is converted to $1,25OH_2D_3$ by the cells of periodontal soft tissues, this conversion could enhance the innate immune defense in the oral cavity. Here we hypothesized that hGF and hPDLC have 1α-hydroxylase activity and can convert $25OHD_3$ to $1,25OH_2D_3$. The objective of this study was to test the above hypothesis.

Results

1α-hydroxylase mRNA was detected in all the cells of the five donors (Fig. 1 and 2). The 1α-hydroxylase protein was detected with an antibody that detects 1α-hydroxylase expression in human osteoblasts, indicating that the 1α-hydroxylase in hGF and hPDLC could be the same CYP27B1 enzyme as that found in osteoblasts [15,16].

After confirming the expression of 1α-hydroxylase in hGF and hPDLC, the function of 1α-hydroxylase was investigated. While 1000 nM $25OHD_3$ did not have a significant cytotoxic effect on any of the cells within 48 h. hGF and hPDLC generated $1,25OH_2D_3$ in response to $25OHD_3$ and the amount of $1,25OH_2D_3$ increased with incubation time (Fig. 3A, B). The fact that extra- and intracellular $1,25OH_2D_3$ was generated in the presence of $25OHD_3$ provides the most convincing evidence of the existence of 1α-hydroxylase in hGF and hPDLC. Although the total amounts of $1,25OH_2D_3$ synthesized by hGF and hPDLC were not significantly different, more $1,25OH_2D_3$ was released by hPDLC 12 h after adding $25OHD_3$. At all other time points, there was no significant difference in the levels of intracellular and extracellular $1,25OH_2D_3$ between the two cell types. Moreover, CYP27B1 mRNA expression peaked at 1 h and no difference was detected between 0 h and any other time point (Fig. 3C). CYP24A1 mRNA expression increased over time and was significant higher at 24 h and 48 h than at 0 h (Fig. 3D).

In addition, exposure to $25OHD_3$ also resulted in an up-regulation of the $1,25OH_2D_3$ responsive genes CYP24A1 and RANKL in hGF and hPDLC (Fig. 4A, B), which is further evidence of 1α-hydroxylase activity in hGF and hPDLC.

Based on this direct evidence for 1α-hydroxylase activity in hGF and hPDLC, we examined the effect of 1α-hydroxylase knock-down. The efficiency of RNA interference against CYP27B1 was over 70% (Fig. 5). The generation of $1,25OH_2D_3$ increased with increasing $25OHD_3$ concentrations but dropped significantly when CYP27B1 was knocked down using specific siRNA (Fig. 6A, B).

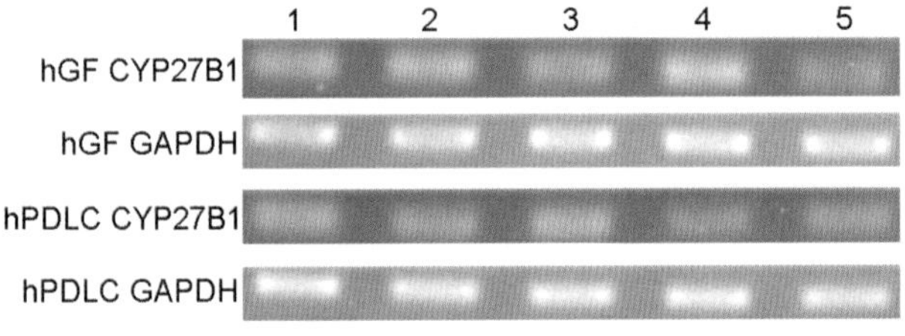

Figure 1. mRNA expression of CYP27B1 in hGF and hPDLC. mRNA expression of CYP27B1 was detected by RT-PCR in hGF and hPDLC from all five donors (each lane represents one donor). GAPDH was used as an internal control.

Although $1,25OH_2D_3$ is the major ligand of VDR, $25OHD_3$ could bind VDR with lower affinity and have a biological effect [22]. To address this issue, we knocked down CYP27B1 and found that the expression of CYP24A1 and RANKL decreased significantly (Fig. 7A, B), which strongly suggests that the effect of $25OHD_3$ in hGF and hPDLC occurs after its conversion to $1,25OH_2D_3$. This is additional evidence for the activity of 1α-hydroxylase in hGF and hPDLC.

After a comprehensive confirmation of 1α-hydroxylase activity in hGF and hPDLC, the regulation of 1α-hydroxylase in hGF and hPDLC was investigated. Parathyroid hormone (PTH), calcium, $1,25OH_2D_3$ and *Porphyromonas gingivalis* lipopolysaccharide (*Pg*-LPS) did not significantly influence CYP27B1 mRNA expression in hGF and hPDLC (Fig. 8A). In contrast, interleukin-1β (IL-1β) and sodium butyrate strongly induced CYP27B1 expression independently of $1,25OH_2D_3$ (Fig. 8B). In addition, no significant differences in the regulation of CYP27B1 was observed between hGF and hPDLC.

Despite the detection of the two kinds of DBP receptor expression, megalin mRNA expression was not detected. Both mRNA and protein expression of cubilin were detected in hGF and hPDLC (Fig. 9, 10).

Discussion

Interestingly, the $1,25OH_2D_3$ produced by hGF and hPDLC can influence vitamin D-responsive gene expression (Fig. 4, 7), an observation that provides a solid indication of an autocrine/paracrine action of vitamin D in periodontal fibroblasts. Because metabolism of $25OHD_3$ and $1,25OH_2D_3$ by CYP24A1 is very important in the autocrine/paracrine action of vitamin D, we investigated the time course of CYP27B1 and CYP24A1 mRNA expression. CYP27B1 was only up-regulated at 1 h, while CYP24A1 mRNA expression increased over time (Fig. 3C, D). The results indicated that as more $1,25OH_2D_3$ was synthesized, CYP24A1 was more robustly expressed, which resulted in more conversion of $1,25OH_2D_3$ to $1,24,25OH_3D_3$ and $25OHD_3$ to $24,25OH_2D_3$, in turn resulting in less substrate for $1,25OH_2D_3$ synthesis. Thus, hGF and hPDLC could regulate their own $1,25OH_2D_3$ generation; this provided further evidence for autocrine/paracrine action of vitamin D.

Vitamin D binding protein (DBP) is the plasma carrier of vitamin D in humans [23]. Nykjaer et al. [24,25] confirmed that vitamin D enters cells by receptor-mediated endocytosis and via the endocytic receptors megalin and cubilin. In the present study, cubilin mRNA and protein were detected in hGF and hPDLC (Fig. 9, 10), however, megalin was not detected despite the use of two pairs of primers. Atkins et al. [16] reported that osteosarcoma cell lines and primary osteoblast-like cells express abundant cubilin mRNA but only osteosarcoma cell lines express megalin mRNA. The cells used in our study were primary cells and their expression of DBP receptors was similar to the DBP receptor expression in primary osteoblast-like cells. Due to the presence of DBP receptors, plentiful $25OHD_3$ around periodontal fibroblasts [20] could be used as a substrate for $1,25OH_2D_3$ synthesis. In addition, extracellular $1,25OH_2D_3$ (Fig. 3A, 6A), generated by hGF and hPDLC, could enter the surrounding cells through cellular uptake associated with DBP, which suggests the possibility of paracrine action of vitamin D.

In the present study, CYP24A1 and RANKL mRNA expression were chosen to test the downstream biological effects of $25OHD_3$. It is striking that the biological effects caused by the locally produced $1,25OH_2D_3$ after 1000 nM $25OHD_3$ treatment were much stronger than those achieved with exogenous 10 nM

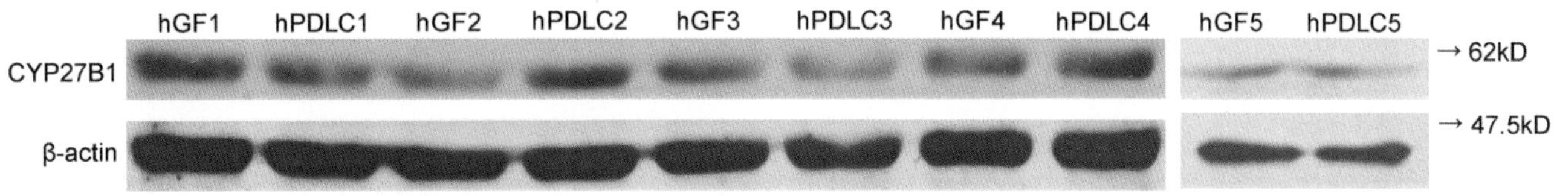

Figure 2. Protein expression of CYP27B1 in hGF and hPDLC. Protein expression of CYP27B1 was detected by Western blot in hGF and hPDLC from all five donors (donors are numbered 1–5). β-actin was used as an internal control.

$1,25OH_2D_3$ (Fig. 4A, B), and those similarly observed in treatment of osteoblasts [15]. After 1000 nM $25OHD_3$ treatment, $1,25OH_2D_3$ concentration in the supernatants of hGF and hPDLC were 120 pM–360 pM and 120 pM–600 pM, respectively, much lower than 10 nM, but the biological effects were much stronger. One reason might be that after $25OHD_3$ treatment, $1,25OH_2D_3$ is found not only in the supernatant but also in the cell lysates, allowing intracellular $1,25OH_2D_3$ to bind VDR and influence the function of these cells directly. On the other hand, exogenous $1,25OH_2D_3$ should enter the cells before eliciting a response. Thus, the direct availability at the site of action might be of great importance.

IL-1β in gingival crevicular fluids of patients with periodontitis reduced significantly after initial periodontal therapy, indicating that IL-1β is associated with periodontitis [20]. *Porphyromonas gingivalis* is an important pathogen of periodontitis and butyrate is its metabolite [26]. In our previous studies [27,28], we demonstrated that the butyrate concentrations in gingival crevicular fluids

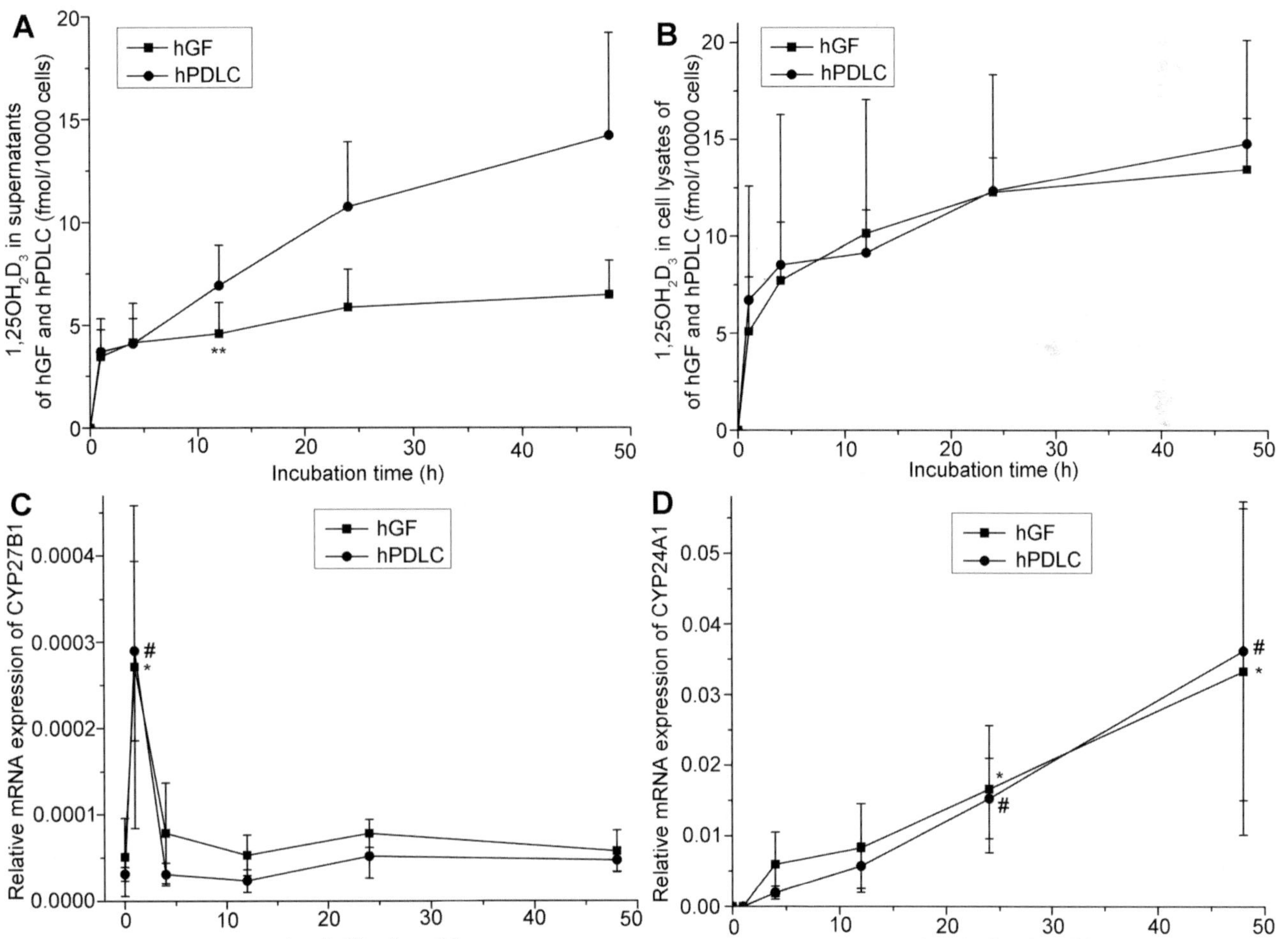

Figure 3. Activity of 1α-hydroxylase in hGF and hPDLC. hGF and hPDLC from donors 2, 3 and 5 were incubated with 1000 nM $25OHD_3$ for the times indicated and the production of $1,25OH_2D_3$ was determined in (A) supernatants and (B) cell lysates. After prolonged incubation, production of $1,25OH_2D_3$ increased. hPDLC released more $1,25OH_2D_3$ than hGF 12 h after incubation with $25OHD_3$. The data is presented as the mean±SE. ** hGF generated significantly less $1,25OH_2D_3$ than hPDLC at the same time point ($p<0.05$). The time course of CYP27B1 (C) and CYP24A1 (D) mRNA expression is also presented. CYP27B1 mRNA expression peaked at 1 h and no difference was detected between 0 h and any other time point. CYP24A1 mRNA expression was significantly higher at 24 h and 48 h than 0 h. * CYP27B1 or CYP24A1 mRNA expression at the time point was significantly different from that at 0 h in hGF ($p<0.05$). # CYP27B1 or CYP24A1 mRNA expression at the time point was significantly different from that at 0 h in hPDLC ($p<0.05$).

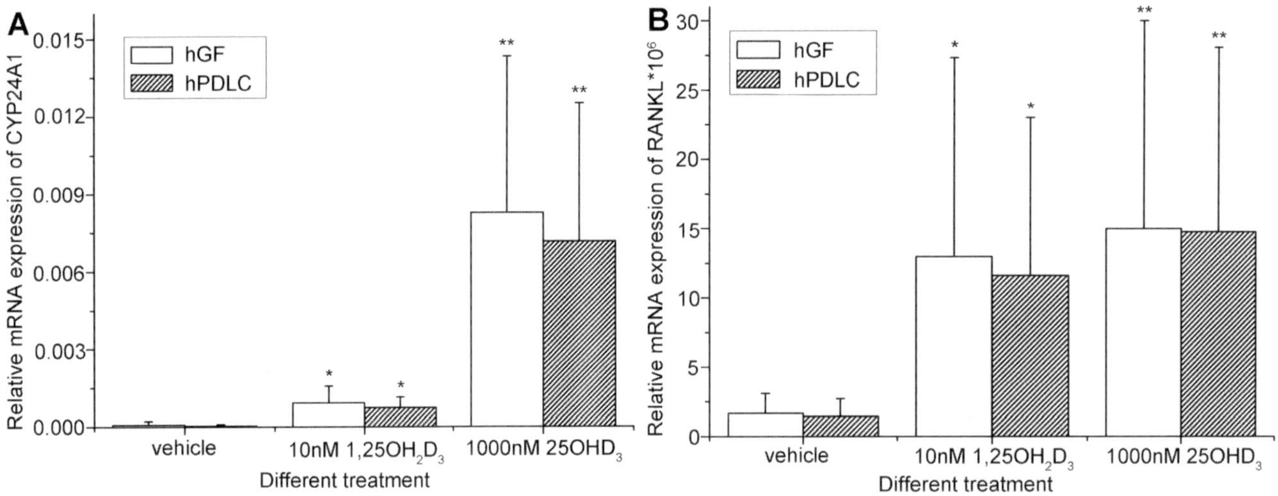

Figure 4. Effect of $25OHD_3$ incubation on gene expression in hGF and hPDLC. hGF and hPDLC from all five donors were treated with 1000 nM $25OHD_3$, 10 nM $1,25OH_2D_3$ or vehicle for 48 h and mRNA expression of (A) CYP24A1 and (B) RANKL was examined by real-time PCR. The up-regulation observed after 1000 nM $25OHD_3$ treatment was significantly stronger than that observed after 10 nM $1,25OH_2D_3$ treatment. The data are presented as the mean±SE. * denotes difference from vehicle ($p<0.05$). ** denotes difference from vehicle and $1,25OH_2D_3$ ($p<0.05$).

of patients with periodontitis were significantly higher than those of healthy controls and butyrate levels in gingival crevicular fluids were significantly correlated with periodontal inflammation. To investigate the regulation of 1α-hydroxylase in hGF and hPDLC, IL-1β, *Pg*-LPS and sodium butyrate were chosen for the current study. However, although stimuli with periodontal characteristics were used here to simulate a periodontitis condition, this does not properly model a chronic disease situation in vivo and can only help to investigate the regulation of CYP27B1 in hGF and hPDLC. We found the NF-κB activator IL-1β to be a potent up-regulator of CYP27B1 mRNA in hGF and hPDLC (Fig. 8), which is in line with the observation in osteoblasts [15]. We also found that sodium butyrate could significantly up-regulate the expression

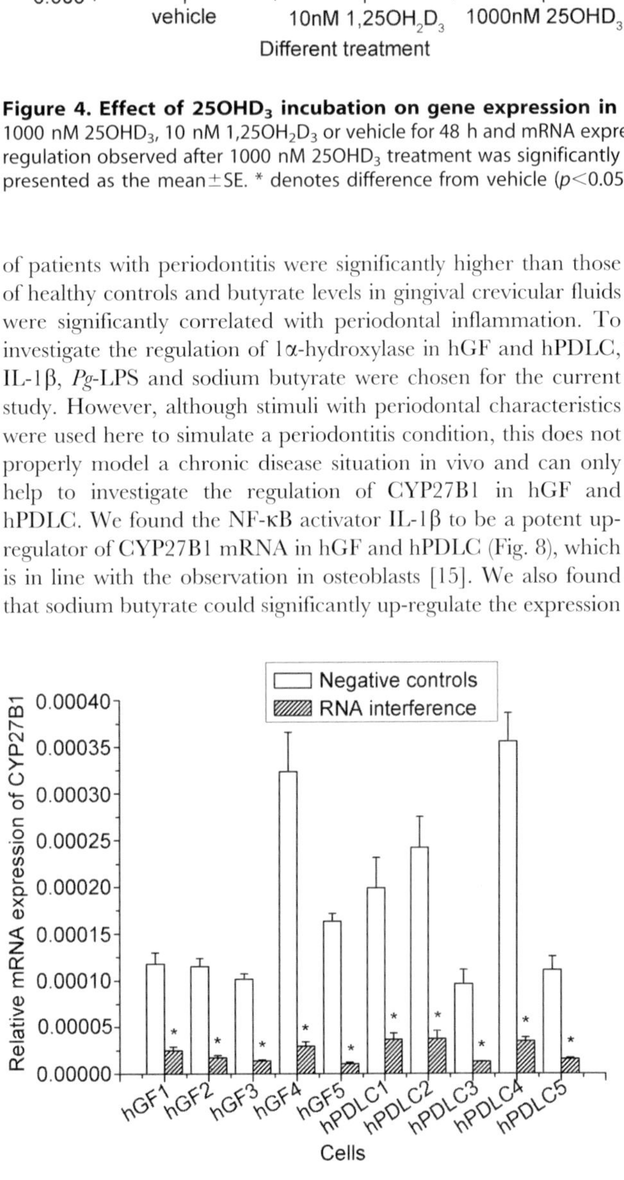

Figure 5. Efficiency of RNA interference against CYP27B1. All cells were transfected with either a siRNA oligonucleotide for CYP27B1 or a non-silencing control. Using real-time PCR as a measure, the efficiency of RNA interference against CYP27B1 was over 70% in hGF and hPDLC from all 5 donors. Donors are numbered 1–5. The data are presented as the mean±SD. * denotes difference from vehicle ($p<0.05$).

of CYP27B1 while *Pg*-LPS could not, an observation which requires further study. Classical renal regulators of 1α-hydroxylase are parathyroid hormone, calcium and $1,25OH_2D_3$ [10,29]. Renal $1,25OH_2D_3$ synthesis is primarily stimulated by low serum calcium, and consequently by parathyroid hormone that up-regulates CYP27B1 expression while $1,25OH_2D_3$ itself down-regulates CYP27B1 by negative feedback [30]. In contrast to this, we found that 1α-hydroxylase expression in hGF and hPDLC was less sensitive to a regulation by these agents (Fig. 8). In addition, $1,25OH_2D_3$ did not significantly change the up-regulation of CYP27B1 by IL-1β and sodium butyrate. A possible explanation might be that the induction of 1α-hydroxylase in hGF and hPDLC involves NF-κB pathways that are different from those involved in renal, cAMP-mediated protein kinase A signaling [31,32] and negative vitamin D response element [33,34]. This concept is similar to that of Hewison [35].

In the present study, each donor supplied both hGF and hPDLC and the CYP27B1 activity of hGF and hPDLC was compared. We demonstrated that hPDLC released more $1,25OH_2D_3$ than hGF 12 h after adding $25OHD_3$. In the study of van D M et al. [15], osteoblasts incubated with 1000 nM $25OHD_3$ also generated $1,25OH_2D_3$ and the concentration of $1,25OH_2D_3$ in the supernatant was about 400–800 pM. In the present study, $1,25OH_2D_3$ concentrations in the supernatants of hGF and hPDLC were 120 pM–360 pM and 120 pM–600 pM, respectively. Thus, osteoblasts might release more $1,25OH_2D_3$ than hGF and hPDLC. hGF and hPDLC are two different types of fibroblasts of periodontal soft tissues. It has previously been demonstrated that hPDLC has a higher degree of similarity with osteoblasts than hGF [36,37,38]. This might be the reason for the higher release of $1,25OH_2D_3$ by hPDLC than by hGF.

In recent years, increasing attention has been paid to the relationship between vitamin D and periodontitis. Dietrich et al. [39] reported that serum $25OHD_3$ concentrations are significantly and inversely associated with attachment loss in people aged over 50 years, however, there is no significant association between serum $25OHD_3$ concentrations and attachment loss in patients younger than 50 years. Dietrich et al. [40] also reported that subjects with high serum $25OHD_3$ concentrations were less likely to have bleeding on probing compared to subjects with low serum

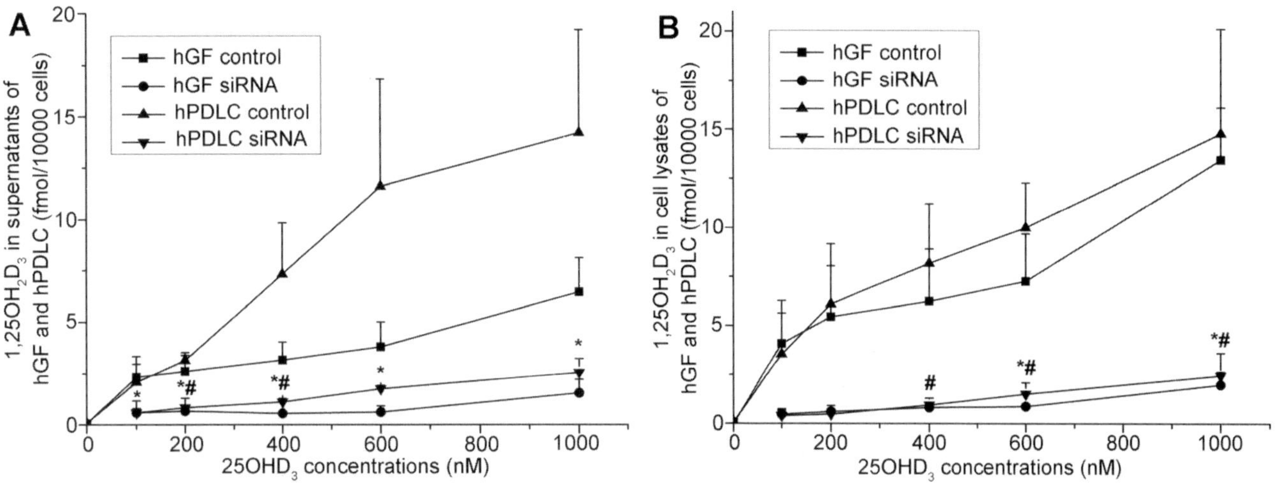

Figure 6. Effect of CYP27B1 silencing on $1,25OH_2D_3$ generation. hGF and hPDLC from donors 2, 3 and 5 were treated with $25OHD_3$ at various concentrations indicated in the figure for 48 h after transfection with the siRNA oligonucleotide for CYP27B1 or a non-silencing control and $1,25OH_2D_3$ production was measured in (A) supernatants and (B) cell lysates. When CYP27B1 was not silenced, production of $1,25OH_2D_3$ increased with increasing concentration of $25OHD_3$. When CYP27B1 was silenced, the generation of $1,25OH_2D_3$ decreased significantly compared with when CYP27B1 was not silenced. The data are presented as the mean±SE. * hGF generated significantly less $1,25OH_2D_3$ with the same amount of $25OHD_3$ when CYP27B1 was knocked down ($p<0.05$). # hPDLC generated significantly less $1,25OH_2D_3$ (with the same amount of added $25OHD_3$) when CYP27B1 was knocked down ($p<0.05$).

$25OHD_3$ concentrations. However, periodontally healthy subjects were not distinguishable from patients with either aggressive periodontitis or chronic periodontitis, and local $25OHD_3$ levels in gingival crevicular fluids were not detected in these studies. Thus, we designed our previous studies and found that patients with aggressive periodontitis had higher plasma $25OHD_3$ concentrations than healthy controls and that after periodontal therapy the higher plasma $25OHD_3$ concentrations were significantly reduced, indicating that $25OHD_3$ might be involved in periodontal inflammation [19,20]. In addition, local $25OHD_3$ levels in gingival crevicular fluids were 300 times higher than plasma levels in patients with aggressive periodontitis [20]. Because $1,25OH_2D_3$ may enhance the antibacterial defense of human gingival epithelial cells [21], the confirmation of 1α-hydroxylase activity in hGF and hPDLC implies that local $25OHD_3$ in gingival crevicular fluids might be metabolized to $1,25OH_2D_3$ by hGF and hPDLC and be involved in the innate immune defense in the oral cavity. From this perspective, 1α-hydroxylase activity in hGF and hPDLC may benefit periodontal health. Recently, it was reported that calcium and vitamin D supplementation have a positive effect on periodontal health [41,42]. However, topical application of vitamin D has not been reported. Since hGF and hPDLC have the ability to synthesize $1,25OH_2D_3$, a topical application of $25OHD_3$ might fulfill the function of $1,25OH_2D_3$. Thus, our data

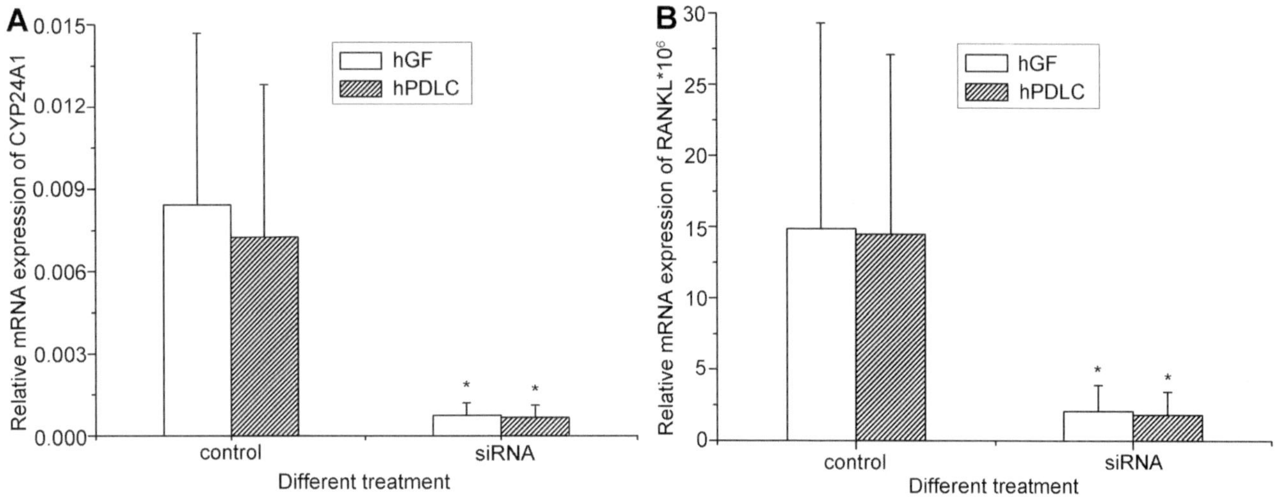

Figure 7. Effect of CYP27B1 silencing on gene up-regulation by $25OHD_3$. hGF and hPDLC from all five donors were treated with 1000 nM $25OHD_3$ for 48 h after transfection with the siRNA oligonucleotide for CYP27B1 or a non-silencing control and mRNA expression of (A) CYP24A1 and (B) RANKL was determined by real-time PCR. Compared with the transfection with a non-silencing control, transfection with the siRNA oligonucleotide for CYP27B1 resulted in a significantly weaker up-regulation of CYP24A1 and RANKL in both hGF and hPDLC. The data are presented as the mean±SE. * denotes difference from control ($p<0.05$).

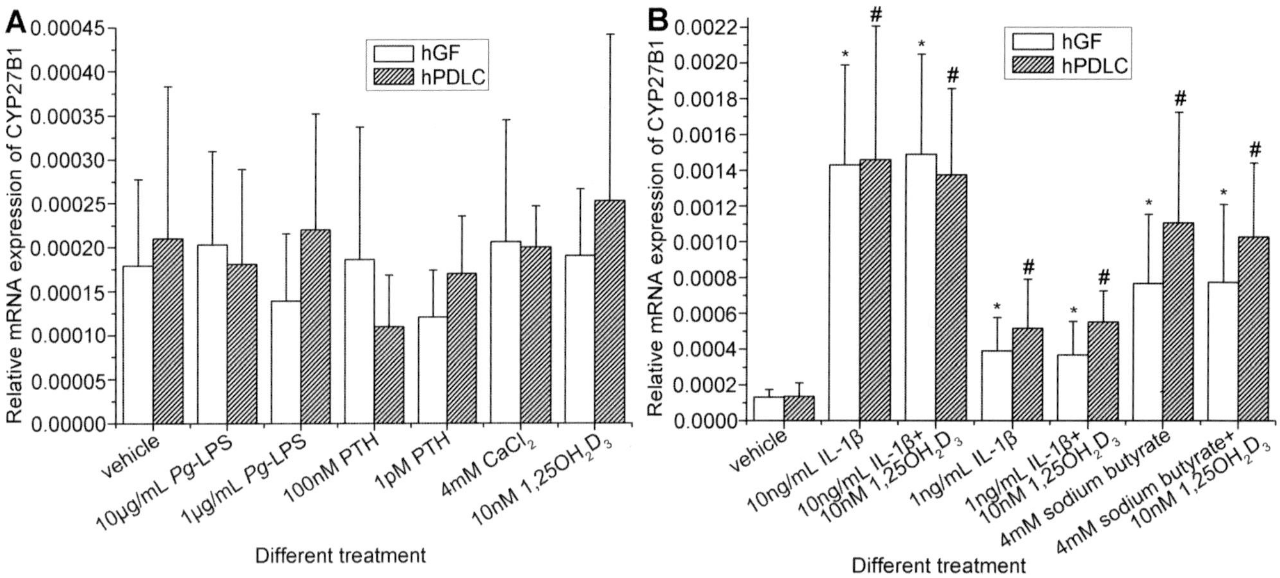

Figure 8. Preliminary investigation of CYP27B1 regulation in hGF and hPDLC. hGF and hPDLC from donors 2, 3, 4 and 5 were stimulated with different treatments indicated in the figure for 24 h and CYP27B1 expression was determined by real-time PCR. (A) *Pg*-LPS, parathyroid hormone, $CaCl_2$ and $1{,}25OH_2D_3$ did not significantly influence CYP27B1 mRNA expression. (B) IL-1β and sodium butyrate significantly up-regulated CYP27B1 mRNA expression independently of $1{,}25OH_2D_3$. Additionally, the characteristics of CYP27B1 regulation in hGF and hPDLC were not significantly different. The data are presented as the mean±SE. * CYP27B1 mRNA expression was significantly different from that of the vehicle group in hGF ($p<0.05$). # CYP27B1 mRNA expression was significantly different from that of the vehicle group in hPDLC ($p<0.05$). IL-1β: interleukin-1β. *Pg*-LPS: *Porphyromonas gingivalis* lipopolysaccharide. PTH: parathyroid hormone.

suggest a potential benefit of topical application of $25OHD_3$ in periodontal therapy.

Because no established cell lines of hGF or hPDLC are available, the cells used in the present study were all obtained from primary culture. Although all data were obtained from cell from at least 3 donors, the existence of individual differences among the cells from primary culture was the limitation of this study.

In conclusion, the results in the current study have identified for the first time hGF and hPDLC as new sites of extrarenal synthesis of $1{,}25OH_2D_3$. Similar to other extrarenal 1α-hydroxylases, periodontal 1α-hydroxylase appears to fulfill an autocrine/paracrine function.

Materials and Methods

Ethics Statement

The study protocol was approved by the institutional review board of Peking University School and Hospital of Stomatology (PKUSSIRB-2011007) and written informed consent was obtained from each participant in accordance with the Declaration of Helsinki.

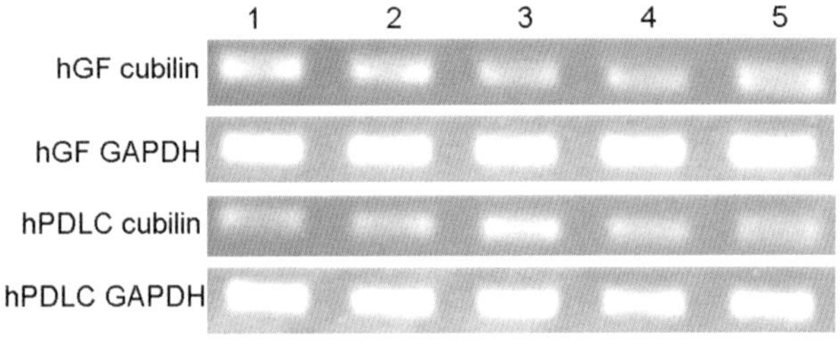

Figure 9. mRNA expression of cubilin in hGF and hPDLC. mRNA expression of cubilin was determined by RT-PCR in hGF and hPDLC from all five donors (each lane represents one donor). GAPDH was used as an internal control.

Cell culture

Primary culture of hGF and hPDLC was carried out according to previously described methods [7,26,36,43]. Briefly, hPDLC were prepared from extracted third molars of 5 young healthy volunteers and hGF were obtained from gingiva of the same 5 donors. The periodontal ligament tissues attached to the middle third of the roots were gently curetted by a surgical scalpel, minced and inoculated into 24-well plates. Gingiva from different donors was also minced and inoculated into 24-well plates. Tissue explants were maintained in Dulbecco's Modified Eagle's Medium (DMEM; Gibco, Grand Island, NY, USA) supplemented with 10% (v/v) fetal bovine serum (FBS; PAA, Coelbe, Germany), 100 U/ml penicillin G and 100 μg/ml streptomycin. Cultures were maintained in a humidified atmosphere of 5% (v/v) CO_2 at 37°C. After reaching 80% confluence, hGF and hPDLC were digested with 0.25% (w/v) trypsin and 0.02% (w/v) EDTA and subcultured at a 1:3 ratio.

DMEM without phenol red (Sigma, St. Louis, MO, USA), 10% dextran-coated charcoal stripped FBS (DCC-FBS; TBD, Tianjin, China) and cells of passage 4 were used in all of the following experiments. Experiments were all conducted in triplicate.

Cytotoxicity test of $25OHD_3$

hGF and hPDLC from three donors were used in the cytotoxicity test. hGF and hPDLC in their logarithmic phase were plated into 96-well plates at a density of 3000 cells/well in DMEM with 10% DCC-FBS. 24 h later, the medium was replaced by DMEM without DCC-FBS. After another 24 h, the medium was changed to DMEM with 10% DCC-FBS and supplemented with 1000 nM $25OHD_3$ or vehicle, respectively. The cytotoxicity test was carried out according to the Cell

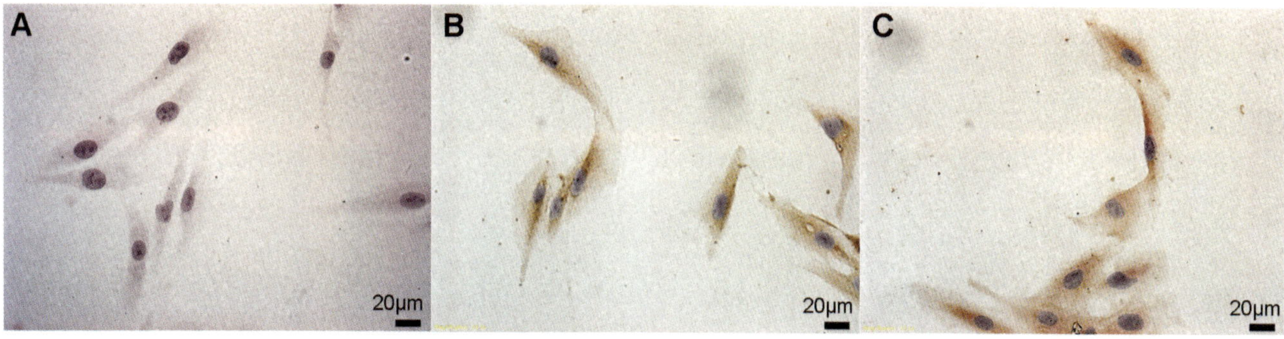

Figure 10. Protein expression of cubilin in hGF and hPDLC. hGF and hPDLC from all five donors were used for immunocytochemical staining of cubilin; expression of cubilin was detected in all the cells examined. Panel A is the negative control for the immunocytochemical staining of cubilin (400×). Panel B and C contain images of the hGF and hPDLC, respectively, from donor 2 (400×). The primary antibody was replaced with PBS for the negative control.

Counting Kit-8 protocol (CCK-8; Dojindo, Kumamoto, Japan). Briefly, at hours 0, 24 and 48, cells were incubated with CCK-8 for the last 3 h of the culture period after which the optical density values (OD values) were determined at 490 nm with a microplate reader (Bio-Rad Model 550, Hercules, CA, USA).

Detection of CYP27B1 expression

Cells from all five donor were seeded into 6-well plates at a density of 5000/cm^2 in DMEM supplemented with 10% DCC-FBS. 4 days later, a portion of the cells were harvested using Trizol agent (Dongsheng Biotech, Guangzhou, China) for RT-PCR. RNA was extracted using Trizol according to the manufacturer's instructions and was reverse transcribed to cDNA using a reverse transcription kit (Bio-Rad, Hercules, CA, USA). PCR reactions were performed using the Taq PCR MasterMix (Tiangen Biotech, Beijing, China) in a Hybaid PCR Thermal Cycler (Thermo Scientific, Boston, Mass, USA). The primers used are listed in Table 1.

The remaining cells were harvested using lysis buffer [20 mM Tris (pH 7.4), 150 mM NaCl, 1 mM EDTA, 1 mM EGTA, 1% (v/v) Triton X-100, 2.5 mM sodium pyrophosphate, 1 mM β-glycerol phosphate and 2 mM Na_3VO_4 supplemented with protease inhibitor cocktail (Roche, Mannheim, Germany)] [43] for Western blotting. Protein concentration was determined using the Bicinchoninic Acid Protein Assay Kit (Applygen, Beijing, China). 20 μg of total protein from each sample was loaded onto a gel comprising a 5% (w/v) stacking gel and a 10% (w/v) running gel. At the end of the electrophoresis, samples were transferred onto nitrocellulose blotting membranes (Hybond^{TM}; Amersham Pharmacia, Little Chalfont, UK). Blots were probed with a sheep polyclonal antibody to CYP27B1 (diluted 1:200; The Binding Site Ltd., Birmingham, UK) or a mouse monoclonal antibody to β-actin (diluted 1:1000; Santa Cruz Biotechnology, Santa Cruz, CA, USA). After washing, blots were incubated with horseradish peroxidase-linked secondary antibody. The secondary antibody against sheep (Kirkegaard & Perry Laboratories, Inc., Maryland, USA) and mouse (Beijing Zhongshan Golden Bridge Biotechnology, Beijing, China) were both diluted 1:2500. Antigen-antibody complexes were detected using the Enhanced Chemiluminescence reagent (Applygen, Beijing, China).

Measurement of $1,25OH_2D_3$ production

Cells from 3 donors were treated with 1000 nM $25OHD_3$ (Sigma, St. Louis, MO, USA) for 1 h, 4 h, 12 h, 24 h or 48 h, after which supernatants were collected and a portion of cells were scraped in PBS containing 0.2% Triton X-100 and stored at −80°C. Prior to use, cell lysates were sonicated on ice in a sonifier cell disrupter for 2×15 s. $1,25OH_2D_3$ levels in cell supernatants and cell lysates were detected using a $1,25OH_2D_3$ radioimmunoassay kit (DiaSorin, Stillwater, MN) according to the manufacturer's instructions. The cross-reactivity with $25OHD_3$ was less than 0.01%.

In addition, a portion of the cells were harvested using Trizol reagent for the detection of the time course of CYP27B1 and CYP24A1 mRNA expression using real-time PCR. Real-time PCR reactions were performed using SYBR® Premix Ex Taq^{TM} II (TaKaRa Biotechnology, Dalian, China) in an ABI 7500 real-time Thermocycler (Applied Biosystems, Foster city, CA, USA).

Table 1. Primer sequences used for PCR or real-time PCR.

Target genes	Forward primer (5′→3′)	Reverse primer (5′→3′)	Products (bp)
CYP27B1	GAAGTGCTAAGACTGTACCCTGT	CCTTGAAGTGGCATAGTGACAC	126
RANKL	GACATCCCATCTGGTTCCCA	CCCAACCCCGATCATGGTA	61
CYP24A1	GACTACCGCAAAGAAGGCTAC	CATCACTTCCCCTGGTTTCATTA	105
megalin	GCCGGCCAGTGGCCAAGAA	ACAGCGCAGCCAATTTCATCC	129
megalin	AAATTGAGCACAGCACCTTTGA	TCTGCTTTCCTGACTCGAATAATG	151
cubilin	TTCTTACGGGGTCTGCTCAAA	TGCAAGCCTTGGAATTTTCTCTC	226
GAPDH	GAAGGTGAAGGTCGGAGTC	GAAGATGGTGATGGGATTTC	226

The primers used are listed in Table 1. The data were analyzed using the SDS software according to the manufacturer's instructions. Glyceraldehyde-3-phosphate-dehydrogenase (GAPDH) was used as an internal control. The data are presented as relative mRNA levels calculated by the equation $2^{-\Delta Ct}$ ($\Delta Ct = Ct$ of target gene minus Ct of GAPDH) [44].

Detection of CYP24A1 and RANKL mRNA expression

Cells from five donors were incubated with 10 nM $1{,}25OH_2D_3$ (Sigma, St. Louis, MO, USA), 1000 nM $25OHD_3$ or vehicle for 48 h before harvesting. Then RNA and cDNA were obtained and real-time PCR reactions were performed as described previously.

RNA interference of CYP27B1

To confirm the dependence of $25OHD_3$ conversion into $1{,}25OH_2D_3$ on CYP27B1, the highly specific technique of RNA interference was utilized. Cells were seeded at a density of 15000/cm^2 in 6-well plates. 8 h later, cells were transfected with either CYP27B1 siRNA (10 nM) or non-silencing control siRNA using Hiperfect™ transfection reagent (Qiagen, Duesseldorf, Germany) according to the manufacturer's instructions. The target sequence of CYP27B1 siRNA was 5′-CTGGTTTACGGTTTCTTATAA-3′ and the non-silencing control was a non-homologous, scrambled sequence equivalent.

60 h after transfection, cells were harvested to confirm the effect of RNAi using real-time PCR. RNA and cDNA were obtained and real-time PCR was performed as described earlier.

After verifying the effect of RNAi, $1{,}25OH_2D_3$ production after RNAi was determined. Cells were first transfected with CYP27B1 siRNA (10 nM) or non-silencing control siRNA and 12 h after transfection, these cells were treated with 200 nM, 400 nM, 600 nM or 1000 nM $25OHD_3$ (Sigma, St. Louis, MO, USA) for another 48 h. Then, the $1{,}25OH_2D_3$ concentrations in the cell supernatants and cell lysates were determined as described earlier.

CYP24A1 and RANKL mRNA expression was also examined after RNAi. Cells were first transfected with CYP27B1 siRNA (10 nM) or non-silencing control siRNA and 12 h after transfection, these cells were treated with 1000 nM $25OHD_3$ for another 48 h. Then, CYP24A1 and RANKL mRNA expression was determined by real-time PCR.

Regulation of CYP27B1 in hGF and hPDLC

A portion of the cells from four donors were incubated with IL-1β (PeproTech, London, UK; 1 ng/mL and 10 ng/mL), parathyroid hormone (PTH; SinoBio, Shanghai, China; 100 nM and 1 pM), *Pg*-LPS (Invivogen, San Diego, CA, USA; 1 μg/mL and 10 μg/mL), sodium butyrate (SCRC, Shanghai, China; 4 mM), $CaCl_2$ (SCRC, Shanghai, China; 4 mM) and $1{,}25OH_2D_3$ (10 nM) for 24 h. The other portion of the donor cells were incubated with IL-1β (1 ng/mL or 10 ng/mL) and $1{,}25OH_2D_3$ (10 nM) or sodium butyrate (4 mM) and $1{,}25OH_2D_3$ (10 nM) for 24 h.

Detection of vitamin D binding protein receptor expression

The mRNA expression of megalin and cubilin were detected by RT-PCR as described earlier and the primers used are listed in Table 1.

Protein expression of cubilin was detected by immunocytochemistry. Cells from five donors were seeded on glass slides at a density of 20000/cm^2 and 8 h later cells on glass slides were incubated with primary antibodies against cubilin (diluted 1:50; Santa Cruz Biotechnology, Santa Cruz, CA, USA). The PV-9000 Polymer Detection System (Zhongshan Golden Bridge Biotechnology, Beijing, China) was used for immunocytochemical staining and a diaminobenzidine (DAB) kit (Zhongshan Golden Bridge Biotechnology, Beijing, China) was used to develop the colour followed by haematoxylin staining. The primary antibody was replaced by PBS for negative controls.

Statistical Methods

The Shapiro-Wilk test was used to determinate the distribution of the variants. The Wilcoxon test and Friedman test were used to compare differences between the mRNA expression levels of CYP24A1 and RANKL in different groups. The effect of RNA interference and the effect of $25OHD_3$ exposure on CYP27B1 mRNA expression was analyzed using the paired samples t-test. Comparison of $1{,}25OH_2D_3$ generation by hGF and hPDLC, comparison of $1{,}25OH_2D_3$ generation with and without knockdown of CYP27B1 and comparison of CYP27B1 up-regulation in hGF and hPDLC were all performed using a paired samples t-test.

Statistical analyses were carried out using the SPSS 11.5 software package (SPSS Inc., Chicago, IL, USA). A p value<0.05 was considered statistically significant.

Author Contributions

Conceived and designed the experiments: HXM KNL JXH. Performed the experiments: KNL. Analyzed the data: KNL JXH. Contributed reagents/materials/analysis tools: HXM JXH. Wrote the paper: KNL HXM JXH.

References

1. Rachez C, Freedman LP (2000) Mechanisms of gene regulation by vitamin D(3) receptor: a network of coactivator interactions. Gene 246: 9–21.
2. von EM, Kongsbak M, Schjerling P, Olgaard K, Odum N, et al. (2010) Vitamin D controls T cell antigen receptor signaling and activation of human T cells. Nat Immunol 11: 344–349.
3. Chen KS, DeLuca HF (1995) Cloning of the human 1 alpha,25-dihydroxyvitamin D-3 24-hydroxylase gene promoter and identification of two vitamin D-responsive elements. Biochim Biophys Acta 1263: 1–9.
4. Haussler MR, Whitfield GK, Haussler CA, Hsieh JC, Thompson PD, et al. (1998) The nuclear vitamin D receptor: biological and molecular regulatory properties revealed. J Bone Miner Res 13: 325–349.
5. Christakos S, Dhawan P, Liu Y, Peng X, Porta A (2003) New insights into the mechanisms of vitamin D action. J Cell Biochem 88: 695–705.
6. Kitazawa S, Kajimoto K, Kondo T, Kitazawa R (2003) Vitamin D3 supports osteoclastogenesis via functional vitamin D response element of human RANKL gene promoter. J Cell Biochem 89: 771–777.
7. Tang X, Meng H (2009) Osteogenic induction and 1,25-dihydroxyvitamin D3 oppositely regulate the proliferation and expression of RANKL and the vitamin D receptor of human periodontal ligament cells. Arch Oral Biol 54: 625–633.
8. Jones G, Strugnell SA, DeLuca HF (1998) Current understanding of the molecular actions of vitamin D. Physiol Rev 78: 1193–1231.
9. Takeyama K, Kitanaka S, Sato T, Kobori M, Yanagisawa J, et al. (1997) 25-Hydroxyvitamin D3 1alpha-hydroxylase and vitamin D synthesis. Science 277: 1827–1830.
10. Bland R, Walker EA, Hughes SV, Stewart PM, Hewison M (1999) Constitutive expression of 25-hydroxyvitamin D3-1alpha-hydroxylase in a transformed human proximal tubule cell line: evidence for direct regulation of vitamin D metabolism by calcium. Endocrinology 140: 2027–2034.
11. Zhang MY, Wang X, Wang JT, Compagnone NA, Mellon SH, et al. (2002) Dietary phosphorus transcriptionally regulates 25-hydroxyvitamin D-1alpha-hydroxylase gene expression in the proximal renal tubule. Endocrinology 143: 587–595.
12. Lehmann B (1997) HaCaT cell line as a model system for vitamin D3 metabolism in human skin. J Invest Dermatol 108: 78–82.
13. Khorchide M, Lechner D, Cross HS (2005) Epigenetic regulation of vitamin D hydroxylase expression and activity in normal and malignant human prostate cells. J Steroid Biochem Mol Biol 93: 167–172.
14. Overbergh L, Stoffels K, Waer M, Verstuyf A, Bouillon R, et al. (2006) Immune regulation of 25-hydroxyvitamin D-1alpha-hydroxylase in human monocytic THP1 cells: mechanisms of interferon-gamma-mediated induction. J Clin Endocrinol Metab 91: 3566–3574.

15. van DM, Koedam M, Buurman CJ, Hewison M, Chiba H, et al. (2006) Evidence for auto/paracrine actions of vitamin D in bone: 1alpha-hydroxylase expression and activity in human bone cells. FASEB J 20: 2417–2419.
16. Atkins GJ, Anderson PH, Findlay DM, Welldon KJ, Vincent C, et al. (2007) Metabolism of vitamin D3 in human osteoblasts: evidence for autocrine and paracrine activities of 1 alpha,25-dihydroxyvitamin D3. Bone 40: 1517–1528.
17. Kramer C, Seltmann H, Seifert M, Tilgen W, Zouboulis CC, et al. (2009) Characterization of the vitamin D endocrine system in human sebocytes in vitro. J Steroid Biochem Mol Biol 113: 9–16.
18. Huang DC, Papavasiliou V, Rhim JS, Horst RL, Kremer R (2002) Targeted disruption of the 25-hydroxyvitamin D3 1alpha-hydroxylase gene in ras-transformed keratinocytes demonstrates that locally produced 1alpha,25-dihydroxyvitamin D3 suppresses growth and induces differentiation in an autocrine fashion. Mol Cancer Res 1: 56–67.
19. Liu K, Meng H, Tang X, Xu L, Zhang L, et al. (2009) Elevated plasma calcifediol is associated with aggressive periodontitis. J Periodontol 80: 1114–1120.
20. Liu K, Meng H, Lu R, Xu L, Zhang L, et al. (2010) Initial periodontal therapy reduced systemic and local 25-hydroxy vitamin D(3) and interleukin-1beta in patients with aggressive periodontitis. J Periodontol 81: 260–266.
21. McMahon L, Schwartz K, Yilmaz O, Brown E, Ryan LK, et al. (2011) Vitamin D-mediated induction of innate immunity in gingival epithelial cells. Infect Immun 79: 2250–2256.
22. Bouillon R, Okamura WH, Norman AW (1995) Structure-function relationships in the vitamin D endocrine system. Endocr Rev 16: 200–257.
23. Haddad JG (1995) Plasma vitamin D-binding protein (Gc-globulin): multiple tasks. J Steroid Biochem Mol Biol 53: 579–582.
24. Nykjaer A, Dragun D, Walther D, Vorum H, Jacobsen C, et al. (1999) An endocytic pathway essential for renal uptake and activation of the steroid 25-(OH) vitamin D3. Cell 96: 507–515.
25. Nykjaer A, Fyfe JC, Kozyraki R, Leheste JR, Jacobsen C, et al. (2001) Cubilin dysfunction causes abnormal metabolism of the steroid hormone 25(OH) vitamin D(3). Proc Natl Acad Sci U S A 98: 13895–13900.
26. Kurita-Ochiai T, Ochiai K, Suzuki N, Otsuka K, Fukushima K (2002) Human gingival fibroblasts rescue butyric acid-induced T-cell apoptosis. Infect Immun 70: 2361–2367.
27. Li QQ, Meng HX, Gao XJ, Wang ZH (2005) Analysis of volatile fatty acids in gingival crevicular fluid of patients with chronic periodontitis. Zhonghua Kou Qiang Yi Xue Za Zhi 40: 208–210.
28. Lu RF, Meng HX, Gao XJ, Feng L, Xu L (2008) Analysis of short chain fatty acids in gingival crevicular fluid of patients with aggressive periodontitis. Zhonghua Kou Qiang Yi Xue Za Zhi 43: 664–667.
29. Bland R, Zehnder D, Hughes SV, Ronco PM, Stewart PM, et al. (2001) Regulation of vitamin D-1alpha-hydroxylase in a human cortical collecting duct cell line. Kidney Int 60: 1277–1286.
30. Cross HS (2007) Extrarenal vitamin D hydroxylase expression and activity in normal and malignant cells: modification of expression by epigenetic mechanisms and dietary substances. Nutr Rev 65: S108–S112.
31. Rost CR, Bikle DD, Kaplan RA (1981) In vitro stimulation of 25-hydroxycholecalciferol 1 alpha-hydroxylation by parathyroid hormone in chick kidney slices: evidence for a role for adenosine 3′,5′-monophosphate. Endocrinology 108: 1002–1006.
32. Henry HL (1985) Parathyroid hormone modulation of 25-hydroxyvitamin D3 metabolism by cultured chick kidney cells is mimicked and enhanced by forskolin. Endocrinology 116: 503–510.
33. Murayama A, Kim MS, Yanagisawa J, Takeyama K, Kato S (2004) Transrepression by a liganded nuclear receptor via a bHLH activator through co-regulator switching. EMBO J 23: 1598–1608.
34. Fujiki R, Kim MS, Sasaki Y, Yoshimura K, Kitagawa H, et al. (2005) Ligand-induced transrepression by VDR through association of WSTF with acetylated histones. EMBO J 24: 3881–3894.
35. Hewison M, Zehnder D, Bland R, Stewart PM (2000) 1alpha-Hydroxylase and the action of vitamin D. J Mol Endocrinol 25: 141–148.
36. Somerman MJ, Archer SY, Imm GR, Foster RA (1988) A comparative study of human periodontal ligament cells and gingival fibroblasts in vitro. J Dent Res 67: 66–70.
37. Ivanovski S, Li H, Haase HR, Bartold PM (2001) Expression of bone associated macromolecules by gingival and periodontal ligament fibroblasts. J Periodontal Res 36: 131–141.
38. Xu Y, Jiang Y (2006) Mineralization effects of human platelet-rich plasma on human periodontium cells. Zhonghua Kou Qiang Yi Xue Za Zhi 41: 743–746.
39. Dietrich T, Joshipura KJ, Dawson-Hughes B, Bischoff-Ferrari HA (2004) Association between serum concentrations of 25-hydroxyvitamin D3 and periodontal disease in the US population. Am J Clin Nutr 80: 108–113.
40. Dietrich T, Nunn M, Dawson-Hughes B, Bischoff-Ferrari HA (2005) Association between serum concentrations of 25-hydroxyvitamin D and gingival inflammation. Am J Clin Nutr 82: 575–580.
41. Garcia MN, Hildebolt CF, Miley DD, Dixon DA, Couture RA, et al. (2011) One-year effects of vitamin D and calcium supplementation on chronic periodontitis. J Periodontol 82: 25–32.
42. Bashutski JD, Eber RM, Kinney JS, Benavides E, Maitra S, et al. (2011) The impact of vitamin D status on periodontal surgery outcomes. J Dent Res 90: 1007–1012.
43. Tang X, Meng H, Han J, Zhang L, Hou J, et al. (2008) Up-regulation of estrogen receptor-beta expression during osteogenic differentiation of human periodontal ligament cells. J Periodontal Res 43: 311–321.
44. Livak KJ, Schmittgen TD (2001) Analysis of relative gene expression data using real-time quantitative PCR and the 2(−Delta Delta C(T)) Method. Methods 25: 402–408.

8

Multiple Single-Cell Genomes Provide Insight into Functions of Uncultured *Deltaproteobacteria* in the Human Oral Cavity

Alisha G. Campbell[1,2], James H. Campbell[2], Patrick Schwientek[3], Tanja Woyke[3], Alexander Sczyrba[3¤], Steve Allman[2], Clifford J. Beall[4], Ann Griffen[4], Eugene Leys[4], Mircea Podar[1,2,5]*

1 Genome Science and Technology Program, University of Tennessee, Knoxville, Tennessee, United States of America, **2** Biosciences Division, Oak Ridge National Laboratories, Oak Ridge, Tennessee, United States of America, **3** DOE Joint Genome Institute, Walnut Creek, California, United States of America, **4** College of Dentistry, Ohio State University, Columbus, Ohio, United States of America, **5** Department of Microbiology, University of Tennessee, Knoxville, Tennessee, United States of America

Abstract

Despite a long history of investigation, many bacteria associated with the human oral cavity have yet to be cultured. Studies that correlate the presence or abundance of uncultured species with oral health or disease highlight the importance of these community members. Thus, we sequenced several single-cell genomic amplicons from *Desulfobulbus* and *Desulfovibrio* (class *Deltaproteobacteria*) to better understand their function within the human oral community and their association with periodontitis, as well as other systemic diseases. Genomic data from oral *Desulfobulbus* and *Desulfovibrio* species were compared to other available deltaproteobacterial genomes, including from a subset of host-associated species. While both groups share a large number of genes with other environmental *Deltaproteobacteria* genomes, they encode a wide array of unique genes that appear to function in survival in a host environment. Many of these genes are similar to virulence and host adaptation factors of known human pathogens, suggesting that the oral *Deltaproteobacteria* have the potential to play a role in the etiology of periodontal disease.

Editor: Matthias Horn, University of Vienna, Austria

Funding: This research was supported by grant R01 HG004857 from the National Human Genome Research Institute (NHGRI) of the National Institutes of Health (NIH) to M.P. and by grant 1R56DE021567 from the National Institute for Dental and Cranial Research (NIDCR) of the NIH to M.P., A.G. and E.L. Oak Ridge National Laboratory is managed by UT-Battelle, LLC, for the U.S. Department of Energy under contract DE681 AC05-00OR22725. P.S., T.W. and A.S. were supported by the U.S. Department of Energy Joint Genome Institute and the Office of Science of the U.S. Department of Energy under Contract No. DE-AC02-05CH11231. The funders had no role in study design, data collection and analysis, decision to publish, or preparation of the manuscript.

Competing Interests: The authors have declared that no competing interests exist.

* E-mail: podarm@ornl.gov

¤ Current address: Center for Biotechnology, Bielefeld University, Bielefeld, Germany

Introduction

Recent large-scale efforts have profiled the large number of microbial communities associated with the human body and the importance of determining the composition and function of these communities and, ultimately, their effects on human health [1–3]. Studies of microbes in the human oral cavity have been ongoing since the discovery of "animalcules" by Antony van Leeuwenhoek in 1676, but despite this long history, over 50% of oral microbes remains uncultured. Likewise, periodontitis, an inflammatory gum disease, has been under investigation since the early 19th century, but the role of microbial communities associated with the disease remains unclear [4,5]. Periodontitis is the leading cause of tooth loss worldwide and has been linked to a number of systemic diseases, including diabetes, cardiovascular disease, osteoporosis and preterm low birth weight [6–11]. Thus, understanding the roles of periodontitis-associated microbial community members is of utmost importance. Genomic information provides an initial way to assess functional potential. Although there are relatively few published analyses using closed genome sequences of cultured bacteria associated with periodontitis [12–14], under the Human Microbiome Project (HMP) there are over 400 ongoing or completed genome sequencing projects for cultured human oral bacteria [2] (http://www.hmpdacc.org/). Combined with the hundreds of oral metagenomic datasets generated by the HMP [15], this vast genomic information for health- and disease-associated microbes should ultimately result in more effective treatments and preventative measures for periodontitis and other oral diseases.

Recent culture-independent studies have associated several uncultured organisms with periodontitis [16–19]. One group of uncultured oral microbes that are of great importance is sulfate-reducing bacteria (SRB). These organisms have been of long-standing interest because of their ability to produce hydrogen sulfide, a compound that can be toxic to human cells. Potential SRB within the oral microbial community include several members of *Deltaproteobacteria*. Both culture-based studies [20,21] as well as quantitative PCR studies based upon dissimilatory sulfate reduction genes (*dsrAB*) [22] have linked SRB to periodontitis, particularly to more clinically severe cases with deeper periodontal pockets.

Several culture-independent studies have linked the deltaproteobacterial genus *Desulfobulbus*, with progressive periodontitis

[17,23]. *Desulfobulbus* sp. oral taxon 041 is present in low levels in most adults [24] but has been found in greater abundance in both healthy and diseased sites of subjects with periodontitis compared to healthy control subjects [16]. Despite these findings, little is known about oral *Desulfobulbus* species because there are no cultured representatives from this environment and only one genome published from this genus [25]. Isolates of *Desulfovibrio fairfieldensis* and closely related species have also been associated with periodontitis [26], and these organisms have been found as the causative agent of several cases of bacteremia [27,28]. Although cultured isolates are available for *Desulfovibrio fairfieldensis*, no genomic information has been published. Obtaining genomic information for these oral *Deltaproteobacteria* would greatly enhance our knowledge and shed light on their potential function in the etiology of progressive periodontitis.

Thus, our aim was to selectively isolate single cells of oral *Deltaproteobacteria* and sequence their genomes. We sequenced both individuals and groups of single-cell amplicons most closely related to the uncultured *Desulfobulbus* sp. oral taxon 041 [3], as well as a group of single-cell amplicons most closely related to the uncultured *Desulfovibrio* sp. oral taxon 040 [3]. Groups of single-cell amplicons were sequenced to provide more complete genomic information for each genus. Genomic data were analyzed and compared to sequenced, environmental isolates of related organisms and other host-associated, *Deltaproteobacteria* genomes.

Results and Discussion

Cell Isolation, Sequencing and Phylogenetic Analysis

Single cells of both oral *Desulfobulbus* ($n = 7$) and *Desulfovibrio* ($n = 5$) were isolated from ethanol-fixed samples using a combination of fluorescence *in situ* hybridization (FISH) and flow cytometric cell sorting. FISH was performed using *Deltaproteobacteria*-specific probes [29,30]. A culture of *Desulfobulbus propionicus* 1pr3 (DSM 2032) was used to test and optimize hybridization conditions, (Figure S1). The genomic DNA of single cells was amplified using multiple displacement amplification (MDA) followed by taxonomic characterization of the single cell amplified genomes (SAGs) by small subunit rRNA (SSU rRNA or 16S rRNA) gene amplification and sequencing. SAGs confirmed to represent target *Deltaproteobacteria* were sequenced individually (Dsb1, Dsb2, Dsb3) or in groups (Dsb4, Dsb5, Dsv1). The confirmed deltaproteobacterial SAGs originated from samples collected from both healthy individuals and individuals with periodontitis (Table 1).

Oral *Desulfobulbus* cells sequenced in this study were chosen for genomic sequencing based on SSU rRNA gene similarity to a previously known oral clone, *Desulfobulbus* sp. oral taxon 041 [3], that has been associated with periodontitis [16]. Comparisons of full-length SSU rRNA genes revealed that amplicons Dsb1– Dsb4 are identical, and these amplicons are over 99% identical to Dsb5 and *Desulfobulbus* sp. oral taxon 041 (Figure 1). However, all the oral taxa form a distinct clade compared to *Desulfobulbus* from other environments.

The full length (1430 nt) SSU rRNA gene of Dsv1 is over 99% identical to *Desulfovibrio* sp. oral taxon 040 [3] and 98% identical to *Desulfovibrio fairfieldensis*, a cultured oral isolate [31]. In addition, the SSU rRNA gene of Dsv1 is also highly similar (>98%) to *Desulfovibrio* sp. 3_1_syn3 and *Desulfovibrio* sp. 6_1_46AFAA, two human-associated, sequenced species from the gut (Figure 1). When comparing the predicted proteins of Dsv1 to those of *D.* sp. 3_1_syn3, BLASTP [32] percent identity between the two organisms was 80% or greater for roughly half the proteins predicted in Dsv1. Only 13% of Dsv1 predicted proteins had the same level of similarity to human-associated *Desulfovibrio piger*, and 3% of genes were this closely related to environmental *Desulfovibrio vulgaris* Hildenborough (Figure S2).

Genome Statistics

After normalization and assembly, the *Desulfobulbus* datasets had 0.45–0.96 Mbp each, with 527-1007 total genes (Table 1). Although Dsb4 and Dsb5 were a combination of two single amplified genomes (SAGs), only Dsb5 showed a noticeable increase in data (Table 1). Higher levels of contamination removal from Dsb4 most likely explain this discrepancy. Analyses comparing average nucleotide identity (ANI) of *Desulfobulbus* data showed that the amplicons were an average of 97.4% similar to one another (Table S1 in File S1). Similarly, comparing tetranucleotide frequencies revealed a 98.7% average similarity between *Desulfobulbus* datasets Dsb1 through Dsb5 (Table S2 in File S1). Although the *Desulfobulbus* cells were isolated from both patients with periodontitis as well as healthy controls, there was no obvious separation between these groups. This similarity is expected since previous studies have shown the same *Desulfobulbus* species present in most adults but increasing in abundance during periodontitis [16,24] In light of these findings, we treated these cells as members of a single operational taxonomic unit (OTU), and all downstream metabolic analyses were performed on a combined assembly of *Desulfobulbus* data. This combined data set will be referred to as Dsb1-5 throughout. After removing redundant data, Dsb1-5 had a total of 1910 unique genes and 1.9 Mbp, with a GC content of 58.6%. Using a genome size estimation based on a conserved single copy gene set, the genome of this oral *Desulfobulbus* OTU is approximately 2.48 Mbp. Thus, we have captured approximately 76% of the complete genome.

For the oral *Desulfovibrio*, five separate and taxonomically confirmed SAGs were combined before sequencing and will be referred to as Dsv1. The combination of genomic DNA from five SAGs provided a large increase of sequence data compared to the single and two-cell assemblies sequenced for the *Desulfobulbus* species. Dsv1 contained 2.6 Mbp of non-redundant data with a total of 2890 predicted genes and a GC content of 59.9%. A genome size estimate of 2.63 Mbp revealed that we were able to capture over 99% of the *Desulfovibrio* genome. Analysis with BLASTCLUST [32] revealed that the genomic dataset of these five cells, all sorted from the same sample, assembled well. Of the 2842 gene clusters formed at a similarity of 95% and an overlapping length of 0.7, 2839 were unique. The three overlapping clusters contained small, hypothetical genes, with at least one cluster having high similarity to integrase/transposase-like proteins.

Metabolism

Although Dsb1-5 is human-associated, several aspects of its metabolism appear to be similar to those found in the most closely related sequenced species, *Desulfobulbus. propionicus*, an isolate from anaerobic mud [33]. Forty four percent of Dsb1-5 predicted proteins had top BLASTP [32] hits to proteins in *D. propionicus*. *D. propionicus* has a complete pathway for glycolysis/gluconeogenesis, and most of these genes are also present in Dsb1-5. Similar genes are also found in the pentose phosphate pathway, although several genes were missing in our partial Dsb1-5 genome. The ability to respire sulfate appears to be present in Dsb1-5. The genes for dissimilatory sulfite reductase (*dsrAB*) are present, as well as dissimilatory adenylylsulfate reductase (*aprAB*). In addition, genes encoding QmoA and B and DsrJ, K, M, O and P [34] are present. A dissimilatory nitrate reductase gene is also present in *D.*

Table 1. Metadata and genome statistics for single and multi-cell oral amplicons.

	Genome Assembly						
	Dsb1	**Dsb2**	**Dsb3**	**Dsb4**	**Dsb5**	**Dsb1-5**	**Dsv1**
Number of cells sequenced	1	1	1	2	2	7	5
Donor health status	Healthy	Healthy	Periodontitis	Periodontitis	Periodontitis	Healthy+ Periodontitis	Periodontitis
Assembly size (bp)	455,123	768,341	798,161	748,829	959,378	1,883,075	2,603,557
DNA scaffolds	64	164	231	70	112	349	259
G+C (%)	56.6	57.6	57.2	59	59.7	58.6	59.9
Estimated genome size (Mbp)	1.39	2.09	2.12	3.75	2.26	2.48	2.63
Estimated genome recovey (%)	32.8	36.8	37.6	20.0	42.4	76.0	99.1
CRISPR	2	0	1	2	0	–	0
Genes total number	527	808	860	781	1007	1936	2890
5S rRNA	1	1	1	1	1	1	1
SSU rRNA	1	1	1	1	1	1	1
23S rRNA	1	1	1	1	0	1	1
tRNA genes	10	9	12	16	15	23	36
Other RNA genes	0	0	1	0	0	0	4
Protein coding genes	514	796	844	762	990	1910	2847

propionicus and Dsb1-5, although Dsb1-5 had no evidence of the nitrogenase found in *D. propionicus*.

Despite the similarities, key differences can be seen in Dsb1-5 compared to some of the characteristics most associated with the *Desulfobulbus* genus. Several genes needed for propionate metabolism and the methylmalonyl pathway are missing in Dsb1-5 (Figure S3). In particular, genes capable of converting propionyl phosphate to propionyl-CoA are present only in the *D. propionicus* genome. However, Dsb1-5 does code for formate C-acetyltransferase (E.C. 2.3.1.54), an enzyme not seen in *D. propionicus*, which would directly convert 2-oxobutyrate to propionyl-CoA.

Fermentation of pyruvate and alcohols has been found to proceed via the methylmalony-CoA pathway in *D. propionicus* [35]. Two of the three essential genes for the methylmalonyl-CoA fermentation pathway (EC 5.1.99.1 and EC 5.4.99.2) were not found in Dsb1-5, and pyruvate dehydrogenase and malate dehydrogenase, proteins that are active in *D. propionicus* [35], were also absent. Key enzymes of an alternative, acetyl-CoA pathway (formyltetrahydrofolate synthetase, carbon monoxide dehydrogenase and acetyl-CoA synthase) were also absent from Dsb1-5. Although this could be due to the incomplete nature of the Dsb1-5, it allows speculation that these capabilities may have been lost in the human-associated species. Additionally, these genes are not localized in *D. propionicus* but are found across the genome, making it even more unlikely that all such genes would be missed by our sequencing efforts. Dsb1-5 also lacks genes involved in butanoate metabolism and lactate utilization. In addition, *D. propionicus* encodes a partial TCA cycle that includes genes for 2-oxoglutarate:ferrodoxin reductase, but Dsb1-5 has only three genes involved in the TCA cycle, leaving its use of this cycle unclear.

Metabolic capabilities of Dsv1 seem to be similar to those found in other human-associated *Desulfovibrio* genomes (especially *Desulfovibrio* sp. 3_1_syn3), and these genomes also share many similarities to sequenced *Desulfovibrio* species from other environmental niches. Using BLASTP [32], 42% of Dsv1 predicted proteins had top hits to the *Desulfovibrio* sp. 3_1_syn3 genome. Approximately 32% of Dsv1 predicted proteins showed greatest similarity to other host-associated Deltaproteobacteria (*Desulfovibrio* sp. 6_1_46AFAA = 22%, *Desulfovibrio piger* = 2%, *Desulfovibrio desulfuricans* subsp. *desulfuricans* str. ATCC 27774 = 2%, *Bilophila wadsworthia* 3_1_6 = 4%, *Bilophila* sp. 4_1_30 = 2%).

All of the human-associated *Desulfovibrio* species, including Dsv1, contain genes for glycolysis/gluconeogenesis and key components of the pentose phosphate pathway, although the gene for glucose-6-phosphate isomerase is missing in Dsv1. Dsv1 also has the genes necessary for sulfate respiration, including *dsrAB*, *aprAB*, *dsrJKMOP* [34], *qmoABC* and *hmc* genes. All three human-associated *Desulfovibrio* genomes harbor the genes needed to reduce nitrate to ammonia that are also found in many environmental *Desulfovibrio* species. Human-associated *Desulfovibrio* all have an F-type ATPase, cytochrome *bd* complex and cytochrome *c* family III, much like environmental *Desulfovibrio* species. However, there is no evidence for a cytochrome *c* oxidase in the human-associated *Desulfovibrio* species. All host-associated *Desulfovibrio* species have a complete (*D. desulfuricans* ATCC 27774, *D. piger*, Dsv1) or partial (*D.* sp. 3_1_syn3) transporter for methionine that is not seen in any sequenced, environmental *Desulfovibrio* species.

Dsv1 contains an RNF-type complex I similar to other *Desulfovibrio* species. In addition, Dsv1 appears to have a partial Nuo-type NADH dehydrogenase (subunits A-D, H-K) that is not present in either of the gut *Desulfovibrio* genomes, and all subunits have top matches to the NADH dehydrogenase genes from *D. propionicus*. The complex appears to lack the NADH binding and oxidizing subunits (NuoEFG) and may transfer electrons from ferredoxin to quinones of the respiratory chain. Similar complexes were found in Dsb1-5, *D. propionicus* and *D. desulfuricans desulfuricans* ATCC 27774, a bacterium isolated from a sheep rumen. Both Dsv1 and *D.* sp. 3_1_syn3 have genes that encode fumarate reductase, an enzyme that functions in anaerobic respiration, but this appears to be absent in *D. piger*.

Chromosome partitioning and cell division. As expected, a gene encoding cell division protein FtsZ was found in Dsb1-5, along with other proteins involved in the cell division protein complex, including FtsA, FtsB, FtsE, FtsK, FtsQ and FtsX. Similar

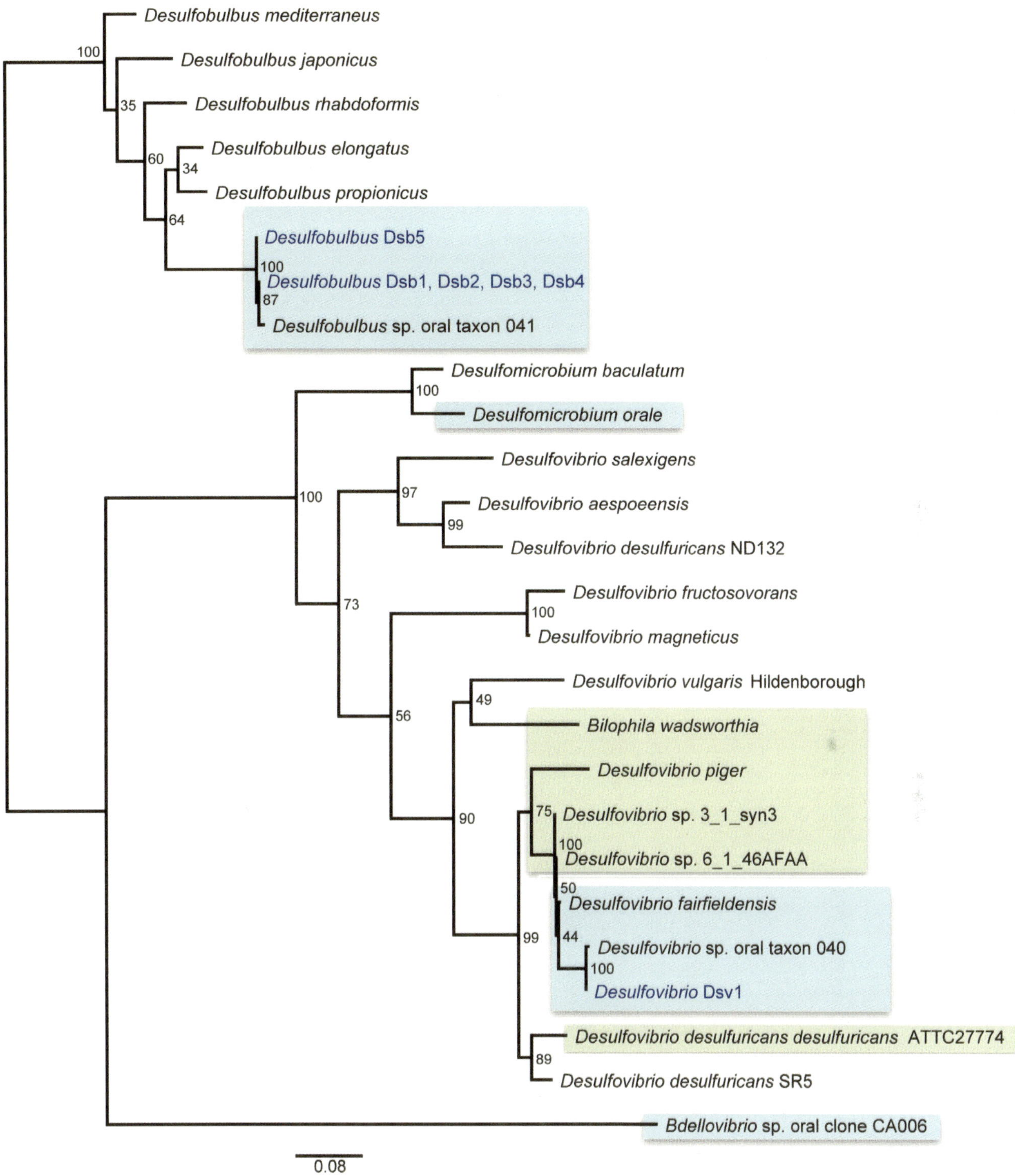

Figure 1. Maximum likelihood phylogenetic tree based on the SSU rRNA gene of select *Deltaproteobacteria* isolates as well as full-length clones from the Human Oral Microbiome Database [3]. The tree was reconstructed using PHYML [84] in the program Geneious® Pro 5.6.5 with a GTR (+ gamma+invariant sites) substitution model. Sequences from the present study are in blue text. Other host-associated sequences are denoted by blue (oral) or green (gut/rumen) boxes. The scale bar indicates 0.08 substitutions per nucleotide position. Numbers given at the nodes represent bootstrap percentages calculated on 100 replicates.

genes encoding the FtsZ system were also found in the Dsv1. In addition, Dsv1 also contained genes encoding the proteins MreB, MreC and RodA, proteins known to be involved in shape determination, particularly for elongated, rod-shaped bacteria.

Phage-related genes. Both Dsb1-5 and Dsv1 have large numbers of phage-related genes including Mu-like proteins. Both Dsv1 and Dsb1-5 harbor killer and antidote proteins of a killer gene system. This system can be used for stress response, cell cycle arrest and maintenance of otherwise disposable genes, such as in an integron [36]. All of the toxin/antitoxin gene pairs found in Dsb1-5 and Dsv1 appear to be chromosomal and are found in close proximity to transposase, integrase and other phage-related genes.

Replication and Repair. Genes functioning in replication and repair were found in Dsb1-5 and Dsv1, including genes involved in DNA replication, homologous recombination and base excision, mismatch and nucleotide excision repair. The top BLASTP hits for Dsb1-5 were variable, with a wide range of *Deltaproteobacteria* and lower overall percent identity. Most proteins in Dsv1 had high BLASTP percent identity to proteins predicted in two HMP *Desulfovibrio* sp. that have been sequenced from the human gut (*D. sp. 3_1_syn3* and *D. sp. 6_1_46AFAA*). Thus, replication and repair machinery in the oral Dsb1-5 are further removed from any of the currently sequenced *Deltaproteobacteria* than that of Dsv1.

Motility. Cell mobility is an important factor of chemotaxis, biofilm formation and oral pathogenicity, and the oral *Deltaproteobacteria* characterized here have the potential for several types of mobility. Dsb1-5 contained proteins for chemotaxis, including methyl-accepting chemotaxis proteins for detection of chemical gradients and chemotactic proteins CheA, CheW and CheY. Dsv1 contained all the chemotaxis proteins found in Dsb1-5, as well as CheB, CheV and CheZ. These chemotactic proteins are involved in a signal transduction system that could control flagellar swimming motility and/or pilin twitching motility.

Evidence for flagellar biosynthetic and motor proteins was present in Dsb1-5 and Dsv1 and included FliG, FliL, FliM, FliN, FliP, FliQ, and motor proteins MotA and MotB. However, only Dsv1 had evidence of flagellar proteins necessary for the formation of the flagellar distal and proximal rods, hook and filament. Although *D. piger* is nonmotile, both Dsv1 and *D.* sp. 3_1_syn3 have all the genes necessary for flagellar motility. *D. propionicus* strains 2pr4 and 3pr10 produce a single polar flagella and are motile while strain 1pr3 was nonmotile without a visible flagellum [33], despite the presence of several flagellar encoding genes. Based on the absence of several flagellar proteins, it is possible that Dsb1-5 has lost the ability to produce flagella, much like *D. propionicus* 1pr3.

In addition to an incomplete set of flagellar proteins, Dsb1-5 also includes a variety of genes for pilin proteins. These genes code for proteins PilA, PilB, PilF, PilO, PilT, PilV, PilW, PilX, and PilY1. The presence of PilT, a protein involved in pilus retraction and disassembly, suggests that Dsb1-5 forms type IV pili that can be used for twitching motility and biofilm formation [37,38]. This is not surprising as twitching motility is found in organisms within Proteobacteria divisions Delta, Beta and Gamma [37]. *D. propionicus* strain 1pr3 also produces pili [33], and many of the pili genes in Dsb1-5 have top BLASTP hits to *D. propionicus*.

Secretion. Several of the genes found in Dsb1-5 for twitching motility also overlap with genes used in type II secretion systems. The presence of additional genes PulD, PulE, PulF and PulO suggest that Dsb1-5 also contain a type II secretion system. Genes that code for both the Sec-dependent protein export as well as twin arginine targeting protein export are present in both Dsb1-5 and Dsv1. A type IV secretion system is also present in both organisms. The type IV proteins match pfam categories that include both virulence and conjugal transfer proteins. The presence of a type IV secretion system potentially allows Dsb1-5 to adapt to environmental changes during periodontitis and to uptake antibiotic resistance genes. It is also possible that conjugative pili could be working to aid colonization and biofilm formation [39]. Both Dsb1-5 and Dsv1 contained a gene encoding a putative homolog of TadD, a Flp pilus assembly protein important for tight, nonspecific adherence of certain bacteria to surfaces [40]. The *tad* locus has been studied in *Aggregatibacter actinomycetemcomitans* and found to be essential for the ability to colonize tooth surfaces [40]. In addition, *tadD* was found to be an important virulence factor in the pathogens *Pasteurella multocida* and *Yersinia ruckeri* [41,42]. The presence of a membrane fusion protein similar to HlyD points to type I secretion capabilities in both Dsb1-5 and Dsv1.

Defense Mechanisms. Several genes in Dsb1-5 are involved in self-defense. It appears that oral *Desulfobulbus* species have both type I and II restriction modification systems in place to protect against bacteriophage. Dsv1 shows evidence of type I and III restriction modification systems. CRISPR regions were found in Dsb1-5, and CRISPR-associated genes were found in both Dsb1-5 and Dsv1. Dsb1-5 and Dsv1 also contain genes that provide a wide range of antibiotic and multi-drug resistance, including both primary and secondary active transporters. Both Multi-Antimicrobial Extrusion (MATE) and Resistance nodulation cell division (RND) families of secondary active transporters were found in Dsb1-5 and Dsv1. One multi-drug efflux pump found in both oral genera had high similarity (0.0e+00 E-value) with the AcrB/D/F family (pfam00873), which is known to have a wide range of substrate specificity and exports most antibiotics in use [43]. In addition, several multidrug and antimicrobial ATP-binding cassette (ABC) transporters are encoded in both Dsb1-5 and Dsv1. Dsb1-5 contains genes for bacteriocin/lantibiotic transporters. Also, oral Dsb1-5 carries class C beta-lactamase genes; thus, it is likely resistant to penicillin and other beta-lactam-containing antibiotics. Finally, Dsb1-5 included an undecaprenyl-diphosphatase gene, which confers resistance to bacitracin.

Oxygen-Tolerance. Although originally thought to be obligate anaerobes, it is now known that many sulfate-reducing bacteria are oxygen tolerant. In fact, both *Desulfobulbus* and *Desulfovibrio* species have been shown to perform aerobic respiration with several electron donors, including sulfur compounds. However, these bacteria were not able to grow with oxygen as the electron acceptor [44], but rather, they seem to use aerobic respiration as a defense mechanism to avoid production of toxic products such as hydrogen peroxide and superoxide radicals [45]. Genes important for oxygen tolerance were found in both Dsb1-5 and Dsv1, suggesting that this trait is also important in the oral environment. A catalase gene was found in Dsb1-5, and this enzyme is able to detoxify certain oxygen species [45]. In addition, rubredoxin and desulfoferrodoxin genes were found in both Dsb1-5 and Dsv1, and a gene encoding rubrerythrin was found in Dsb1-5. Homologous genes in *Desulfarculus baarsii* were found to protect against damage caused by reactive oxygen species [46]. The ability to deal with oxygen stress efficiently would be an important trait for successful pathogens.

Pathogen-associated Genes

Both Dsb1-5 and Dsv1 carry genes that are beneficial for a pathogen lifestyle. Some of these genes are in common with *Desulfovibrio* species found in the environment, but several genes seem to be uniquely associated with a host-associated niche. Pathogen-associated genes provide a microbe with a competitive advantage in a host environment. Putative virulence factors for oral pathogens include genes for adherence, defense, uptake of limited nutrients, stress adaptation and interactions with both host cells and other microbial cells found within a biofilm. Categories of putative virulence factors that were found in Dsb1-5 and Dsv1 are listed in Table 2 and discussed below.

Iron is an essential element used in several metabolic processes; however, bio-available forms of iron are often limited in the

Table 2. Categories of putative virulence factors found in Dsb1-5 and Dsv1.

Category	Annotation	Dsb1-5	Dsv1
Acquisition of iron	FeoB ferrous iron uptake	+	+
	ABC-type Fe^{3+}-siderophore transport system	+	+
	Hemolysin	+	+
	ferrous iron transport protein A	+	+
	Fur family ferric uptake regulator	+	+
	TonB-dependent receptor	+	+
Secretion	Sec system	+	+
	Type I secretion	+	+
	Type II secretion	+	
	Type IV secretion	+	+
Stress Response	Universal stress protein UspA	+	+
	Clp proteins	+	+
	RelA/SpoT family protein	+	+
	5′/3′-nucleotidase SurE	+	+
	Crp/Fnr family transcriptional regulator	+	+
	desulfoferrodoxin	+	+
	rubredoxin	+	+
	Rubrerythrin	+	
	Catalase	+	
	Peroxiredoxin		+
Evasion	2-dehydro-3-deoxyphosphooctonate aldolase	+	
	Acetyltransferase	+	+
	alginate o-acetyltransferase	+	
	Beta-glucosidase-related glycosidases		+
	CMP-2-keto-3-deoxyoctulosonic acid synthetase		+
	dTDP-4-dehydrorhamnose 3,5-epimerase		+
	dTDP-4-dehydrorhamnose reductase	+	
	dTDP-glucose 4,6-dehydratase		+
	glucose 1-phosphate thymidylyltransferase	+	
	glycoside hydrolase family protein		
	Glycosyltransferase	+	+
	lytic transglycosylase	+	
	membrane-bound lytic murein transglycosylase		+
	N-acetylmuramoyl-L-alanine amidase	+	+
	NAD-dependent epimerase/dehydratase	+	
	nucleotide sugar dehydrogenase	+	+
	pantetheine-phosphate adenylyltransferase, bacterial		+
	peptidoglycan O-acetyltransferase PacA	+	
	GDP:alpha-D-mannose-1-phosphate guanylyltransferase	+	
	putative exopolysaccharide biosynthesis protein		+
	UDP-N-acetylglucosamine 2-epimerase	+	
	undecaprenyl-phosphate galactose phosphotransferase	+	
Defense mechanism	ABC-type bacteriocin/lantibiotic exporter	+	
	ABC-type multidrug transport system	+	+
	acriflavin resistance protein	+	+
	choline/carnitine/betaine transporter family	+	
	Cation/multidrug efflux pump	+	+
Protease/Peptidase	Clp protease	+	+
	La protease	+	+

Table 2. Cont.

Category	Annotation	Dsb1-5	Dsv1
	carboxyl-terminal protease	+	
	Collagenase and related proteases		+
	FtsH protease	+	
	Membrane proteins related to metalloendopeptidases		+
	O-sialoglycoprotein endopeptidase	+	
	signal peptide peptidase SppA	+	+
	Trypsin-like serine proteases, typically periplasmic		+
	Xaa-Pro aminopeptidase		+
	putative glycoprotease GCP		+
	periplasmic serine protease, Do/DeqQ family		+
	outer membrane protease	+	
Adhesion	Type IV pili	+	
	TPR repeat-containing protein	+	+
	YD repeat-containing protein	+	
	Surface antigens	+	+
	Lipoproteins	+	+

The presence of a gene is noted by (+).

environment [47]. The ability to acquire iron is a particularly important trait for human-associated bacteria, where iron can be even more limited by iron-binding proteins of host cells. In the oral environment, most iron is bound to the host protein lactoferrin [47]. Thus, successful human pathogens often have several genes that give them an advantage in acquiring iron. In addition to several iron transport systems, both Dsb1-5 and Dsv1 also contain hemolysin. Using IMG, these genes can also found in many environmental *Deltaproteobacteria* genomes and have likely persisted in Dsb1-5 and Dsv1 because of their continued benefits in the host environment.

In order to be successful pathogens, bacteria must cope with environmental changes and harmful molecules. Both Dsb1-5 and Dsv1 encode a wide range of transporters and efflux systems to protect against drugs and antibiotics. In addition, Dsb1-5 and Dsv1 contain oxygen-tolerance genes discussed above, universal stress protein UspA and a suite of Clp proteins. The Clp proteins in *Porphyromonas gingivalis* have been shown to be important for stress response, as well as biofilm formation and entry into host epithelial cells [48]. Knockouts of ClpB resulted in reduced virulence in both *Leptospira interrogans* and *Enterococcus faecalis* and reduced general stress resistance in *L. interrogans* [49,50]. Further, ClpAP mutants in *Helicobacter pylori* showed increased sensitivity to antibiotics and oxidative stress and disrupted colonization of macrophages [51].

Another important aspect of pathogenicity includes the ability to attach to other cells. The type IV pili found in Dsb1-5 are likely important for its adhesion [38,52]. Additional surface proteins that may play a role in binding to cells include tetratrico peptide repeat (TPR) and YD dipeptide repeat-containing domains, surface antigens and lipoproteins [14]. Additionally, both Dsb1-5 and Dsv1 contain several proteases and peptidases that often serve as virulence factors that degrade host proteins for nutrients and may contribute to the cytotoxicity of periodontitis [14,53].

Lastly, both genomes had several genes for polysaccharide metabolism, including an abundance of glycosyl transferases [14,53]. Both genomes had a large number of genes involved in lipopolysaccharide biosynthesis, and there were also genes present in Dsb1-5 (UDP-N-acetylglucosamine 2-epimerase and polysaccharide biosynthesis protein CapD) that are putatively involved in extracellular polysaccharide (EPS) or capsular production. At least two scaffolds in Dsb1-5 include genes that may be involved in EPS or capsular production, and the majority of genes on these scaffolds appear to be horizontally transferred, with most genes having top BLASTP hits to genomes other than *D. propionicus* (Table S3 in File S1). The presence of a capsule would be beneficial to a pathogen in the oral environment by providing adherence to oral surfaces and other biofilm members and resistance to both specific and nonspecific host immune systems [54].

COG Comparisons to Other *Deltaproteobacteria* Genomes

To further understand the unique properties of the oral *Deltaproteobacteria* characterized here, comparisons were done with other sequenced *Deltaproteobacteria* using the presence/absence of COGs. Overall percentages of genes in each COG category for Dsb1-5 and Dsv1 were similar to those seen in other sequenced *Deltaproteobacteria*. Comparisons of Dsb1-5 to *D. propionicus* closely matched initial comparisons made with BLASTP hits and revealed a large overlap of genes. Dsb1-5 shares 920 COGS with *D. propionicus*, whereas only 222 COGs (19%) were unique to the oral genomes (Figure 2A). A complete Dsb1-5 genome would likely show an even greater overlap with *D. propionicus*. Several of the unique COGs in Dsb1-5 were for related functions. Nine COGS included components of a type IV secretion system found in Dsb1-5, whereas only components of the type II secretion system were found in *D. propionicus*. Dsb1-5 also encodes an array of unique COGS for transporters, including those that transport dipeptides/oligopeptides, bacteriocins/lantibiotics, monosaccharides, betaine and cobalt. Dsb1-5 contained COGs for both Na^+/alanine and Na^+/H^+-dicarboxylate symporters, while *D. propionicus* contains a unique multi-subunit, Na^+/H^+ antiporter. Many of the Dsb1-5 specific COGs contain proteins discussed above that may be used for host evasion and possible capsular production. Other

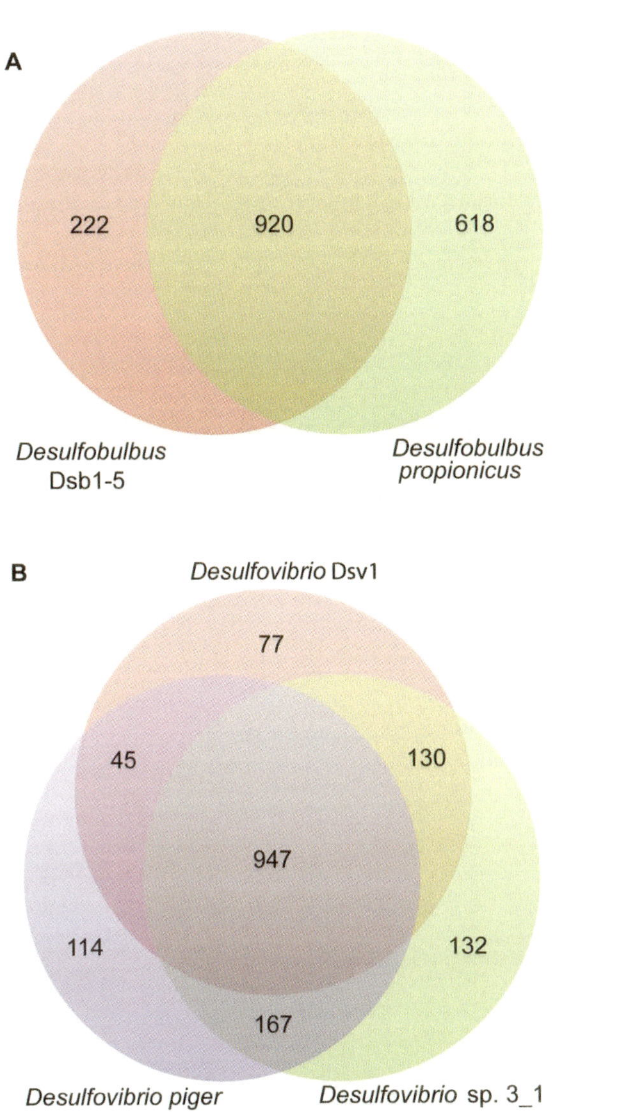

Figure 2. Comparison of COG categories (presence/absence) for human-associated and free living *Deltaproteobacteria*. (A). *Desulfobulbus* Dsb1-5 and *Desulfobulbus propionicus*. (B) *Desulfovibrio* Dsv1, *D.* sp. 3_1_syn3 and *D. piger*.

differences include unique COGs in each genome for phage-related proteins and outer membrane proteins.

COG categories were also used to compare the oral Dsv1 genome to other available human-associated species, *D.* sp. 3_1_syn3 and *D. piger* (Figure 2B). Again, the COGs were similar to BLASTP results and largely overlapped, with 947 COGs found in all three species. An additional 130 COGs overlapped in both Dsv1 and *D.* sp. 3_1_syn3. COGs that were unique to Dsv1 included six NADH dehydrogenase subunits, a toxin/antitoxin growth regulation system, an ABC-type sulfate/molybdate transporter and an organic solvent tolerance protein. The large number of overlapping COGs found in all species included many metabolic genes, genes for cell division, DNA replication and repair and a large number of ABC-type transporters and Na^+ symporters and antiporters.

A broader comparison of genomes within the *Desulfovibrio* genus found COGs that are specific to either host-associated or environmental organisms (Table S4 in File S1). Unfortunately, genes for four of the differential, human-associated COGs were predicted to encode uncharacterized proteins, leaving the function of these proteins unclear. Both pfam and top BLASTP hits for the uncharacterized COG proteins shed light on their potential function. The genes that fall into COG3735 also fall into pfam PF01963, the TraB family of proteins. In *Enterococcus faecalis*, TraB is an important regulator for the peptide pheromone cAD1 that is encoded on a hemolysin/bacteriocin plasmid and used to control both clumping and plasmid transfer between cells containing plasmids and those that do not [55]. COG2326-associated proteins are likely similar to polyphosphate kinase 2, an enzyme converts AMP to ADP. Another uncharacterized COG contained a protein that is found, in every host-associated genome analyzed, between a tripartite ATP-independent periplasmic (TRAP) transporter solute receptor protein and a TRAP fused permease component and may be involved in this secondary transport system. The final human-specific COG was a putative amino acid racemase.

In addition to these differential genes, eight additional genes fell into COG categories that were present in both human-associated and sheep rumen-associated *Desulfovibrio*, but absent in environmental *Desulfovibrio*. Interesting genes in this group include hits to COG2011 and COG1464. Further investigation of pfam and KO modules revealed these two proteins are likely used as a D-methionine transport system, and BLASTP results show that the closest hits outside of the host-associated *Desulfovibrio* are to clostridia. An additional COG (1897) that includes homoserine O-succinyltransferase, the first step in the biosynthesis of methionine, was found in all host-associated Deltaproteobacteria, except the incomplete, Dsb1-5 genome. Both COG0214 and COG0311 contain proteins that are part of the pyridoxine (vitamin B_6) biosynthesis pathway.

Twenty-five COGs were detected only in the environmental *Desulfovibrio* species, eight of which are uncharacterized proteins. Two COGs encoded proteins similar to FtsE and FtsX, proteins involved in cell divison and important under low osmotic conditions [56]. Additional differential COGs include a distinct endocuclease III and IV and Fe-S oxidoreductase.

A comparison of all available *Deltaproteobacteria* genomes in IMG ($n = 53$) revealed two COG categories (COG4457, COG4458) that were found in all human-associated Deltaproteobacteria as well as *D. desulfuricans* ATCC 27774 but were not represented in any of the environmental Deltaproteobacteria genomes. These COGs included *srfB* and *srfC*, two genes of the SrfABC operon originally found in *Salmonella enterica* [57]. Although initially thought to be activated by SsrB, the transcriptional activator of a two-part regulatory system that controls gene activity of *Salmonella* pathogenicity island 2 (SPI2) [57], more recent work did not support this finding [58]. Additional studies have linked regulation of this operon to genes responsible for flagella production [59] and oxygen sensing [60]. Ultimately, the function of these genes is still unclear. BLASTP was used within IMG to find closely related predicted proteins in other genomes. When top hits were aligned and a phylogenetic tree was made, the most closely related proteins were found in a wide range of plant and animal-associated microbes, including both commensal and pathogenic bacteria (Figures S4, S5). Similar matches were found for a neighboring gene that encodes a putative *Haemophilus* adhesion and penetration (Hap)-like protein that is important for biofilm formation and adherence and entry into epithelial cell [61].

In addition to putative SrfABC and Hap encoding genes, all host-associated *Deltaproteobacteria* genomes share at least 3 other genes (*tagQ, ppkA and ligA*) in the same gene neighborhood. The majority of host-associated *Deltaproteobacteria* contained 3 additional

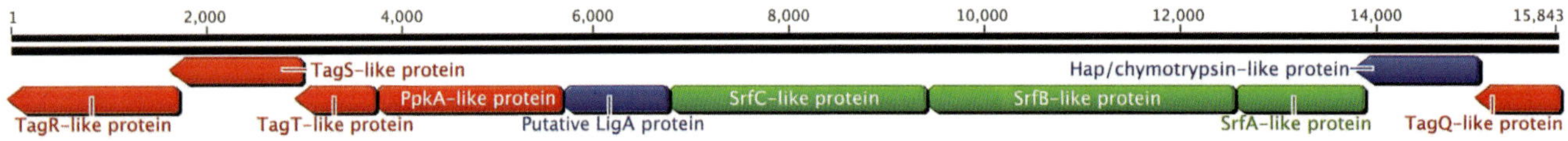

Figure 3. Gene neighborhood that includes two genes (*srfB* and *srfC*) unique to host-associated deltaproteobacterial genomes and with low similarity to *Deltaproteobacteria* from other environments. Genes are color-coded based on an association with the *srf* operon (green), type VI secretion (T6SS) post-translational control (red) or unknown association (blue). Genes encoding TagR, TagT and TagS were not found in Dsv1 or *B. wadsworthia*.

homologous genes (*tagR, tagS, tagT*), resulting in a neighborhood of 10 genes with low homology to deltaproteobacterial genomes from other environments (Figure 3). Five of these genes (TagQ, TagR, TagS, TagT and PpkA) have been linked to type VI secretion (T6SS) post-translational control proteins in the threonine phosphorylation pathway (TPP) [62]. These genes act as part of a transmembrane signaling pathway that promotes T6SS activity under optimal conditions. Despite this, only *Desulfovibrio* sp. 3_1 contains genes necessary for type VI secretion machinery.

PpkA is a threonine protein kinase responsible for the phosphorylation of T6SS component Fha1, an event that triggers the export of an effector protein [62] Thus, it is possible that PpkA could trigger the export of SrfC, which was also predicted to be an effector protein [57]. TagQ is an outer membrane lipoprotein and is suspected to be involved in signal detection, due to its similarity to a 17kDa *Rickettsia* surface antigen [63]. TagR is proposed to be a co-receptor for the environmental signal that activates T6SS (Hsu, Schwarz et al. 2009). TagT and TagS form an ABC transporter that falls into a family of transporters that interacts with membrane-integrated histidine kinases and seem to play a role in regulated responses to external environment (Casabona, Silverman et al. 2012). All of the host-associated deltaproteobacterial genomes have TPP genes that are most closely related to those found in *Pseudomonas* species. This system in *Pseudomonas aeruginosa* has been shown to be an important virulence component [62].

One additional gene in this gene neighborhood encodes for a protein of unknown function. However, it was annotated as a LigA protein in at least one genome, and top BLASTP hits included *Taylorella asinigenitalis*, *Xenorhabdus bovienii* SS-2004, and *Proteus penneri* ATCC 35198, all host-associated organisms. Although it is remains unclear how these genes function, they are likely important to survival in the host and interactions with both host and other bacterial cells.

Conclusion

The genomes of Dsb1-5 and Dsv1 enabled the first insight into the potential functions of these *Deltaproteobacteria* within the oral environment (Figure 4). Even with an extreme environmental change, both groups still had considerable metabolic overlap with related environmental organisms. Although no other host-associated *Desulfobulbus* species have been sequenced, comparisons of Dsv1 with gut-associated *Desulfovibrio* revealed that there is good congruence in these genomes. However, it is clear that some oral and gut-associated species are more closely related than others (Dsv1 and *D.* sp_3_1_syn3 versus Dsv1 and *D. piger*). Further, analyzing distinct genes of Dsb1-5 and Dsv1 revealed a suite of genes that is essential for a host-adapted lifestyle. These unique genes are associated with adhesion, stress resistance, defense mechanisms and possible host-cell interactions and degradation. Thus, it is possible that associations of these organisms with disease are due to these virulent properties. This insight into the potential importance of uncultured, low-abundance members of microbial communities to disease will hopefully encourage similar genomic studies of other putative pathogens.

Materials and Methods

Ethics Statement

Human subjects enrollment and sample collection protocols were approved by the Ohio State University Institutional Review Board and by the Oak Ridge Site-Wide Institutional Review Board. Signed informed written consent was obtained from all human subjects that provided samples for this study.

Sample Collection

We acquired three single-cells (Dsb1, Dsb2, Dsb3) and two combined pools (Dsb4, Dsb5) of a *Desulfobulbus* species, as well as one pool (Dsv1) of a *Desulfovibrio* species. Samples came from both periodontally healthy subjects and subjects with periodontitis. Patients were identified as having periodontitis based upon previously published criteria [16]. Dsb1 and Dsb2 were retrieved from a subgingival paper point sample taken from a healthy volunteer. Dsb3 was retrieved from a mixture of paper point samples taken from affected teeth from two subjects with periodontitis, and Dsb4 was retrieved from samples obtained by curette from a subject with periodontitis. Dsb5 and Dsv1 were retrieved from a mixture of paper point samples taken from affected teeth from four subjects with periodontitis. In all cases, samples were taken and immediately stored in 1 × PBS at 4°C and transported on ice to the lab within 24 hours. When samples arrived at the lab, each was vortexed vigorously for one minute, and the PBS from each sample was combined as noted above. Samples were then fixed in 50% ethanol and stored at −20°C for one to three days before *in situ* hybridization.

Fluorescence *in situ* Hybridization

For fluorescence *in situ* hybridization (FISH) we used the *Deltaproteobacteria*-specific probes DELTA495a [30] and SRB385 [29]. These are group-specific probes that have been shown to capture a large percentage of known *Desulfobulbus* and *Desulfovibrio* species [64]. Hybridization and wash buffers were prepared as previously described, and previous hybridization protocols were slightly adapted to work in-solution [65]. Briefly, 500 uL of ethanol-fixed samples were centrifuged (3000 g, 5:00 min), and the resulting pellet was resuspended in 50 uL of a 1:10 probe (50 ng/μL): hybridization buffer solution. Hybridization buffer contained 35% formamide [30]. This mixture was hybridized at 46°C for 3 hrs or overnight (~20 hrs). Based on control hybridizations using *D. propionicus* and *D. piger*, the signal was enhanced by overnight incubations and that condition was applied to the oral samples. Following centrifugation, the cells were washed using standard FISH solution and resuspended in PBS for cell sorting. Both Alexa488-labeled DELTA495a probe alone and Alexa488-labeled DELTA495a mixed with Cy5-dual-labeled SRB385 [66] probe combinations were used. When samples were

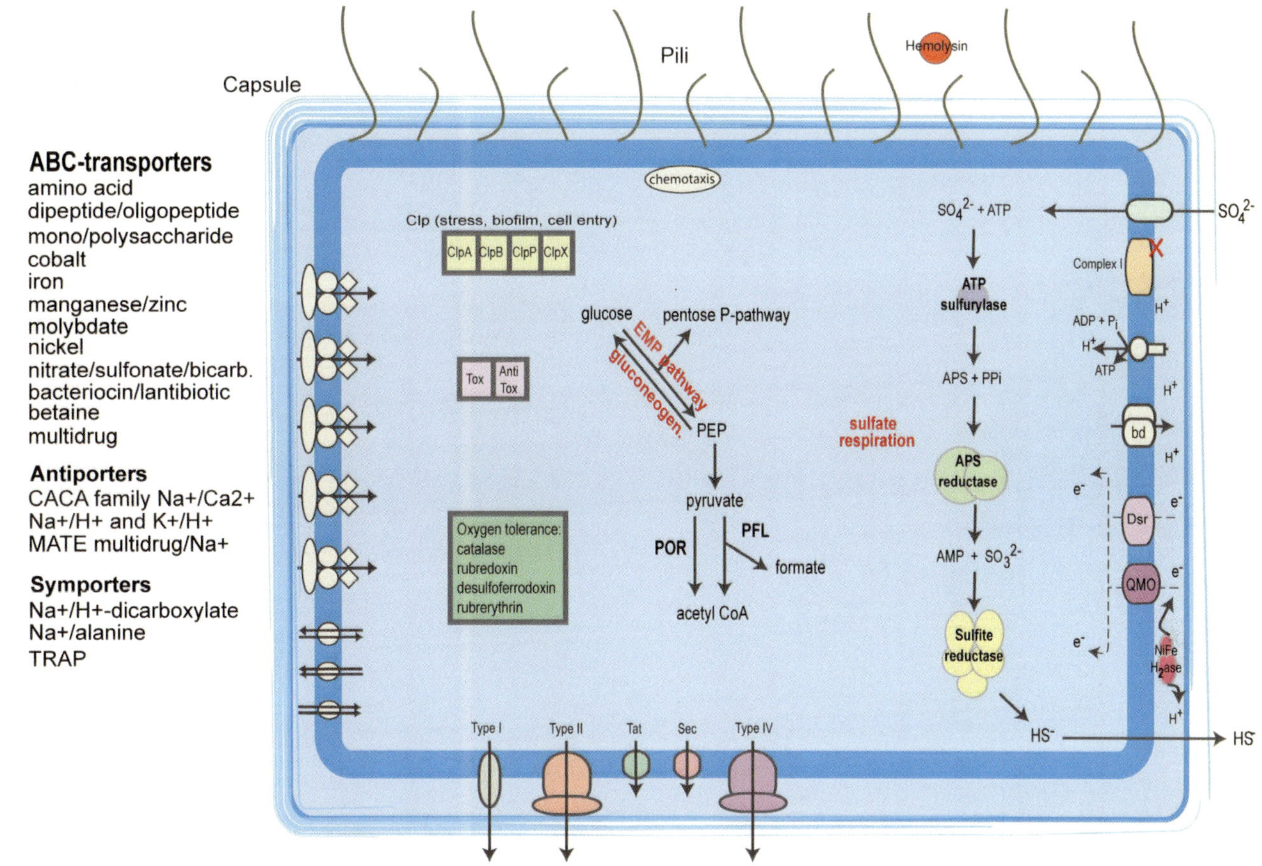
Capsule
Pili
Hemolysin
ABC-transporters
amino acid
dipeptide/oligopeptide
mono/polysaccharide
cobalt
iron
manganese/zinc
molybdate
nickel
nitrate/sulfonate/bicarb.
bacteriocin/lantibiotic
betaine
multidrug
Antiporters
CACA family Na+/Ca2+
Na+/H+ and K+/H+
MATE multidrug/Na+
Symporters
Na+/H+-dicarboxylate
Na+/alanine
TRAP
chemotaxis
Clp (stress, biofilm, cell entry)
ClpA ClpB ClpP ClpX
Tox Anti Tox
glucose
pentose P-pathway
EMP pathway
gluconeogen.
PEP
pyruvate
POR
PFL
formate
acetyl CoA
Oxygen tolerance: catalase rubredoxin desulfoferrodoxin rubrerythrin
sulfate respiration
SO_4^{2-} + ATP
ATP sulfurylase
APS + PPi
APS reductase
AMP + SO_3^{2-}
Sulfite reductase
HS^-
SO_4^{2-}
Complex I
ADP + P_i
ATP
H^+
bd
Dsr
QMO
NiFe H_2ase
e^-
Type I
Type II
Tat
Sec
Type IV

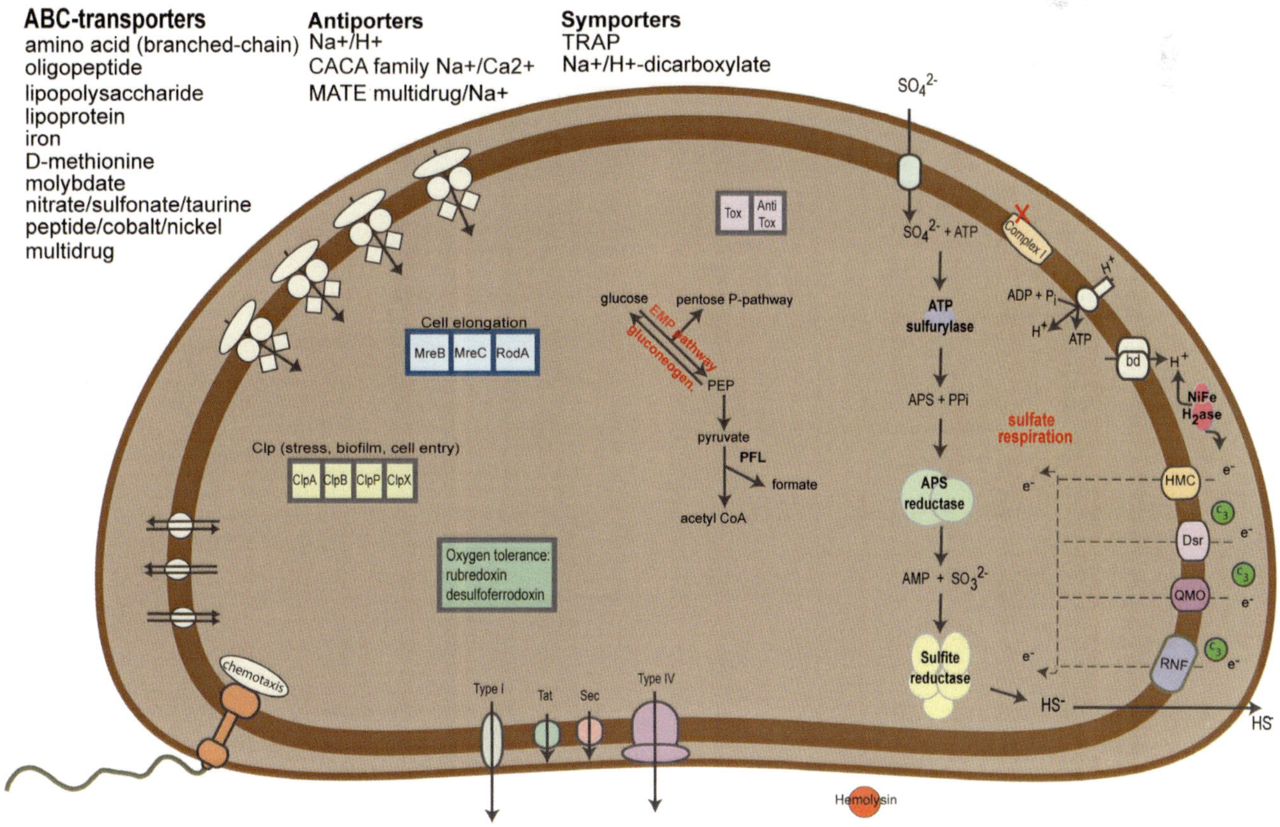
ABC-transporters
amino acid (branched-chain)
oligopeptide
lipopolysaccharide
lipoprotein
iron
D-methionine
molybdate
nitrate/sulfonate/taurine
peptide/cobalt/nickel
multidrug
Antiporters
Na+/H+
CACA family Na+/Ca2+
MATE multidrug/Na+
Symporters
TRAP
Na+/H+-dicarboxylate
SO_4^{2-}
Tox Anti Tox
Cell elongation
MreB MreC RodA
Clp (stress, biofilm, cell entry)
ClpA ClpB ClpP ClpX
glucose
pentose P-pathway
EMP pathway
gluconeogen.
PEP
pyruvate
PFL
formate
acetyl CoA
Oxygen tolerance: rubredoxin desulfoferrodoxin
SO_4^{2-} + ATP
ATP sulfurylase
APS + PPi
APS reductase
AMP + SO_3^{2-}
Sulfite reductase
HS^-
Complex I
ADP + P_i
ATP
H^+
bd
NiFe H_2ase
sulfate respiration
HMC
Dsr
QMO
RNF
C_3
e^-
chemotaxis
Type I
Tat
Sec
Type IV
Hemolysin

Figure 4. Brief overview of inferred metabolic and transport capabilities of *Desulfobulbus* Dsb1-5 (top panel) and *Desulfovibrio* Dsv1 (bottom panel). EMP, Embden-Meyerhof pathway. APS, adenosine 5′-phosphosufate. Bd, cytochrome bd. C_3, cytochrome family III. Hmc, high-molecular-weight cytochrome c. Dsr, complex DsrMKJOP. QMO, QmoABC complex. RNF, Rnf-type complex I. Complex I, Nuo-type complex I (missing periplasmic components are denoted by a red X. H2ase, hydrogenase. PEP, phosphoenolpyruvatye. PFL, pyruvate formate lyase. POR, pyruvate ferredoxin oxidoreductase. TRAP, tripartite ATP-independent periplasmic. MATE, multidrug and toxic compound extrusion. Tox/AntiTox, killer gene system.

hybridized with the combined probes, cells had both red and green fluorescence.

Cell Sorting

For cell sorting we used a Cytopeia Influx cell sorter (BD, Franklin Lakes, NJ, USA). The instrument was cleaned prior to use in a similar manner to those described earlier [67,68]. Briefly, the fluidic lines were cleaned with 10% bleach for 45 min and rinsed with 0.2 µm filtered ddH_20 for 30 min, followed by rinsing with sheath fluid for an additional hour prior to sorting. 1× PBS was used as sheath fluid, and the reservoir tank and sheath fluid were UV-sterilized overnight. Between successive samples, fluidic lines were flushed with 10% bleach, followed by sheath fluid. Ethanol-fixed oral samples from periodontitis patients were first passed through a CellTrics 30 µm disposable filter (Partec, Görlitz, Germany). Prior to sorting, samples were labeled by FISH as described above, or stained with 5 µM of nucleic acid-binding dyes SYTO 9 (green) and SYTO 62 (red) (Life Technologies, Grand Island, NY USA) for 15 min. Cells labeled by FISH probes were sorted only once, as single cells. Samples labeled with nucleic acid dyes were sorted twice, using SYTO9 emission for the first sort and SYTO62 emission for the final sort, to further dilute any possible contaminating free DNA found in the original sample [68]. Cells sorted in the final round were deposited as single cells into 3 µL UV-sterilized TE buffer. Three *Desulfobulbus* cells (Dsb1, Dsb2, Dsb3) were obtained by random sorting using nucleic acid-binding dyes.

Multiple Displacement Amplification

Single-cells retrieved by sorting were used for multiple displacement amplification (MDA). All plasticware, water and reagents used for MDA reactions (except the primers, dNTPs and enzyme) were UV treated as described [69]. Reactions were set up in a manner similar to [68]. Briefly, cells were subjected to lysis by addition of 3 µL of buffer that consisted of 0.13 M KOH, 3.3 mM EDTA pH 8.0 and 27.7 mM DTT, heated to 95°C for 30 sec, and immediately placed on ice for 10 min. 3 µL neutralization buffer (0.13 M HCl, 0.42 M Tris pH 7.0, 0.18 M Tris 8.0) was added followed by 11 µL of MDA master mix: 90.9 µM random hexamers with two protective, phosporothioate bonds on the 3′ end (Integrated DNA Technologies, Coralville, IA, USA), 1.09 mM dNTPs (Roche Indianapolis, IN, USA), 1.8× phi29 DNA polymerase buffer (New England BioLabs, Ipswich, MA, USA), 4 mM DTT (Roche) and ~100 U phi29 DNA polymerase enzyme (purified in house) [70]. Amplification was performed for 10 hrs at 30°C followed by inactivation at 80°C for 20 min and storage at −20C.

Target Identification

A small aliquot of each single cell amplified genomic product (SAG) was diluted (1:150) in PCR-grade water (Ambion, Austin, TX, USA), and the remainder product was stored at −80°C. Dilutions were used for SSU rRNA gene PCR amplifications using universal bacterial primer 27fm (5′-AGA GTT TGA TYM TGG CTC AG-3′) [71] and *Deltaproteobacteria*-specific primer Delta495a (5'-AGT TAG CCG GTG CTT CCT-3′) (Loy, Lehner et al. 2002). Fifty microliter reactions contained the following: 1× polymerase buffer, 200 µM each dNTP (Roche, Indianapolis, IN USA), 2 mM MgCl2 (Ambion), 5 µg BSA (New England BioLabs), 300 µM each primer (Integrated DNA Technologies), 1 U of either *Taq* or *Pfu* polymerase and 1 µL diluted MDA product. PCR reactions ran under the following thermal conditions: 94°C for 2 min, followed by 30 cycles of 94°C for 30 sec, 55°C for 30 sec, 72°C for 1.5 min and a final extension at 72°C for 5 min. MDA products that gave amplicons were visualized by gel electrophoresis with 1% (w/v) agarose gels. All PCRs that produced clean bands were purified with PCR filtration plates (Millipore, Billerica, MA, USA) and sequenced directly on an ABI3730 DNA Analyzer (Applied Biosystems) using the primer 27 fm. Resulting chromatograms were manually edited and the sequences used for phylogenetic identifications with the RDP Classifier [72]. Samples for which the chromatograms were not homogeneous and that denoted potential heterogeneous template DNA (more than one sorted cell) were not further used. All confirmed deltaproteobacterial MDA products were used to generate secondary MDA products. Five secondary MDA reactions were set up for each SAG, and each reaction used 1 uL of a 1:10 dilution of the original MDA product. All buffers and amplification mixes were constructed as described above for the primary MDA reactions. Secondary MDAs were only amplified for 6 hrs before heat inactivation.

MDA Purification and Sequencing

Secondary deltaproteobacterial SAGs were purified by phenol:-chloroform:isoamyl alcohol extraction and alcohol precipitation before being sent for sequencing. Illumina Hi-Seq 100-bp paired-end libraries were constructed and sequenced at the Hudson Alpha Institute for Biotechnology (Huntsville, AL, USA).

Genome Assembly and Annotation

SAG libraries Dsb2 and Dsb3 were submitted to the Joint Genome Institute's single-cell assembly and QC pipeline, similar to Illumina SAG libraries described previously [73]. Dsb1, Dsb4, Dsb5 and Dsv1 genomic data were normalized and assembled in-house using digital normalization [74] and Velvet assembly [75]. Briefly, for digital normalization, the following parameters were used: coverage threshold (C) = 30, k-mer size (k) = 30, n hashes (N) = 4 and minimum hash size (x) = 1e+09. In Velvet, each genome was computed from hash length 59 to 65 with a step of two. The number of nodes, n50, maximum number of bases in a scaffold and total number of bases for each hash length were compared to select the final assembled dataset. Assembled genomes were subjected to the JGI/ORNL automated annotation pipeline, which uses Prodigal for ORF calling [76], before submission into IMG [77] and RAST [78] for further analysis and for comparisons with genomes sequenced under the Human Microbiome Project [2]. The search for potentially contaminating DNA contigs (human and non-deltaproteobacterial) was conducted using BLASTP [32] as well as by GC content and tetramer analysis [79] of each scaffold. Contigs that were aberrant based on all these analyses were removed from further analysis but represented a small fraction of the dataset.

Combined Non-redundant Assembly

To assess the phylogenetic relationships between the multiple Dsb SAGs, Dsb1-Dsb5 were compared using average nucleotide identity (ANI) and tetranucleotide frequency. Both ANI and tetranucleotide frequencies were calculated using the software JSpecies [80]. In order to discuss the potential function of oral *Desulfobulbus* as a whole, all datasets were combined (Dsb1-5). Repetitive regions between amplicons were removed iteratively with the aid of custom perl scripts. A region was considered redundant if it exhibited more than 95% identity over a region of at least 1000 bp. Remaining overlaps were assessed using BLASTCLUST [32] (S = 95, L = 0.7) as well as Mauve [81] and the *de novo* assembler within Geneious® Pro 5.6.5 and removed by hand. The final individual and combined assemblies were submitted to GenBank under BioProject accession numbers PRJNA188735-PRJNA188740. They are also readily available with full annotations under the public IMG portal at http://img.jgi.doe.gov/cgi-bin/w/main.cgi (taxon IDs: 2517572070, 3400000002, 3400000008, 3400000010–3400000012).

Genome Size Estimation

Genome size and coverage was estimated using a conserved single copy gene (CSCG) set that has been determined from all 1516 finished bacterial genome sequences in the IMG database [77]. The set consists of 138 CSCG that were found to occur only once in at least 90% of all genomes by analysis of an abundance matrix based on hits to the protein family (Pfam) database [82]. Hidden Markov models of the identified Pfams were used to search assemblies by means of the HMMER3 software [83]. Resulting best hits above pre-calculated cutoffs were counted and the coverage was estimated as the ratio of found CSCG to total CSCGs in the set after normalization to 90%. Based thereon, the estimated complete genome size was calculated by division of the estimated genome coverage by the total assembly size.

Supporting Information

Figure S1 Optimization of sample hybridization times. Panel A shows the scatterplot pattern of a *Desulfobulbus propionicus* culture after 3 (top) or 20 (bottom) hours of hybridization. Panel B shows actual sorting gates for an oral sample after 20 hour hybridization. All images of 528-38 emission (left) were samples hybridized with Alexa488-labeled DELTA495a. All images of 670-30 emission (right) were samples hybridized with Cy5-dual labeled SRB385.

Figure S2 Number of Dsv1 genes with homologs in gut species *Desulfovibrio* sp. 3_1_syn3, *D. piger* or environmental species *D. vulgaris* Hildenborough. The search for homologous genes was performed in IMG [85] with increasing minimum percent identity requirements. A total of 2890 Dsv1 genes were analyzed.

Figure S3 Map of enzymes used in propionate metabolism and the methylmalonyl pathway. Genes found in Dsb1-5 (based on E.C. number) are shown in blue. Genes in *Desulfobulbus propionicus* are shown in red.

Figure S4 Maximum likelihood tree of putative *srfB* genes. The tree was constructed using PHYML [86] in the program Geneious® Pro 5.6.5 with a JTT (+ gamma+invariant sites) substitution model. Predicted proteins from host-associated *Deltaproteobacteria* are denoted by a blue box. The scale bar indicates 0.3 substitutions per nucleotide position. Numbers given at the nodes represent bootstrap percentages calculated on 100 replicates.

Figure S5 Maximum likelihood tree of putative *srfC* genes. The tree was constructed using PHYML [86] in the program Geneious® Pro 5.6.5 with a JTT (+ gamma+invariant sites) substitution model. Predicted proteins from host-associated *Deltaproteobacteria* are denoted by a blue box. The scale bar indicates 0.8 substitutions per nucleotide position. Numbers given at the nodes represent bootstrap percentages calculated on 100 replicates.

File S1

Acknowledgments

We thank the NIH Human Microbiome Project research community for making available sequence data used for comparative analyses. We also thank Dr. Paul Blainey for the phi29 polymerase overexpression clone, Sarah Kauffman for technical assistance with the project, Dr. Matt Heaton and Dr. Jeffrey Becker for advice and help with sample collection and processing.

Author Contributions

Conceived and designed the experiments: AGC PS TW AS AG EL MP. Performed the experiments: AGC SA CB. Analyzed the data: AGC JHC PS AS CB. Wrote the paper: AGC PS MP.

References

1. Arumugam M, Raes J, Pelletier E, Le Paslier D, Yamada T, et al. (2011) Enterotypes of the human gut microbiome. Nature 473: 174–180.
2. Methe B, Nelson KE, Pop M, Creasy HH, Giglio MG, et al. (2012) Structure, function and diversity of the healthy human microbiome. Nature 486: 207–214.
3. Dewhirst FE, Chen T, Izard J, Paster BJ, Tanner ACR, et al. (2010) The Human Oral Microbiome. J Bacteriol 192: 5002–5017.
4. Darveau RP (2010) Periodontitis: a polymicrobial disruption of host homeostasis. Nature Rev Microbiol 8: 481–490.
5. Hajishengallis G, Lamont RJ (2012) Beyond the red complex and into more complexity: the polymicrobial synergy and dysbiosis (PSD) model of periodontal disease etiology. Mol Oral Microbiol 27: 409–419.
6. Humphrey LL, Fu RW, Buckley DI, Freeman M, Helfand M (2008) Periodontal Disease and Coronary Heart Disease Incidence: A Systematic Review and Meta-analysis. J Gen Int Med 23: 2079–2086.
7. Kuo LC, Poison AM, Kang T (2008) Associations between periodontal diseases and systemic diseases: A review of the inter-relationships and interactions with diabetes, respiratory diseases, cardiovascular diseases and osteoporosis. Pub Health 122: 417–433.
8. Preshaw PM, Alba AL, Herrera D, Jepsen S, Konstantinidis A, et al. (2012) Periodontitis and diabetes: a two-way relationship. Diabetologia 55: 21–31.
9. Ramirez-Tortosa MC, Quiles JL, Battino M, Granados S, Morillo JM, et al. (2010) Periodontitis is associated with altered plasma fatty acids and cardiovascular risk markers. Nut Metab Cardiovasc Dis 20: 133–139.
10. Scannapieco FA DA, Chhun N (2010) Does periodontal therapy reduce the risk for systemic diseases? Dent Clin North Am 54: 18.
11. Kinane D, Bouchard P, European Workshop P (2008) Periodontal diseases and health: Consensus Report of the Sixth European Workshop on Periodontology. J Clin Periodont 35: 333–337.
12. Kapatral V, Anderson I, Ivanova N, Reznik G, Los T, et al. (2002) Genome sequence and analysis of the oral bacterium Fusobacterium nucleatum strain ATCC 25586. J Bacteriol 184: 2005–2018.
13. Nelson KE, Fleischmann RD, DeBoy RT, Paulsen IT, Fouts DE, et al. (2003) Complete genome sequence of the oral pathogenic bacterium *Porphyromonas gingivalis* strain W83. J Bacteriol 185: 5591–5601.
14. Seshadri R, Myers GS, Tettelin H, Eisen JA, Heidelberg JF, et al. (2004) Comparison of the genome of the oral pathogen *Treponema denticola* with other spirochete genomes. Proc Natl Acad Sci U S A 101: 5646–5651.

15. Huttenhover C, Gevers d, Knight R, Abubucker S, Badger JH, et al. (2012) Structure, function and diversity of the healthy human microbiome. Nature 486: 207–214.
16. Griffen AL, Beall CJ, Campbell JH, Firestone ND, Kumar PS, et al. (2011) Distinct and complex bacterial profiles in human periodontitis and health revealed by 16S pyrosequencing. ISME J 6: 1176–1185.
17. Kumar PS, Griffen AL, Moeschberger ML, Leys EJ (2005) Identification of candidate periodontal pathogens and beneficial species by quantitative 16S clonal analysis. J Clin Microbiol 43: 3944–3955.
18. Wade WG (2012) The oral microbiome in health and disease. Pharmacol Res S1043–6618(12)00227–7. doi: 10.1016/j.phrs.2012.11.006. [Epub ahead of print].
19. Abusleme L, Dupuy AK, Dutzan N, Silva N, Burleson JA, et al. (2013) The subgingival microbiome in health and periodontitis and its relationship with community biomass and inflammation. ISME J doi: 10.1038/ismej.2012.174. [Epub ahead of print].
20. Boopathy R, Robichaux M, LaFont D, Howell M (2002) Activity of sulfate-reducing bacteria in human periodontal pocket. Canadian J Microbiol 48: 1099–1103.
21. Langendijk PS, Hanssen JTJ, Van der Hoeven JS (2000) Sulfate-reducing bacteria in association with human periodontitis. J Clin Periodont 27: 943–950.
22. Vianna ME, Holtgraewe S, Seyfarth I, Conrads G, Horz HP (2008) Quantitative analysis of three hydrogenotrophic microbial groups, methanogenic archaea, sulfate-reducing bacteria, and acetogenic bacteria, within plaque biofilms associated with human periodontal disease. J Bacteriol 190: 3779–3785.
23. Wade WG, Munson MA, de Lillo A, Weightman AJ (2005) Specificity of the oral microflora in dentinal caries, endodontic infections and periodontitis. Int Cong Ser 1284: 150–157.
24. Kumar PS, Griffen AL, Barton JA, Paster BJ, Moeschberger ML, et al. (2003) New bacterial species associated with chronic periodontitis. J Dent Res 82: 338–344.
25. Pagani I, Lapidus A, Nolan M, Lucas S, Hammon N, et al. (2011) Complete genome sequence of *Desulfobulbus propionicus* type strain (1pr3(T)). Stand Gen Sci 4: 100–110.
26. Langendijk PS, Kulik EM, Sandmeier H, Meyer J, van der Hoeven JS (2001) Isolation of Desulfomicrobium orale sp nov and Desulfovibrio strain NY682, oral sulfate-reducing bacteria involved in human periodontal disease. Int J Sys Evol Microbiol 51: 1035–1044.
27. Loubinoux J, Mory F, Pereira IAC, Le Faou AE (2000) Bacteremia caused by a strain of Desulfovibrio related to the provisionally named *Desulfovibrio fairfieldensis*. J Clin Microbiol 38: 1707–1707.
28. Pimentel JD, Chan RC (2007) *Desulfovibrio fairfieldensis* bacteremia associated with choledocholithiasis and endoscopic retrograde Cholangiopancreatography. J Clin Microbiol 45: 2747–2750.
29. Amann RI, Binder BJ, Olson RJ, Chisholm SW, Devereux R, et al. (1990) Combination of 16S rRNA-targeted oligonucleotide probes with flow cytometry for analyzing mixed microbial populations. Appl Environ Microbiol 56: 1919–1925.
30. Loy A, Lehner A, Lee N, Adamczyk J, Meier H, et al. (2002) Oligonucleotide microarray for 16S rRNA gene-based detection of all recognized lineages of sulfate-reducing prokaryotes in the environment. Appl Environ Microbiol 68: 5064–5081.
31. Loubinoux J, Bisson-Boutelliez C, Miller N, Le Faou AE (2002) Isolation of the provisionally named Desulfovibrio fairfieldensis from human periodontal pockets. Oral Microbiol Immunol 17: 321–323.
32. Altschul SF, Gish W, Miller W, Meyers EW, Lipman DJ (1990) Basic local alignment search tool. J Mol Biol 215: 403–410.
33. Widdel F, Pfennig N (1982) Studies on dissimilatory sulfate-reducing bacteria that decompose fatty-acids II. Incomplete oxidation of propionate by *Desulfobulbus propionicus* gen. nov., sp. nov. Arch Microbiol 131: 360–365.
34. Pires RH, Venceslau SS, Morais F, Teixeira M, Xavier AV, et al. (2006) Characterization of the Desulfovibrio desulfuricans ATCC 27774 DsrMKJOP complex - A membrane-bound redox complex involved in the sulfate respiratory pathway. Biochemistry 45: 249–262.
35. Tasaki M, Kamagata Y, Nakamura K, Okamura K, Minami K (1993) Acetogenesis from pyruvate by *Desulfotomaculum thermobenzoicum* and differences in pyruvate metabolism among 3 sulfate-reducing bacteria in the absence of sulfate. FEMS Microbiol Letters 106: 259–264.
36. Van Melderen L, Saavedra De Bast M (2009) Bacterial Toxin-Antitoxin Systems: More Than Selfish Entities? PLoS Genet 5: e1000437.
37. Mattick JS (2002) Type IV pili and twitching motility. Ann Rev Microbiol 56: 289–314.
38. Li YX, Hao GX, Galvani CD, Meng YZ, De la Fuente L, et al. (2007) Type I and type IV pili of *Xylella fastidiosa* affect twitching motility, biofilm formation and cell-cell aggregation. Microbiol 153: 719–726.
39. Cascales E, Christie PJ (2003) The versatile bacterial type IV secretion systems. Nature Rev Microbiol 1: 137–149.
40. Clock SA, Planet PJ, Perez BA, Figurski DH (2008) Outer membrane components of the tad (tight adherence) secreton of *Aggregatibacter actinomycetemcomitans*. J Bacteriol 190: 980–990.
41. Fernandez L, Marquez I, Guijarro JA (2004) Identification of specific in vivo-induced (ivi) genes in Yersinia ruckeri and analysis of ruckerbactin, a catecholate siderophore iron acquisition system. Appl Environ Microbiol 70: 5199–5207.
42. Fuller TE, Kennedy MJ, Lowery DE (2000) Identification of Pasteurella multocida virulence genes in a septicemic mouse model using signature-tagged mutagenesis. Microb Pathogen 29: 25–38.
43. Murakami S, Nakashima R, Yamashita E, Yamaguchi A (2002) Crystal structure of bacterial multidrug efflux transporter AcrB. Nature 419: 587–593.
44. Dannenberg S, Kroder M, Dilling W, Cypionka H (1992) Oxidation of H-2, organic compounds and inorganic sulfur compounds coupled to reduction of O-2 or nitrate by sulfate-reducing bacteria. Arch Microbiol 158: 93–99.
45. Cypionka H (2000) Oxygen respiration by *Desulfovibrio* species. Ann Rev Microbiol 54: 827–848.
46. Sun H, Spring S, Lapidus A, Davenport K, Del Rio TG, et al. (2010) Complete genome sequence of *Desulfarculus baarsii* type strain (2st14(T)). Stand Gen Sci 3: 276–284.
47. Wang RK, Kaplan A, Guo LH, Shi WY, Zhou XD, et al. (2012) The influence of iron availability on human salivary microbial community composition. Microb Ecol 64: 152–161.
48. Capestany CA, Tribble GD, Maeda K, Demuth DR, Lamont RJ (2008) Role of the Clp system in stress tolerance, Biofilm formation, and intracellular invasion in *Porphyromonas gingivalis*. J Bacteriol 190: 1436–1446.
49. Lourdault K, Cerqueira GM, Wunder EA, Picardeau M (2011) Inactivation of clpB in the Pathogen *Leptospira interrogans* Reduces Virulence and Resistance to Stress Conditions. Infect Immun 79: 3711–3717.
50. de Oliveira NEM, Abranches J, Gaca AO, Laport MS, Damaso CR, et al. (2011) *clpB*, a class III heat-shock gene regulated by CtsR, is involved in thermotolerance and virulence of *Enterococcus faecalis*. Microbiol 157: 656–665.
51. Loughlin MF, Arandhara V, Okolie C, Aldsworth TG, Jenks PJ (2009) *Helicobacter pylori* mutants defective in the clpP ATP-dependant protease and the chaperone clpA display reduced macrophage and murine survival. Microb Pathogen 46: 53–57.
52. Winther-Larsen HC, Hegge FT, Wolfgang M, Hayes SF, van Putten JPM, et al. (2001) *Neisseria gonorrhoeae* PilV, a type IV pilus-associated protein essential to human epithelial cell adherence. Proc Natl Acad Sci U S A 98: 15276–15281.
53. Ajdic D, McShan WM, McLaughlin RE, Savic G, Chang J, et al. (2002) Genome sequence of Streptococcus mutans UA159, a cariogenic dental pathogen. Proc Natl Acad Sci U S A 99: 14434–14439.
54. Roberts IS (1996) The biochemistry and genetics of capsular polysaccharide production in bacteria. Annual Review of Microbiology 50: 285–315.
55. An FY, Clewell DB (1994) Characterization of the determinant (traB) encoding sex pheromone shutdown by the hemolysin/bacteriocin plasmid pAD1 in *Enterococcus faecalis*. Plasmid 31: 215–221.
56. Reddy M (2007) Role of FtsEX in cell division of *Escherichia coli*: viability of ftsEX mutants is dependent on functional SufI or high osmotic strength. J Bacteriol 189: 98–108.
57. Worley MJ, Ching KHL, Heffron F (2000) *Salmonella* SsrB activates a global regulon of horizontally acquired genes. Molec Microbiol 36: 749–761.
58. Garcia-Calderon CB, Casadesus J, Ramos-Morales F (2007) Rcs and PhoPQ regulatory overlap in the control of *Salmonella enterica* virulence. J Bacteriol 189: 6635–6644.
59. Frye J, Karlinsey JE, Felise HR, Marzolf B, Dowidar N, et al. (2006) Identification of new flagellar genes of *Salmonella enterica* serovar *typhimurium*. J Bacteriol 188: 2233–2243.
60. Fink RC, Evans MR, Porwollik S, Vazquez-Torres A, Jones-Carson J, et al. (2007) FNR is a global regulator of virulence and anaerobic metabolism in Salmonella enterica serovar typhimurium (ATCC 14028s). J Bacteriol 189: 2262–2273.
61. Meng GY, Spahich N, Kenjale R, Waksman G, St Geme JW (2011) Crystal structure of the *Haemophilus influenzae* Hap adhesin reveals an intercellular oligomerization mechanism for bacterial aggregation. EMBO J 30: 3864–3874.
62. Mougous JD, Gifford CA, Ramsdell TL, Mekalanos JJ (2007) Threonine phosphorylation post-translationally regulates protein secretion in *Pseudomonas aeruginosa*. Nature Cell Biol 9: 797–U121.
63. Casabona MG, Silverman JM, Sall KM, Boyer F, Couté Y, et al. (2012) An ABC transporter and an outer membrane lipoprotein participate in posttranslational activation of type VI secretion in *Pseudomonas aeruginosa*. Environmental microbiology: no-no.
64. Lucker S, Steger D, Kjeldsen KU, MacGregor BJ, Wagner M, et al. (2007) Improved 16S rRNA-targeted probe set for analysis of sulfate-reducing bacteria by fluorescence in situ hybridization. J Microbiol Meth 69: 523–528.
65. Fuchs BM, Pernthaler J, Amann R (2007) Single cell identification by fluorescence *in situ* hybridization. In: Reddy CA, Beveridge TJ, Breznak JA, Marzluf G, Schmidt TM et al., editors. Methods for General and Molecular Microbiology. 3rd ed. Washington, D.C.: ASM Press. 886–896.
66. Stoecker K, Dorninger C, Daims H, Wagner M (2010) Double Labeling of Oligonucleotide Probes for Fluorescence In Situ Hybridization (DOPE-FISH) Improves Signal Intensity and Increases rRNA Accessibility. Appl Environ Microbiol 76: 922–926.
67. Stepanauskas R, Sieracki ME (2007) Matching phylogeny and metabolism in the uncultured marine bacteria, one cell at a time. Proc Natl Acad Sci U S A 104: 9052–9057.
68. Rodrigue S, Malmstrom RR, Berlin AM, Birren BW, Henn MR, et al. (2009) Whole genome amplification and de novo assembly of single bacterial cells. PLoS One 4: e6864.

69. Tamariz J, Voynarovska K, Prinz M, Caragine T (2006) The application of ultraviolet irradiation to exogenous sources of DNA in plasticware and water for the amplification of low copy number DNA. J Forensic Sci 51: 790–794.
70. Blainey PC, Quake SR (2011) Digital MDA for enumeration of total nucleic acid contamination. Nucl Acids Res 39.
71. Weisburg WG, Barns SM, Pelletier DA, Lane DJ (1991) 16S ribosomal DNA amplification for phylogenetic study. J Bacteriol 173: 697–703.
72. Wang Q, Garrity GM, Tiedje JM, Cole JR (2007) Naive Bayesian classifier for rapid assignment of rRNA sequences into the new bacterial taxonomy. Appl Environ Microbiol 73: 5261–5267.
73. Swan BK, Martinez-Garcia M, Preston CM, Sczyrba A, Woyke T, et al. (2011) Potential for Chemolithoautotrophy Among Ubiquitous Bacteria Lineages in the Dark Ocean. Science 333: 1296–1300.
74. Brown CT, Howe A, Zhang Q, Pyrkosz AB, Brom TH (2012) A Reference-Free Algorithm for Computational Normalization of Shotgun Sequencing Data. arXiv 1203.4802 [q-bio.GN].
75. Zerbino DR, Birney E (2008) Velvet: Algorithms for de novo short read assembly using de Bruijn graphs. Genome Res 18: 821–829.
76. Hyatt D, Chen G-L, LoCascio PF, Land ML, Larimer FW, et al. (2010) Prodigal: prokaryotic gene recognition and translation initiation site identification. BMC Bioinformatics 11: 1–11.
77. Markowitz VM, Chen I-MA, Palaniappan K, Chu K, Szeto E, et al. (2012) IMG: the integrated microbial genomes database and comparative analysis system. Nucl Acids Res 40: D115–D122.
78. Aziz RK, Bartels D, Best AA, DeJongh M, Disz T, et al. (2008) The RAST Server: rapid annotations using subsystems technology. BMC Genomics 9: 75.
79. Woyke T, Xie G, Copeland A, Gonzalez JM, Han C, et al. (2009) Assembling the marine metagenome, one cell at a time. PLoS One 4: e5299.
80. Richter M, Rossello-Mora R (2009) Shifting the genomic gold standard for the prokaryotic species definition. Proc Natl Acad Sci U S A 106: 19126–19131.
81. Darling ACE, Mau B, Blattner FR, Perna NT (2004) Mauve: Multiple alignment of conserved genomic sequence with rearrangements. Genome Res 14: 1394–1403.
82. Punta M, Coggill PC, Eberhardt RY, Mistry J, Tate J, et al. (2012) The Pfam protein families database. Nucl Acids Res 40: D290–D301.
83. Eddy SR (2011) Accelerated Profile HMM Searches. PLoS Comput Biol 7: e1002195.
84. Guindon S, Dufayard JF, Lefort V, Anisimova M, Hordijk W, et al. (2010) New algorithms and methods to estimate maximum-likelihood phylogenies: assessing the performance of PhyML 3.0. Syst Biol 59: 307–321.

9

Interactions of Adiponectin and Lipopolysaccharide from *Porphyromonas gingivalis* on Human Oral Epithelial Cells

Dominik Kraus[1,2], Jochen Winter[2,3], Søren Jepsen[2,3], Andreas Jäger[2,4], Rainer Meyer[5], James Deschner[2,6*]

1 Department of Prosthodontics, Preclinical Education, and Material Sciences, University of Bonn, Bonn, Germany, **2** Clinical Research Unit 208, University of Bonn, Bonn, Germany, **3** Department of Periodontology, Operative and Preventive Dentistry, University of Bonn, Bonn, Germany, **4** Department of Orthodontics, University of Bonn, Bonn, Germany, **5** Institute of Physiology II, University of Bonn, Bonn, Germany, **6** Experimental Dento-Maxillo-Facial Medicine, University of Bonn, Bonn, Germany

Abstract

Background: Periodontitis is an inflammatory disease caused by pathogenic microorganisms, such as *Porphyromonas gingivalis*, and characterized by the destruction of the periodontium. Obese individuals have an increased risk for periodontitis and show decreased serum levels of adiponectin. This in-vitro study was established to examine whether adiponectin modulates critical effects of lipopolysaccharide (LPS) from *P. gingivalis* on oral epithelial cells (OECs).

Methodology/Principal Findings: The presence of adiponectin and its receptors in human gingival tissue samples and OECs was analyzed by immunohistochemistry and PCR. Furthermore, OECs were treated with LPS and/or adiponectin for up to 72 h, and the gene expression and protein synthesis of pro- and anti-inflammatory mediators, matrix metalloproteinases (MMPs) and growth factors were analyzed by real-time PCR and ELISA. Additionally, cell proliferation, differentiation and in-vitro wound healing were studied. The nuclear translocation of NFκB was investigated by immunofluorescence. Gingival tissue sections showed a strong synthesis of adiponectin and its receptors in the epithelial layer. In cell cultures, LPS induced a significant up-regulation of interleukin (IL) 1β, IL6, IL8, MMP1 and MMP3. Adiponectin abrogated significantly the stimulatory effects of LPS on these molecules. Similarly, adiponectin inhibited significantly the LPS-induced decrease in cell viability and increase in cell proliferation and differentiation. Adiponectin led to a time-dependent induction of the anti-inflammatory mediators IL10 and heme oxygenase 1, and blocked the LPS-stimulated NFκB nuclear translocation.

Conclusions/Significance: Adiponectin may counteract critical actions of *P. gingivalis* on oral epithelial cells. Low levels of adiponectin, as observed in obese individuals, may increase the risk for periodontal inflammation and destruction.

Editor: Markus M. Heimesaat, Charité, Campus Benjamin Franklin, Germany

Funding: This study was supported by a grant from the German Research Foundation (KFO 208/TP4/TP9) and the University of Bonn, Germany. The funders had no role in study design, data collection and analysis, decision to publish, or preparation of the manuscript.

Competing Interests: The authors have declared that no competing interests exist.

* E-mail: james.deschner@uni-bonn.de

Introduction

Periodontitis is a chronic inflammatory disease and characterized by the progressive destruction of the tooth-supporting tissues, i.e. periodontium. The disease is caused by pathogenic bacteria embedded in a biofilm on the tooth surface and leads to epithelial proliferation in combination with periodontal pocket formation, increased tooth mobility and even tooth loss [1]. Based on data from the National Health and Nutrition Examination Survey (NHANES) III, which assessed the health and nutritional status in the United States, it is estimated that half of the US population aged over 30 years suffers from periodontitis [2]. Periodontitis has a significant negative impact on a wide range of physical, psychological and social aspects of quality of life in affected individuals [3,4]. Furthermore, periodontal infections are associated with cardiovascular diseases, diabetes mellitus, arthritis, preterm low birth weight and other systemic diseases and conditions [5].

Although a variety of microorganisms have been associated with periodontitis, *Porphyromonas gingivalis* represents one of the main etiologic agents in the initiation and progression of periodontal diseases, and is found more frequently and in higher numbers at sites of periodontal inflammation [6]. *P. gingivalis* is characterized by a great number of virulence factors with proteases, such as gingipains, being the most important ones [7]. Another key virulence factor of *P. gingivalis* is lipopolysaccharide (LPS) [8]. LPS is the major macromolecule on the outer surface of gram-negative microorganisms and binds to a Toll-like receptor (TLR) 4–MD-2–CD14 protein complex. However, LPS of *P. gingivalis* is different from those of enterobacteria in that LPS of *P. gingivalis* also signals through TLR2 and is less potent in inducing an inflammatory reaction [8–10]. The oral epithelium is the first physical barrier, which periodontopathogenic bacteria encounter [6]. By the release of pro-inflammatory and chemotactic cytokines, matrix-degrading enzymes and prostaglandins, oral epithelial cells, which express TLRs, function as non-professional inflammatory cells and help professional cells of the innate and adaptive immune system to clear the bacterial infection [11–13]. Therefore, oral epithelial cells can actively participate in periodontal inflammation. However, a balance between pro- and anti-inflammatory mediators is critical. If the inflammatory response is exaggerated, irreversible loss of periodontal tissues occurs [14,15]. Levels of pro-inflammatory cytokines, such as interleukin (IL) 1β, IL6, and IL8, which promote recruitment and activation of professional inflammatory cells, are increased at inflamed sites [16–18]. Although anti-inflammatory mediators, such as IL10, antagonize the pro-inflammatory activities, the balance between pro- and anti-inflammatory mediators is shifted towards inflammation [14,15]. In response to pathogenic microorganisms and inflammatory mediators, resident cells and infiltrated inflammatory cells of the periodontium release enzymes, such as matrix metalloproteinases (MMPs). MMPs can cleave all components of the extracellular matrix and, additionally, activate, deactivate, or modify non-matrix bioactive molecules [19]. In periodontitis, the balance between matrix synthesis and degradation is disrupted and shifted towards periodontal tissue destruction [19].

As mentioned above, periodontitis has been shown to affect systemic health. Conversily, systemic diseases, such as diabetes mellitus, can also increase the risk of periodontitis. Recent meta-analyses have revealed that obesity is also significantly associated with periodontitis, and it has been suggested that adipokines, such as adiponectin, which are cytokines released from the adipose tissue, might be a critical pathomechanistic link in this association [20–22]. Adipokines not only regulate food intake and energy expenditure, but also immune, inflammatory and wound healing processes. For example, adiponectin plays an anti-inflammatory role in the pathophysiology of several chronic inflammatory diseases [23,24]. Heme oxygenase 1 (HMOX1) has recently been identified as an important downstream mediator for the anti-inflammatory actions of adiponectin in primary cultures of Kupffer cells [25]. HMOX1 catabolizes heme into carbon monoxide, biliverdin and free iron, which then exert the anti-inflammatory, anti-apoptotic and anti-proliferative effects of HMOX1 [26]. Besides its effects on inflammatory mediators, adiponectin has also been shown to be involved in cell proliferation and differentiation [27]. A common marker of keratinocyte differentiation is involucrin, which first appears in the cytoplasm of differentiating cells in the stratum spinosum and is then cross-linked to membrane proteins in the stratum granulosum by the action of transglutaminase enzymes, which provides structural support to the cells [28–30].

Since serum levels of adiponectin have been shown to be negatively correlated with overweight and obesity, the beneficial effects of adiponectin are significantly reduced in overweight and obese individuals [31]. Whether adiponectin regulates the function of periodontal cells and inflammatory processes in periodontitis is as yet unknown. This in-vitro study was established to examine whether adiponectin inhibits the response of oral epithelial cells to LPS from *P. gingivalis* and, thereby, to test the hypothesis that decreased levels of adiponectin may confer an increased risk of periodontal destruction.

Materials and Methods

Isolation and culture of human oral epithelial cells

Healthy gingival tissues were obtained from six donors, who underwent tooth extraction and/or dentoalveolar surgery. Written informed parental consent and approval of the Ethics Committee of the University of Bonn were obtained. The gingival specimens were washed twice with phosphate buffered saline (PBS; PAA Laboratories, Cölbe, Germany) supplemented with 1% antibiotic and antimycotic solution (PAA Laboratories) and subsequently digested with collagenase 2 solution (PAA Laboratories) at 37°C for 2.5 h. Afterwards, the epithelium was mechanically separated from the underlying connective tissue layer with sterile forceps. In order to obtain a single cell suspension, the epithelium was then dissociated with 0.05% trypsin in 0.02% EDTA solution (PAA Laboratories) at 37°C for 15 min. After centrifugation, epithelial cells were resuspended in serum-free keratinocyte growth medium (KGM2; Promocell, Heidelberg, Germany) supplemented with 1% antibiotic and antimycotic solution, and grown at 37°C in a humidified atmosphere of 5% CO_2. Cells were used at passage three and medium was changed every other day. For evaluation of cell viability, epithelial cells were stained with trypan blue solution (Sigma-Aldrich, Munich, Germany) and, subsequently, live and dead cells were counted.

Cell stimulation

Cells were stimulated with ultrapure LPS from *P. gingivalis* (2 μg/ml; Cayla-InvivoGen, Toulouse, France) and/or recombinant human full-length adiponectin (1 μg/ml; R&D Systems, Wiesbaden, Germany) for up to 72 h. The concentrations applied were based on the results from other studies to ensure that data are comparable [11,13,32]. Furthermore, pre-experiments showed that these concentrations had a significant stimulatory effect on pro- and anti-inflammatory cytokines and, therefore, allowed to examine the interactions of LPS and adiponectin on epithelial cells (data not shown).

Reverse transcription-PCR

Total RNA was isolated using the RNeasy Protect Mini Kit (Qiagen, Hilden, Germany) and quantified using the NanoDrop®ND-1000 Spectrophotometer (NanoDrop Technologies, Wilmington, DE, USA). A total of 1 μg of RNA was reversely transcribed using iScript™ Select cDNA Synthesis Kit (Bio-Rad Laboratories, Munich, Germany) with oligo(dT)-primers according to the manufacturer's protocol. The gene expression of adiponectin and its receptors AdipoR1 and AdipoR2, IL1β, IL6, IL8, IL10, heme oxygenase 1 (HMOX1), MMP1, MMP3, transforming growth factor (TGF) β1, keratinocyte growth factor (KGF), and involucrin was detected by real-time PCR using the iCycler iQ detection system (Bio-Rad Laboratories), SYBR Green (Bio-Rad Laboratories), and specific primers (Metabion, Martinsried, Germany). Primer sequences, annealing temperatures and efficiencies are presented in Table 1. Real-time PCR was performed by adding 50 ng cDNA to a master mix containing primers and iQ™ SYBR® Green Supermix (Bio-Rad Laboratories). Cloned PCR-products derived from the specific primers served as positive controls, whereas water was used as negative control. PCR conditions were defined as follows: 5 min preceding denaturation step at 95°C was succeeded by 50 cycles of 15 s at 95°C, 30 s at annealing temperatures specific for the primers, and 30 s at 72°C for elongation. Relative differential gene expression was calculated using the method described by Pfaffl [33] with β-actin serving as house-keeping gene. Additionally, the PCR products for adiponectin, AdipoR1 and AdipoR2 were visualized by 2% agarose gel electrophoresis and ethidium bromide staining.

ELISA

The concentrations of IL1β, IL8 and MMP1 in culture supernatants at 24 h and 72 h were analyzed by a commercially available enzyme-linked immunoassay (ELISA) kit (RayBiotech, Norcross, USA) according to the manufacturer's instructions. The absorbance was measured with a microplate reader (Bio-Rad Laboratories) at 450 nm. The data were normalized by the cell number, which was measured with an automatic cell counter (Moelab, Hilden, Germany).

Table 1. Sequences, efficiency and annealing temperature of primers.

Gene		Primer sequences	Efficiency	Annealing temperature
Adiponectin	sense antisense	5′-GCCTCTTCAAGAAGGACAAGGCTATG -3′ 5′-CAGTTGGTGTCATGGTAGAGAAG -3′	1.93	69°C
AdipoR1	sense antisense	5′-ACTGGAGCTGGCCTTTATGCTGC -3′ 5′-AGAGAAGGGTGTCATCAGTACAGC -3′	2.04	69°C
AdipoR2	sense antisense	5′-CCATAGGGCAGATAGGCTGGTTGA -3′ 5′-CAGTGCATCCTCTTCACTGCAGC -3′	1.97	69°C
β-actin	sense antisense	5′-CATGGATGATGATATCGCCGCG-3′ 5′-ACATGATCTGGGTCATCTTCTCG-3′	1.84	69°C
HMOX1	sense antisense	5′-CCAGGCAGAGAATGCTGAGTTCAT-3′ 5′-CCGTACCAGAAGGCCAGGTCC-3′	1.97	69°C
IL1β	sense antisense	5′-ATGGCAGAAGTACCTGAGCTCGC-3′ 5′-TTAGGAAGACACAAATTGCATGGTG-3′	1.83	68°C
IL6	sense antisense	5′-ATGAACTCCTTCTCCACAAGC-3′ 5′-CTACATTTGCCGAAGAGCCC-3′	2.12	68°C
IL8	sense antisense	5′-ATGACTTCCAAGCTGGCCGTGG-3′ 5′-TGAATTCTCAGCCCTCTTCAAAAAC-3′	2.02	68°C
IL10	sense antisense	5′-TTAAGGGTTACCTGGGTTGC-3′ 5′-GCCTTGCTCTTGTTTTCACA-3′	1.94	65°C
MMP1	sense antisense	5′-ATGCACAGCTTTCCTCCACTGC-3′ 5′-CACTGGGCCACTATTTCTCCGC-3′	2.05	69°C
MMP3	sense antisense	5′-ATCGATGCAGCCATTTCTGATAAGG-3′ 5′-TCAACAATTAAGCCAGCTGTTACT-3′	2.06	69°C
Involucrin	sense antisense	5′-CCCAGCAACACACACTGCCAGT-3′ 5′-GCTCAGGCAGTCCCTTTACAGCA-3′	1.98	69°C
TGFβ1	sense antisense	5′-GAGCCCTGGACACCAACTAT-3′ 5′-GACCTTGCTGTACTGCGTGT-3′	1.94	69°C
KGF	sense antisense	5′-AGTTGGAATTGTGGCAATCA-3′ 5′-CCGTTGTGTGTCCATTTAGC-3′	1.84	65°C

Proliferation assay

The epithelial cell proliferation was determined by using the PromoKine XTT Cell Proliferation Kit (Promocell). Following stimulation with LPS and/or adiponectin for 24 h and 48 h, cells were incubated with XTT reaction solution for 4 h. Finally, the absorbance was measured by using a microplate reader at 490 nm.

In-vitro wound healing assay

In order to study the wound fill rate in vitro, we used an established in-vitro wound healing model [34,35]. Briefly, epithelial cells were seeded onto 35 mm culture dishes (Greiner Bio-One, Frickenhausen, Germany) and grown until confluence. Then, defined cell-free areas were created by disrupting the monolayers with sterile instruments in a standardized manner. Subsequently, medium was changed and cells were stimulated, as described above. Pictures of the wounded area were taken on an inverted microscope (Axiovert 25 C, AxioCam, Zeiss, Oberkochen, Germany) immediately after wounding and at 1 d, 2 d and 3 d. The wound areas were then measured and analyzed with the freely available image-processing software ImageJ 1.43 (http://rsb.info.nih.gov/ij). In order to determine the percentage of wound fill, the recovered wound areas at 1 d, 2 d, and 3 d were related to the wound areas measured at baseline.

Immunohistochemistry

Gingival tissues were derived from patients who underwent wisdom tooth extraction in the Dept. of Oromaxillofacial Surgery of the University of Bonn. The tissue samples were fixed in 4% buffered formalin (Sigma-Aldrich) and embedded in paraffin. In order to assess the presence of adiponectin, 4 µm thick tissue slices were prepared and immunostaining for adiponectin in the epithelial and subepithelial layers of the gingiva was performed. Briefly, selected sections were deparaffinized, rehydrated and rinsed with tris-buffered saline (TBS, Sigma-Aldrich) for 10 min. Endogenous peroxidase was blocked in a methanol/H_2O_2 (Merck, Darmstadt, Germany) solution in the dark for 45 min. Sections were blocked with 1% bovine serum albumin (BSA, Sigma-Aldrich) at room temperature (RT) for 20 min and incubated with rabbit anti-adiponectin (Santa Cruz Biotechnology, Heidelberg, Germany) in a 1:50 dilution in a humid chamber overnight. Antigen–antibody binding was visualized using the EnVision Detection System Peroxidase/DAB (Dako, Hamburg, Germany) and slides were counterstained with Mayer's haematoxylin.

Immunofluorescence

Oral epithelial cells were grown on coverslips and cultured for 24 h. Cells were fixed in 4% paraformaldehyde (Sigma-Aldrich) for 15 min, washed in PBS and treated with PBS containing 0.1% Triton X-100 (Sigma-Aldrich) for 15 min. Then, cells were washed, blocked with 10% BSA for 1 h at RT and incubated with a rabbit anti-adiponectin antibody (Santa Cruz Biotechnology) in a 1:75 dilution. After washing, cells were incubated with a Cy3-conjugated goat anti-rabbit IgG secondary antibody (1:500; Dianova, Hamburg, Germany) at RT for 1 h. For nuclear staining, cells were treated with DAPI for 5 min. Finally, slides were washed and mounted with Mowiol/DABCO (Roth, Karlsruhe, Germany) for fluorescence microscopic analysis. Cells treated with LPS and/or adiponectin for 2 h were processed in the same manner, except incubation with a rabbit anti-NFκB (p65) antibody (1:100; BioLegend GmbH, Fell, Germany). For quantification, all nuclei were counted in five fields of vision at a primary magnification of 40×. NFκB positive nuclei were plotted as percentage of all nuclei.

Statistical Analysis

Mean ± SEM (n = 6) were calculated. One-way ANOVA and the post-hoc Tukey's multiple comparison test were applied using a statistical software program (GraphPad Software, San Diego, CA, USA). P-values less than 0.05 were considered to be statistically significant.

Results

Presence of adiponectin in oral epithelial cells

Healthy human gingival tissue sections showed a strong adiponectin synthesis in oral epithelial cells, as analyzed by immunohistochemistry. By contrast, only weak staining was found in the subepithelial layer (Fig. 1A and B). The presence of adiponectin in oral epithelium was also confirmed at transcriptional and protein levels in cultured oral epithelial cells, as shown in Fig. 1C–F. Furthermore, oral epithelial cells expressed both receptors for adiponectin (Fig. 1E and F). Taken together, these findings suggest that epithelial cells are a significant source and target of adiponectin in gingival tissues.

Actions of adiponectin on pro- and anti-inflammatory mediators in oral epithelial cells

Adiponectin down-regulated significantly the constitutive mRNA expression of IL1β at 4 h and 24 h, as analyzed by real-time PCR (Fig. 2A). Moreover, adiponectin inhibited significantly the mRNA expression of IL6 at 24 h and of IL8 at 4 h (Fig. 2A). Interestingly, anti-inflammatory mediators were also subject to regulation by adiponectin: After an initial adiponectin-induced down-regulation of IL10 mRNA at 4 h and 8 h, the levels of this anti-inflammatory molecule were significantly increased at 24 h. In addition, the HMOX1 expression was significantly enhanced by adiponectin at 4 h and 8 h (Fig. 2B). In summary, these data suggest that adiponectin regulates the expression of pro- and anti-inflammatory mediators in oral epithelial cells.

Effect of adiponectin on the LPS-stimulated nuclear translocation of NFκB

As shown in Fig. 3A and B, LPS from *P. gingivalis* induced a pronounced nuclear translocation of NFκB at 2 h, whereas no such effect was observed for adiponectin. Interestingly, adiponectin abolished the LPS-stimulated NFκB translocation, as visualized by immunofluorescence (Fig. 3A and B).

Effects of adiponectin on the LPS-induced expression of pro- and anti-inflammatory cytokines

LPS caused a significant up-regulation of the IL1β mRNA expression at 4 h and 8 h but had no stimulatory effect on this cytokine at 24 h (Fig. 4A). Interestingly, adiponectin significantly

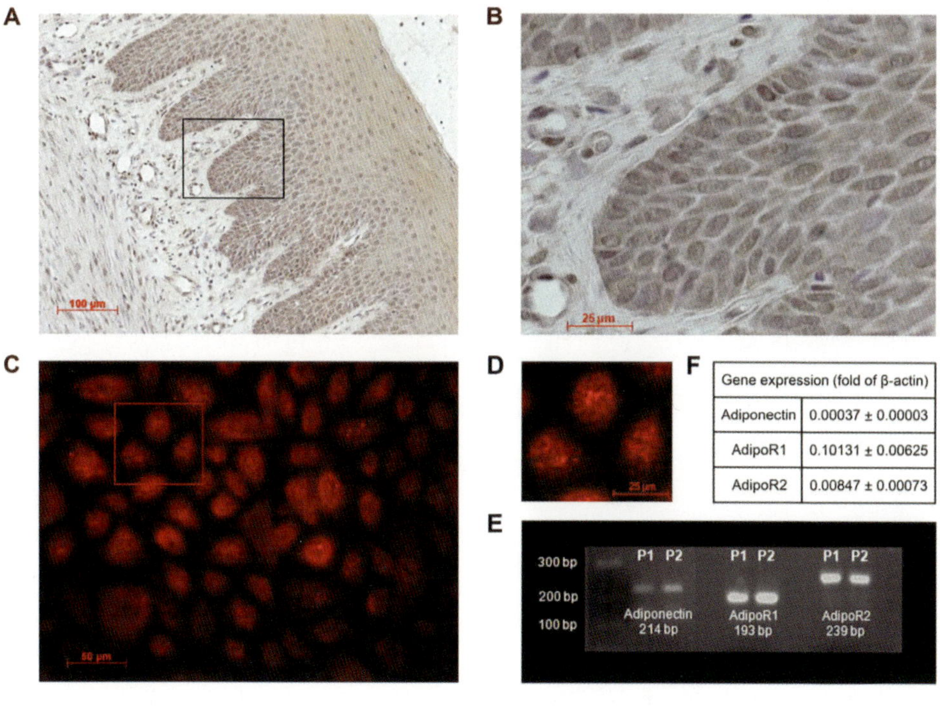

Gene expression (fold of β-actin)	
Adiponectin	0.00037 ± 0.00003
AdipoR1	0.10131 ± 0.00625
AdipoR2	0.00847 ± 0.00073

Figure 1. Adiponectin in gingival tissues and cultured oral epithelial cells. (A) Representative gingival tissue section from one out of 6 patients exhibiting adiponectin distribution assessed by immunohistochemistry with DAB-staining (brown color). (B) Higher magnification of the rectangular area shown in (A). (C) Immunofluorescence staining of adiponectin in cultured oral epithelial cells from one out of 6 patients. (D) Higher magnification of the rectangular area shown in (C). (E) Gene expression of adiponectin and its receptors AdipoR1 and AdipoR2 from oral epithelial cells of 2 patients (P1 and P2), as demonstrated by gel electrophoresis. (F) Gene expression of adiponectin and its receptors AdipoR1 and AdipoR2 from oral epithelial cells from 6 patients, as demonstrated by real-time PCR.

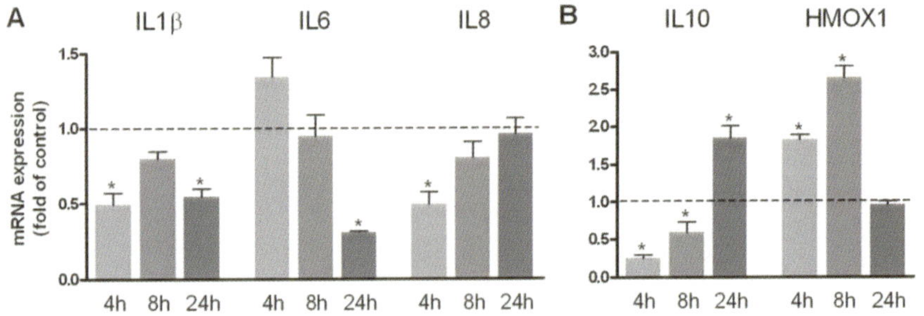

Figure 2. Effects of adiponectin on pro- and anti-inflammatory mediators. Effects of adiponectin (1 μg/ml) on IL1β, IL6 and IL8 (A) as well as IL10 and HMOX1 (B) in oral epithelial cells at 4 h, 8 h, and 24 h. Mean ± SEM; n = 6; * $p<0.05$ difference between adiponectin-treated and control cells.

down-regulated the LPS-induced IL1β expression at 4 h and 8 h, and also led to a significant decrease in the constitutive IL1β expression at 4 h and 24 h (Fig. 4A). Similar findings were observed at protein level at 24 h, as determined in the supernatants by ELISA (Fig. 4B). Furthermore, LPS significantly increased the IL6 mRNA expression at 4 h, 8 h, and 24 h. As observed for IL1β, IL6 was significantly down-regulated by adiponectin in LPS-stimulated cells (Fig. 4C). Although adiponectin did not affect the constitutive IL6 mRNA expression at 4 h and 8 h, this adipokine caused a significant reduction of the constitutive IL6 expression at 24 h (Fig. 4C). The chemokine IL8 was also significantly up-regulated by LPS at 8 h and 24 h (Fig. 4D). The LPS-induced IL8 mRNA expression was significantly reduced by adiponectin at 8 h and 24 h. Additionally, the constitutive mRNA expression of IL8 was down-regulated by adiponectin at 4 h (Fig. 4D). The transcriptional data on IL8 were paralleled by findings at protein level (Fig. 4E). LPS also up-regulated significantly the mRNA expression of the anti-inflammatory cytokine IL10 at 8 h (Fig. 4F). However, adiponectin abrogated the stimulatory effects of LPS on IL10 expression at this time point. Moreover, adiponectin inhibited significantly the constitutive IL10 expression at 4 h and stimulated significantly the constitutive expression of IL10 mRNA at 24 h (Fig. 4F). In summary, these results suggest that adiponectin may dampen inflammatory processes in periodontitis by regulation of pro- and anti-inflammatory cytokines.

Effects of adiponectin on the LPS-induced up-regulation of MMPs

LPS also affected the production of the matrix-degrading proteases MMP1 and MMP3 in epithelial cells (Fig. 5A–C). In the presence of LPS, MMP1 and MMP3 were significantly up-regulated at 8 h and 24 h and at 4 h, 8 h, and 24 h, respectively (Fig. 5A and C). At all time points, adiponectin diminished significantly the LPS-induced mRNA expression of MMP1 and MMP3 (Fig. 5A and C). The stimulatory effect of LPS on MMP1 and the inhibition of the LPS action by adiponectin were also observed at protein level (Fig. 5B). Our data suggest that adiponectin exerts matrix-protective effects by down-regulation of MMPs.

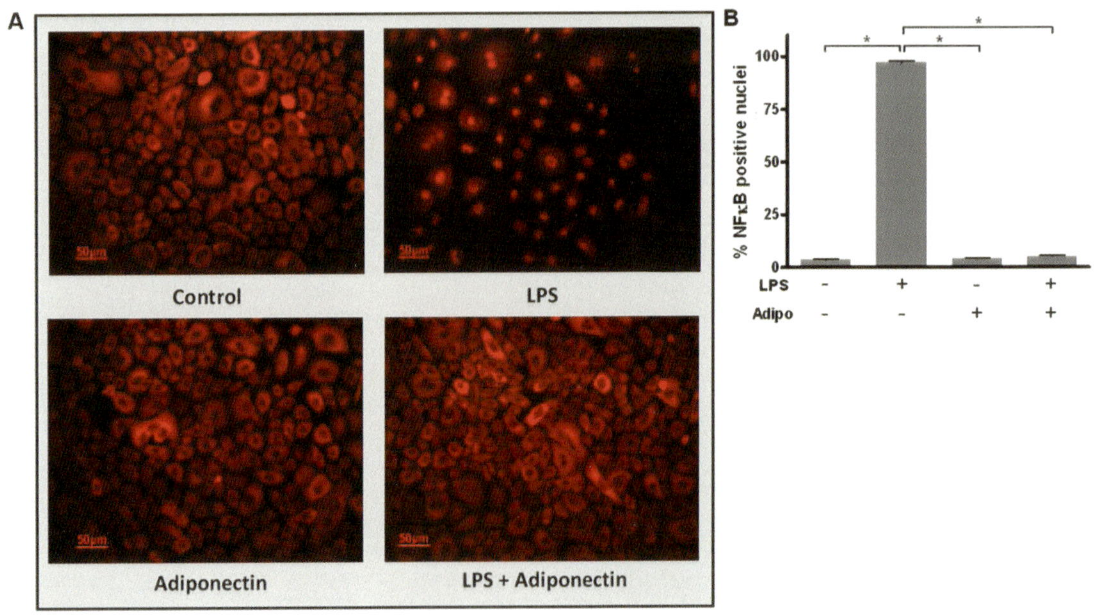

Figure 3. Effect of lipopolysaccharide and/or adiponectin on NFκB signaling. Effect of lipopolysaccharide (LPS; 2 μg/ml) and/or adiponectin (Adipo; 1 μg/ml) on the nuclear translocation of NFκB at 2 h. NFκB visualized by immunofluorescence (A). Quantitative analysis of immunofluorescence samples; evaluation as % NFκB positive nuclei (B).

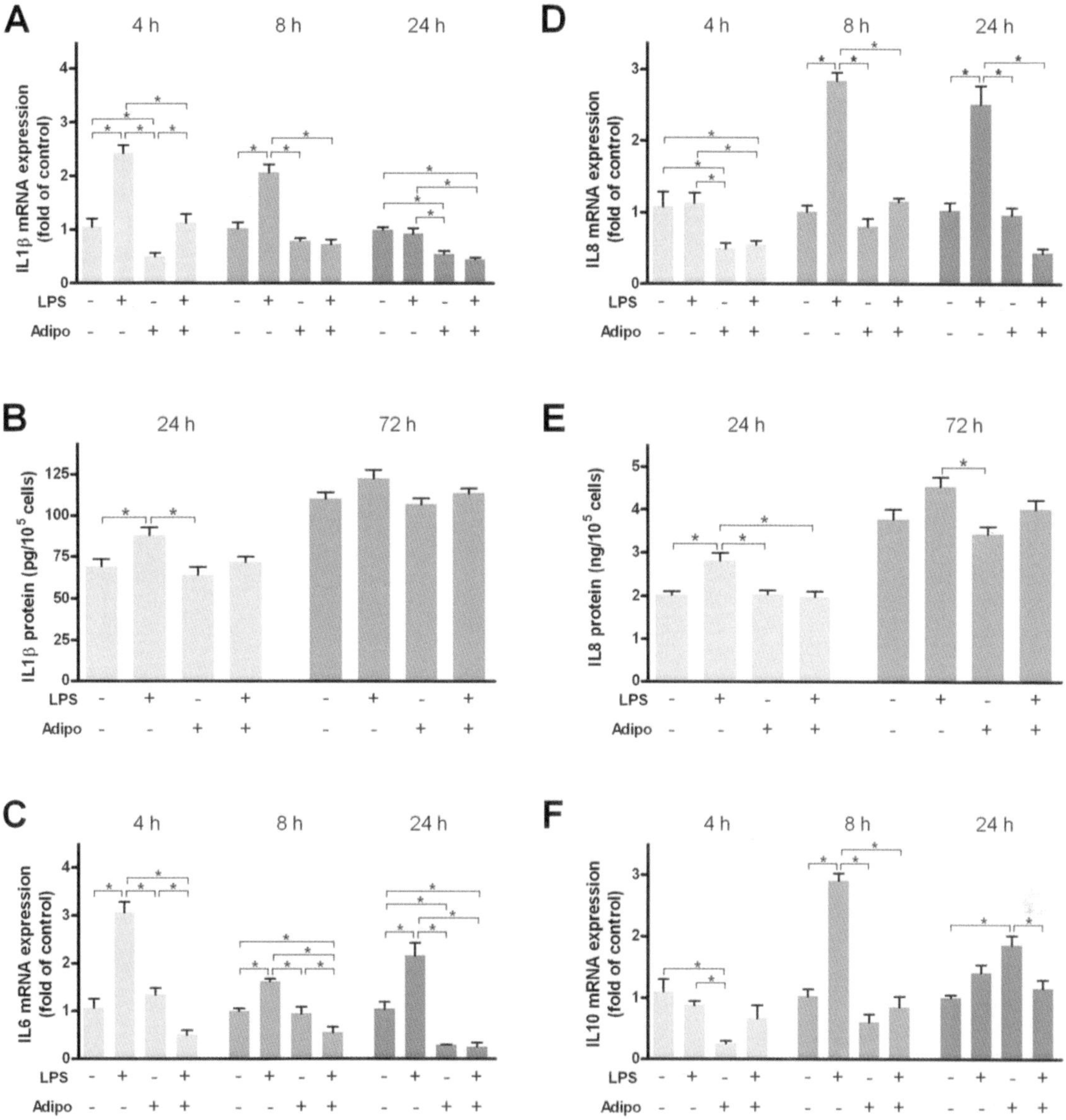

Figure 4. Interactions of lipopolysaccharide and adiponectin on pro- and anti-inflammatory mediators. Effects of lipopolysaccharide (LPS; 2 μg/ml) and/or adiponectin (Adipo; 1 μg/ml) on the mRNA expression of IL1β (A), IL6 (C), IL8 (D), and IL10 (F) at 4 h, 8 h, and 24 h and on the protein level of IL1β (B) and IL8 (E) in supernatants at 24 h and 72 h. Mean ± SEM; n = 6; * $p<0.05$ difference between groups.

Effects of LPS and/or adiponectin on proliferation, cell viability and wound fill rate

Although the epithelial cell proliferation was not strongly affected by LPS and/or adiponectin, the stimulatory effect of LPS was significant at 24 h (Fig. 6A). Interestingly, the LPS-induced increase in epithelial cell proliferation was significantly counter-regulated by adiponectin at this time point. These findings suggest that adiponectin may inhibit the formation of pocket epithelium in the presence of periodontal infection. Furthermore, our experiments revealed, that LPS significantly reduced the percentage of viable cells over a time period of 72 h and that the LPS-induced decrease in cell viability was significantly abolished in the presence of adiponectin (Table 2), indicating that adiponectin may protect against infection-induced damage of epithelial cells and, thereby, increased permeability of the epithelial barrier. Next we studied whether LPS and/or adiponectin modulated the wound closure in an in-vitro wound healing assay over 3 days. The wound closure in cell cultures treated either with LPS or adiponectin alone was not significantly different from that of control cells. However, when cells were simultaneously exposed to LPS and adiponectin, the wound closure was significantly delayed as compared to control (Fig. 6B). These findings suggest that adiponectin, when combined with LPS from *P. gingivalis*, may inhibit the wound fill rate in LPS-treated epithelial cells.

Inhibition of the LPS-induced involucrin expression by adiponectin

LPS increased significantly the involucrin mRNA expression in epithelial cells at 4 h and 8 h. An LPS-induced up-regulation of involucrin was also observed at 24 h but the increase did not reach significance (Table 3). When LPS-treated cells were exposed to adiponectin, the involucrin mRNA expression was significantly reduced (Table 3). These data suggest that adiponectin may inhibit the formation of a pocket epithelium by both inhibition of the

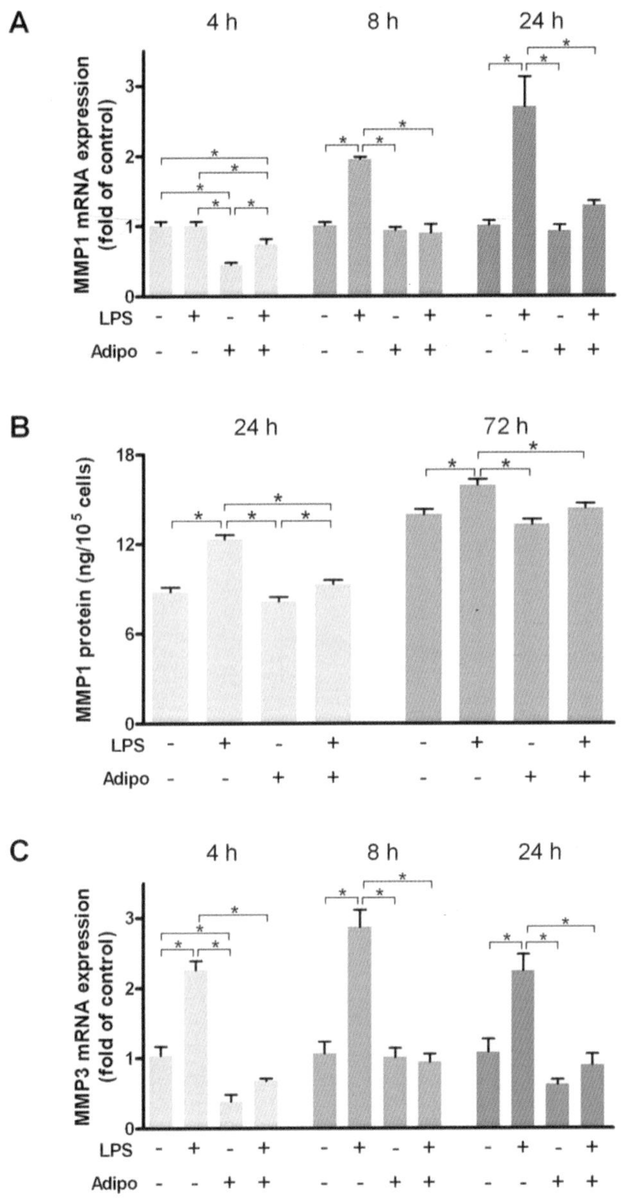

Figure 5. Interactions of lipopolysaccharide and adiponectin on matrix metalloproteinases. Effects of lipopolysaccharide (LPS; 2 μg/ml) and/or adiponectin (Adipo; 1 μg/ml) on the mRNA expression of MMP1 (A) and MMP3 (C) at 4 h, 8 h, and 24 h and on the protein level of MMP1 (B) in supernatants at 24 h and 72 h. Mean ± SEM; n = 6; * $p<0.05$ difference between groups.

LPS-induced proliferation and, additionally, the LPS-stimulated epithelial differentiation.

Regulation of TGFβ1 and KGF by adiponectin and/or LPS

Although the constitutive TGFβ1 expression was not significantly regulated by LPS, adiponectin caused a significant TGFβ1 down-regulation at 4 h and 24 h (Table 3). Adiponectin did not significantly affect TGFβ1 levels in LPS-treated cells (Table 3). Furthermore, LPS significantly up-regulated KGF at 8 h and significantly down-regulated this growth factor at 24 h. Although adiponectin abolished the LPS-increased KGF expression at 8 h, this adipokine had no significant influence on the LPS-down-regulated KGF expression at 24 h. In addition, adiponectin decreased significantly the constitutive KGF mRNA expression at 4 h and 8 h in epithelial cells. In summary, these data suggest that adiponectin may exert inhibitory effects on KGF expression and, therefore, formation of pocket epithelium.

Discussion

Our experiments demonstrated that LPS from *P. gingivalis*, which is considered one of the main etiological agents of periodontal diseases, elicits synthesis of pro-inflammatory cytokines and matrix-degrading enzymes and promotes proliferation and differentiation of oral epithelial cells, emphasizing the pathogenic role of this microorganism in periodontal inflammation, destruction and pocket formation. However, more importantly, our study shows that the LPS-induced effects on oral epithelial cells are counteracted by adiponectin, which is a novel finding and might, at least partially, explain how overweight and obesity can increase the risk of periodontitis.

LPS, which is a major macromolecule on the outer surface of *P. gingivalis*, has been shown to bind to TLR2 and TLR4 [8,10]. Upon receptor engagement, LPS triggers an intracellular signaling cascade, which involves the nuclear transactivation of NFκB [8].

The gingival epithelium is the first physical barrier, which periodontopathogenic bacteria, such as *P. gingivalis*, encounter [6]. Our experiments revealed that *P. gingivalis*-LPS induces the expression and release of pro-inflammatory cytokines in oral epithelial cells, which underlines the detrimental role of this pathogen in periodontal diseases. These findings are in line with several other in-vitro studies, which have also demonstrated a stimulatory effect of *P. gingivalis*-LPS on the synthesis of these inflammatory mediators in oral epithelial cells [11,13,36]. In one of these studies, it was also analyzed whether LPS from *P. gingivalis* induces the release of proteases [36]. *P. gingivalis*-LPS did not affect the secretion of MMP2 and MMP9 in oral epithelial cells. Since MMP1 and MMP3 have also been implicated in periodontal destruction, we studied their expression in oral epithelial cells in response to *P. gingivalis* [37–39]. Interestingly, both MMPs were up-regulated by LPS, suggesting that LPS from *P. gingivalis* can promote periodontal destruction via stimulation of both inflammation and matrix-degradation. In one study, oral epithelial cells were exposed to *P. gingivalis*-derived membrane vesicles, which retain the full components of the outer membrane constituents, including LPS [12]. The expression of IL6, IL8, MMP1, and MMP3 were significantly up-regulated in the vesicle-stimulated cells, which is in accordance with our data for LPS. The most important and novel finding of our study is that the pro-inflammatory and matrix-degrading effects of LPS on oral epithelial cells were significantly reduced in the presence of adiponectin. This observation is in accordance with several studies on monocytes and macrophages [25,32,40]. However, periodontopathogens, such as *P. gingivalis*, will usually first encounter oral epithelial cells, which are present in the gingiva in great numbers. Therefore, our finding, that the protective actions of adiponectin are not limited to immunoinflammatory cells in the gingiva, might be of utmost importance.

A few studies have suggested that adiponectin also exerts pro-inflammatory and tissue-destructive effects [41,42]. It has even been speculated that an initial up-regulation of pro-inflammatory mediators by adiponectin might also be the cause for the subsequent anti-inflammatory effects of this adipokine [43,44]. Moreover, this initial pro-inflammatory effect might result from contamination of adiponectin with LPS during the manufacture process [45]. Interestingly, such an initial adiponectin-induced increase of pro-inflammatory cytokines was not observed in our

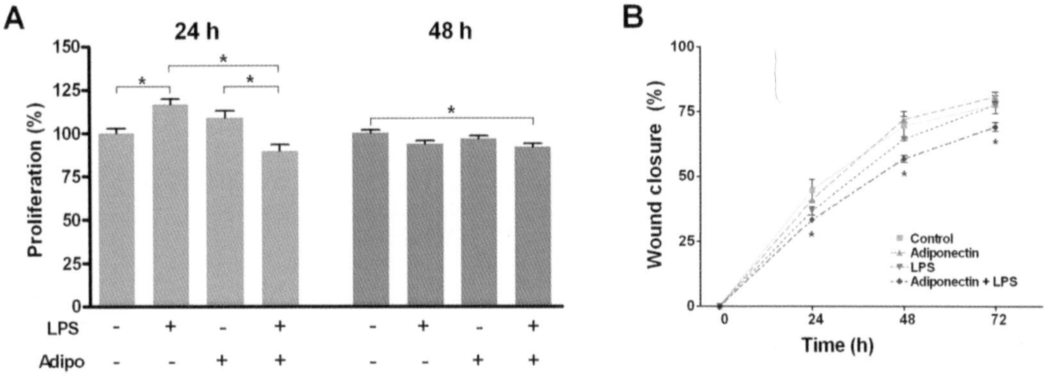

Figure 6. Interactions of lipopolysaccharide and adiponectin on proliferation and wound closure. Effects of lipopolysaccharide (LPS; 2 μg/ml) and/or adiponectin (Adipo; 1 μg/ml) on the proliferation at 24 h and 48 h (A) and wound closure over 72 h (B). Mean ± SEM; * $p<0.05$ difference between groups (A) and difference between cells simultaneously treated with LPS and adiponectin, and control (A).

study. Furthermore, IL10 has been shown to mediate some of the anti-inflammatory effects of adiponectin [25,40,43]. In the present study, we did not perform blocking experiments for IL10. However, the pro-inflammatory cytokines were already down-regulated by adiponectin at 4 h, when the IL10 expression was not yet increased by LPS and/or adiponectin, indicating that IL10 may not play a role in the anti-inflammatory actions of adiponectin at this early time point. Whether adiponectin mediates anti-inflammatory effects via up-regulation of IL10 at later time points, as observed at 24 h, needs to be further determined. Recently, HMOX1 has been identified as another important downstream mediator for the anti-inflammatory actions of adiponectin in primary cultures of Kupffer cells [25]. Interestingly, HMOX1 was significantly up-regulated by adiponectin in oral epithelial cells, suggesting that HMOX1 might be responsible, at least in part, for the anti-inflammatory effects of adiponectin in our study. Finally, adiponectin might interfere with the binding of LPS to its receptor because of the high binding affinity of adiponectin to LPS, suggesting an additional extracellular mode of anti-inflammatory action for adiponectin [46]. If this mechanism also contributed to the anti-inflammatory effects of adiponectin in our experiments remains to be elucidated.

In the circulation, adiponectin occurs as full-length and globular adiponectin. Full-length adiponectin exists as low, middle and high molecular weight oligomeric complexes. In addition, full-length adiponectin can be proteolytically cleaved to globular adiponectin, which consists of the C-terminal domain of the full-length protein. Both forms of adiponectin are biologically active and bind to the adiponectin receptors. Upon receptor engagement, adiponectin triggers several intracellular signaling pathways [23,47,48]. Different forms of adiponectin have been used in in-vitro studies, and although these forms often have similar effects, some actions are different, which could also explain controversial results among studies [47]. As mentioned above, LPS triggers an intracellular signaling cascade, which involves the nuclear translocation of NFκB [8]. Our experiments revealed that adiponectin inhibits the LPS-induced NFκB nuclear translocation in oral epithelial cells. This observation concurs with findings in other cells, where adiponectin inhibited the LPS-stimulated IκB degradation, thus preventing NFκB activation and DNA binding activity of NFκB [49–52]. Whether adiponectin also affects other LPS-triggered signaling pathways, such as ERK1/2, as it has been suggested, needs to be determined in further studies [52,53].

Since epithelial cell migration, proliferation, and differentiation are critical to periodontal pocket formation in periodontitis, we

Table 2. Interactions of lipopolysaccharide and adiponectin on cell viability.

Cell viability (%)			
Group	**24 h**	**48 h**	**72 h**
Control	93.30±0.96	95.63±0.58	96.79±0.64
LPS	79.25±2.80*	84.03±0.47*	80.49±0.90*
Adipo	99.81±1.02* †	99.73±0.32* †	99.78±0.77†
LPS + Adipo	95.22±0.36†	90.97±0.30* † #	96.06±0.11† #

Effects of lipopolysaccharide (LPS; 2 μg/ml) and/or adiponectin (Adipo; 1 μg/ml) on the cell viability, as assessed by trypan blue exclusion test, at 24 h, 48 h, and 72 h. Mean ± SEM; n = 6;
*$p<0.05$ different from control,
†different from LPS-treated cells,
#different from adiponectin-treated cells.

Table 3. Interactions of lipopolysaccharide and adiponectin on involucrin and growth factors.

Target gene	Group	4 h	8 h	24 h
Involucrin	LPS	2.91±0.12*	4.86±0.34*	1.58±0.24
	Adipo	0.87±0.13†	2.50±0.21* †	0.97±0.23
	LPS + Adipo	0.89±0.21†	2.02±0.14* †	0.69±0.10†
TGFβ1	LPS	1.06±0.07	0.77±0.07	0.83±0.19
	Adipo	0.28±0.04* †	1.03±0.06	0.52±0.09*
	LPS + Adipo	0.96±0.14#	0.75±0.04* #	0.84±0.05
KGF	LPS	0.63±0.16	2.01±0.11*	0.59±0.03*
	Adipo	0.19±0.04* †	0.64±0.06* †	1.02±0.10†
	LPS + Adipo	0.49±0.09*	0.68±0.08†	0.41±0.05* #

Effects of lipopolysaccharide (LPS; 2 μg/ml) and/or adiponectin (Adipo; 1 μg/ml) on the mRNA expression of involucrin, TGFβ1, and KGF at 4 h, 8 h, and 24 h expressed as fold of control. Mean ± SEM; n = 6;
*$p<0.05$ different from control,
†different from LPS-treated cells,
#different from adiponectin-treated cells.

also studied the actions of LPS and adiponectin on these parameters [1]. In an in-vitro wound healing assay, which mainly assesses cell migration and proliferation, adiponectin alone had no significant effect on epithelial cells. However, when these cells were exposed to adiponectin in the presence of LPS, the wound closure was significantly delayed, suggesting that adiponectin may inhibit cell migration in the presence of periodontal infection. At 1 day, adiponectin also inhibited the proliferation of oral epithelial cells exposed to LPS, suggesting that adiponectin may have, at least initially, some anti-proliferative effects in the presence of periodontal infection. Interestingly, adiponectin also reduced the LPS-induced cell proliferation and migration in a study on adventitial fibroblasts, supporting our results in oral epithelial cells [54]. The cell viability was significantly reduced by LPS but the LPS-induced decrease in cell viability was abrogated by adiponectin, indicating that adiponectin may protect against infection-induced damage of epithelial cells. However, another study did not observe *P. gingivalis*-induced changes in oral epithelial cell viability and numbers, but the controversial results could be explained by the different sources, strains and/or concentrations of LPS [11]. In studies on cancer cells, it has been shown that the anti-proliferative effect of adiponectin involves inhibition of cell cycle and activation of cell apoptosis [27,55]. Whether *P. gingivalis*-LPS and adiponectin also affect apoptosis of oral epithelial cells remains to be examined in further studies. The epithelium acts as a protective barrier against physical, chemical, and microbial insults. In order to fulfill this function, epithelial cells undergo differentiation and express a number of structural proteins, such as involucrin [28–30]. Our experiments revealed that LPS from *P. gingivalis* up-regulates involucrin, whereas adiponectin counteracts the stimulatory effects of LPS on this differentiation marker, suggesting that adiponectin may prevent epithelial cell differentiation and, thereby, formation of pocket epithelium, in the presence of periodontal infection.

Since epithelial proliferation and migration are regulated by growth factors, we also studied the expression of KGF1 and TGFβ1 in oral epithelial cells. KGF1 belongs to the heparin-binding fibroblast growth factor family, binds to the epithelial-specific KGF receptor and stimulates epithelial cell proliferation and migration [56–58]. Moreover, KGF1 has been shown to inhibit tumor necrosis factor-α- and LPS-induced epithelial cell apoptosis [59]. Although KGF is usually expressed by connective tissues, this growth factor has also been detected in epithelial cells, where it seems to act in an autocrine manner [60,61]. It has been hypothesized that the KGF1 up-regulation in periodontal diseases is associated with the onset and progression of periodontal pocket formation. The increased KGF1 protein production in epithelial cells may reduce apoptosis and maintain the integrity of the epithelium despite bacterial infection [62]. Although epithelial cell proliferation is a hallmark of periodontitis, the regulation of this proliferation is only partially unraveled. Our experiments revealed that LPS from *P. gingivalis* transiently up-regulated KGF at 8 h and decreased the KGF expression at 24 h. More importantly, adiponectin down-regulated significantly the constitutive KGF expression at 4 h and 8 h and also inhibited significantly the LPS-induced KGF expression at 8 h. Thus, the anti-proliferative effect of adiponectin in the presence of LPS may be, at least in part, mediated by inhibition of the KGF expression. TGFβ1 is another important growth factor, which regulates cell proliferation and migration, matrix synthesis, angiogenesis, and wound healing processes. TGFβ1 has both pro-inflammatory and immunosuppressive effects [63]. Increased TGFβ1 concentrations in gingival tissues and GCF from sites with deeper periodontal pockets have been reported [64]. In the present study, LPS had no effect on TGFβ1, and the addition of adiponectin to LPS-stimulated cells caused only minor changes in TGFβ1 expression. Thus, the anti-proliferative effects of adiponectin on LPS-treated cells do not seem to be dependent on TGFβ1.

In summary, our experiments demonstrated that adiponectin abrogates the *P. gingivalis*-LPS-induced up-regulation of pro-inflammatory cytokines and matrix-degrading enzymes as well as proliferation and differentiation of oral epithelial cells. Therefore, low levels of adiponectin, as observed in overweight and obese individuals, may confer an increased risk for periodontal inflammation, destruction and pocket formation.

Author Contributions

Conceived and designed the experiments: JD DK JW SJ AJ RM. Performed the experiments: DK JW. Analyzed the data: JD DK JW SJ AJ RM. Contributed reagents/materials/analysis tools: JD DK JW SJ AJ RM. Wrote the paper: JD DK JW SJ AJ RM.

References

1. Pihlstrom BL, Michalowicz BS, Johnson NW (2005) Periodontal diseases. Lancet 366: 1809–1820.
2. Albandar JM (2011) Underestimation of periodontitis in NHANES surveys. J Periodontol 82: 337–341.
3. Beikler T, Flemmig TF (2011) Oral biofilm-associated diseases: trends and implications for quality of life, systemic health and expenditures. Periodontol 2000 55: 87–103.
4. O'Dowd LK, Durham J, McCracken GI, Preshaw PM (2010) Patients' experiences of the impact of periodontal disease. J Clin Periodontol 37: 334–339.
5. Seymour GJ, Ford PJ, Cullinan MP, Leishman S, Yamazaki K (2007) Relationship between periodontal infections and systemic disease. Clin Microbiol Infect 13 Suppl 4: 3–10.
6. Kinane DF, Galicia JC, Gorr SU, Stathopoulou PG, Benakanakere M (2008) *P. gingivalis* interactions with epithelial cells. Front Biosci 13: 966–984.
7. Fitzpatrick RE, Wijeyewickrema LC, Pike RN (2009) The gingipains: scissors and glue of the periodontal pathogen, *Porphyromonas gingivalis*. Future Microbiol 4: 471–487.
8. Jain S, Darveau RP (2010) Contribution of *Porphyromonas gingivalis* lipopolysaccharide to periodontitis. Periodontol 2000 54: 53–70.
9. Jotwani R, Moonga BS, Gupta S, Cutler CW (2010) Nuclear factor-kappaB p50 subunits in chronic periodontitis and *Porphyromonas gingivalis* lipopolysaccharide-pulsed dendritic cells. Ann N Y Acad Sci 1192: 278–285.
10. Kocgozlu L, Elkaim R, Tenenbaum H, Werner S (2009) Variable cell responses to *P. gingivalis* lipopolysaccharide. J Dent Res 88: 741–745.
11. Johnson GK, Guthmiller JM, Joly S, Organ CC, Dawson DV (2010) Interleukin-1 and interleukin-8 in nicotine- and lipopolysaccharide-exposed gingival keratinocyte cultures. J Periodontal Res 45: 583–588.
12. Kou Y, Inaba H, Kato T, Tagashira M, Honma D, et al. (2008) Inflammatory responses of gingival epithelial cells stimulated with *Porphyromonas gingivalis* vesicles are inhibited by hop-associated polyphenols. J Periodontol 79: 174–180.
13. Takahashi N, Honda T, Domon H, Nakajima T, Tabeta K, et al. (2010) Interleukin-1 receptor-associated kinase-M in gingival epithelial cells attenuates the inflammatory response elicited by *Porphyromonas gingivalis*. J Periodontal Res 45: 512–519.
14. Garlet GP (2010) Destructive and protective roles of cytokines in periodontitis: a re-appraisal from host defense and tissue destruction viewpoints. J Dent Res 89: 1349–1363.
15. Taylor JJ (2010) Cytokine regulation of immune responses to *Porphyromonas gingivalis*. Periodontol 2000 54: 160–194.
16. Engebretson SP, Grbic JT, Singer R, Lamster IB (2002) GCF IL-1β profiles in periodontal disease. J Clin Periodontol 29: 48–53.
17. Hönig J, Rordorf-Adam C, Siegmund C, Wiedemann W, Erard F (1989) Increased interleukin-1β (IL-1β) concentration in gingival tissue from periodontitis patients. J Periodontal Res 24: 362–367.
18. Tsai CC, Ho YP, Chen CC (1995) Levels of interleukin-1β and interleukin-8 in gingival crevicular fluids in adult periodontitis. J Periodontol 66: 852–859.
19. Sorsa T, Tjäderhane L, Konttinen YT, Lauhio A, Salo T, et al. (2006) Matrix metalloproteinases: contribution to pathogenesis, diagnosis and treatment of periodontal inflammation. Ann Med 38: 306–321.
20. Chaffee BW, Weston SJ (2010) Association between chronic periodontal disease and obesity: a systematic review and meta-analysis. J Periodontol 81: 1708–1724.

21. Preshaw PM, Foster N, Taylor JJ (2007) Cross-susceptibility between periodontal disease and type 2 diabetes mellitus: an immunobiological perspective. Periodontol 2000 45: 138–157.
22. Suvan J, D'Aiuto F, Moles DR, Petrie A, Donos N (2011) Association between overweight/obesity and periodontitis in adults. A systematic review. Obes Rev 12: 381–404.
23. Brochu-Gaudreau K, Rehfeldt C, Blouin R, Bordignon V, Murphy BD, et al. (2010) Adiponectin action from head to toe. Endocrine 37: 11–32.
24. Lago F, Dieguez C, Gómez-Reino J, Gualillo O (2007) Adipokines as emerging mediators of immune response and inflammation. Nat Clin Pract Rheumatol 3: 716–724.
25. Mandal P, Park PH, McMullen MR, Pratt BT, Nagy LE (2010) The anti-inflammatory effects of adiponectin are mediated via a heme oxygenase-1-dependent pathway in rat Kupffer cells. Hepatology 51: 1420–1429.
26. Otterbein LE, Soares MP, Yamashita K, Bach FH (2003) Heme oxygenase-1: unleashing the protective properties of heme. Trends Immunol 24: 449–455.
27. Dieudonne MN, Bussiere M, Dos Santos E, Leneveu MC, Giudicelli Y, et al. (2006) Adiponectin mediates anti-proliferative and apoptotic responses in human MCF7 breast cancer cells. Biochem Biophys Res Commun 345: 271–279.
28. Eckert RL, Crish JF, Efimova T, Dashti SR, Deucher AB, et al. (2004) Regulation of involucrin gene expression. J Invest Dermatol 123: 13–22.
29. Kalinin AE, Kajava AV, Steinert PM (2002) Epithelial barrier function: assembly and structural features of the cornified cell envelope. Bioessays 24: 789–800.
30. Presland RB, Dale BA (2000) Epithelial structural proteins of the skin and oral cavity: function in health and disease. Crit Rev Oral Biol Med 11: 383–408.
31. Inadera H (2008) The usefulness of circulating adipokine levels for the assessment of obesity-related health problems. Int J Med Sci 5: 248–262.
32. Kamio N, Akifusa S, Yamaguchi N, Nonaka K, Yamashita Y (2009) Anti-inflammatory activity of a globular adiponectin function on RAW 264 cells stimulated by lipopolysaccharide from *Aggregatibacter actinomycetemcomitans*. FEMS Immunol Med Microbiol 56: 241–247.
33. Pfaffl MW (2001) A new mathematical model for relative quantification in real-time RTPCR. Nucleic Acid Res 29: 2002–2007.
34. Katz RW, Teng SY, Thomas S, Landesberg R (2002) Paracrine activation of extracellular signal-regulated kinase in a simple in-vitro model of wounded osteoblasts. Bone 31: 288–295.
35. Lackler KP, Cochran DL, Hoang AM, Takacs V, Oates TW (2000) Development of an in-vitro wound healing model for periodontal cells. J Periodontol 71: 226–237.
36. Andrian E, Grenier D, Rouabhia M (2005) *Porphyromonas gingivalis* lipopolysaccharide induces shedding of syndecan-1 expressed by gingival epithelial cells. J Cell Physiol 204: 178–183.
37. Soell M, Elkaim R, Tenenbaum H (2002) Cathepsin C, matrix metalloproteinases, and their tissue inhibitors in gingiva and gingival crevicular fluid from periodontitis-affected patients. J Dent Res 81: 174–178.
38. Tüter G, Kurtiş B, Serdar M (2002) Effects of phase I periodontal treatment on gingival crevicular fluid levels of matrix metalloproteinase-1 and tissue inhibitor of metalloproteinase-1. J Periodontol 73: 487–493.
39. Tüter G, Kurtiş B, Serdar M, Yücel A, Ayhan E, et al. (2005) Effects of phase I periodontal treatment on gingival crevicular fluid levels of matrix metalloproteinase-3 and tissue inhibitor of metalloproteinase-1. J Clin Periodontol 32: 1011–1015.
40. Park PH, McMullen MR, Huang H, Thakur V, Nagy LE (2007) Short-term treatment of RAW264.7 macrophages with adiponectin increases tumor necrosis factor-α (TNF-α) expression via ERK1/2 activation and Egr-1 expression: role of TNF-α in adiponectin-stimulated interleukin-10 production. J Biol Chem 282: 21695–21703.
41. Choi HM, Lee YA, Lee SH, Hong SJ, Hahm DH, et al. (2009) Adiponectin may contribute to synovitis and joint destruction in rheumatoid arthritis by stimulating vascular endothelial growth factor, matrix metalloproteinase-1, and matrix metalloproteinase-13 expression in fibroblast-like synoviocytes more than pro-inflammatory mediators. Arthritis Res Ther 11: R161.
42. Ogunwobi OO, Beales IL (2006) Adiponectin stimulates proliferation and cytokine secretion in colonic epithelial cells. Regul Pept 134: 105–113.
43. Huang H, Park PH, McMullen MR, Nagy LE (2008) Mechanisms for the anti-inflammatory effects of adiponectin in macrophages. J Gastroenterol Hepatol 23: 50–53.
44. Tsatsanis C, Zacharioudaki V, Androulidaki A, Dermitzaki E, Charalampopoulos I, et al. (2005) Adiponectin induces TNF-α and IL-6 in macrophages and promotes tolerance to itself and other pro-inflammatory stimuli. Biochem Biophys Res Commun 335: 1254–1263.
45. Turner JJ, Smolinska MJ, Sacre SM, Foxwell BM (2009) Induction of TLR tolerance in human macrophages by adiponectin: does LPS play a role? Scand J Immunol 69: 329–336.
46. Peake PW, Shen Y, Campbell LV, Charlesworth JA (2006) Human adiponectin binds to bacterial lipopolysaccharide. Biochem Biophys Res Commun 341: 108–115.
47. Neumeier M, Weigert J, Schäffler A, Wehrwein G, Müller-Ladner U, et al. (2006) Different effects of adiponectin isoforms in human monocytic cells. J Leukoc Biol 79: 803–808.
48. Stofkova A (2009) Leptin and adiponectin: from energy and metabolic dysbalance to inflammation and autoimmunity. Endocr Regul 43: 157–168.
49. Ajuwon KM, Spurlock ME (2005) Adiponectin inhibits LPS-induced NF-κB activation and IL-6 production and increases PPARγ2 expression in adipocytes. Am J Physiol Regul Integr Comp Physiol 288: 1220–1225.
50. Folco EJ, Rocha VZ, López-Ilasaca M, Libby P (2009) Adiponectin inhibits pro-inflammatory signaling in human macrophages independent of interleukin-10. J Biol Chem 284: 25569–25575.
51. Jortay J, Senou M, Delaigle A, Noel L, Funahashi T, et al. (2010) Local induction of adiponectin reduces lipopolysaccharide-triggered skeletal muscle damage. Endocrinology 151: 4840–4851.
52. Park PH, Huang H, McMullen MR, Mandal P, Sun L, et al. (2008) Suppression of lipopolysaccharide-stimulated tumor necrosis factor-α production by adiponectin is mediated by transcriptional and post-transcriptional mechanisms. J Biol Chem 283: 26850–26858.
53. Wulster-Radcliffe MC, Ajuwon KM, Wang J, Christian JA, Spurlock ME (2004) Adiponectin differentially regulates cytokines in porcine macrophages. Biochem Biophys Res Commun 316: 924–929.
54. Cai XJ, Chen L, Li L, Feng M, Li X, et al. (2010) Adiponectin inhibits lipopolysaccharide-induced adventitial fibroblast migration and transition to myofibroblasts via AdipoR1-AMPK-iNOS pathway. Mol Endocrinol 24: 218–228.
55. Dos Santos E, Benaitreau D, Dieudonne MN, Leneveu MC, Serazin V, et al. (2008) Adiponectin mediates an anti-proliferative response in human MDA-MB 231 breast cancer cells. Oncol Rep 20: 971–977.
56. Finch PW, Rubin JS, Miki T, Ron D, Aaronson SA (1989) Human KGF is FGF-related with properties of a paracrine effector of epithelial cell growth. Science 245: 752–755.
57. Ornitz DM, Itoh N (2001) Fibroblast growth factors. Genome Biol 2: REVIEWS3005.
58. Rubin JS, Osada H, Finch PW, Taylor WG, Rudikoff S, et al. (1989) Purification and characterization of a newly identified growth factor specific for epithelial cells. Proc Natl Acad Sci U S A 86: 802–806.
59. Firth JD, Putnins EE (2004) Keratinocyte growth factor 1 inhibits wound edge epithelial cell apoptosis in vitro. J Invest Dermatol 122: 222–231.
60. Ka H, Spencer TE, Johnson GA, Bazer FW (2000) Keratinocyte growth factor: expression by endometrial epithelia of the porcine uterus. Biol Reprod 62: 1772–1778.
61. Steele IA, Edmondson RJ, Bulmer JN, Bolger BS, Leung HY, et al. (2001) Induction of FGF receptor 2-IIIb expression and response to its ligands in epithelial ovarian cancer. Oncogene 20: 5878–5887.
62. Li M, Firth JD, Putnins EE (2005) Keratinocyte growth factor-1 expression in healthy and diseased human periodontal tissues. J Periodontal Res 40: 118–128.
63. Mantel PY, Schmidt-Weber CB (2011) Transforming growth factor-β: recent advances on its role in immune tolerance. Methods Mol Biol 677: 303–338.
64. Skaleric U, Kramar B, Petelin M, Pavlica Z, Wahl SM (1997) Changes in TGF-β 1 levels in gingiva, crevicular fluid and serum associated with periodontal inflammation in humans and dogs. Eur J Oral Sci 105: 136–142.

10

Dissemination of Periodontal Pathogens in the Bloodstream after Periodontal Procedures

Anna Carolina Ratto Tempestini Horliana, Leandro Chambrone, Adriana Moura Foz, Hilana Paula Carillo Artese, Mariana de Sousa Rabelo, Cláudio Mendes Pannuti, Giuseppe Alexandre Romito*

Department of Stomatology, School of Dentistry, University of São Paulo, São Paulo, Brazil

Abstract

Background: To date, there is no compilation of evidence-based information associating bacteremia and periodontal procedures. This systematic review aims to assess magnitude, duration, prevalence and nature of bacteremia caused by periodontal procedures.

Study Design: Systematic Review

Types of Studies Reviewed: MEDLINE, EMBASE and LILACS databases were searched in duplicate through August, 2013 without language restriction. Observational studies were included if blood samples were collected before, during or after periodontal procedures of patients with periodontitis. The methodological quality was assessed in duplicate using the modified Newcastle-Ottawa scale (NOS).

Results: Search strategy identified 509 potentially eligible articles and nine were included. Only four studies demonstrated high methodological quality, whereas five were of medium or low methodological quality. The study characteristics were considered too heterogeneous to conduct a meta-analysis. Among 219 analyzed patients, 106 (49.4%) had positive bacteremia. More frequent bacteria were *S. viridans, A. actinomycetemcomitans P. gingivalis, M. micros* and species *Streptococcus and Actinomyces*, although identification methods of microbiologic assays were different among studies.

Clinical Implications: Although half of the patients presented positive bacteremia after periodontal procedures, accurate results regarding the magnitude, duration and nature of bacteremia could not be confidentially assessed.

Editor: Michael Glogauer, University of Toronto, Canada

Funding: The authors have no support or funding to report.

Competing Interests: The authors have declared that no competing interests exist.

* E-mail: garomito@usp.br

Introduction

Bacteremia is defined as the transient, intermittent, or continuous presence of bacteria in the bloodstream [1]. It has been argued that the periodontal microbiota in intimate contact with the ulcerated epithelium of gingival sulcus/periodontal pockets is capable of reaching the bloodstream [2,3].

Molecular techniques have identified DNA sequences from periodontopathogens (e.g. *A. actinomycetemcomitans, P. gingivalis, P. intermedia*) in different organs and systems of the body [4–7]. In a recent systematic review [8] authors reported that biofilm accumulation and gingival inflammation increased prevalence of bacteremia after toothbrushing. Moreover, bacteremia is related to the magnitude of tissue trauma, density of bacterial microbiota and inflammation or infection at the site of trauma [9]. The association between periodontal treatment and bacteremia have been reported in several publications [10–27] and ranged from 13% [16] to 80.9% [18]; periodontal probing 20% [16] to 43% [24] and periodontal surgery 60% [26]. This wide variation may be attributed to the different employed laboratorial and clinical methods. For detection of bacteremia, culture plates were the most disseminated method [26] but compared with the current techniques it become obsolete. Some authors [13,17,28] have reported lysis filtration a very sensitive method that permit to access magnitude whereas conventional broth-based methods are the most commonly used procedure [11,12,16,19,20,24,25,29] because of the relative convenience and speed of the outcome. However, the principal disadvantage is the diversity of complementary methods for identification.

Recently, the polymerase chain reaction (PCR) has been cited as a more sensitive and specific test that does not depend on bacterial growth, detecting dead organisms degraded by the host immune [16,21–23]. Therefore, diverse microbiological analyses have been performed and do not allow for accurate comparisons to be made, which, in practical terms, can lead to misrepresentative findings. To date, and to our knowledge, there have been no evidence-based compilation studies documenting the association between periodontal procedures and bacteremia. Thus, the purpose of this systematic review was to assess magnitude, duration prevalence and nature of bacteremia induced by periodontal procedures.

Methods and Materials

Criteria for considering studies for this review

Type of studies. Because our research question was based on dissemination of periodontal bacteria into the bloodstream following periodontal procedures, the most adequate design to answer this question was a systematic review of observational studies. Thus, case series, case-control, cross-sectional and prospective cohort studies were eligible for inclusion. In addition, to reduce potential biases within the review process and to describe a standardized study, this systematic review was prepared in accordance with the MOOSE [30], PRISMA [31] and Check Review [32] checklists (Figure S1).

Types of participants and inclusion/exclusion criteria. Minimum sample size of 10 patients healthy patients with aggressive or chronic periodontitis [33] who underwent periodontal procedures: probing pocket depth, prophylaxis, scaling and root planing (hand curettes/scalers or with ultrasonic devices) or periodontal surgery (e.g., open flap debridement, guided tissue regeneration) were included. They must describe at least two blood samples (baseline and one more during/or after periodontal procedures) analyzed by molecular or culture-based methods. Patients submitted to any treatment (i.e. antibiotic treatment), were not included.

Outcome measure. A positive diagnosis of oral or non-oral bacteria in the bloodstream following periodontal procedures.

Search strategy

Search strategies were developed for the MEDLINE, EMBASE and LILACS databases. MesH terms, key words and other free terms were used for searching, and Boolean operators were used to combine searches. Databases were searched through April, 2013, without language restrictions based on the following search strategy developed for MEDLINE (via PubMed): ((((periodontal diseases OR chronic periodontitis OR aggressive periodontitis OR periodontitis OR periodontal pocket)) OR (subgingival curettage OR scaling OR dental scaling OR root planning OR tooth root scaling OR periodontal procedures OR periodontal basic procedures OR periodontal debridement))) AND (bacteremia OR bacteremia OR blood-borne pathogens). Reference lists of previous reviews and potential studies were examined (i.e., hand searching).

Assessment of validity, data extraction, and methodological quality in included studies

Three review authors did the acquisition of data (A.C.R.T.H., A.M.F. and H.P.C.A.) independently screened titles, abstracts and full texts of the search results. Full text was obtained for all studies that appeared to meet the inclusion criteria or in instances where there was insufficient information from the title or abstract to make a clear decision. Disagreement was resolved by revising it critically for important intellectual content (G.A.R., L.C. and C.M.P.). Data was extracted and recorded in duplicate (A.C.R.T.H., A.M.F., H.P.C.A. and M.S.R.) using specially designed data-extraction forms: citation, publication status, year of publication; study location; characteristics of participants; type of periodontal procedures; method used to assess bacteremia; outcome measures; methodological quality of the study; and source of funding or conflicts of interest. Methodological quality was conducted using The Newcastle–Ottawa scale (NOS scale) [34] modified by others authors [35,36]. The following topics represented areas of focus: 1) Selection of study groups: sample size calculation; representativeness of the patients with periodontitis; assessment of periodontal conditions; method used to assess bacteremia; calibration of assessors of outcomes; and clear inclusion/exclusion criteria 2) Comparability of patients and management of confounders 3) Outcome of interest: criteria applied to evaluate bacteremia and assessment of outcomes 4) Statistical analysis: appropriateness and unit of analysis. If all criteria of methodological quality were fulfilled within the domains, points ("stars") were assigned to the respective study. The NOS Scale was adapted for the purpose of this review, and each included study receives a maximum of 12 points. Studies with 9–12 points were considered as high methodological quality, 6–8 points medium and those with <6 points were considered to be of low methodological quality.

Data synthesis

Data were combined into evidence tables and grouped according to the type of study. A descriptive summary was performed to determine the quantity of the data by further evaluating study variations in terms of the study characteristics and outcomes.

Results

Search results and description of included studies

The search strategy identified 509 potentially eligible articles, of which 479 were excluded after the title and/or the abstract, were reviewed and duplicate removed (Figure 1). Subsequently, 30 of the full texts considered potentially relevant were screened. Of these, 18 [37–54] did not fulfill the inclusion criteria (Table 1). The main characteristics of the 9 included studies are listed in the Tables 2, 3 and 4. One study was reported in three different publications [21–23], represented by a single study name [18]. In total, 219 patients were assessed within nine cross-sectional studies included in this review, and positive bacteremia were identified in 106 [16–20,24–26,55] of these cases (49.4%).

Bacteremia following periodontal procedures

Periodontal probing. Generally, the prevalence of bacteremia after probing was 33,7% (27/80) [16,24,25]. Daly et al., (1997) [25], found 43% (13/30) [25] in patients with periodontal disease. In a different sample, Daly et al., (2001) [24] related 40% (8/20) [24] after periodontitis and 10% (2/20) [24] after gingivitis probing. Kinane et al., (2005) [16] found 20% (6/30) for periodontitis patients with culture and 16% (5/30) with PCR methodology. Some of the most common species in pos-probing period were *Micrococcus* [16], *Streptococcus* [24], *Corynebacterium* [24,25], *Bacteroides* [24,25], *Desulfomonas* [24,25], *Peptostreptococcus* [24.25], Gemella [25], *and bacteria S. viridans* [25,16], *S. milleri* [25] *N. pharynges* [16], *P. intermedia* [16], *A. naeslundii* [16], *H. aphrophilus* [16].

Non-surgical periodontal therapy (NSPT). NSPT led to a total degree of 46% of positive bacteremia [16–20,23,55] and frequent microorganisms were *A. actinomycetemcomitans* [20,23,19] *P. gingivalis* [20,19,23], *M. micros* [20,19], S. viridans [55], *S. sanguis* [16] A. *naeslundii* [16], *S. parasanguis* [16], and species *Actinomyces*

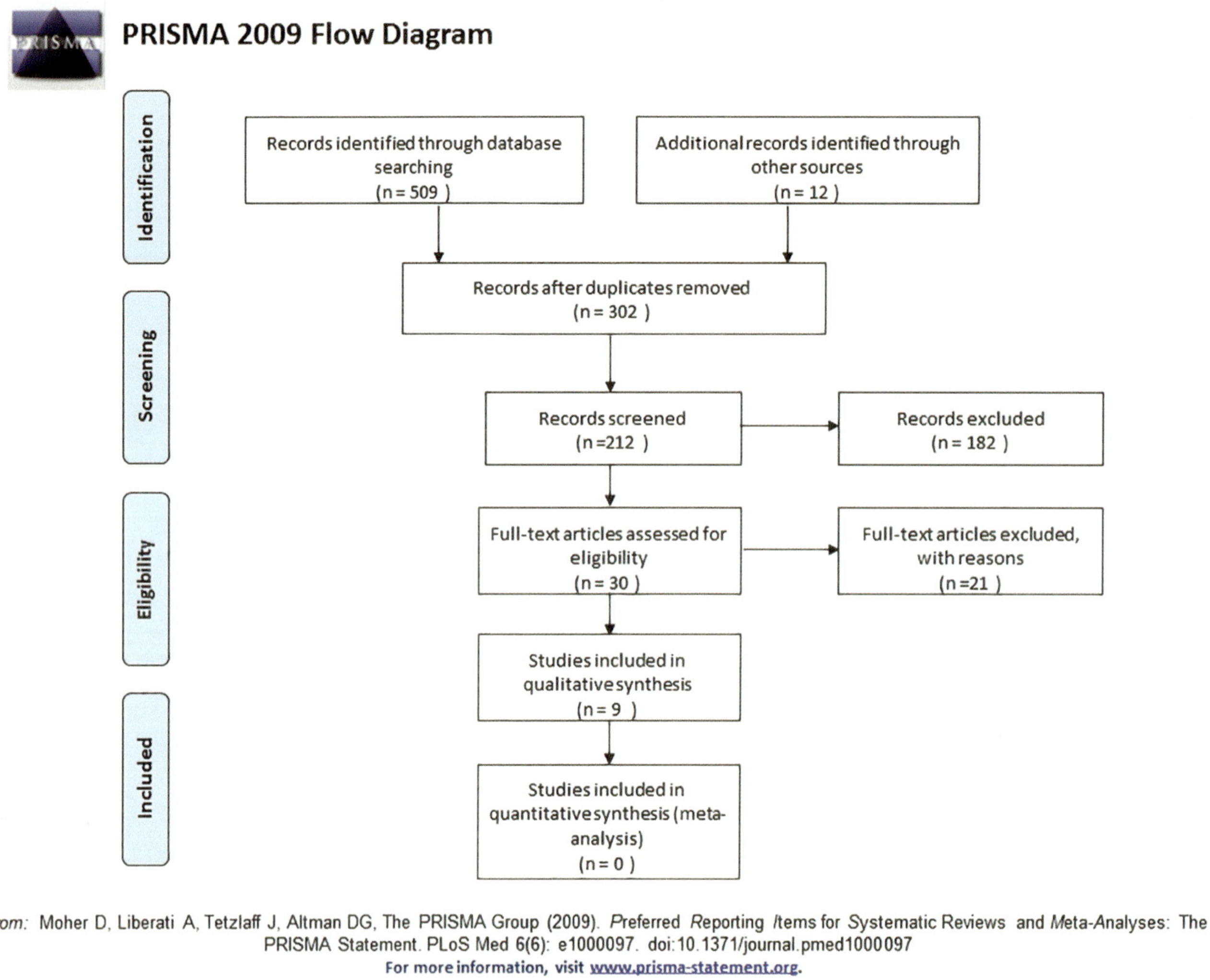

Figure 1. Flow chart of manuscripts screened through the review process.

[19,55,16], *Streptococcus* [17,16,20], *Enterococcus* [16], and one isolate of *Candida* [16]. In one study [23] was found 19% of positive bacteremia with nested PCR and 47.6% with anaerobic culture. Some high detected bacteria in subgingival plaque samples (i.e. *T. forsythia, P. intermedia*) were low detected in blood samples [23]. Zhang et al., (2013) [55] found 43.3% of positive bacteremia (13/30) and magnitude of 2±2.0 CFU/mL after NSPT. The highest prevalence was at 5 minutes (10/30) 33.3%. For *S. viridans*, 26.7% (8/30) of samples were positive after NSPT. Kinane et al., (2005) [16] found prevalence of 13% (4/30) for culture and 23% (7/30) for PCR. Forner et al., (2006) [17] found 75% (15/20) and magnitude of 0.78 [0.111–0.67] CFU/mL after 0,5 minutes of NSPT and 35% (7/20) and magnitude of 0.22 [0.11–0.67] CFU/mL in 10 minutes and 10% (2/20) and [0.11–0.11] after 30 minutes. In gingivitis group, all values were minor than in periodontitis. Padilla et al., (2007) [19] found 41,6% (5/12) for healthy and 16% (2/12) for atherosclerosis patients. In Maestre-Vera et al., (2008) [20] study, the prevalence was 76,9% (10/13).

Periodontal surgery. Lineberger et al., (1973) [26] found 60% (6/10) of positive bacteremia after diverse surgical procedures: gengivectomy, osteoplasty, and/or flap operation. One of the most prevalent microorganisms was S. *viridans* (22.9%) for the whole sample.

Overall, the characteristics of the nine included studies (i.e., technique of blood sampling, the point of sampling, time of sampling after periodontal procedure, the type of analysis conducted and treatment provided), were considered too heterogeneous to be combined in a meta-analysis (Table 5). Individual outcomes were reported in Tables 2, 3 and 4. Basically three techniques were used to assess bacteremia: hemoculture, lysis filtration and PCR and all of them detect positive bacteremia, ranging from 13% [16] to 80.9% [18] for NSPT 43 [24] to 20% [16] for probing by culturing and 16% with by PCR analysis [16]. For periodontal surgery [26] a sum of 60% (6/10) positive cases.

Risk of bias (quality assessment)

Of the nine included studies, one received an 11-point score (of a total of 12) one a 10-point score, two a 9-point score, two a 7-point score, two a 6-point score, and the last one receive a 4-point score (Figure 2). Thus, 4 studies were considered of high

Table 1. Excluded studies and the reason for exclusion.

Study	Reason for exclusion
Lacassin F, Hoen B, Leport C, Selton-Suty C, Delahaye F et al., 1995 [37]	Case control with no bacteremia outcomes
Lieberman MB, 1992 [38]	Case report
Lofthus JE, Waki MY, Jolkovsky D Otomo-Corgel J, Newman MG et al., 1991 [39]	Inclusion of patients undergo periodontal maintenance
Font Buxo J, 1985 [40]	Review
Trivedi DN, 1984 [41]	Review
Wank HA, Levison ME, Rose LF, Cohen DW, 1976 [42]	There was no periodontal treatment
Ewart NP, 1971 [43]	Review
Kraal JH, 1970 [44]	Review
Montanari G, 1957 [45]	not fulfill inclusion criteria of methodology
Bandt, C.L., Korn, N.A., Schaffer, E.M, 1964 [52]	not fulfill inclusion criteria of methodology
Winslow MB, Kobernick SD, 1960 [53]	not fulfill inclusion criteria of methodology
Raetzke P, O'Leary DMD, Miller CH, 1981 [54]	not fulfill inclusion criteria of methodology
Baltch, AL, Shaffer C, Hammer MC 1982 [50]	not fulfill inclusion criteria of methodology
Bayliss R, Clarke C, Oakley et al., 1983 [49]	Case control with no bacteremia outcomes
Conner HD, Haberman S, Collings CK, 1967 [48]	not fulfill inclusion criteria of methodology
Korn NA, EM Schaffer, 1962 [51]	not fulfill inclusion criteria of methodology
Rogosa M, Hamppeg, Nevinta, 1960 [47]	not fulfill inclusion criteria of methodology
Lazansky JP, Robinson L, Rodofsky L., 1949 [46]	not fulfill inclusion criteria of methodology

methodological quality [16–18,55], 2 were of medium [24,25], and 3 were of low methodological quality [19,20,26]. In all of the included studies, descriptions of the inclusion/exclusion criteria and unit of analysis (number of patients per group) were considered adequately addressed (i.e., received a star). With exception of one study [26], all of them described standardized methods for the assessment of bacteremia and microbiological analysis. Only one study reported sample size calculations [55], and two [16,55] presented trained/calibrated assessment of periodontal outcomes, but not a description of a blind examiner. One study [55] reported a blinded assessment for microbiological analysis. Some of the studies had relatively representativeness of patients with periodontitis, [16–18,24,25,55] the management of confounders,[16–18,55] and the assessment of periodontal conditions (diagnosis based on full mouth probing measurements or full mouth radiographic evaluation) [16–18,55].

Discussion

Summary of the main results

The outcomes of this systematic review reinforce that studies of bacteremia after periodontal procedures in general are poorly designed, and too different in terms of reported methodologies. Despite the heterogeneity related to the time point of blood collection, periodontal diagnosis and microbiological techniques, the prevalence of positive cases of bacteremia after periodontal procedures was 49.4%. More frequent species are not coincident, but in general were *Actinomyces* spp. [19,55] *Streptococcus* spp [17,16] and bacteria were *A. actinomycetemcomitans* [20,23] *P. gingivalis* [20,19,23], *M. micros* [20,19], S. viridans [55]. The duration and magnitude of bacteremia could not be adequately estimated.

Agreements and disagreements with previous studies

Although a large amount of microorganisms (10^8 to 10^{12} of Gram-negative bacteria) [57] may be found in untreated periodontal pockets, dental bacteremia is associated with a low magnitude (1–100 CFU/mL) [58]. Therefore, sensitivity of microbiological tests are crucial in bacteremia studies. Traditional broth-based methods (liquid, solid, and biphasic media) are widely used. Some authors [13,17,59] considered lysis filtration a more sensitive method compared to hemoculture. Although hemoculture is considered the gold standard [18] and an important diagnostic method to detect alive microorganisms [60], presents some disadvantages. There are two phases to complete the process: detecting bacteria after incubation time and identifying them. The problem really lies with the different methods used for identification. Also, this method can lead to false-negative results because some species (*Prevotella*, *Neisseria*, *Veilonella*) are difficult to cultivate [60,23] and identify [61], also peculiar oral microbiota requires different culture mediums [2,17,59]. This methodology does not detect bacteria degraded by the immune system nor estimate the magnitude of bacteremia [2,62]. On the other hand, allow rapid response (±10 hours) [62] compared to lysis filtration (2 to 10 days) [13,17,62] fundamental in detecting life-threatening septicemia [62].

Culture methods are suitable for detecting alive infective endocarditis microorganisms (i.e S. viridans [55], HANEK - group of fastidious organisms including A. actinomycetemcomitans). As partial solution to these problems, molecular probe-based identification methods (universal 16S rRNA genes or other specific bacterial gene markers) are becoming more popular because of its sensitivity, do not discriminate between live and dead bacteria [16,23] and identify some uncultivable oral species (i.e. *Prevotella*) [2]. Moreover cannot be utilized in studies for prophylaxis of bacteremia [63] (i.e. antibiotics). A link is being

Table 2. Characteristics of the included studies: periodontal probing procedures.

Study	Participants	PD definition	Methods	Outcomes	Conclusion
Daly and colleagues, 2001 [25]	40 patients, 21 males and 19 females, mean age 41,8 years, submitted to periodontal probing	Periodontitis group were selected based on radiographic evidence of interproximal alveolar bone loss on a dental panoramic tomography.	BS was collected before and immediately following periodontal probing and were analyzed via aerobic and anaerobic media culture bottles. Gram stained and subculture to appropriate media and isolates identified to genus level.	Microorganisms were identified in the peripheral blood after probing in 40% (8/20) periodontitis patients and in 10% (2/20) gingivitis patients. Frequent MO: *Streptococcus* spp. were the most common isolates in both groups.	"Patients with untreated adult periodontitis are at greater risk of bacteremia due to periodontal probing than patients with gingivitis "
Daly and colleagues, 2001 [24]	30 patients, 15 males and 15 females, mean age 42.7 years, submitted to periodontal probing	Periodontitis group were selected when exhibit radiographic evidence of periodontitis.	BS was collected before and immediately following periodontal probing and were analyzed via aerobic and anaerobic media culture bottles. Gram stained and subculture to appropriate media and isolates identified to genus or species level.	Microorganisms were identified in the peripheral blood before probing in 3 patients (2 of these grew skin commensals and one of these, *Prevotella*). Before (3/30) 10% Immediately after (13/30) 43% Frequent MO: S. *viridans* were the most common isolates.	"The results indicate that periodontal probing can cause bacteremia in patients with periodontitis "
Kinane and colleagues, 2005 [16]	30 patients, 18 male and 12 female, mean age 42,3 years submitted to periodontal probing	Periodontal disease was defined as having all quadrants with at least one pocket >6 mm, and ≥20 teeth	BS was collected before and immediately after (range 30 s to 1 min) this procedure via blood culture bottles (aerobic/anaerobic) and PCR assay.	Culture methods: Baseline 6% (2/30) Probing (20%) (6/30), PCR analysis: Baseline: (9%) 3/30), Probing 16% (5/30)	"Detectable dental bacteremias induced by periodontal procedures are at a lower level than previously reported"

MO – microorganisms; BS – blood sample; mm – millimeters; PCR – polymerase chain reaction.
Studies of Daly [24,25] and Kinane [16] are University-based (University of Sydney and United Kingdon respectively)

made between *P. gingivalis* and systemic complications [21] including cardiovascular diseases, stroke, lung inflammation, arthritis rheumatoid [64,21]. This bacterium is capable of binding its fimbriae to endothelial cells [65] and also probably evades the immune system exploiting red blood cells as a transport vehicle rendering it inaccessible to attack by phagocytes [64].

Although it has been identified by culture methods [18], PCR is indicated [21] once red blood cells are lysed as part of the process. Summarizing, it is important to establish bacteria involved in systemic disease, its survival conditions, incubation time, and pathogenicity (alive or dead bacteria) before choose the microbiology test to be used in the study. Four studies using hemoculture detected 73.8% (31/42),[18] 13% (4/30),[16] 76% (10/13) [20] and 29% (7/24) [19] of positive bacteremia. The wide range of prevalence may be attributed to diverse periods of incubations (14 [18], 15 [16], 21 [20] and 35 [19] days) and diversity of time point of blood collection: immediately [16,18] one [20] and five [19] minutes after NSPT.

Discrepancies must be considered even for the same sample for hemoculture (47.6% – 20/42) [23] and nested PCR (19% - 8/42) [23]. When specific time point was analyzed (immediately after NSPT), hemoculture detect 38% (16/42) [23] whereas nested PCR 21.4% (9/42) [23]. In the same study group [18], 73.8% (31/42) of patients had positive bacteremia immediately after periodontal treatment using hemoculture bottles. PCR would increase the sensitivity and specificity of the detection of periodontal pathogens [16,23] in this sense, Kinane et al. (2006) [16] found 23% (7/30) of positive bacteremia using PCR and 13% (4/30) with culture method. Some authors [16,23] used both hemoculture and PCR. It seems techniques would complement each other [23]. Related to molecular methods, newer DNA-DNA hybridization microarrays (bacteremias $>10^4$) [63] or 16SrDNA pyrosequencing should be tested [18] in the future, in order to access both more accurate magnitude and diversity of nature of bacteremia. Only one of the included studies uses lysis filtration method [17]. After 30 seconds of NSPT, 75% of patients with periodontitis, 20% gingivitis and 10% with healthy periodontal gum presented bacteremia. These findings seem to be linked to the bacterial load related to the disease; however, no other study using lysis filtration could be included in the review.

Some authors [61] suggested extractions are most likely among dental procedures to cause bacteremia, however periodontal procedures and daily oral activities potentially cause disruption of a larger surface area of inflamed juntional epithelium. Although both procedures have the same access via to the bloodstream, the intensity of trauma is quite different, and also a review of bacteremia in daily oral procedures was performed recently [8]. So we decide to include all periodontal procedures that cause bacteremia via junctional epithelium. Regard to NSPT, some authors [55] suggested that ultrasonic scaler may remove part of bacteria by the flushing action of the water irrigation but others disagree [16] suggesting higher tissue trauma. In included studies, procedures are diverse: full mouth ultrasonic scaling [16,17] a combination with hand instruments [17,19,20] and 10 minutes of scaling and root planning [18] hampering comparison of results.

All the included studies performed baseline blood sampling. In healthy patient that do not realize oral daily activities (at least one hour before the study) [55,56], and in no contaminated samples (i.e. skin microorganisms) , the results were expected to be null. It is not clear why low-level of transient bacteremia may occur in the absence of therapeutic intervention [18,16] and clinical relevance

Table 3. Characteristics of the included studies: non-surgical periodontal therapy.

Study	Participants	PD definition	Methods	Outcomes	Conclusion
Lafaurie and colleagues, 2007 [18]	42 patients, 25 males and 17 females, mean age 38,15 years, submitted to periodontal treatment	PD was defined as at least 10 pockets with PPD≥7 mm requiring periodontal surgery after SRP	BS was collected before and after SRP (immediately, 15 min, 30 min) and were analyzed via blood culture bottles (anaerobic)	Microorganisms growing under anaerobic conditions were identified in the peripheric blood after SRP in 80.9% (34/42) patients. Evaluation times: T1 - 2,4% (1/42) patients T2 - 73.8% (31/42) patients, T3 - 38% (16/42) patients, T4 - 19% (8/42) patients, Frequent MO *P. gingivalis*, and *M. micros in peripheral blood*	"Scaling and root planning induced bacteremia associated with anaerobic bacteria, especially in patients with periodontal disease"
Maestre and colleagues, 2008 [20]	13 patients, 8 males and 5 females, mean age 58.6 years submitted to periodontal treatment	PD was defined as PPD≥4 mm.	BS was collected before and after SRP (1 min) and were analyzed via blood culture bottles (aerobic/anaerobic)	Baseline: 0% (0/13) After treatment 76.9% (10/13) Predominate anaerobic bacteria of the genus *Prevotella*, followed *M. micros and F. nucleatum.*	"Periodontal procedures induce bacteremia and may represent risk of developing systemic complications. The use of antibiotic prophylaxis is crucial for its prevention".
Padilla and colleagues, 2007 [21]	24 patients, 14 males and 10 females, mean age 63,5 years submitted to periodontal treatment	PD was defined as CAL≥5 mm.	BS was collected before and after (5 min.) SRP. Via blood culture bottles (anaerobics)	Baseline 0%. After treatment 29,1% (7/12) of patients with and without atherosclerosis. The most prevalent bacteria in both groups was *A. actinomycetemcomitans*	"Bacteremia occurred in 7/24 patients after SRP. In 4 patients, the same species found in periodontic pockets and blood cultures were selected in atherosclerotic plaques obtained one week after the dental procedure"
Forner and colleagues, 2006 [17]	60 patients (20 with periodontitis), 5 males and 15 females, mean age 43,75 years submitted to periodontal treatment	PD was defined as at least 10 sites with PPD>5 mm.	BS was collected before and after (0.5, 10, and 30 min.) SRP. Via lysis filtration (aerobic/anaerobic)	Baseline 0%, 0,5 min: 75% (15/20), 10 min 35% (7/20) , 30 min: 10% (2/20). The isolated bacteria represented a larger variety of species reflecting the increased complexity of the microflora of periodontal pocket	"Patients with periodontitis as compared with healthy individuals and gingivitis patients are at increased risk of experiencing bacteremia in association with scaling" .
Kinane and colleagues, 2006 [16]	30 patients, 18 male and 12 female, mean age 42,3 years submitted to periodontal treatmet	Periodontal disease was defined as having all quadrants with at least one pocket >6 mm, and ≥20 teeth	BS was collected before and after (immediately) via blood culture bottles (aerobic/anaerobic) and PCR assay.	Baseline: Culture methods: Baseline - 3% (1/30), SRP - 13% (4/30), PCR analysis Baseline: 13% (4/30), SRP 23% (7/30)	"Detectable dental bacteremias induced by periodontal procedures are at a lower level than previously reported
Zhang and colleagues, 2013 [55]	30 patients, 12 males and 18 females, mean age 47 (±9,5) years submitted to periodontal treatment	Periodontal disease was defined as having at list one quadrant (qualified quadrant) with a minimum of five teeth with probing depths ≥5 mm not at the same tooth.	BS was collected before, five minutes 30 seconds and 10 min after periodontal treatment and plated onto chromogenic agar, chocolate agar, and brain heart infusion agar supplemented with vitamin K plates. Any grow was subcultured and identified to at least genus level.	Culture methods: Baseline - 3% (1/30), SRP - 13% (4/30), PCR analysis: Baseline: 13% (4/30), SRP 23% (7/30)	"Detectable dental bacteremias induced by periodontal procedures are at a lower level than previously reported"

SRP – scaling and root planning, PPD Periodontal probing depth, CAL -clinical attachment level, PD – periodontal disease, MO – microorganisms; BS – blood sample; mm – millimeters; PCR – polymerase chain reaction

Lafaurie [18] - University-based (Colombia) This study was supported by the Instituto Colombiano para la Ciencia y la Tecnologia Francisco Jose de Caldas; Maestre Vera [20] - University-based (Spain); Padilla [21] -University-based (Chile); Forner [17] - University-based (Denmark) This study was supported by the Danish Dental Association, Colgate–Palmolive and the Danish Foundation for Mutual Efforts in Dental Care; Kinane [16] - University- based (United Kingdom), Zhang [55] – University-based (Australia).

Table 4. Characteristics of the included studies for periodontal surgery.

Study	Participants	PD definition	Methods	Outcomes	Conclusion
Lineberger, De Marco, 1973 [28]	21 patients, 8 males and 13 females, mean age 41,8 years, submitted to gingivectomy, flap procedures, and or osteoplasty	Generalized periodontitis group were selected with pocket depth greater than 3 mm in all quadrants	BS was collected before and after the operator had judge maximal trauma from the procedure and were analyzed via aerobic and anaerobic cultured agar pour plates and were characterized on the basis of the morphologic description of the colony, gran staining and biochemical tests.	MO were identified in the peripheral blood after surgical procedures in 60% (6/10) in untreated periodontitis patients and in 40% (4/10) in patients with prior dental prophylaxis and plaque control patients. Frequent MO: Anaerobic/anaeróbic *Diphtheroids, S. viridans and Staphylococcus epidermitis* were the most common isolates in both groups.	"A significant incidence of bacteremia occurred during the manipulation of gingival tissues. The use of stimudents, or periodontal surgery in untreated patients and periodontal surgery in treated patients will produce a significant incidence of bacteremia"

MO –microorganisms, BS – blood sample, mm- millimeters, mm – millimeters
Lineberger [28]- University-based (Ohio)

of such condition remains unknown. The "pumping action" created by movement of the tooth within the socket [66] (bruxism) should be investigated. In an immune person, the nonspecific host defense (phagocytes and complement) provides the first line protection. In a bacteremic episode, macrophages of the reticuloendotelial system, provide efficient and rapid clearance [16], after blood circulate through the liver [67]. Thus, bacteremia of oral origin is normally fast [58], once repetitive aggressions who's this immune barrier has a strong adapted to attack [16]. Some confounders for bacteremia duration are: heart rate, blood volume and proximity of blood collection to the source of bacteremia [56]. In immunosuppressed patients (i.e. poorly controlled diabetes, leukemia) or treated with immunosuppressing (rheumatoid arthritis, organ transplant) [61,68] there would be an increased incidence and magnitude of bacteremia [69] and very often attenuated inflammation signs and symptoms. Antibiotic prophylaxis should be individually evaluated. Overall, in questionable cases, balancing of the known risks (i.e. drug reactions, resistant strains) against the possible benefits of antimicrobial regimen (i.e. antibiotics, oral antiseptics), should be evaluated [58,56].

Plaque accumulation and gingival inflammation significantly increase the prevalence of bacteremia after toothbrushing [8]. There are superficial bacterial effect of mouthrinse in undisturbed dental biofilm [70,71] and essential oils seems to reduced amount of bacteremia in subjects with gingivitis [15]. They could diminish total load of bacteria before periodontal procedures, especially together with oral hygiene procedures when antibiotic prophylaxis is not indicated. On the other hand, bacterial colonization causing infective endocarditis must be prevented for high susceptible individual undergo invasive procedures [9].

Quality of the evidence and potential biases in the review process

Heterogeneity of high methodological quality studies [16–18,55] did not allowed comparisons between results, thus meta-analyses of such data may be questionable due to potential bias and the lack of control of confounders [35]. Thus, the most transparent approach was a systematic review of observational studies. Mainly different diagnosis of periodontitis, clinical and microbiological methods, could explain, discrepancies between studies. Also, periodontal treatment should be standardized (i.e. duration of treatment, ultrasonic or hand instruments, scaling or scaling and root planning, full mouth or conventional treatment). Another important issue is the sample size calculations [55], which could underestimated outcomes, once low prevalence of bacteremia require larger samples to achieve statistical differences. Also, a clear description of a blind and calibrated assessment of periodontal outcomes should be cited.

Conclusions

Almost half of attended patients may present positive bacteremia after periodontal procedures. However, confident results on the magnitude, duration and nature of bacteremia could not be assessed because of the poor design of included studies. Thus, these conditions should be taken into consideration when interpreting the results of this review. Prospective cohort studies and RTCs (comparing different types of procedures) may provide more accurate outcomes on the dissemination of periodontal pathogens into the bloodstream.

Table 5. Heterogeneity in methodology and results obtained in different studies selected for this review.

Study	Technique of blood sampling	The point of sampling	Time of sampling	Type of analysis conducted	Type of treatment conducted
Lafaurie and colleagues, 2007 [18]	After 1% povidone-iodine disinfection, cannulation was performed by a nurse with 18 GA IV catheter. An injection site adapter was positioned and attached to a sterile multiple sample needle. 5 ml of blood was collected in each sampling	Blood samples were drawn from antecubital vein	T1 = before periodontal procedure; T2 = immediately after periodontal procedure; T3 = 15 min after periodontal procedure; T4 = 30 min after periodontal procedure	blood culture bottles (anaerobic)	Periodontal treatment
Maestre and colleagues, 2008 [20]	The technique of blood sample was not described. 20 ml of blood was collected in each sampling	It was not described	T1 = before periodontal procedure; T2 = 1 minute after completion of periodontal treatment	blood culture bottles (aerobic/anaerobic)	Periodontal treatment
Padilla and colleagues, 2007 [19]	The blood collection procedure was performed according to the classical aseptic standards. The technique of blood sample was not described. 10 ml of blood was collected in each sampling	It was not described	T1 = before periodontal procedure; T2 = 5 minutes after completion of periodontal treatment	blood culture bottles (anaerobic)	Periodontal treatment
Forner and colleagues, 2006 [17]	After 0.5% clorexidina ethanol disinfection, an indwelling catheter was used. This catheter was rinsed with saline after insertion and after obtaining each blood sample. The site of venepuncture was covered by a sterile pad. Two millilitres of blood was discarded before drawing the blood for the bacteremia analysis. 9 ml of blood was collected in each sampling	Blood samples were drawn from antecubital veins	T1 = before periodontal procedure; T2 = 0.5 minutes after completion of periodontal treatment;T3 = 10 minutes after completion of periodontal treatment; T4 = 30 minutes after completion of periodontal treatment	lysis filtration (aerobic/anaerobic)	Periodontal treatment
Kinane and colleagues, 2006 [16]	The puncture site was disinfected with isopropyl. Each sample comprised 28 ml of blood using a butterfly (19G) and safety lock blood collection set, 20 ml syringe and vacutainer holder, which were all attached to a Connecta TH three-way stopcock. Two 4.4 ml vacutainer tubes containing ethylenedia-minetetraacetic acid (EDTA) were used for the collection of samples required for PCR analysis.	Blood samples were drawn from veins in antecubital fossa	T1 = before periodontal procedure; T2 = immediately (30 s to 1 min) following periodontal treatment. There are other procedures (toothbrushing and periodontal probing depths)	blood culture bottles (aerobic/anaerobic) and PCR assay	Periodontal treatment
Zhang and colleagues, 2013 [55]	Blood samples was obtained using a 25/22 G cannula, which was left in place during each experimental visit to avoid multiple insertions of a needle. The venipuncture technique utilized has been described previously. A 20 ml blood sample was obtained in each sample	Blood samples were drawn from a vein in the antecubital fossa	T1 = before periodontal procedure; T2 = 30 s after periodontal treatment; T3 = 5 min after periodontal treatment; T2 = 10 min. after periodontal treatment	Samples was plated onto chromogenic agar, chocolate agar, and brain heart infusion agar supplemented with vitamin K plates. Any grow was subcultured and identified to at least genus level.	Periodontal treatment
Lineberger and colleagues, 1973 [26]	Thirty second application of 2% iodine and then wiped with a sterile 70% alcohol sponge. Each sample consisted of ten milliliters of blood, which was drawn into a vacuntainer using a 20 G needle.	Blood samples were drawn from the median basilica vein in the antecubital fossa to either right or left arm.	T1 = before periodontal procedure;T2 = after the operator had judged maximal trauma from the procedure to have occurred but while the specific procedure was still being carried out.	Were analyzed via aerobic and anaerobic cultured agar pour plates and were characterized on the basis of the morphologic description of the colony, gran staining and biochemical tests	Periodontal surgery (gengivectomy, osteoplasty, and/or flap operation)
Daly and colleagues, 1997 [25]	The skin was wiped with polvidone-iodine and 70% alcohol.A 20 ml blood sample was obtained in each sample.	Blood samples were obtained by means of venipuncture.	T1 = before periodontal probing; T2 = immediately following periodontal probing.	Were analyzed via aerobic and anaerobic media culture bottles. Gram stained and subculture to appropriate media and isolates identified to genus or species level.	Periodontal probing
Daly and colleagues, 2001 [24]	The skin was wiped with polvidone-iodine and 70% alcohol. A 20 ml blood sample was obtained in each sample.	Blood samples were obtained by means of venipuncture.	T1 = prior periodontal probing; T2 = immediately following periodontal probing	Were analyzed via aerobic and anaerobic media culture bottles. Gram stained and subculture to appropriate media and isolates identified to genus or species level.	Periodontal probing

G- Gauge, IV –Intravascular, T- time, ml-milliliters, PCR –polymerase chain reaction.

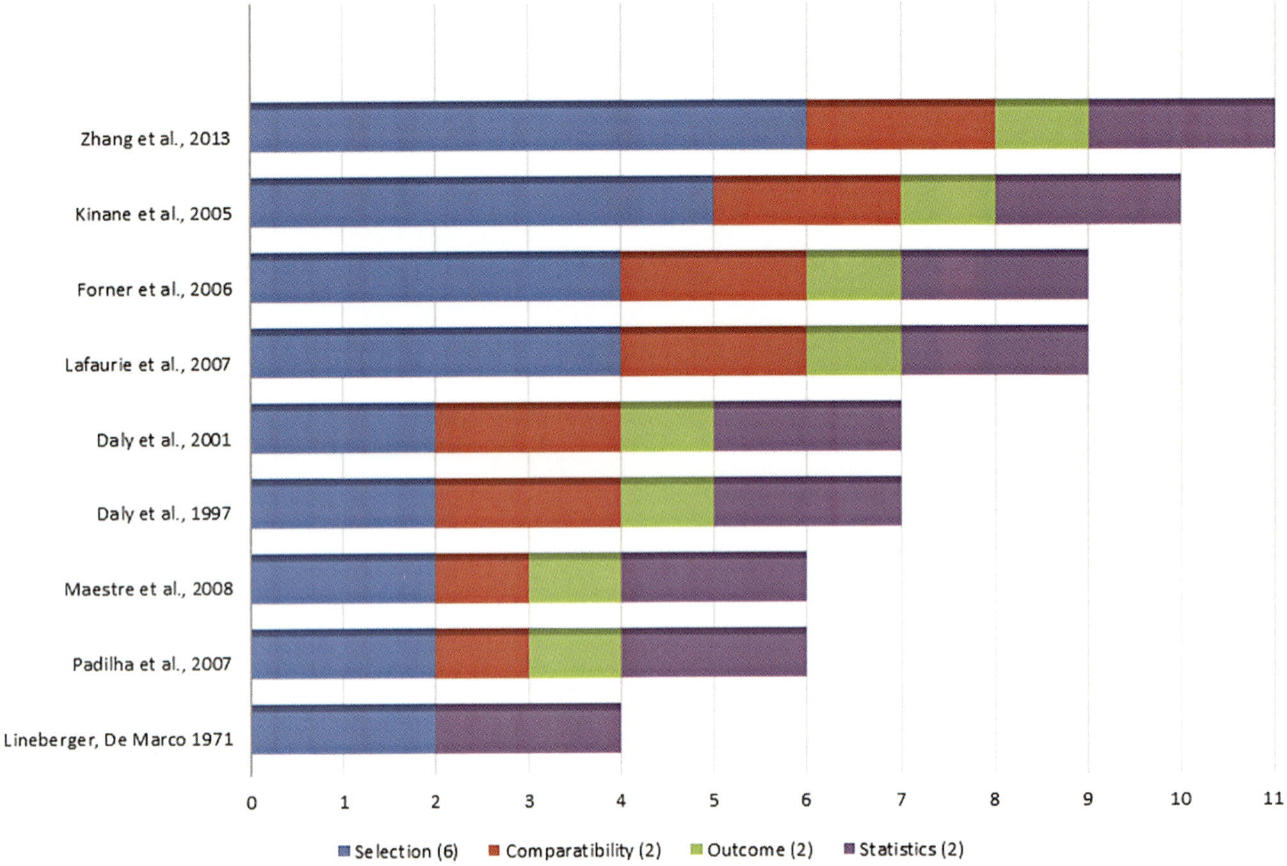

Figure 2. Methodological quality of included observational studies (stars assigned to respective study).

Author Contributions

Analyzed the data: GAR LC CMP. Contributed reagents/materials/analysis tools: LC CMP. Wrote the paper: ACRTH. Designed the search strategy: LC. Data extraction and record in duplicate: ACRTH HPCA AMF MdSR. Conception and design of the work: LC ACRTH. Acquisition of data: ACRTH HPCA AMF. Analysis and interpretation of data: LC CMP. Drafted the article or revised it critically for important intellectual content: GAR LC CMP. Final approval of the version to be published: GAR LC CMP.

References

1. American Academy of Periodontology. (2001) Glossary of Periodontal terms. 4th ed. Chicago: The American Academy of Periodontology pp.5.
2. Parahitiyawa NB, Jin LJ, Leung WK, Yam WC, Samaranayake LP. (2009) Microbiology of odontogenic bacteremia: beyond endocarditis. Clin Microbiol Rev 2:46–64.
3. Pizzo G, Guiglia R, Lo Russo L, Campisi G. (2010) Dentistry and internal medicine: from the focal infection theory to the periodontal medicine concept. Eur J Intern Med 21:496–502.
4. Herzberg MC, Weyer MW. (1998) Dental plaque, platelets, and cardiovascular diseases. Ann Periodontol:151–60.
5. Millar BC, Moore JE. (2004) Emerging issues in infective endocarditis. Emerg Infect Dis 10:1110–6.
6. Tonetti MS, D'Aiuto F, Nibali L, Donald A, Storry C, et al. (2007) Treatment of periodontitis and endothelial function. N Engl J Med 356:911–20.
7. Fisher MA, Taylor GW, Papapanou PN, Rahman M, Debanne SM. (2008) Clinical and serologic markers of periodontal infection and chronic kidney disease. *J Periodontol* :1670–8.
8. Tomás I, Diz P, Tobías A, Scully C, Donos N. (2012) Periodontal health status and bacteraemia from daily oral activities: systematic review/meta-analysis. J Clin Periodontol 39:213–28.
9. Wilson W, Taubert KA, Gewitz M, Lockhart PB, Baddour LM, et al. (2007) Prevention of infective endocarditis: guidelines from the American Heart Association. Circulation :1736–54.
10. Madsen KL. (1974) Effect of chlorhexidine mouthrinse and clinical periodontal procedures upon bacteremia produced by oral hygiene procedures. Scand J Dent Res 82:1–7.
11. Witzenberger T, O'Leary TJ, Gillette WB. (1982) Effect of a local germicide on the occurrence of bacteremia during subgingival scaling. J Periodontol;53(3):172–9.
12. Reinhardt RA, Bolton RW, Hlava G. (1982) Effect of nonsterile versus sterile water irrigation with ultrasonic scaling on postoperative bacteremias. J Periodontol :96–100.
13. Heimdahl A, Hall G, Hedberg M, Sandberg H, Söder PO, et al. (1990) Detection and quantitation by lysis-filtration of bacteremia after different oral surgical procedures. J Clin Microbiol 28:2205–9.
14. Allison C, Simor AE, Mock D, Tenenbaum HC (1993) Prosol-chlorhexidine irrigation reduces the incidence of bacteremia during ultrasonic scaling with the Cavi-Med: a pilot investigation. J Can Dent Assoc 59: 676–82.
15. Fine DH, Furgang D, McKiernan M, Tereski-Bischio D, Ricci-Nittel D, et al. (2010) An investigation of the effect of an essential oil mouthrinse on induced bacteraemia: a pilot study. J Clin Periodontol 37:840–7.
16. Kinane DF, Riggio MP, Walker KF, MacKenzie D, Shearer B. (2005) Bacteraemia following periodontal procedures. J Clin Periodontol 32:708–13.
17. Forner L, Larsen T, Kilian M, Holmstrup P. (2006) Incidence of bacteremia after chewing, tooth brushing and scaling in individuals with periodontal inflammation. J Clin Periodontol 33:401–7.

18. Lafaurie GI, Mayorga-Fayad I, Torres MF Castillo DM, Aya MR, et al. (2007) Periodontopathic microorganisms in peripheric blood after scaling and root planing. J Clin Periodontol 34:873–9.
19. Padilla EC, Lobos GO, Jure OG, Matus FS, Descouvieres CC, et al. (2007) Isolation of periodontal bacteria from blood samples and atheromas in patients with atherosclerosis and periodontitis (article in Spanish). Rev Med Chil 135:1118–24.
20. Maestre JR, Mateo M, Sánchez P. (2008) Bacteremia after periodontal procedures (article in Spanish). Rev Esp Quimioter 2:153–6.
21. Pérez-Chaparro PJ, Gracieux P, Lafaurie GI, Donnio PY, Bonnaure-Mallet M (2008) Genotypic characterization of *Porphyromonas gingivalis* isolated from subgingival plaque and blood sample in positive bacteremia subjects with periodontitis. J Clin Periodontol 35:748–53.
22. Pérez-Chaparro PJ, Lafaurie GI, Gracieux P, Meuric V, Tamanai-Shacoori Z, et al. (2009) Distribution of *Porphyromonas gingivalis* fimA genotypes in isolates from subgingival plaque and blood sample during bacteremia. *Biomedica* 29:298–306.
23. Castillo DM, Sánchez-Beltrán MC, Castellanos JE, Sanz I, Mayorga-Fayad I, et al. (2011) Detection of specific periodontal microorganisms from bacteraemia samples after periodontal therapy using molecular-based diagnostics. J Clin Periodontol 38:418–27.
24. Daly CG, Mitchell DH, Highfield JE, Grossberg DE Stewart D (2001) Bacteremia due to periodontal probing: a clinical and microbiological investigation. J Periodontol 72:210–4.
25. Daly CG, Mitchell DH, Highfield JE, Grossberg DE, Stewart D (1997) Bacteraemia caused by periodontal probing. Aust Dent J 42:77–80.
26. Lineberger LT, De Marco TJ. (1973) Evaluation of transient bacteremia following routine periodontal procedures. J Periodontol 44:757–62.
27. Morozumi T, Kubota T, Abe D, Shimizu T, Komatsu Y, et al. (2010) Effects of irrigation with an antiseptic and oral administration of azithromycin on bacteremia caused by scaling and root planning. J Periodontol 81:1555–63.
28. Loockhart PB. (2000) The risk for endocarditis in dental practice. Periodontology 2000;23:127–135.
29. Appleman MD, Sutter VL, Sims TN. (1982) Value of antibiotic prophylaxis in periodontal surgery. J Periodontol 53:319–24.
30. Stroup DF, Berlin JA, Morton SC, Olkin I, Williamson GD, et al. (2000) Meta-analysis of observational studies in epidemiology: a proposal for reporting. Meta-analysis of Observational Studies in Epidemiology (MOOSE) group. JAMA 283:2008–12.
31. Moher D, Liberati A, Tetzlaff J, Altman DG, PRISMA Group (2009) Preferred reporting items for systematic reviews and meta-analyses: the PRISMA Statement. J Clin Epidemiol 62:1006–1012.
32. Chambrone L, Faggion CM, Pannuti CM, Chambrone LA (2010) Evidence-based periodontal plastic surgery: an assessment of quality of systematic reviews in the treatment of recession-type defects. J Clin Periodontol 37:1110–1118.
33. Armitage GC. (1999) American Academy of Periodontology. Development of a classification system for periodontal diseases and conditions. Ann Periodontol 4:1–6.
34. Wells G A, Shea B, O'Connell D. The Newcastle–Ottawa Scale (NOS) for Assessing the Quality of Non randomised Studies in Meta-Analyses. University of Ottawa, 2001 Available at http://www.ohri.ca/pro grams/clinical_epidemiology/oxford.htm. Accessed December 12th, 2012.
35. Chambrone L, Chambrone D, Lima LA, Chambrone LA (2010) Predictors of tooth loss during long term periodontal maintenance: a systematic review of observational studies. J Clin Periodontol 37:675–684.
36. Chambrone L, Guglielmetti MR, Pannuti CM, Chambrone LA (2011) Evidence grade associating periodontitis to preterm birth and/or low birth weight: I. A systematic review of prospective cohort studies. J Clin Periodontol 38:795–808.
37. Lacassin F, Hoen B, Leport C Selton-Suty C, Delahaye F, et al. (1995) Procedures associated with infective endocarditis in adults. A case control study. Eur Heart J 16:1968–74.
38. Lieberman MB. (1992) A life-threatening, spontaneous, periodontitis-induced infective endocarditis. J Calif Dent Assoc:20:37–9.
39. Lofthus JE, Waki MY, Jolkovsky DL, Otomo-Corgel J, Newman MG, et al. (1991) Bacteremia following subgingival irrigation and scaling and root planing. J Periodontol 62:602–7.
40. Font Buxo J. (1985) Bacteremia (article in Spanish). Rev Actual Estomatol Esp 45:58–60.
41. Trivedi DN. (1984) Bacteraemia due to operative procedure. J Indian Dent Assoc 56:447–52.
42. Wank HA, Levison ME, Rose LF, Cohen DW (1976) A quantitative measurement of bacteremia and its relationship to plaque control. J Periodontol 47:683–6.
43. Ewart NP. (1971) Bacteraemia from periodontal disease. Bull N Z Soc Periodontol 32:15–8.
44. Kraal JH. (1970) Bacteremia due to dental intervention (article in Dutch). Ned Tijdschr Tandheelkd 77:5–14.
45. Montanari G. (1967) Studies on bacteremia caused by hand instruments and ultrasonic instruments in periodontal therapy: (preliminary study restricted to the aerobic flora) (article in Italian). Mondo Odontostomatol 9:570–4.
46. Lazansky IP, Robinson L, Rodofsky I. (1949) Factors influencing the incidence of bacteremias following surgical procedures in the oral cavity. J Dent Res 28:533–43.
47. Rogosa M, Hampp EG, Nevin TA, Wagner HN Jr, Driscoll EJ, et al. (1960) Blood sampling and cultural studies in the detection of postoperative bacteremias. J Am Dent Assoc 60:171–80.
48. Conner HD, Haberman S, Collings CK, Winford TE (1967) Bacteremias following periodontal scaling in patients with healthy appearing gingiva. J Periodontol 38:466–72.
49. Bayliss R, Clarke C, Oakley C, Somerville W, Whitfield AG (1983) The teeth and infective endocarditis. Br Heart J 50:506–512.
50. Baltch AL, Schaffer C, Hammer MC. (1982) Bacteremia following dental cleaning in patients with and without penicillin prophylaxis. Am Heart J 104:1335–9.
51. Korn NA, Schaffer EM. (1962) A comparison of the postoperative bacteremias induced following different periodontal procedures. J Periodontol 33:226–231.
52. Bandt, CL Korn NA, Schaffer EM. (1964) Bacteremias from ultrasonic and hand instrumentation. J Periodontol 35:214–215.
53. Winslow MB, Kobernick SD. (1960) Bacteremia after prophylaxis. J Am Dent Assoc 61:69–72.
54. Raetzke P, O'Leary TJ, Miller CH. (1981) Appearance of transitory bacteremia during human periodontal flap operations. Dtsch Zahnarztl Z 36:121–5.
55. Zhang W, Daly CG, Mitchell D, Curtis B. (2013) Incidence and magnitude of bacteraemia caused by flossing and by scaling and root planing. J Clin Periodontol;40:41–52.
56. Lockhart PB, Brennan MT, Sasser HC, Fox PC, Paster BJ, et al. (2008) Bacteremia associated with toothbrushing and dental extraction. Circulation 117:3118–25.
57. Friedewald VE, Kornman KS, Beck JD, Genco R, Goldfine A, et al. (2009) The American Journal of Cardiology and Journal of Periodontology editors' consensus: periodontitis and atherosclerotic cardiovascular disease. J Periodontol 80:1021–32.
58. Que YA, Moreillon P. (2011) Infective endocarditis. Nat Rev Cardiol;8:322–36.
59. Olsen I. Update on bacteraemia related to dental procedures. Transfus Apher Sci. 2008;39(2):173–8.
60. Fenollar F, Raoult D. (2007) Molecular diagnosis of bloodstream infections caused by non-cultivable bacteria. Int J Antimicrob Agents;30 Suppl 1:S7–15.
61. Lockhart PB, Durack DT. (1999) Oral microflora as a cause of endocarditis and other distant site infections. Infect Dis Clin North Am 13:833–50.
62. Lucas VS, Lytra V, Hassan T, Tatham H, Wilson M, et al. (2002) Comparison of lysis filtration and an automated blood culture system (BACTEC) for detection, quantification, and identification of odontogenic bacteremia in children. J Clin Microbiol. 40:3416–20.
63. Bahrani-Mougeot FK, Paster BJ, Coleman S, Ashar J, Barbuto S, et al. (2008) Diverse and novel oral bacterial species in blood following dental procedures. J Clin Microbiol 46:2129–32.
64. Belstrøm D, Holmstrup P, Damgaard C Borch TS, Skjødt MO, et al. (2011) The atherogenic bacterium *Porphyromonas gingivalis* evades circulating phagocytes by adhering to erythrocytes. Infect Immun;79:1559–65.
65. Deshpande RG, Khan M, Genco CA. (1998) Invasion strategies of the oral pathogen *Porphyromonas gingivalis*: implications for cardiovascular disease. Invasion Metastasis;18:57–69.
66. Murphy AM, Daly CG, Mitchell DH, Stewart D, Curtis BH (2006) Chewing fails to induce oral bacteremia in patients with periodontal disease. J CLin Periodontol33:730–6.
67. Cates KL. (1983) Host factors in bacteremia. Am J Med. 28:19–25.
68. Gendron R, Grenier D, Maheu-Robert L. (2000) The oral cavity as a reservoir of bacterial pathogens for focal infections. Microbes Infect 2:897–906.
69. Coburn B, Morris AM, Tomlinson G, Detsky AS. (2012) Does this adult patient with suspected bacteremia require blood cultures? JAMA 308:502–11.
70. Zanatta FB, Antoniazzi RP, Rösing CK. (2007) The effect of 0.12% chlorhexidine gluconate rinsing on previously plaque-free and plaque-covered surfaces: a randomized, controlled clinical trial. J Periodontol 78:2127–34.
71. Zaura-Arite E, van Marle J, ten Cate JM. (2001) Conofocal microscopy study of undisturbed and chlorhexidine-treated dental biofilm. J Dent Res 80:1436–40.

Prevalence of *Porphyromonas gingivalis* Four *rag* Locus Genotypes in Patients of Orthodontic Gingivitis and Periodontitis

Yi Liu[1], Yujie Zhang[2], Lili Wang[3], Yang Guo[2], Shuiqing Xiao[2]*

1 Pediatric Research Institute, Qilu Children's Hospital of Shandong University, Ji'nan, Shandong, China, **2** Department of Orthodontic, Jinan Stomatological Hospital, Jinan, Shandong, China, **3** Clinical Laboratory, Jinan Central Hospital of Shandong University, Jinan, Shandong, China

Abstract

Porphyromonas gingivalis is considered as a major etiological agent in periodontal diseases and implied to result in gingival inflammation under orthodontic appliance. *rag* locus is a pathogenicity island found in *Porphyromonas gingivalis.* Four *rag* locus variants are different in pathogenicity of *Porphyromonas gingivalis.* Moreover, there are different racial and geographic differences in distribution of *rag* locus genotypes. In this study, we assessed the prevalence of *Porphyromonas gingivalis* and *rag* locus genotypes in 102 gingival crevicular fluid samples from 57 cases of gingivitis patients with orthodontic appliances, 25 cases of periodontitis patients and 20 cases of periodontally healthy people through a 16S rRNA-based PCR and a multiplex PCR. The correlations between *Porphyromona.gingivalis/rag* locus and clinical indices were analyzed. The prevalence of *Porphyromonas gingivalis* and *rag* locus genes in periodontitis group was the highest among three groups and higher in orthodontic gingivitis than healthy people ($p<0.01$). An obviously positive correlation was observed between the prevalènce of *Porphyromonas gingivalis/rag* locus and gingival index. *rag*-3 and *rag*-4 were the predominant genotypes in the patients of orthodontic gingivitis and mild-to-moderate periodontitis in Shandong. *Porphyromonas.gingivalis* carrying *rag-1* has the strong virulence and could be associated with severe periodontitis.

Editor: Krzysztof Pyrc, Jagiellonian University, Poland

Funding: This work was funded by Jinan Science and Technology Research Project (JK200905034) from Jinan Science and Technology Committee. The funders had no role in study design, data collection and analysis, decision to publish, or preparation of the manuscript.

Competing Interests: The authors have declared that no competing interests exist.

* E-mail: shqxiao@126.com

Introduction

Malocclusion is one of the most common oral-maxillofacial diseases that bring some negative effects on facial aesthetics, oral physical function and health as well. In China, morbidity of malocclusion in teenagers is as high as 67.82% [1]. Orthodontic treatment is currently the preferred and most common method for the reason of solving above the problems, but it also holds some potentials of harming teeth and periodontal tissues due to plaque accumulation and gingival inflammation that are induced by the changes of oral internal environment after wearing fixed orthodontic appliance, therefore lead to changing of host physiology and the composition of the oral microflora [2,3]. The inflammatory reaction of gingival tissue can often be detected in patients wearing fixed orthodontic appliances. The overall morbidity of gingivitis was higher as 56.8% and 34.4% in adolescent group and adult group respectively during fixed orthodontic treatment in China [4]. Primary pathogenic micro-organisms strongly implicated in gingival inflammation and posterior periodontal destruction, such as *Porphyromonas gingivalis*, *Prevotella intermedia/nigrescens*, *Aggregatibacter actinomycetemcomitans*, *Tannerella forsythia*, *Treponema denticola*, and *Fusobacterium* species have been found elevated in patients after bracket placement [5–7]. Our previous research showed that the percentage of *bacilli*, esp. *Porphyromonas gingivalis*, *Aggregatibacter actinomycetemcomitans*, *Fusobacterium nucleatum* increased significantly after wearing orthodontic appliance and the increase of those pathogens was significantly related with the development of gingivitis in orthodontic treatment [8–9].

Porphyromonas gingivalis is a gram-negative oral anaerobe and considered as a major etiological agent in periodontal diseases by producing a number of virulence factors and extracellular proteases, such as lipopolysaccharide, capsule, gingipain, fimbria and so on, resulting in the destruction of periodontal tissues [10–13]. The pathogenicity of *P.gingivalis* has been investigated in a variety of experimental animal models, such as rat [14–15], mouse [16–17], rabbit [18], drosophila [19], and cell models [20–23], showing complicated mechanisms of *P.gingivalis*-host interactions in development of periodontal diseases. Three gingipains referred to be the important virulence factors, Arg-x-specific proteinase and adhesins (RgpA), Arg-x-specific proteinase (RgpB), and a Lys-x-specific proteinase and adhesins (Kgp) have been well known and studied in details with properties of activating and/or degrading a wide range of host proteins through different mechanisms [20–23].

Pathogenicity island is a large unstable chromosome DNA region encoding virulence determinants of pathogenic bacteria and was first described in human pathogens of the species *Escherichia coli* by Hacker et al.[24]. The island has been also detected in other pathogens, such as *Klebsiella pneumoniae*, *Enterobacter aerogenes*, and *Citrobacter koseri* isolates with high conservative property among these species and is in association with the yersiniabactin determinant [25]. In 1999, Curtis et al [26] found a novel pathogenicity island in a proportion of *P.gingivalis* strains named *rag* locus and it was more frequently detected in deep periodontal pockets in periodontal patients. It was reported that the *rag* locus of *P.gingivalis* might arise from *Bacteriodes* via horizontal gene transfer and encodes *RagA* and *RagB*. *RagA* is a 115-kDa TonB-dependent outer membrane receptor, and *RagB* is a 55-kDa lipoprotein constituting an immunodominant outer antigen. Both proteins of *RagA* and *RagB* constitute a membrane transporter system. Further study demonstrated that four *rag* locus variants with different pathogenicity were detected from clinical isolates of *P.gingivalis* [26–28]. A significant correlation was observed between prevalence of *rag-1* allele and a highly virulent phenotype in a murine model of soft tissue destruction [29]. In addition, there are different racial and geographic differences in distribution of *rag* locus genotypes [28]. Wang et al.[30] investigated the distribution of *rag* genotypes in chronic periodontitis patients in Northeast of China and found *P.gingivalis* carrying *rag-1*, *rag-3* was more predominant in chronic periodontitis so that might be associated with the development of pediodontitis.

There have been reports about the association between prevalence of *P.gingivalis* and gingival inflammation during orthodontic treatment [31–35]. Our previous research showed that the prevalence of *P. gingivalis* was totally higher as 40.62% two months after orthodontics detected by using traditional anaerobic culture [9]. While there have been no investigations about the correlation between *P.gingivalis rag* locus and periodontal health status in orthodontic gingivitis patients. Therefore, we assessed the prevalence of *P.gingivalis* and *rag* locus genotypes in gingival crevicular fluid samples from the gingivitis lesions of orthodontic patients and compared them with periodontitis patients as well as periodontally healthy people who showed healthy periodontal tissues before wearing orthodontic appliances.

Materials and Methods

Subjects

The study subjects consisted of three groups who visited Jinan stomatological hospital for orthodontic or periodontitis treatment from 2010 to 2011. Of three groups, orthodontic group (OG) included 57 patients, 38 females and 19 males, aged between 10 and 30 years (mean 16.3) who got gingival inflammation during orthodontic treatment; control group (CG) contained 20 periodontally healthy people, 12 females and 8 males, aged between 10 and 30 years (mean 16.05) before orthodontic treatment; periodontitis group (PG) was composed of 25 periodontitis patients, 10 females and 15 males, aged from 20 to 60 years (mean 25) who came to hospital for periodontitis treatment. The patients who are having any systemic diseases, antibiotics therapy within the last 3 months and pregnant or lactating females were excluded.

Ethics statement

This work was approved by the Medical Ethics Committee of the Jinan Stomatological Hospital. All patients or their parents gave their verbal followed by written informed consent before the examination was performed. The relevant regulations and institutional polices were followed strictly.

Bacteria strains

The reference strains of *P.gingivalis* ATCC33277, *F.nucleatum* ATCC25586 and *A.actinomycetemcomitans* ATCC29522 were from the West-China Dental School of Sichun University and *P.gingivalis* W83 was from Beijing Oral Research Institute of Capital Medical University.

Clinical examination

We selected the gingivitis or periodontal sites that exhibited the deepest pocket depth of every subject. The clinical parameters included gingival index (GI), plaque index (PI), sulcus bleeding index (SBI) and probing depth (PD) of each person were examined and recorded. All clinical examinations were carried out by the same dentist.

Sample collection and DNA extraction

Gingival crevicular fluid (GCF) was obtained from the two deepest periodontal pockets in the maxilla according to Rüdin et al [36]. In brief, before collecting, saline solution was used to rinse out food debris and then each site was cleaned by cotton rolls. Sterile filter paper strips were placed for 30 seconds into the packet until a minimum of resistance. The paper points were placed into a sterile microcentrifuge tube containing 0.5 ml of 1×PBS immediately. The tubes were mixed thoroughly and stored at −20°C until analyzed. The bacterial DNA was extracted by the boiling method [37]. In short, a 10 μl aliquot of each stored sample was added to 10 μl of 2 ×lysis buffer (2 mM EDTA, 1% X-100). The mixture was boiled for 10 minutes and then placed on ice. The supernatant was used as the template for PCR amplification.

The 16S rRNA-based PCR and multiplex PCR amplification

The 16S rRNA gene specific primers were used to determine the prevalence of *P.gingivalis* in GCF, while four different *rag* locus variants primers were utilized to amplify the rag locus variants genes from GCF samples containing *P.gingivalis*. The 16S rRNA-based PCR was first performed on DNA extracts from GCF samples using primers of 16S rRNA-F (5′-AGG CAG CTT GCC ATA CTG CG-3′) and 16S rRNA-R (5′-ACT GTT AGC AAC TAC CGA TGT-3′) that amplify a 404-bp region of the 16S rRNA gene[38]. The specificity of this PCR was confirmed by sequencing and amplifying *P.gingivalis* ATCC33277, W83, as well as unrelated pathogens *F.nucleatum* ATCC25586 and *A.actinomycetemcomitans* ATCC29522. Then the multiplex PCR was utilized to amplify *rag* locus genes from the positive *P.gingivalis* samples. Amplification reaction was run in a Tetrad Thermal Cycler (MJ Research, South San Francisco, USA) in a 25 μl reaction mixture containing 4.5 μl 10×PCR buffer (100 mM Tris-HCl, 500 mM KCl, and 15 mM MgCl2), 0.25 mM of each deoxynucleoside triphosphate (dNTP), 10 μM of each primers, 5 μl of DNA extracts from GCF samples, and 1.5 units of Taq DNA

Table 1. Primers of *rag* locus genotypes used for PCR.

Primers	Sequences(5′→3′)	Sizes (bp)
rag-1F	5′-CGCGACCCCGAAGGAAAAGATT-3′	628
rag-1R	5′-CACGGCTCACATAAAGAACGCT-3′	
rag-2F	5′-GCTTTGCCGCTTGTGACTTGG-3′	979
rag-2R	5′-CCACCGTCACCGTTCACCTT-3′	
rag-3F	5′-CCGGAAGATAAGGCCAAGAAAGA-3′	423
rag-3R	5′-ACGCCAATTCGCCAAAGCT-3′	
rag-4F	5′-CCGGATGGAAGTGATGAACAGA-3′	739
rag-4R	5′-CGCGGTAAACCTCAGCAAATT-3′	

Table 2. Prevalence of P.gingivalis among three groups.

Groups	Cases (n)	Prevalence of P.gingivalis	
		P.gingivalis counts	P.gingivalis(%)
OG	57	35	61.40*
CG	20	7	35.00
PG	25	23	92.00**
Total	102	65	63.73

**P<0.01 between PG and CG; * P<0.05 between OG and CG (Chi-squared test).

polymerase (Transgen Biotech, Beijing) for 5 min at 94°C and 33 cycles, with each cycle consisting of denaturation at 94°C for 30 sec, annealing at 57°C for 30 sec, extension at 72°C for 1 min, and final extension for 10 min. Nucleotide sequences of the forward and reverse primers for *rag* locus genes were listed in Table 1 [39].

The amplified PCR products were then electrophoreses on 1.5% agarose gel in Tris-acetate buffer (40 mM Tris acetate, 1 mM EDTA, pH 8.0). The products were visualized with ethidium bromide by UV transillumination.

Statistical analysis

The differences in the prevalence of *rag* locus genes were analyzed using the Chi square test. The Spearman Correlation Test was utilized to analyze the correlation between prevalence of *P.gingivalis/rag* locus genes and clinical indices in three research groups. All statistical analyses were done by using a statistical software package (SPSS for Windows 13.0).

Results

Detection and confirmation of 16S rRNA-based PCR for *P.gingivalis*

The reference stains were first amplified by the 16S rRNA-based PCR to evaluate the specificity of it. The positive product appeared only from *P.gingivalis* ATCC33277 and W83, not from *F.nucleatum* ATCC25586 and *A.actinomycetemcomitans* ATCC29522.

Sixty-five *P.gingivalis* was detected in 65 (63.73%) cases of GCF samples from 102 cases of three groups, thirty-five (61.40%) from orthodontic group (OG), Seven (35%) from control group (CG), and 23 (92%) from periodontitis group (PG). Prevalence of

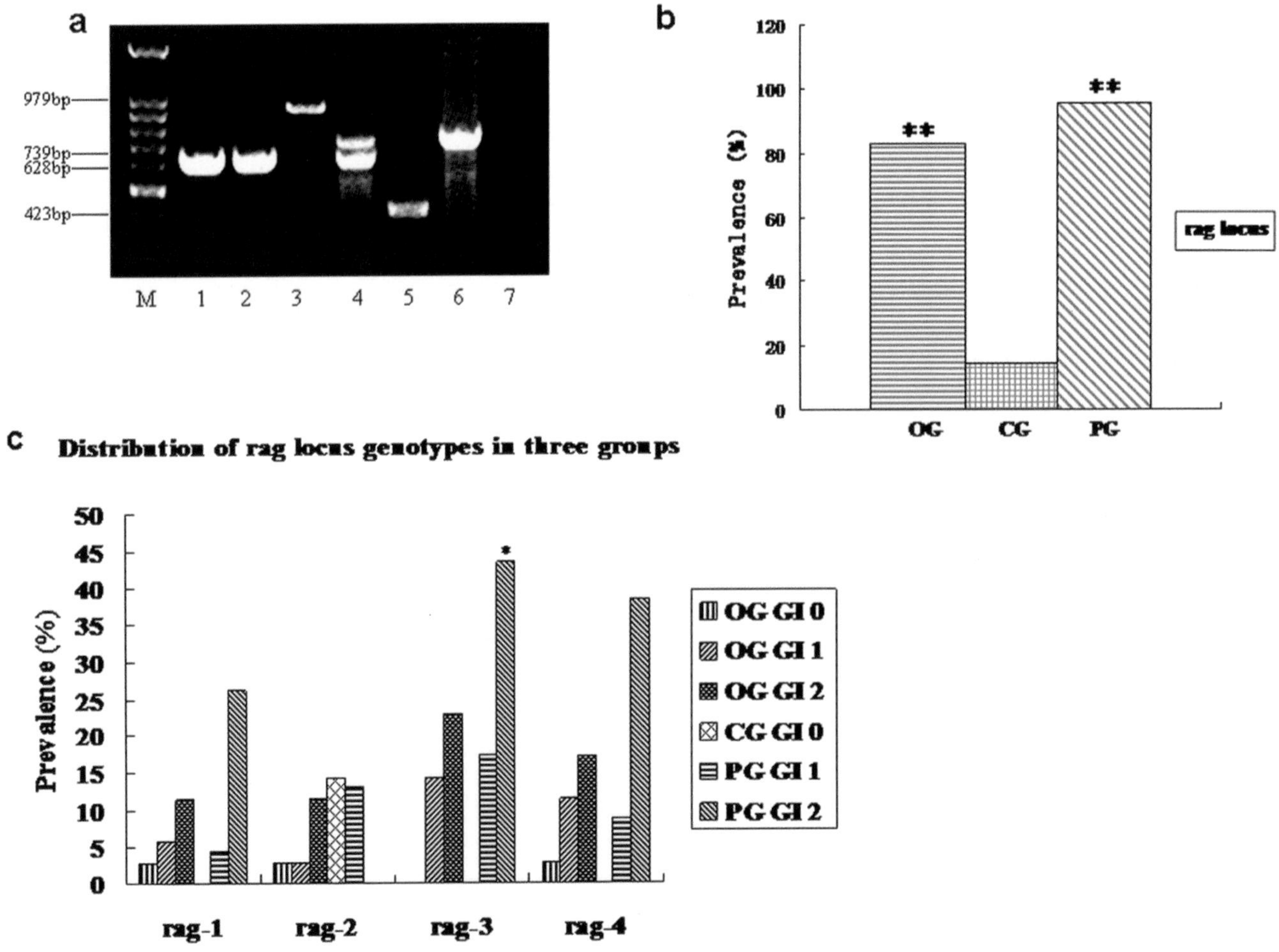

Figure 1. Detection and distribution of *rag* locus genes. a. Detection of rag locus genes in clinical GCF samples. M DNA Marker; Lane1 positive control of *P.gingivalis* W83; Lane 2–7 clinical GCF samples, showing *rag-1* (lane 2), *rag-2* (lane3), *rag-1* combined with *rag-4* (lane4), *rag-3* (lane5), *rag-4* (lane6), and negative (lane 7). b. The prevalence of *rag* locus genes in clinical GCF samples of three groups. ** P<0.01 between OG/PG and CG (Chi-squared test). c. Distribution of four *rag* locus genes among three groups.

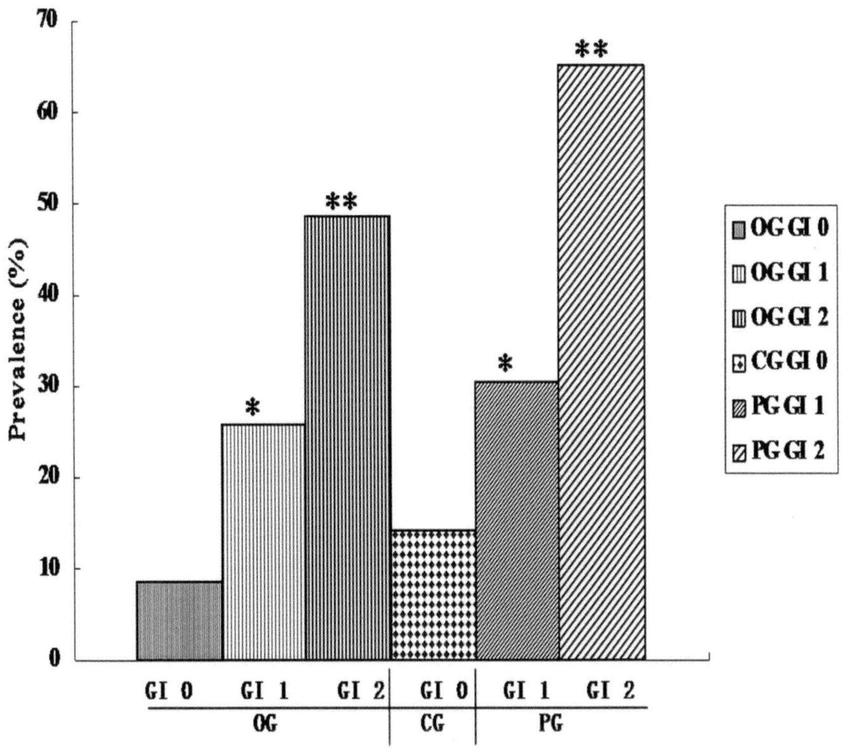

Figure 2. Correlation of rag locus genes and gingival indices (GI). ** P<0.01 between GI 2 and GI 0; * P<0.05 between GI 1 and GI 0, # P<0.05 between GI 2 and GI 1 in PG (Chi-squared test).

P.gingivalis was found significantly different in three groups: *P.gingivalis* was the highest prevalence in PG (P<0.01) and higher level in OG than CG (P<0.05) (Table 2). Of 65 *P.gingivalis* positive samples, 10 were randomly sequenced by a 3730 DNA sequencer in Invitrogen Company (Invitrogen, Shanghai) and confirmed the validity of the 16S rRNA-based PCR for clinical GCF samples (date were not showed).

The correlation of patients' age and prevalence of *P.gingivalis* was analyzed. The average age of patients with positive *P.gingivalis* in GCF was 25.54 years, while patients with negative *P.gingivalis* was 16.19 years, and there was statistical difference between the patients' ages of both positive and negative *P.gingivalis* (P<0.05).

Table 3. Prevalence of *rag* locus under different gingival index (GI) among three groups.

Groups	GI (n)	rag locus(%)	rag-1 (%)	rag-2 (%)	rag-3 (%)	rag-4 (%)
OG	0 (16)	8.57	2.86	2.86	0	2.86
	1 (20)	25.72*	5.72	2.86	14.29	11.43
	2 (21)	48.57**	11.43	11.43	22.86	17.14
CG	0 (20)	14.29	0	14.29	0	0
PG	1 (10)	30.43*	4.35	13.04	17.39	8.70
	2 (15)	65.22**	26.09	0	43.48#	38.46

**P<0.01 between GI 2 and GI 0; * P<0.05 between GI 1 and GI 0, #P<0.05 between GI 1 and GI 0 (Chi-squared test).

Multiplex-PCR amplification of *rag* locus genes

Multiplex-PCR was firstly used to detect *rag* locus genes from the high virulent *P.gingivalis* W83 and low virulent *P.gingivalis* ATCC33277. It showed that *rag-1* gene was amplified from *P.gingivalis* W83 and *rag-4* was from ATCC33277, which were consistent with previous documents [40,41].

There were 52 (80%) positive *rag* locus genes detected from the 65 GCF samples which were *P.gingivalis* positive, twenty-nine (82.86%) from those in OG, 22 (95.65%) from those in PG, only one case (14.29%) from healthy people. The prevalence of *rag* locus was significantly higher in PG and OG than in CG (P<0.01), while no significant difference between PG and OG (P>0.05) (Fig. 1).

Among *P.gingivalis*-positive GCF samples from three groups, the most prevalent rag gene was rag-3 (51.92%), followed by rag-4(38.26%) and rag-1(26.92%). While in those of PG, rag-3 (60.87%), rag-4 (39.13%), rag-1(30.43%) were much higher than those in CG (only rag-2 positive); Similar to those of periodontitis group, in those of OG, the proportion of *rag* genotypes were: *rag-3* 44.83%, *rag-4* 37.93%, *rag-2* 20.69%; but in CG: only one case of *rag-2* (14.29%) was detected.

Correlation of *rag* locus genes and clinical indices

It was noticed that clinical indices were all higher in OG and PG than CG (P<0.05). The prevalence of *rag* locus genes, except rag-2, elevated directly with increases of GI values in both OG and PG. The significant positive correlation between *rag* locus and GI was showed by using Spearman Correlation Test (P<0.01) (Fig. 2). However, there were no statistical difference between *rag* locus and PD/PI/SBI, while we detected the increase of *rag* locus in OG and PG with higher GI and higher PD/PI/SBI. *rag-1* often appeared from the deeper periodontal pocket with higher PD/PI/SBI values and 10/14 of *rag-1* positive cases accompanied with *rag-3* and/or *rag-4*. Interestingly, an exception was found that one case of *rag-1* gene was from a patient of GI 0 lever in orthodontic group, so further research would be done for the possible variation of *rag-1* gene. The prevalence of four *rag* locus genes among three groups showed in table 3.

Discussion

P.gingivalis has been known to be a risk factor for periodontal diseases though the exact roles of it in the initiation and progression of the oral diseases remain unclear. Mouse model tests have indicated difference in the virulence of *P.gingivalis* with and without *rag* locus [28,29]. Shi et al. mutated *rag* locus genes in *P.gingivalis* by using an allele replacement strategy and clearly showed that inactivation of the rag locus reduced the virulence of *P.gingivalis* in a mouse model of soft tissue destruction [29]. In a collection of 168 isolates of *P.gingivalis* from western European countries, including the Netherlands, Romania, Sweden, the United Kindom, Kenya and Germany, Hall et al. found different prevalence and geographic differences in distribution of four *rag* alleles [28]. In this case, we detected prevalence of *P.gingivalis* and *rag* locus genotypes in local patients of orthodontic gingivitis, periodontitis and periodontally healthy people to evaluate the distribution of *P.gingivalis* and predominant genotypes of *rag* locus in different periodontal health statuses, then further deduce the pathogenicity of *P.gingivalis* carrying different rag locus during orthodontic treatment.

In periodontal disease, gingival crevicular fluid (GCF) is an inflammatory exudate. GCF contains substances from supra-and subgingival located bacteria. Analysis of microflora in GCF becomes more and more important in diagnosis and therapy of periodontal diseases. There are a large number of periodonto-pathic bacteria including *P.gingivalis* in GCF [42]. Considering the method of filter paper strips is recommended to collect the microflora from GCF for microbiological analysis in dental practice [35]. With sterile filter paper strips, we collected GCF samples divided into orthodontic gingivitis, periodontally healthy control and periodontitis groups from 102 patients to investigate the prevalence of *P.gingivalis* in above three groups. The occurrence of *P.gingivalis* was 61.40% in OG, 35% in CG, and 92% in PG, respectively. There was a statistically higher prevalence of *P.gingivalis* in PG followed by OG than CG. Furthermore, a significantly strong positive correlation was observed between the prevalence of *P.gingivalis* and GI by Spearman Correlation Test ($P<0.01$), which was consistent with previous reports [31–33,43]. While once wearing fixed appliance, oral hygiene will turns bad if teeth cleaning can not be paid special attention, as a result, dental plaque will accumulate and gingival inflammation will happen. By then, one side, anaerobic environment will be created due to swollen gum, deeper gingival sulcus, and pseudo periodontal pocket; on the other side, the gum will be susceptible to bleeding and therefore it will be more conductive for periodontal anaerobic *P.gingivalis* to survive. *P.gingivalis* may play a similar role in orthodontic gingivitis and periodontitis.

P.gingivalis has been reported to be related with adult periodontitis [10,12]. In this study, we analyzed correlation of patients' age and occurrence of *P.gingivalis* and found the age of both *P.gingivalis* positive and negative was statistically different; implying the prevalence of *P.gingivalis* may increase as patients'age increased.

In order to further explore whether the *P.gingivalis rag* locus was associated with gingival inflammation under orthodontic appliance,we detected the distribution of *rag* locus in three groups and discovered 52 (80%) of positive *rag* locus genes from 65 *P.gingivalis*-positive GCFs. The prevalence of *rag* locus was higher in those of PG and OG than those of CG. The *P.gingivalis* without *rag* locus was mostly detected from periodontally healthy control and GI 0 level OG patients, demonstrating that they present the avirulent or weak virulence genotype of *P.gingivalis*. A clear positive correlation was indicated between the gingival index and *rag* locus genes, implying *rag* locus genes may play a pathogenic and similar role in the development of gum inflammation during orthodontic in comparison with periodontitis.

The prevalence of *rag-3* (27 cases) was the most detected followed by *rag-4* (20 cases) and *rag-1* (14 cases); the lowest occurrence was *rag-2* (10 cases) with lower GI and PD/PI/SBI values, showing the *rag-3* and *rag-4* locus genes might be the predominant genotypes in the patients of orthodontic gingivitis and mild-to-moderate periodontitis in the populations of Shandong region. Besides, we found *rag-1* was detected from 14 cases, mostly with higher GI and PD/PI/SBI, and often combined with *rag-3* and/or *rag-4*, suggesting the *P.gingivalis* carrying *rag-1* is the strong virulent genotype and can be closely associated with severe periodontitis, which is consistent with Hanley et al[44].

In summary, *P.gingivalis* carrying *rag-3*, *rag-4* locus is one of the risk factors that are responsible for gingivitis during orthodontic treatment. Thus monitoring *P.gingivalis* is highly recommended following the placement of orthodontic appliances. In addition, appropriate oral hygiene is necessary to reduce invasion of pathogens and exerts a beneficial effect to oral tissues.

Author Contributions

Conceived and designed the experiments: YL SX. Performed the experiments: YZ LW YG. Analyzed the data: YZ SX. Contributed reagents/materials/analysis tools: YZ SX. Wrote the paper: YL SX.

References

1. Fu M, Zhang D, Wang B, Deng Y, Wang F, et al. (2002) The prevalence of malocclusion in China-an investigation of 25 392 children. Chin J Stomatol, 37(5):371-373.
2. Bollen AM, Cunha-Cruz J, Bakko DW, Huang GJ, Hujoel PP (2008) The effects of orthodontic therapy on periodontal health: a systematic review of controlled evidence. J Am Dent Assoc, 139(4):413-422.
3. Lara-Carrillo E, Montiel-Bastida NM, Sanchez-Perez L, Alanis-Tavira J (2010) Effect of orthodontic treatment on saliva, plaque and the levels of Streptococcus mutans and Lactobacillus. Med Oral Patol Oral Cir Bucal, 15(6):e924-929.
4. Chen Jiapeng (2011) Effects of oral education on the incidence of gingivitis during fixed orthodontic treatment in adults and adolescents. J Anhui Med 32(5):604-606.
5. Lee SM, Yoo SY, Kim HS, Kim KW, Yoon YJ, et al. (2005) Prevalence of putative periodontopathogens in subgingival dental plaques from gingivitis lesions in Korean orthodontic patients. J Microbiol 43(3):260-265.
6. Naranjo AA, Trivino ML, Jaramillo A, Betancourth M, Botero JE (2006) Changes in the subgingival microbiota and periodontal parameters before and 3 months after bracket placement. Am J Orthod Dentofacial Orthop 130(3):275.e17-22.
7. Ristic M, Vlahovic Svabic M, Sasic M, Zelic O (2007) Clinical and microbiological effects of fixed orthodontic appliances on periodontal tissues in adolescents. Orthod Craniofac Res 10(4):187-195.
8. Huang X, Xiao S (2010) The impact of fixed orthodontic appliance on gum conditions and bacteria of gingival crevicular fluid. China Clin Prac Med 4(1):26-27.
9. Wang J, Zhang Y, Xiao S (2011) The changes of the bacterial ecology and ALP activity in gingival crevicular fluid during orthodontic treatment. Stomatology 31(9):531-535.
10. Decaillet F, Giannopoulou C, Cionca N, Almaghlouth A, Mombelli A (2012) Microbial profiles of patients seeking treatment for periodontitis. Influence of origin, smoking and age? Schweiz Monatsschr Zahnmed 122(3):198-204.
11. Bostanci N, Belibasakis GN (2012) Porphyromonas gingivalis: an invasive and evasive opportunistic oral pathogen. FEMS Microbiol Lett 331(1):1-9.

12. Hayashi F, Okada M, Oda Y, Kojima T, Kozai K (2012) Prevalence of Porphyromonas gingivalis fimA genotypes in Japanese children. J Oral Sci 54(1):77-83.
13. Perez-Chaparro PJ, Lafaurie GI, Gracieux P, Meuric V, Tamanai-Shacoori Z, et al. (2009) Distribution of Porphyromonas gingivalis fimA genotypes in isolates from subgingival plaque and blood sample during bacteremia. Biomedica 29(2):298-306.
14. Evans RT, Klausen B, Ramamurthy NS, Golub LM, Sfintescu C,et al.(1992) Periodontopathic potential of two strains of Porphyromonas gingivalis in gnotobiotic rats. Arch Oral Biol 37(10):813-819.
15. Katz J, Ward DC, Michalek SM (1996) Effect of host responses on the pathogenicity of strains of Porphymonas gingivalis. Oral Microbiol Immunol 11(5):309-318.
16. O'Brien-Simpson NM, Paolini RA (2001) Hoffmann B, Slakeski N, Dashper SG, Reynolds EC. Role of RgpA, RgpB, and Kgp proteinases in virulence of Porphyromonas gingivalis W50 in a murine lesion model. Infect Immun 69(12):7527-7534.
17. Gibson FC, 3rd, Genco CA (2001) Prevention of Porphyromonas gingivalis-induced oral bone loss following immunization with gingipain R1. Infect Immun 69(12):7959-7963.
18. Hasturk H, Jones VL, Andry C, Kantarci A (2007) 1-Tetradecanol complex reduces progression of Porphyromonas gingivalis-induced experimental periodontitis in rabbits. J Periodontol 78(5):924-932.
19. Igboin CO, Moeschberger ML, Griffen AL, leys EJ (2011) Porphyromonas gingivalis virulence in a Drosophila melanogaster model. Infect Immun 79(1):439-448.
20. Sheets SM, Potempa J, Travis J, Casiano CA, Fletcher HM (2005) Gingipains from porphyromonas gingivalis W83 induce cell adhesion molecule cleavage and apoptosis in endothelial cells. Infect Immun 73(3):1543-1552.
21. Fitzpatrick RE, Aprico A, Wijeyewickrema LC, Pagel CN, Wong DM, et al. (2009) High molecular weight gingipains from porphyromonas gingivalis induce cytokine responses from human mcrophage-like cells via a nonproteolytic mechanism. J Innate Immun 1(2):109-117.
22. Haruyama K, Yoshimura A, Naito M, Kishimoto M, Shoji M, et al. (2009) Identification of a gingipain-sensitive surface ligand of porphyromonas gingivalis that induces Toll-like recepotor 2- and 4- independent NF-kappaB activation in CHO cells. Infect Immun 77(10):4414-4420.
23. Grenier D, Tanabe S (2010) Porphyromonas gingivalis gingipains trigger a proinflammatory response in human monocyte-derived macrophages through the p38α mitogen-activated protein kinase signal transduction pathway. Toxins (Basel) 2(3):341-352.
24. Hacker J, Ott M, Blum G, Marre R, Heesemann J, et al. (1992) Genetics of Escherichia coli uropathogenicity: analysis of the O6:K15:H31 isolate 536. Zentralbl Bakteriol 276(2):165-175.
25. Putze J, Henneguin C, Nougayrede JP, Zhang W, Homburg S, et al. (2009) Genetic structure and distribution of the colibactin genomic island among members of the family Enterobacteriaceae. Infect Immun 77(11):4696-4703.
26. Curtis MA, Hanley SA, Aduse-Opoku J (1999) The rag locus of porphyromonas gingivalis: a novel pathogenicity island. J Periodontal Res 34(7):400-405.
27. Su Z, Kong F, Wang S, Chen J, Yin R, et al. (2010) The rag locus of porphyromonas gingivalis might arise from Bacterioides via horizontal gene transfer. Eur J Clin Microbiol Infect Dis 29(4):429-437.
28. Hall LM, Fawell SC, Shi X, Faray-Kele MC, Aduse-Opoku J, et al. (2005) Sequence diversity and antigenic variation at the rag locus of Porphyromonas gingivalis. Infect Immun 73(7):4253-4262.
29. Shi X, Hanley SA, Faray-Kele MC, Fawell SC, Aduse-Opoku J, et al. (2007) The rag locus of Porphyromonas gingivalis contributes to virulence in a murine model of soft tissue destruction. Infect Immun 75(4):2071-2074.
30. Wang GH, Zhang DM, Pan YP (2009) Distribution of rag genotypes of Porphyromonas gingivalis in patients with chronic periodontitis. Hua Xi Kou Qiang Yi Xue Za Zhi 27(2):168-171.
31. Sallum EJ, Nouer DF, Klein MI, Goncalves RB, Machion L, et al. (2004) Clinical and microbiologic changes after removal of orthodontic appliances. Am J Orthod Dentofacial Orthop 126(3):363-366.
32. Naranjo AA, Trivino ML, Jaramillo A, Betancourth M, Botero JE (2006) Changes in the subgingival microbiota and periodontal parameters before and 3 months after bracket placement. Am J Orthod Dentofacial Orthop 130(3):275.
33. Liu H, Sun J, Dong Y, Lu H, Zhou H, et al. (2011) Periodontal health and relative quantity of subgingival Porphyromonas gingivalis during orthodontic treatment. Angle Orthod 81(4):609-615.
34. Cardoso-Silva C, Barberia E, Ramos Atance JA, Maroto M, Hernandez A, et al. (2011) Microbiological analysis of gingivitis in pediatric patients under orthodontic treatment. Eur J Paediatr Dent 12(4):210-214.
35. Guentsch A, Kramesberger M, Sroka A, Pfister W, Potempa J, et al. (2011) Comparison of gingival crevicular fluid sampling methods in patients with severe chronic periodontitis. J Periodontol 82(7):1051-1060.
36. Rudin HJ, Overdiek HF, Rateitschak KH (1970) Correlation between sulcus fluid rate and clinical rate and clinical and histological inflammation of the marginal gingival. Helv Odontol Acta 14(1):21-26.
37. Lee SM, Yoo SY, Kim HS, Kim KW, Yoon YJ, et al. (2005) Prevalence of putative periodontopathogens in subgingival dental plaques from gingivitis lesions in Korean orthodontic patients. J Microbol 43(3):260-265.
38. Ashimoto A, Chen C, Bakker I, Slots J (1996) Polymerase chain reaction detection of 8 putative periodontal pathogens in subgingival plaque of gingivitis and advanced periodontitis lesions. Oral Microbiol Immunol 11(4):266-273.
39. Hall LM, Fawell SC, Shi X, Faray-Kele MC, Aduse-Opoku J, et al. (2005) Sequence diversity and antigenic variation at the rag locus of Porphyromonas gingivalis. Infect Immun 73(7):4253-4262.
40. Lin L, Li C, Liu J, Zhang D, Zhao J, et al. (2009) Virulence genes of Porphyromonas gingivalis W83 in chronic periodontitis. Acta Odontol Scand 67(5):258-264.
41. Lin L, Pan Y, Li C (2006) Comparison between genes of highly toxic strain and minimally toxic strain of porphyromonas gingivalis. Chin J Stomatol 41(12):734-738.
42. Lopez N (2000) Occurrence of Actinobacillus actinomycetemcomitans, Porphyromonas gingivalis, and prevotella intermedia in progressive adult periodontitis. J Periodontol 71(6):948954.
43. Klein MI, Goncalves RB (2003) Detection of Tannerella forsythensis (Bacteriodes forsythus) and porphyromonas gingivalis by polymerase chain reaction in subjects with different periodontal status. J Periodontol 74(6):798-802.
44. Hanley SA, Aduse-Opoku J, Curtis MA (1999) A 55-kilodalton immunodominant antigen of Porphyromonas gingivalis W50 has arisen via horizontal gene transfer. Infect Immun 67(3):1157-1171.

Modulation of Wnt5a Expression by Periodontopathic Bacteria

Hiromi Nanbara[1,2], Nawarat Wara-aswapati[3], Toshiyuki Nagasawa[1¤a], Yasuhiro Yoshida[4]*, Reiko Yashiro[1¤b], Yukiko Bando[1¤c], Hiroaki Kobayashi[1], Janjura Khongcharoensuk[3], Doosadee Hormdee[3], Waranuch Pitiphat[5], Jason A. Boch[6], Yuichi Izumi[1,2]

1 Department of Periodontology, Tokyo Medical and Dental University, Tokyo, Japan, **2** Global Center of Excellence Program, International Research Center for Molecular Science in Tooth and Bone Diseases, Tokyo Medical and Dental University, Tokyo, Japan, **3** Department of Periodontology, Faculty of Dentistry, Khon Kaen University, Khon Kaen, Thailand, **4** Department of Immunology, School of Medicine, University of Occupational and Environmental Health, Fukuoka, Japan, **5** Department of Community Dentistry, Faculty of Dentistry, Khon Kaen University, Khon Kaen, Thailand, **6** Department of Oral Medicine, Infection and Immunity, Harvard School of Dental Medicine, Boston, Massachusetts, United States of America

Abstract

Wingless proteins, termed Wnt, are involved in embryonic development, blood cell differentiation, and tumorigenesis. In mammalian hematopoiesis, Wnt signaling is essential for stem-cell homeostasis and lymphocyte differentiation. Recent studies have suggested that these molecules are associated with cardiovascular diseases, rheumatoid arthritis, and osteoarthritis. Furthermore, Wnt5a signaling is essential for the general inflammatory response of human macrophages. Periodontitis is a chronic inflammatory disease caused by gram-negative periodontopathic bacteria and the resultant host immune response. Periodontitis is characterized by loss of tooth-supporting structures and alveolar bone resorption. There have been no previous reports on Wnt5a expression in periodontitis tissue, and only few study reported the molecular mechanisms of Wnt5a expression in LPS-stimulated monocytic cells. Using RT-PCR, we demonstrated that Wnt5a mRNA expression was up-regulated in chronic periodontitis tissue as compared to healthy control tissue. *P. gingivalis* LPS induced Wnt5a mRNA in the human monocytic cell line THP-1 with a peak at 4 hrs after stimulation. *P. gingivalis* LPS induced higher up-regulation of Wnt5a mRNA than *E. coli* LPS. The LPS receptors TLR2 and TLR4 were equally expressed on the surface of THP-1 cells. *P. gingivalis* LPS induced IκBα degradation and was able to increase the NF-κB binding activity to DNA. *P. gingivalis* LPS-induced Wnt5a expression was inhibited by NF-κB inhibitors, suggesting NF-κB involvement. Furthermore, IFN-γ synergistically enhanced the *P. gingivalis* LPS-induced production of Wnt5a. Pharmacological investigation and siRNA experiments showed that STAT1 was important for *P. gingivalis* LPS-induced Wnt5a expression. These results suggest that the modulation of Wnt5a expression by *P. gingivalis* may play an important role in the periodontal inflammatory process and serve a target for the development of new therapies.

Editor: Roy Martin Roop II, East Carolina University School of Medicine, United States of America

Funding: This study was supported by Grant-in-Aid for Scientific Research 21390553, grant from Global Center of Excellence (GCOE) Program, International Research Center for Molecular Science in Tooth and Bone Diseases Program, from the Ministry of Education, Culture, Sports, Science, and Technology of Japan; the National Research Council of Thailand (NRCT); Japan Society for the Promotion of Science (JSPS) grant, JSPS Invitation Fellowship for Research in Japan (NW), and Khon Kaen University grant. http://www.mext.go.jp/. The funders had no role in study design, data collection and analysis, decision to publish, or preparation of the manuscript.

Competing Interests: The authors have declared that no competing interests exist.

* E-mail: freude@med.uoeh-u.ac.jp

¤a Current address: Department of Periodontology and Endodontology, Health Sciences University of Hokkaido, Hokkaido, Japan
¤b Current address: Department of Preventive Dentistry, School of Dental Medicine, University of Geneva, Geneva, Switzerland
¤c Current address: Clinical Research Center for Diabetes, Tokushima University Hospital, Tokushima, Japan

Introduction

Wingless, a second chromosome recessive mutation in *Drosophila*, was first reported by Sharma and Chopra in 1975 [1]. It was characterized as a segment polarity gene in *Drosophila*, which is essential for embryonic segmentation and patterning [2]. Various homologs of the Wingless protein, termed Wnt, are involved in embryonic development, blood cell differentiation during mammalian hematopoiesis, and tumorigenesis [3]. In mammalian hematopoiesis, Wnt signaling is essential for stem-cell homeostasis [4] and lymphocyte differentiation [5,6].

Of particular interest is Wnt5a, which was first identified in the mouse [7]. It is secreted by activated antigen-presenting cells and by inflammatory synoviocytes from rheumatoid arthritis joints [8] and atherosclerotic lesions [9]. Wnt5a expression is induced by mycobacterial cell wall components and endotoxin in human antigen-presenting cells [10], and Wnt5a signaling is essential for the general inflammatory response of human macrophages during sepsis [11].

Wnt5a expression is dependent on Toll-like receptor (TLR) signaling and activation of the central inflammatory regulator NF-κB in human antigen-presenting cells [10]. Furthermore, interleukin (IL)-6 family members activate the gp130-JAK-signal transducer and activator of transcription 3 (STAT3) signaling cascade to up-regulate Wnt5a transcription in chronic persistent inflammation and rheumatoid arthritis [12]. However, little is known about the expression and modulation of Wnt homologs in inflammatory settings, such as periodontitis.

Periodontal diseases are infections caused by gram negative periodontopathic bacteria [13] which colonize on the tooth surface at or below the gingival margin. In severe cases, these are accompanied by inflammation of the gingiva and destruction of periodontal tissues, leading to alveolar bone loss. Periodontopathic bacteria produce many virulence factors, such as lipopolysaccharide (LPS) and peptidoglycan those induce host immune responses, including the production of inflammatory cytokines. High levels of several inflammatory cytokines, such as IL-1α, IL-1β, IL-6, interferon-γ (IFN-γ), and tumor necrosis factor α (TNF-α), have been found in the tissue and gingival crevicular fluid of patients with advanced periodontitis [14,15]. These inflammatory cytokines are reported to stimulate the production of receptor activator for nuclear factor κB ligand (RANKL) [16,17], which binds to receptor activator for nuclear factor κB (RANK) on the surface of preosteoclasts. This binding stimulates both the differentiation of osteoclast progenitors and the activity of mature osteoclasts leading to alveolar bone resorption [18–21].

The purpose of this study was to evaluate the levels of Wnt5a expression in chronic periodontitis tissue and investigate the modulation of Wnt5a expression by periodontopathic bacteria. We show that Wnt5a mRNA was significantly up-regulated in chronic periodontitis tissue when compared to non-periodontitis tissue. The expression of Wnt5a was dependent on the NF-κB pathway and was partly mediated by the STAT1 signaling pathway in response to *P. gingivalis* LPS/IFN-γ in the human monocytic cell line THP-1. This result suggests that the modulation of Wnt5a expression by *P. gingivalis* may play an important role in the periodontal inflammatory process.

Results

Wnt5a was significantly up-regulated in chronic periodontitis tissues

Wnt5a signaling is known to be essential for the general inflammatory response [11] and it is secreted in chronic inflamed site such as inflammatory synoviocytes [8], the atherosclerotic lesions [9], and the serum and bone marrow of patients with severe sepsis [11]. Table 1 summarizes the characteristics of the study subjects and sampling sites. Subjects in the periodontitis group were significantly older, and had higher mean PD, mean CAL and proportion of BOP-positive sites as compared with the control group. Production of Wnt5a mRNA was detected in all gingival tissue samples (Fig. 1). The mean relative mRNA level of Wnt5a was significantly higher in the periodontitis group (1.44±0.26) than in the control group (1.00±0.22; $p<0.001$). Additional regression analysis controlling for the effect of age confirmed these results that chronic periodontitis was associated with increased mRNA levels of Wnt5a ($p<0.001$).

Wnt5a mRNA was expressed by the human monocytic cell line THP-1 in response to *P. gingivalis* LPS

The human gingival fibroblast cell line HGF-1 and the human monocytic cell line THP-1 were stimulated with *A. actinomycetemcomitans* sonicated extract, *P. gingivalis* sonicated extract, *P. gingivalis* LPS, or TNF-α for 4 hrs. Our results showed that the expression of Wnt5a mRNA in HGF-1 cells was constant in response to different treatments (Fig. 2A). However, in THP-1 cells, Wnt5a

Table 1. Characteristics of the Study Subjects.

Charactereistic	Comparison group		
	Control group (n = 14)	Periodontitis group (n = 13)	p-value*
Age in years (mean ± SD)	31.0±13.1	43.5±13.0	0.02
Female n (%)	12 (85.7)	10 (76.9)	0.65
Probing depth** (mm; mean ± SD)	2.0±0.9	9.5±1.9	<0.001
Clinical attachment level** (mm; mean ± SD)	0.8±0.7	10.5±2.6	<0.001
Bleeding on probing* n (%)	3 (21.4)	13 (100)	<0.001

*Mann-Whitney U test for continuous data, and Fisher's exact test for binary data.
**Measured at the sampling sites.

mRNA was strongly induced by *P. gingivalis* LPS but was only slightly increased by *P. gingivalis* sonicated extracts or a high concentration of TNF-α. Live *P. gingivalis* also significantly increased the expression of Wnt5a mRNA in THP-1 (Fig. 2E). When THP-1 cells were stimulated with various concentrations of *P. gingivalis* LPS or *E. coli* LPS (Fig. 2C), the maximum Wnt5a mRNA expression occurred after stimulation with 1 μg/ml of *P. gingivalis* LPS. *P. gingivalis* LPS could induce more potent Wnt5a mRNA expression than *E. coli* LPS. When THP-1 cells were

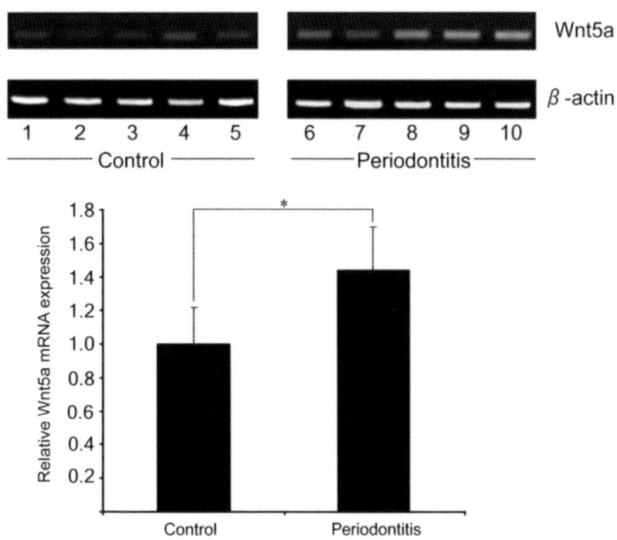

Figure 1. The levels of Wnt5a mRNA were significantly up-regulated in chronic periodontitis tissues. Upper panel; Total RNA was extracted from periodontitis tissues, and the expression of Wnt5a mRNA was detected by RT-PCR. PCR products were electrophoresed on a 1.5% agarose gel and visualized by UV illumination. β-actin served as the internal control. Results are representative of five patients (right panel). Lower panel; The relative mRNA levels of Wnt5a. The horizontal line within each box represents the median expression level in each group.

stimulated with 1 μg/ml of *P. gingivalis* LPS for 0.5, 2, 4, 12, and 24 hrs, the maximum expression of Wnt5a mRNA occurred at 4 hrs after stimulation (Fig. 2B). Flow cytometry demonstrated that TLR2 and TLR4 were equally expressed on the surface of THP-1 cells stimulated by *P. gingivalis* LPS and *E. coli* LPS, suggesting that the expression of these receptors were not changed by the stimulation (Fig. 2D). *P. gingivalis* LPS-induced Wnt5a mRNA was significantly reduced by either TLR2 siRNA or TLR4 siRNA (Fig. 2H), suggesting that *P. gingivalis* LPS used in this study utilized both TLR2 and TLR4.

In primary human gingival fibroblasts (HGF), the expression of Wnt5a mRNA was rather constant after stimulation with *P. gingivalis* LPS (Fig. 2F). On the contrary, in primary monocytes, Wnt5a mRNA expression was significantly increased by *P. gingivalis* LPS and was reduced by using NF-κB inhibitor MG132 (Fig. 2G). These results suggest that monocytes, but not HGF, play an important role in Wnt5a up-regulation at inflamed site.

The *P. gingivalis*-LPS induced Wnt5a expression is dependent upon NF-κB signaling

A recent study showed that Wnt5a expression is dependent on the activation of the central inflammatory regulator NF-κB [10]. We examined the degradation of IκBα in THP-1 cells stimulated with *P. gingivalis* LPS. After 30 mins or 4 hrs, whole cell lysates were subjected to Western blot. In unstimulated THP-1 cells, IκBα was abundant. In contrast, stimulation with *P. gingivalis* LPS markedly reduced the cytosolic level of IκBα (Fig. 3A). To examine *P. gingivalis* LPS-induced NF-κB activity, THP-1 cells were transfected with a luciferase reporter plasmid containing the NF-κB binding site for 18 hrs. After treatment with *P. gingivalis* LPS, the luciferase activity was measured with a luminometer. *P. gingivalis* LPS-induced NF-κB activity was significantly upregulated in THP-1 cells (Fig. 3B). Further, the ability of NF-κB to bind to DNA was analyzed by electrophoretic mobility shift assay (EMSA). The [γ-^{32}P]-labeled probe, which contained the NF-κB binding consensus sequence, was incubated with the nuclear extract of THP-1 cells stimulated with *P. gingivalis* LPS for 40 minutes. Protein-DNA complex bands (Fig. 3C, lower arrow) were super-shifted by the addition of anti-p65 antibody (Fig. 3C, upper arrow). This result suggests that *P. gingivalis* LPS is able to increase the NF-κB binding activity to DNA.

The addition of wedelolactone or IKK inhibitor VII, which act as selective irreversible inhibitors of IKKα or IKKβ kinase activities, inhibited *P. gingivalis* LPS-induced Wnt5a mRNA in a dose-dependent manner expression (Fig. 4A, 4B). Moreover, the effect of an expression vector for a dominant-negative form of IκBα was investigated. The expression of *P. gingivalis* LPS-induced Wnt5a mRNA was inhibited by transfection with a dominant-negative IκBα plasmid (Fig. 4C). Taken together, our results indicate that the induction of Wnt5a mRNA expression by *P. gingivalis* LPS is dependent upon NF-κB signaling.

The induction of Wnt5a is partly mediated via the JAK/STAT signaling pathway

Tandem STAT3-binding sites in the *Wnt5a* gene have been identified [22]. We examined the role of the JAK/STAT pathway in the regulation of Wnt5a mRNA expression. AG490 (JAK/STAT inhibitor), fludarabine (STAT1 inhibitor), and STA21 (STAT3 inhibitor) were used to inhibit the JAK/STAT pathway 1 hr prior to *P. gingivalis* LPS stimulation. Pretreatment with either AG490 or fludarabine significantly decreased Wnt5a mRNA expression in THP-1 cells in a dose-dependent manner (Fig. 5A, B). Additionally, STAT1 siRNA was able to suppress the induction of Wnt5a by *P. gingivalis* LPS as compared to control siRNA (Fig. 5C). However, the *P. gingivalis* LPS-induced Wnt5a mRNA expression was augmented by a STAT3 inhibitor, STA21 (Fig. 5D). Our results suggest that STAT1 positively regulated induction of Wnt5a by *P. gingivalis* LPS.

Wnt5a mRNA expression was increased by co-stimulation with *P. gingivalis* LPS and IFN-γ

To investigate the role of the JAK/STAT pathway in detail, we examined the expression of Wnt5a mRNA after co-stimulation with *P. gingivalis* LPS and either IL-6, IFN-β, or IFN-γ. IL-6, IFN-β, or IFN-γ alone did not elicit the induction of Wnt5a mRNA when compared to the control. Wnt5a mRNA levels were up-regulated in the presence of *P. gingivalis* LPS alone. Furthermore, *P. gingivalis* LPS together with IFN-γ synergistically activated Wnt5a mRNA expression (Fig. 6A).

IFN-γ induces the phosphorylation of STAT1, which forms STAT1 homodimers. The effects of an expression vector for wild-type STAT1 on Wnt5a expression were investigated. After transfection, THP-1 cells were co-stimulated with *P. gingivalis* LPS and IFN-γ. The expression of Wnt5a mRNA was markedly increased by transfection with a wild-type STAT1 expression plasmid (Fig. 6B). Additionally, STAT1 siRNA significantly suppressed the Wnt5a mRNA expression induced by *P. gingivalis* LPS and IFN-γ (Fig. 6C). These results suggest that the induction of Wnt5a mRNA by co-stimulation with *P. gingivalis* LPS and IFN-γ is partly mediated via STAT1 signaling.

Discussion

In this study, we investigated the levels of Wnt5a expression in chronic periodontitis tissues, and the modulation of Wnt5a expression by periodontopathic bacteria. Wnt5a mRNA was significantly up-regulated in chronic periodontitis tissues as compared to healthy control tissues. Chronic inflammatory periodontitis tissue comprises of epithelial cells, gingival fibroblasts and inflammatory cells including PMNs, monocytes and macrophages. The expression of Wnt5a was dependent upon the NF-κB signaling pathway and was partly mediated by the STAT1 signaling pathway in response to *P. gingivalis* LPS/IFN-γ in the human monocytic cell line THP-1.

Wnt5a is secreted by activated antigen-presenting cells [8,10,11] and said to be induced by *M. tuberculosis*, *M. avium*, *S. aureus* or *S. typhimurium* [10,23]. The expression of Wnt5a mRNA in response to periodontopathic bacterial stimuli was also observed in periodontal tissue cells. Whereas the expression of Wnt5a was constant in response to different treatments in HGF-1 cells, it was specifically up-regulated by *P. gingivalis* LPS and was slightly increased by *P. gingivalis* sonicated extracts in the human monocytic cell line THP-1. Sonicated extract of *P. gingivalis* comprises of various components including protein, lipid, LPS and other factors, which have different properties to stimulate host immune responses. But *P. gingivalis* LPS from InvivoGen is ultra-pure LPS (according to the manufacturer) and thus possesses a high concentration of LPS. In our study, primary cells including monocytes and gingival fibroblasts responded to *P. gingivalis* LPS in a similar manner to the cell lines (THP-1 and HGF-1).

P. gingivalis is considered to be an important member of the periodontopathic bacteria involved in periodontal disease [24,25] leading to inflammation and destruction of alveolar bone and the supporting connective tissue surrounding teeth. *P. gingivalis* is a gram-negative obligate anaerobic rod bacterium that has virulence factors such as LPS [24]. Although TLR4 has been reported to function as an LPS signaling receptor, *P. gingivalis* LPS is less

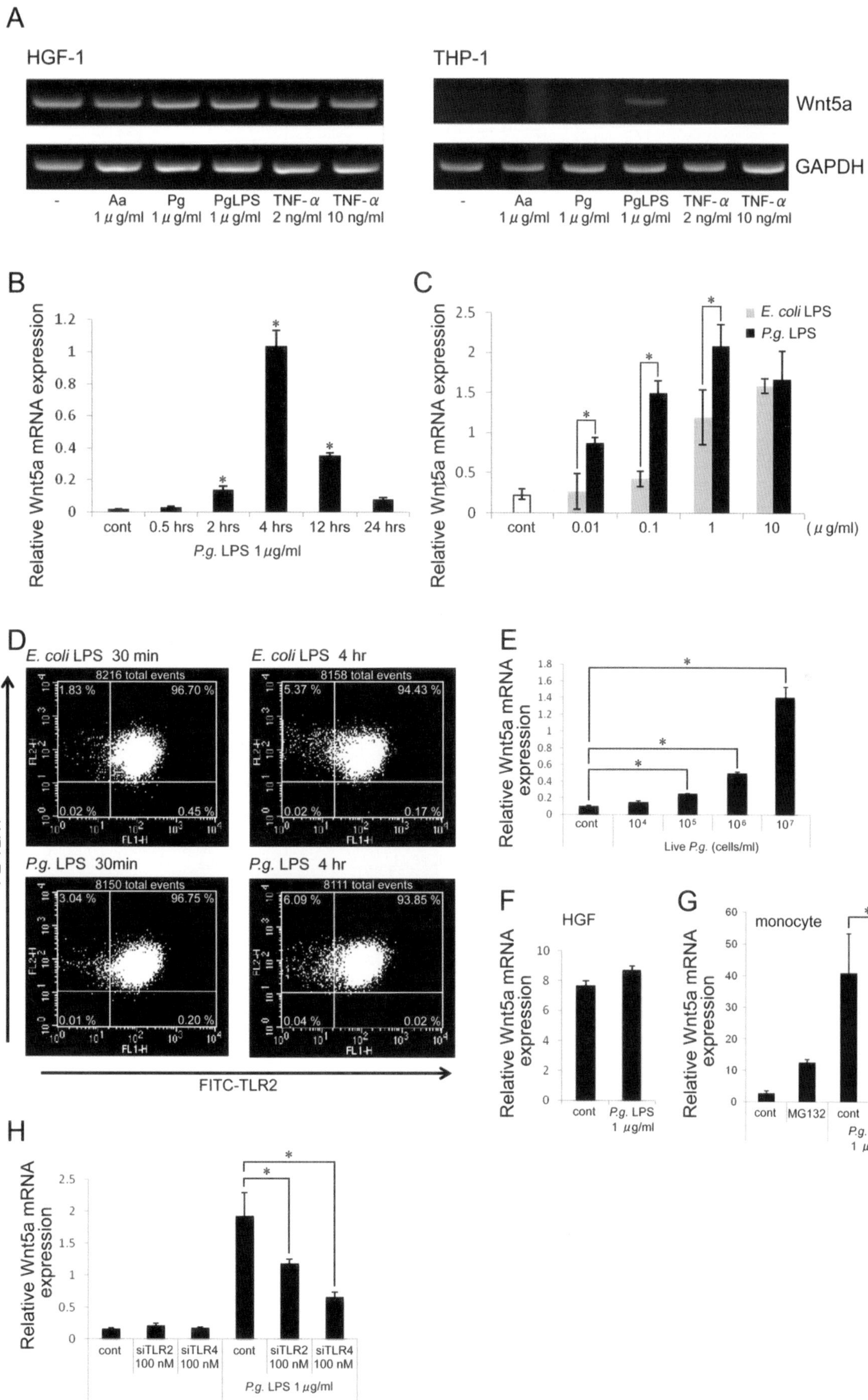
A
HGF-1
THP-1
Wnt5a
GAPDH
- Aa 1 μg/ml Pg 1 μg/ml PgLPS 1 μg/ml TNF-α 2 ng/ml TNF-α 10 ng/ml
B
Relative Wnt5a mRNA expression
cont 0.5 hrs 2 hrs 4 hrs 12 hrs 24 hrs
P.g. LPS 1 μg/ml
C
E. coli LPS
P.g. LPS
cont 0.01 0.1 1 10 (μg/ml)
D
E. coli LPS 30 min
E. coli LPS 4 hr
P.g. LPS 30min
P.g. LPS 4 hr
8216 total events
8158 total events
8150 total events
8111 total events
1.83 % 96.70 % 0.02 % 0.45 %
5.37 % 94.43 % 0.02 % 0.17 %
3.04 % 96.75 % 0.01 % 0.20 %
6.09 % 93.85 % 0.04 % 0.02 %
PE-TLR4
FITC-TLR2
E
Relative Wnt5a mRNA expression
cont 10⁴ 10⁵ 10⁶ 10⁷
Live P.g. (cells/ml)
F
HGF
cont P.g. LPS 1 μg/ml
G
monocyte
cont MG132 cont MG132
P.g. LPS 1 μg/ml
H
Relative Wnt5a mRNA expression
cont siTLR2 100 nM siTLR4 100 nM cont siTLR2 100 nM siTLR4 100 nM
P.g. LPS 1 μg/ml

Figure 2. Wnt5a was specifically up-regulated in THP-1 cells by *P. gingivalis* LPS. (A) HGF-1 and THP-1 cells were stimulated with *A. actinomycetemcomitans* sonicated extract, *P. gingivalis* sonicated extract, *P. gingivalis* LPS, and TNF-α for 4 hrs, and the expression of Wnt5a mRNA was detected by RT-PCR. PCR products were electrophoresed on a 1.5% agarose gel and visualized by UV illumination. GAPDH served as the internal control. (B) THP-1 cells were stimulated with 1 μg/ml of *P. gingivalis* LPS for 0.5, 2, 4, 12, or 24 hrs, and the expression of Wnt5a mRNA was detected by real-time PCR. Relative expression levels of Wnt5a are shown. (C) THP-1 cells were stimulated with 0.01–10 μg/ml of *P. gingivalis* LPS (black bars) or *E. coli* LPS (gray bars) for 4 hrs, and then the expression of Wnt5a mRNA was detected by real-time PCR. Relative expression levels of Wnt5a are presented. (D) THP-1 cells were stimulated with *E. coli* 055:B5 LPS (middle and right upper panels) or *P. gingivalis* LPS (middle and right lower panels) for 30 min or 4 hrs, and then the expression of surface TLR2 and TLR4 protein was determined by flow cytometry. Left upper panel shows no-staining condition, and left lower panel shows un-stimulated condition with staining. (E, F, G, H) The expression of Wnt5a mRNA was detected by real-time PCR. Relative expression levels of Wnt5a mRNA are shown. (E) THP-1 cells were stimulated with 10^4–10^7 cells/ml of live *P. gingivalis* for 4 hrs. (F, G) Primary human gingival fibroblasts (HGF) and human monocytes were stimulated with 1 μg/ml of *P. gingivalis* LPS for 4 hrs. Monocytes were pretreated with the NF-κB inhibitor MG132 for 1 hr. Here we describe typical dates of three samples. (H) THP-1 cells were stimulated with *P. gingivalis* LPS for 4 hrs after being transfected with TLR2 siRNA, TLR4 siRNA or control siRNA for 72 hrs. *$p<0.05$.

dependent on TLR4 signaling than *Escherichia coli* LPS [26]. Lipid A of *P. gingivalis* differs both structurally and functionally from *E. coli* lipid A [24], and *P. gingivalis* LPS utilizes either TLR2 and TLR4 to mediate inflammatory signaling [27]. Indeed, in this study, the expression of Wnt5a mRNA was down-regulated by

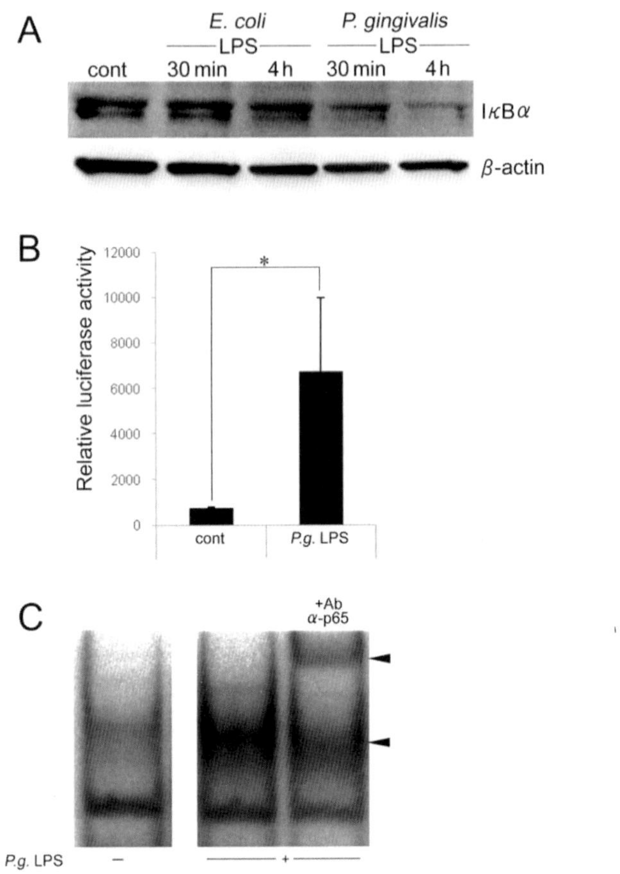

Figure 3. Induction of Wnt5a expression is NF-κB dependent. (A) THP-1 cells were stimulated with *E. coli* LPS or *P. gingivalis* LPS for 30 mins or 4 hrs. Whole cell extracts were prepared and analyzed by Western blot by using antibodies against IκBα. β-actin served as the protein loading control. (B) THP-1 cells were stimulated with *P. gingivalis* LPS for 4 hrs after being transfected with NF-κB reporter plasmid for 12 hrs, and the transcription activity was assessed by luminometer. The activity is represented by the relative luciferase activity. (C) Nuclear extracts were prepared and EMSA was performed with γ^{32}P-labeled oligonucleotides representing the NF-κB consensus sequence as a probe. Anti-p65 antibody was used for supershift assays. The lower arrow shows the DNA-protein complex, and the upper arrow shows the supershifted band. *$p<0.05$.

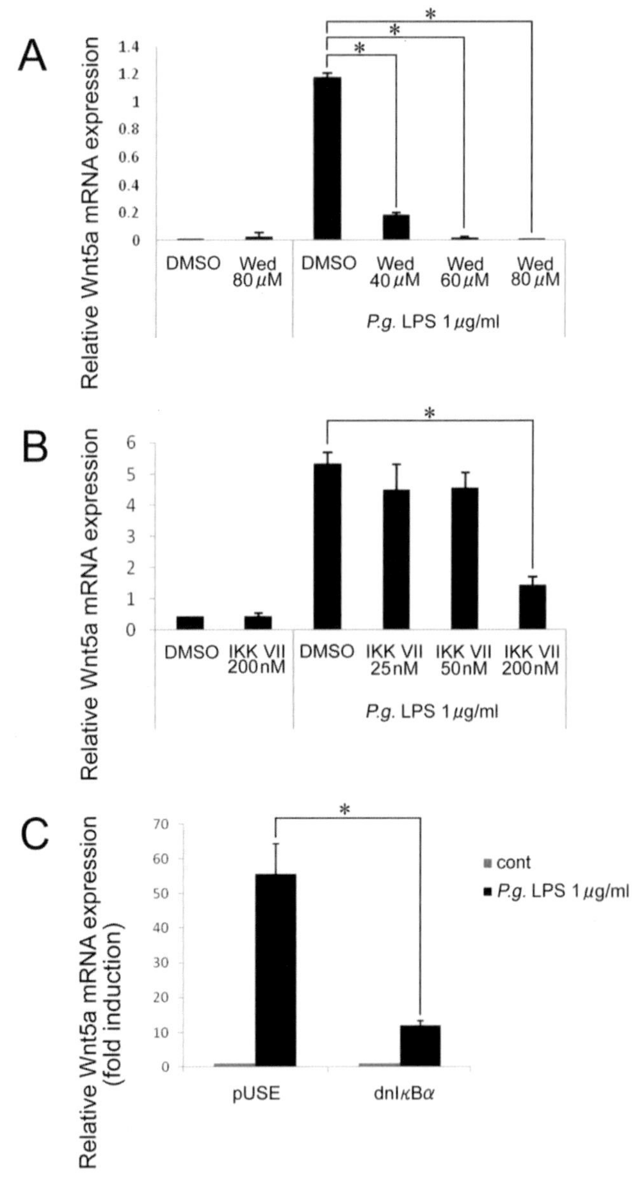

Figure 4. *P. gingivalis* LPS-induced Wnt5a expression was inhibited by wedelolactone or dnIκBα. (A, B) THP-1 cells were pre-treated with the IKK inhibitor wedelolactone or the IKK inhibitor VII for 1 hr. The expression of Wnt5a mRNA was detected by real-time PCR. Relative expression levels of Wnt5a are presented. DMSO is a solvent control for both inhibitors. (C) THP-1 cells were transfected with a dominant-negative form of IκBα (dnIκBα) or the parent plasmid (pUSE) for 12 hrs. Fold induction of Wnt5a mRNA expression is shown. *$p<0.05$.

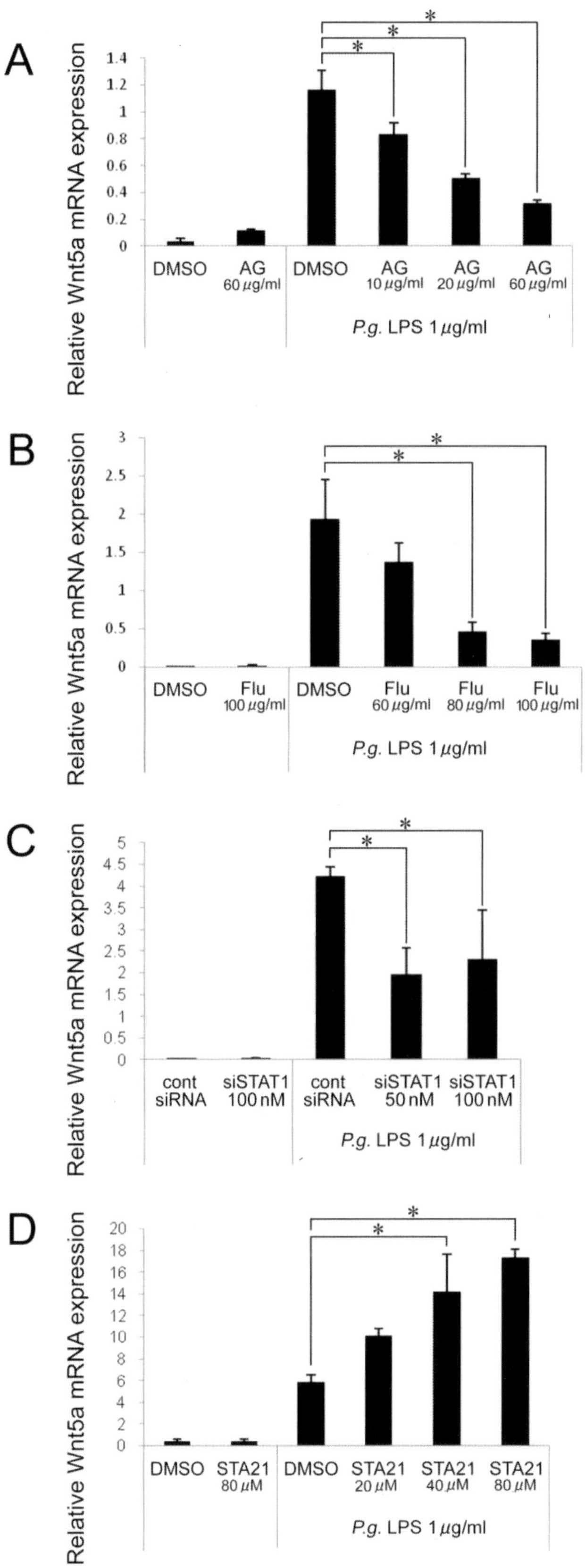

Figure 5. Induction of Wnt5a expression is partly JAK/STAT dependent. (A–D) The expression of Wnt5a mRNA was detected by real-time PCR. Relative expression levels of Wnt5a are presented. (A, B) THP-1 cells were pre-treated with AG490 (A) or fludarabine (B) for 1 hr and then stimulated with *P. gingivalis* LPS for 4 hrs. DMSO is a solvent control for both inhibitors. (C) THP-1 cells were stimulated with *P. gingivalis* LPS for 4 hrs after transfection with STAT1 siRNA or control siRNA for 18 hrs. (D) THP-1 cells were pre-treated with STA21 for 1 hr and stimulated with *P. gingivalis* LPS for 4 hrs. *p<0.05.

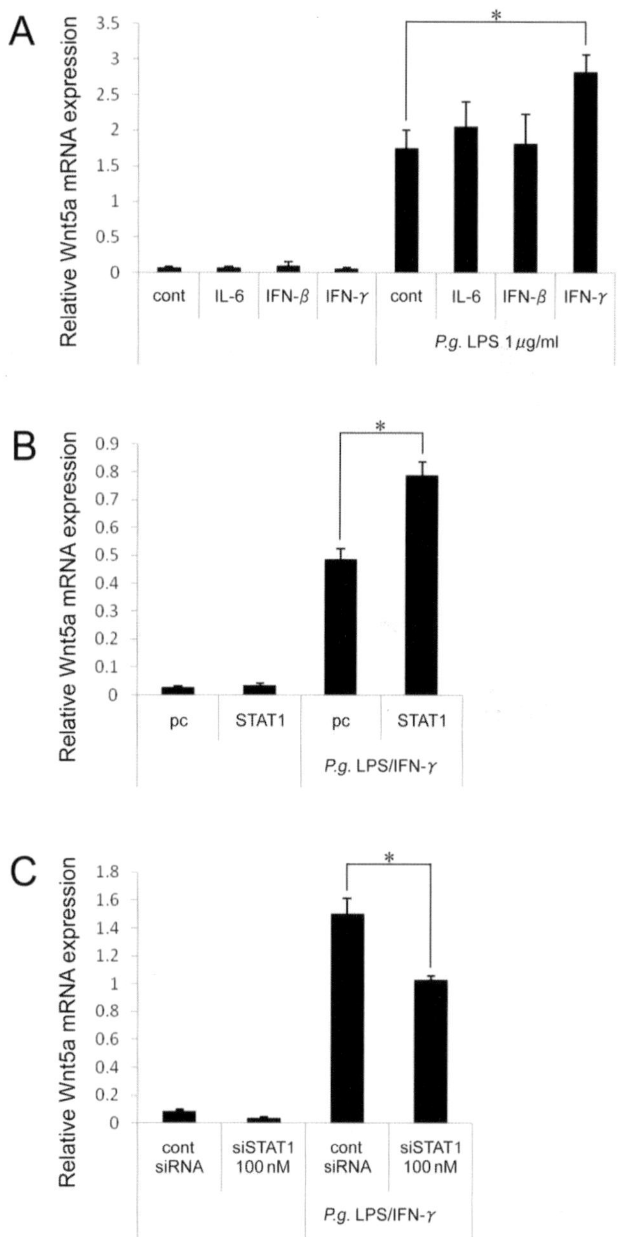

Figure 6. The expression of Wnt5a was increased by co-stimulation with *P. gingivalis* LPS and IFN-γ. (A–C) The expression of Wnt5a mRNA was detected by real-time PCR. Relative expression levels of Wnt5a are presented. (A) THP-1 cells were stimulated with 10 ng/ml of IL-6, 10 ng/ml of IFN-β or 10 ng/ml of IFN-γ with or without *P. gingivalis* LPS for 4 hrs. (B) THP-1 cells were transfected with wild-type STAT1 expression vector or parent plasmid 12 hrs prior to stimulation with *P. gingivalis* LPS/IFN-γ for 4 hrs. (C) THP-1 cells were stimulated with *P. gingivalis* LPS for 4 hrs after being transfected with STAT1 siRNA or control siRNA for 18 hrs. *p<0.05.

TLR2 siRNA and TLR4 siRNA. The engagement of TLR activates a variety of intracellular signaling pathways that ultimately activate the transcriptional factor NF-κB [28]. In this study, the expression of Wnt5a mRNA induced by *P. gingivalis* LPS was higher than the expression induced by *E. coli* LPS. However, the expression of TLR2 and TLR4 receptors on the surface of THP-1 cells was not changed after stimulation with *P. gingivalis* LPS or *E. coli* LPS. These results suggest that the difference in Wnt5a mRNA expression level between *P. gingivalis* LPS and *E. coli* LPS is not dependent upon the expression of TLR. Generally, activated NF-κB induces IκBα de novo, then IκBα will be comparable level to no stimulation as seen in *E. coli* LPS (Fig. 3A). It is not clear but there might be some involvement in strong induction of Wnt5a by *P. gingivalis* LPS in comparison with *E. coli* LPS. In addition, *P. gingivalis* LPS is said to induce lower IL-10 than *E. coli* LPS in dendritic cells generated from human peripheral monocytes [29] suggesting that down-regulation of Wnt5a by *P. gingivalis* LPS-induced IL-10 may be weaker than *E. coli* LPS.

In this study, we found that AG490 and Fludarabine, but not STA21, were capable of suppressing *P. gingivalis* LPS-mediated Wnt5a up-regulation in THP-1 cells. Fludarabine is used in the treatment of various hematological malignancies, particularly B-cell chronic lymphocytic leukemia. It has also been shown that Fludarabine reduces STAT1 phosphorylation and suppress STAT1 protein and transcript levels [30,31]. On the other hand, the expression of Wnt5a was significantly augmented by pretreatment with STA21 compared to *P. gingivalis* LPS alone. This suggests that STAT3 plays some role in the expression of Wnt5a.

Wnt5a might be up-regulated by *P. gingivalis* LPS and IFN-γ via NF-κB and STAT1 pathways, and induce various cellular functions. Wnt5a activates the non-canonical pathway which results in up-regulation of inflammatory cytokines such as IL-6, IL-8, IL-1β and MIP-1β [11] and these cytokines ultimately induce bone resorption [16,17]. Moreover, increased levels of Wnt5a and cytokines may affect other mono nuclear cells including T-cells leading sustained inflammation [10] and affect surrounding resident tissue cells, including vascular smooth muscle cells and endothelial cells [32–34]. Taken together, Wnt5a may play an important role in periodontal inflammation.

Inflammatory reactions are regulated by cytokines. IFN-γ orchestrates immune response cross-talk with other cytokines or extracellular stimuli such as LPS. For example, pro-inflammatory genes such as inducible nitric-oxide synthase [35,36] and intercellular adhesion molecule 1 [37] were induced by co-stimulation with IFN-γ and LPS. Here, we also show a synergistic effect of *P. gingivalis* LPS and IFN-γ but not IL-6 or type I IFN (IFN-β) on Wnt5a expression in the human monocytic cell line THP-1. These synergistic effects might be mediated by transcription factors such as NF-κB and STAT1, although additional experiments are needed. Ohmori et al. demonstrated a synergistic effect of NF-κB and STAT1 on iNOS gene induction in Raw264 cells that was activated by LPS or IFN-α, respectively [36]. On the contrary, in our system, we could not observe a synergistic effect of LPS and IFN-α on Wnt5a induction, suggesting that the autocrine loop of LPS-induced IFN-α is not involved in Wnt5a induction. Previously, we reported that NF-κB and STAT3 co-operative role on several genes [38]. In this paper, we used a pharmacological approach to examine STAT3 involvement in Wnt5a induction. Unexpectedly, an inhibitor of STAT3 increased the Wnt5a mRNA level. Furthermore, STAT3 phosphorylation was not observed until 4 hrs after stimulation in THP-1 cells (data not shown). These results suggest that STAT3 does not positively regulate Wnt5a expression, while it is still unclear if STAT3 plays a role as a negative regulator. The relationship between Wnt5a and STAT3 is cell specific [22,39]. We conclude that Wnt5a gene expression is regulated by NF-κB and STAT1 with different regulatory mechanisms.

Materials and Methods

Study population, clinical examination, and sampling of gingival tissue

The Khon Kaen University review committee approved the protocol for human subjects. Twenty-seven subjects were enrolled in this study. All subjects had at least 10 natural teeth and were systemically healthy. After having signed informed consent forms, samples of gingival tissues were obtained from 14 periodontally healthy individuals (control group) and 13 patients with generalized moderate to severe chronic periodontitis [40] during extraction of teeth. Each subject had at least one tooth which was planned for extraction due to severe periodontal destruction and inflammation (chronic periodontitis patient) or for orthodontic treatment or crown lengthening procedure (control subject). The PD, CAL, and bleeding on probing (BOP) of the sampling sites were evaluated using a periodontal probe (Hu-Friedy, Leimen, Germany).

Human monocyte and human gingival fibroblast

The Tokyo Medical and Dental University review committee approved the protocol for human subjects. After acquiring informed consent, peripheral blood was obtained by venipuncture from 3 healthy volunteers. Peripheral blood mononuclear cells (PBMCs) were isolated by density-gradient centrifugation using Lymphoprep (Axis-Shield, Oslo, Norway). Monocytes were purified by using the MACS Monocyte Isolation Kit II (Miltenyi Biotec, Bergisch Gladbach, Germany). Human gingival fibroblasts (HGF) were isolated from three systemically healthy patients with periodontitis. Three healthy gingival samples were collected during flap surgery. The washed explants were placed in a sterile dish and minced into smaller pieces with a sterile scalpel blade. Attempts were made to remove the epithelium and leave only connective tissue. Fibroblastic cells were allowed to grow out from the explant at 37°C in a humidified atmosphere with 5% CO_2 in the air until they formed a confluent layer, at which point they were subcultured. Cells subcultured to the fifth passage.

Cell culture

The human monocytic cell line THP-1 and the human gingival fibroblast cell line HGF-1 were obtained from the American Type Culture Collection (ATCC, Rockville, MD). THP-1 cells and HGF-1 cells were cultured in RPMI 1640 (Lonza, Basel, Switzerland) and DMEM (ATCC) supplemented with 10% heat-inactivated fetal bovine serum (FBS, Hyclone, Logan, UT) and 1% antibiotics (100 U/ml of penicillin and 100 μg/ml of streptomycin). All cells were grown at 37°C in a humid incubator with 5% CO_2.

Bacteria, reagents, and antibodies

Aggregatibacter actinomycetemcomitans ATCC 43718 and *Porphyromonas gingivalis* 381 were cultured, and sonicated extracts were prepared as described previously [41]. Live *P. gingivalis* 381 (kindly gifted from Dr. Takeuchi), *P. gingivalis* LPS (InvivoGen, San Diego, CA), *E. coli* 055:B5 LPS (Sigma, Taufkirchen, Germany), IL-6, IFN-β, and IFN-γ (R&D systems, Minneapolis, MN) were purchased from the respective companies. Unless otherwise stated, *A. actinomycetemcomitans* and *P. gingivalis* were added to cell cultures at a final concentration of 1 μg/ml. TNF-α was added at a final concentration of 2 ng/ml or 10 ng/ml. IL-6, IFN-β, and IFN-γ were added at a final concentration of 10 ng/ml.

In some experiments, specific signal transduction inhibitors for JAK/STAT (AG490, Calbiochem, San Diego, CA), STAT1 (fludarabine, WAKO, Osaka, Japan), STAT3 (STA21, Santa Cruz Biotechnology, Santa Cruz, CA), NF-κB (MG132, Calbiochem) and IKK (wedelolactone, IKK inhibitor VII, Calbiochem) were added 1 hr prior to stimulation with *P. gingivalis* LPS. When necessary, inhibitors were diluted in DMSO or ethanol. Cell viability was measured by using the Cell Counting Kit-8 (DOJINDO, Kumamoto, Japan). To all unstimulated and control samples, equal amounts of inhibitor solvent were added. Neither DMSO nor ethanol at the concentrations used to prepare inhibitors affected THP-1 cell viability (data not shown).

Antibody for inhibitor κBα (IκBα, sc-371) was purchased from Santa Cruz Biotechnology (Santa Cruz). Anti-β-actin antibody (A5441) was generated by Sigma. HRP-conjugated anti-rabbit IgG (#458) and HRP-conjugated anti-mouse IgG (NA931VS) were purchased from MBL (Nagoya, Japan) and Amersham Pharmacia Bioscience (Buckinghamshire, U.K).

RNA extraction and RT-PCR

Total RNA from gingival tissues and cells was isolated by using an RNeasy Mini kit (Qiagen) according to the manufacturer's instructions, and concentrations were measured by spectrophotometry. RNA quality was assessed by measuring the ratio of absorbance at 260 nm to the absorbance at 280 nm. Reverse transcription-polymerase chain reaction (RT-PCR) was performed with an RT-PCR kit (One-step RT-PCR kit, Qiagen) using a thermal cycler (GeneAmp® PCR system 2400, Perkin Elmer, Roche, NJ, USA). Specific oligonucleotides were synthesized (Qiagen) based on the published sequences of Wnt5a, forward 5′ TTT TTC TCC TTC GCC CAG GTT GT 3′, reverse 5′ GGC TCA TGG CGT TCA CCA C 3′; β-actin, forward 5′ TGA CGG GGT CAC CCA CAC TGT GCC CAT CTA 3′, reverse, 5′ CTA GAA GCA TTT GCG GTG GAC GAT GGA GGG-3′; and GAPDH forward, 5′ ACC ACA GTC CAT GCC ATC AC 3′, reverse 5′ ACC ACC CTG TTG CTG TA 3′. Real-time RT-PCR was performed with a QuantiTect PrimerAssay and SYBR Green PCR Master Mix (Qiagen) with LightCycler technology (Roche Diagnosis, Mannheim, Germany) and StepOne (Applied Biosystems, Foster City, CA). Wnt5a mRNA expression was displayed as relative expression normalized to β-actin or GAPDH.

Flow cytometry

Cell surface expression of TLR2 and TLR4 on THP-1 cells was determined by flow cytometry. After washing, cells were stained with FITC anti-mouse/human TLR2 (Abcam, Cambridge, UK) and PE anti-human TLR4 (eBioscience, San Diego, CA). Data were analyzed by the FACS Calibur (Becton Dickinson, San Jose, CA).

Western blotting

THP-1 cells were lysed with RIPA lysis buffer (1% Nonidet P-40, 0.5% sodium deoxycholate, 0.1% SDS, and protease inhibitor cocktail) for preparation of whole cell extracts. Equivalent amounts of protein (10 μg) were resolved on SDS-PAGE gels, transferred and immobilized on nitrocellulose membranes (Amersham, Little Chalfont, UK), and probed with appropriate primary and secondary antibodies.

Transfection and luciferase assay

THP-1 cells were transfected with the transfection reagent Lipofectamine™2000 (Invitrogen, Carlsbad, CA) at 3 μl of reagent per one μg of DNA as previously reported [38]. IκB dominant-negative vectors (S32A, S36A double mutant) and pUSE control vectors were obtained from Upstate Biotechnology (Lake Placid, NY). STAT1 vectors were constructed by inserting PCR-amplified STAT1 cDNA fragments into the pcDNA3.1 expression vector (Invitrogen). All plasmids for transfections were prepared by means of the EndoFree Plasmid Maxi Kit (Qiagen). NF-κB luciferase reporter construct [38] and expression vectors were added to 90% confluent cells in 24-well culture plates. At 18 hrs after transfection, cells were stimulated with *P. gingivalis* LPS. After an additional 4 hrs of incubation, the cells were lysed with Passive Lysis Buffer (Promega, Madison, WI). Luciferase activity was measured by using a luminescencer-JNR-II.

siRNA transfection

RNA interference for STAT1 (Cell Signaling, Danvers, MA), TLR2, TLR4 (Santa Cruz) and negative control siRNA (Cell Signaling) were used. STAT1 siRNA (Cell Signaling, Danvers, MA) and negative control siRNA (Cell Signaling) were used. THP-1 cells were transfected with Lipofectamine™ RNAiMAX Reagent (Invitrogen) according to the manufacturer's protocol and incubated for 18 hrs. A 42% knockdown of STAT1 mRNA was measured. Following transfection, THP-1 cells were stimulated with *P. gingivalis* LPS for 4 hrs.

Electrophoretic mobility-shift assay (EMSA)

EMSA was performed as described previously [38]. Cells were lysed with NucBuster protein Extraction Kit according to the manufacturer's instructions (Novagen, Darmstadt, Germany). Murine NF-κB oligonucleotide, 5′-AGTTGAGGGGACTTTCC-CAGGC-3′, was purchased from Promega. Ten μg of extract was pre-incubated for 20 min at room temperature in 15 μl of buffer (10 mM Tris–HCl pH 7.5, 1 mM EDTA, 1 mM β-mercaptoethanol, 4% glycerol, and 40 mM NaCl) containing 1 μg of poly (dI-dC) and the oligonucleotide labeled with T4 polynucleotide kinase (New England Biolabs, Beverly, MA) and [γ-^{32}P]ATP (111 TBq mmol-1, Amersham Pharmacia Biotech, Little Chalfont, UK). Protein–DNA complexes were resolved on 4% TBE polyacrylamide gels and analyzed with a specific antibody.

Statistical analysis

Data are represented as means ± SD for replicate experiments. The Mann-Whitney U test was used to compare the Wnt5a/β-actin ratios between periodontitis tissue and non-periodontitis tissue. Data were subjected to one-way analysis of variance (ANOVA) using StatView. Fisher's prospected least significance test was used for the post hoc comparison of specific groups. A value of $p<0.05$ was considered statistically significant.

Author Contributions

Conceived and designed the experiments: NW TN YY YI. Performed the experiments: HN RY. Analyzed the data: WP. Contributed reagents/materials/analysis tools: YB HK JK DH JAB. Wrote the paper: HN.

References

1. Sharma RP, Chopra VL (1976) Effect of the Wingless (wg1) mutation on wing and haltere development in Drosophila melanogaster. Dev Biol 48: 461–465.
2. Klingensmith J, Nusse R (1994) Signaling by wingless in Drosophila. Dev Biol 166: 396–414.

3. Nusse R (2005) Wnt signaling in disease and in development. Cell Res 15: 28–32.
4. Reya T, Duncan AW, Ailles L, Domen J, Scherer DC, et al. (2003) A role for Wnt signalling in self-renewal of haematopoietic stem cells. Nature 423: 409–414.
5. Reya T, O'Riordan M, Okamura R, Devaney E, Willert K, et al. (2000) Wnt signaling regulates B lymphocyte proliferation through a LEF-1 dependent mechanism. Immunity 13: 15–24.
6. Staal FJ, Clevers HC (2003) Wnt signaling in the thymus. Curr Opin Immunol 15: 204–208.
7. Gavin BJ, McMahon AP (1992) Differential regulation of the Wnt gene family during pregnancy and lactation suggests a role in postnatal development of the mammary gland. Mol Cell Biol 12: 2418–2423.
8. Sen M, Lauterbach K, El-Gabalawy H, Firestein GS, Corr M, et al. (2000) Expression and function of wingless and frizzled homologs in rheumatoid arthritis. Proc Natl Acad Sci U S A 97: 2791–2796.
9. Christman MA, 2nd, Goetz DJ, Dickerson E, McCall KD, Lewis CJ, et al. (2008) Wnt5a is expressed in murine and human atherosclerotic lesions. Am J Physiol Heart Circ Physiol 294: H2864–2870.
10. Blumenthal A, Ehlers S, Lauber J, Buer J, Lange C, et al. (2006) The Wingless homolog WNT5A and its receptor Frizzled-5 regulate inflammatory responses of human mononuclear cells induced by microbial stimulation. Blood 108: 965–973.
11. Pereira C, Schaer DJ, Bachli EB, Kurrer MO, Schoedon G (2008) Wnt5A/CaMKII signaling contributes to the inflammatory response of macrophages and is a target for the antiinflammatory action of activated protein C and interleukin-10. Arterioscler Thromb Vasc Biol 28: 504–510.
12. Katoh M (2007) STAT3-induced WNT5A signaling loop in embryonic stem cells, adult normal tissues, chronic persistent inflammation, rheumatoid arthritis and cancer (Review). Int J Mol Med 19: 273–278.
13. Costerton JW, Stewart PS, Greenberg EP (1999) Bacterial biofilms: a common cause of persistent infections. Science 284: 1318–1322.
14. Bickel M, Axtelius B, Solioz C, Attstrom R (2001) Cytokine gene expression in chronic periodontitis. J Clin Periodontol 28: 840–847.
15. Rasmussen L, Hanstrom L, Lerner UH (2000) Characterization of bone resorbing activity in gingival crevicular fluid from patients with periodontitis. J Clin Periodontol 27: 41–52.
16. Hofbauer LC, Lacey DL, Dunstan CR, Spelsberg TC, Riggs BL, et al. (1999) Interleukin-1beta and tumor necrosis factor-alpha, but not interleukin-6, stimulate osteoprotegerin ligand gene expression in human osteoblastic cells. Bone 25: 255–259.
17. Nakashima T, Kobayashi Y, Yamasaki S, Kawakami A, Eguchi K, et al. (2000) Protein expression and functional difference of membrane-bound and soluble receptor activator of NF-kappaB ligand: modulation of the expression by osteotropic factors and cytokines. Biochem Biophys Res Commun 275: 768–775.
18. Burgess TL, Qian Y, Kaufman S, Ring BD, Van G, et al. (1999) The ligand for osteoprotegerin (OPGL) directly activates mature osteoclasts. J Cell Biol 145: 527–538.
19. Hsu H, Lacey DL, Dunstan CR, Solovyev I, Colombero A, et al. (1999) Tumor necrosis factor receptor family member RANK mediates osteoclast differentiation and activation induced by osteoprotegerin ligand. Proc Natl Acad Sci U S A 96: 3540–3545.
20. Lacey DL, Timms E, Tan HL, Kelley MJ, Dunstan CR, et al. (1998) Osteoprotegerin ligand is a cytokine that regulates osteoclast differentiation and activation. Cell 93: 165–176.
21. Matsuzaki K, Udagawa N, Takahashi N, Yamaguchi K, Yasuda H, et al. (1998) Osteoclast differentiation factor (ODF) induces osteoclast-like cell formation in human peripheral blood mononuclear cell cultures. Biochem Biophys Res Commun 246: 199–204.
22. Fujio Y, Matsuda T, Oshima Y, Maeda M, Mohri T, et al. (2004) Signals through gp130 upregulate Wnt5a and contribute to cell adhesion in cardiac myocytes. FEBS Lett 573: 202–206.
23. Bansal K, Trinath J, Chakravortty D, Patil SA, Balaji KN (2011) Pathogen-specific TLR2 protein activation programs macrophages to induce Wnt-beta-catenin signaling. J Biol Chem 286: 37032–37044.
24. Holt SC, Ebersole JL (2005) Porphyromonas gingivalis, Treponema denticola, and Tannerella forsythia: the "red complex", a prototype polybacterial pathogenic consortium in periodontitis. Periodontol 2000 38: 72–122.
25. Loesche WJ, Grossman NS (2001) Periodontal disease as a specific, albeit chronic, infection: diagnosis and treatment. Clin Microbiol Rev 14: 727–752.
26. Pulendran B, Kumar P, Cutler CW, Mohamadzadeh M, Van Dyke T, et al. (2001) Lipopolysaccharides from distinct pathogens induce different classes of immune responses in vivo. J Immunol 167: 5067–5076.
27. Darveau RP, Arbabi S, Garcia I, Bainbridge B, Maier RV (2002) Porphyromonas gingivalis lipopolysaccharide is both agonist and antagonist for p38 mitogen-activated protein kinase activation. Infect Immun 70: 1867–1873.
28. Medzhitov R (2001) Toll-like receptors and innate immunity. Nat Rev Immunol 1: 135–145.
29. Kanaya S, Nemoto E, Ogawa T, Shimauchi H (2004) Porphyromonas gingivalis lipopolysaccharides induce maturation of dendritic cells with CD14+CD16+ phenotype. Eur J Immunol 34: 1451–1460.
30. Frank DA, Mahajan S, Ritz J (1999) Fludarabine-induced immunosuppression is associated with inhibition of STAT1 signaling. Nat Med 5: 444–447.
31. Plosker GL, Figgitt DP (2003) Oral fludarabine. Drugs 63: 2317–2323.
32. Cheng CW, Yeh JC, Fan TP, Smith SK, Charnock-Jones DS (2008) Wnt5a-mediated non-canonical Wnt signalling regulates human endothelial cell proliferation and migration. Biochem Biophys Res Commun 365: 285–290.
33. Masckauchan TN, Agalliu D, Vorontchikhina M, Ahn A, Parmalee NL, et al. (2006) Wnt5a signaling induces proliferation and survival of endothelial cells in vitro and expression of MMP-1 and Tie-2. Mol Biol Cell 17: 5163–5172.
34. Yang DH, Yoon JY, Lee SH, Bryja V, Andersson ER, et al. (2009) Wnt5a is required for endothelial differentiation of embryonic stem cells and vascularization via pathways involving both Wnt/beta-catenin and protein kinase Calpha. Circ Res 104: 372–379.
35. Lowenstein CJ, Alley EW, Raval P, Snowman AM, Snyder SH, et al. (1993) Macrophage nitric oxide synthase gene: two upstream regions mediate induction by interferon gamma and lipopolysaccharide. Proc Natl Acad Sci U S A 90: 9730–9734.
36. Ohmori Y, Hamilton TA (2001) Requirement for STAT1 in LPS-induced gene expression in macrophages. J Leukoc Biol 69: 598–604.
37. Jahnke A, Johnson JP (1994) Synergistic activation of intercellular adhesion molecule 1 (ICAM-1) by TNF-alpha and IFN-gamma is mediated by p65/p50 and p65/c-Rel and interferon-responsive factor Stat1 alpha (p91) that can be activated by both IFN-gamma and IFN-alpha. FEBS Lett 354: 220–226.
38. Yoshida Y, Kumar A, Koyama Y, Peng H, Arman A, et al. (2004) Interleukin 1 activates STAT3/nuclear factor-kappaB cross-talk via a unique TRAF6- and p65-dependent mechanism. J Biol Chem 279: 1768–1776.
39. Dissanayake SK, Olkhanud PB, O'Connell MP, Carter A, French AD, et al. (2008) Wnt5A regulates expression of tumor-associated antigens in melanoma via changes in signal transducers and activators of transcription 3 phosphorylation. Cancer Res 68: 10205–10214.
40. Armitage GC (1999) Development of a classification system for periodontal diseases and conditions. Ann Periodontol 4: 1–6.
41. Wang D, Kawashima Y, Nagasawa T, Takeuchi Y, Kojima T, et al. (2005) Elevated serum IgG titer and avidity to Actinobacillus actinomycetemcomitans serotype c in Japanese periodontitis patients. Oral Microbiol Immunol 20: 172–179.

13

Chronic Oral Infection with *Porphyromonas gingivalis* Accelerates Atheroma Formation by Shifting the Lipid Profile

Tomoki Maekawa[1,2]⁹, Naoki Takahashi[1,2]⁹, Koichi Tabeta[1], Yukari Aoki[1,2], Hirotaka Miyashita[1,2], Sayuri Miyauchi[1,2], Haruna Miyazawa[1,2], Takako Nakajima[1,3], Kazuhisa Yamazaki[1,2]*

1 Center for Transdisciplinary Research, Niigata University, Niigata, Japan, **2** Laboratory of Periodontology and Immunology, Division of Oral Science for Health Promotion, Niigata University Graduate School of Medical and Dental Sciences, Niigata, Japan, **3** General Dentistry and Clinical Education Unit, Niigata University Medical and Dental Hospital, Niigata, Japan

Abstract

Background: Recent studies have suggested that periodontal disease increases the risk of atherothrombotic disease. Atherosclerosis has been characterized as a chronic inflammatory response to cholesterol deposition in the arteries. Although several studies have suggested that certain periodontopathic bacteria accelerate atherogenesis in apolipoprotein E-deficient mice, the mechanistic link between cholesterol accumulation and periodontal infection-induced inflammation is largely unknown.

Methodology/Principal Findings: We orally infected C57BL/6 and C57BL/6.KOR-*Apoe*^{shl} (B6.Apoeshl) mice with *Porphyromonas gingivalis*, which is a representative periodontopathic bacterium, and evaluated atherogenesis, gene expression in the aorta and liver and systemic inflammatory and lipid profiles in the blood. Furthermore, the effect of lipopolysaccharide (LPS) from *P. gingivalis* on cholesterol transport and the related gene expression was examined in peritoneal macrophages. Alveolar bone resorption and elevation of systemic inflammatory responses were induced in both strains. Despite early changes in the expression of key genes involved in cholesterol turnover, such as liver X receptor and ATP-binding cassette A1, serum lipid profiles did not change with short-term infection. Long-term infection was associated with a reduction in serum high-density lipoprotein (HDL) cholesterol but not with the development of atherosclerotic lesions in wild-type mice. In B6.Apoeshl mice, long-term infection resulted in the elevation of very low-density lipoprotein (VLDL), LDL and total cholesterols in addition to the reduction of HDL cholesterol. This shift in the lipid profile was concomitant with a significant increase in atherosclerotic lesions. Stimulation with *P. gingivalis* LPS induced the change of cholesterol transport via targeting the expression of LDL receptor-related genes and resulted in the disturbance of regulatory mechanisms of the cholesterol level in macrophages.

Conclusions/Significance: Periodontal infection itself does not cause atherosclerosis, but it accelerates it by inducing systemic inflammation and deteriorating lipid metabolism, particularly when underlying hyperlidemia or susceptibility to hyperlipidemia exists, and it may contribute to the development of coronary heart disease.

Editor: Pere-Joan Cardona, Fundació Institut Germans Trias i Pujol; Universitat Autònoma de Barcelona CibeRES, Spain

Funding: This work was supported by grants from the Ministry of Education, Science, Sports and Culture of Japan (19390536, 19592384, 19791610, and 20592426)(http://www.jsps.go.jp/) and the Promotion of Niigata University Research Project (http://www.niigata-u.ac.jp/). The funders had no role in study design, data collection and analysis, decision to publish, or preparation of the manuscript.

Competing Interests: The authors have declared that no competing interests exist.

* E-mail: kaz@dent.niigata-u.ac.jp

⁹ These authors contributed equally to this work.

Introduction

Coronary heart disease (CHD) is the leading cause of death in Japan and other developed countries. The major pathway underlying CHD pathology is atherosclerosis. Several risk factors for atherosclerosis have been identified, including smoking, hypertension, hyperglycemia, hypercholesterolemia and genetic factors. However, atherosclerosis can develop in the absence of these classic risk factors [1]. Recent epidemiological studies have suggested a link between atherosclerosis and infection/inflammation. Associations have been reported with *Chlamydia pneumoniae*, *Helicobacter pylori*, and cytomegalovirus [2,3], as well as with dental infections, particularly those associated with periodontitis [4,5].

Periodontitis is a chronic infectious disease initiated by a group of periodontopathic bacteria, such as *Porphyromonas gingivalis*. Periodontitis destroys the tooth-supporting tissues and leads to tooth loss if not adequately treated. Of the several hypotheses proposed to account for the effect of chronic infections on the development of atherosclerosis [6], one—the induction of low-grade systemic inflammation by periodontal infection—is particularly important. In fact, case-control and intervention studies [7,8] have clearly demonstrated that high-sensitivity C-reactive protein (hs-CRP) and interleukin (IL)-6 protein levels are higher in cases of periodontitis and that successful treatment of periodontitis decreases the levels of both mediators. However, despite inferential evidence of an association between periodontitis and CHD, no precise underlying mechanism linking these two diseases has been elucidated.

Several animal studies have assessed the effects of periodontopathic bacterial infection on atherogenesis and documented the formation of atheromatous plaques and elevated systemic inflammatory markers [9,10,11]. Though, there are several points to consider before these findings can be extrapolated to link human periodontitis to atherosclerosis. First, intravenous inoculation with bacteria, rather than the natural route of human periodontitis (i.e., via oral tissues), was used in some experiments. Although transient bacteremia is common in association with the manipulation of the teeth and periodontal tissues, the magnitude of bacteremia resulting from a dental procedure is relatively low ($<10^4$ colony-forming units (CFUs) of bacteria per milliliter) [12]. Moreover, there is no information about the relationship between the severity and extent of the disease and the magnitude of bacteremia. Therefore, the findings observed with direct inoculation of bacteria may not reflect the effects of naturally occurring periodontitis. Second, most studies used apolipoprotein E (ApoE)-deficient mice that spontaneously develop hyperlipidemia, which is a well-characterized risk factor for atherosclerosis. In patients with periodontitis, total cholesterol and low-density lipoprotein (LDL) cholesterol levels were increased and high-density lipoprotein (HDL) cholesterol levels were decreased compared to those in healthy subjects [13,14,15]. Therefore, it is reasonable to investigate the mechanism by which periodontal infection may affect and modify existing risk factors. However, the ways in which periodontal infection affects tissues and organs related to atherogenesis have not been elucidated, primarily because of the limitations of the experimental design described above and the use of short-term infection models rather than chronic infection models.

Here, we compared short-term and long-term infections in normocholesterolemic and hyperlipidemic mice. We found that oral inoculation of *P. gingivalis* affected the gene expression profiles in the aorta and liver, irrespective of abnormalities in the serum lipid profile. Additionally, infection accelerated the development of atheromatous plaques, and the serum lipid profile became more proatherogenic in the presence of preexisting hyperlipidemia.

Results

Alveolar bone loss due to oral Infection with *P. gingivalis*

Gross visual inspection of *P. gingivalis*-infected and sham-infected wild-type mice under a stereoscopic microscope (Fig. 1A–D) revealed the alveolar bone pathology. The distance between the cement-enamel junction (CEJ) and the alveolar bone crest (ABC) in the mandibular molars (measured by micro-CT) was significantly different between the infected mice and the control mice. *P. gingivalis* infection significantly increased the distance between the CEJ and the ABC in the interdental region ($P<0.005$ compared to sham-infected mice; Fig. 1E). The effect of *P. gingivalis* infection tended to be greater in B6.Apoeshl mice compared wild-type mice ($P<0.01$).

Systemic response to oral Infection with *P. gingivalis*

Oral infection with *P. gingivalis* induced a significant elevation in serum IL-6 levels during short-term infection, regardless of whether hyperlipidemia was present (Fig. 2A). During short-term infection, serum amyloid A (SAA) was increased in infected mice compared with those subjected to sham infection, but this difference did not reach a statistically significant level. Further elevation of IL-6 and SAA was observed during long-term infection, and significant differences were observed in both wild-type and B6.Apoeshl mice (Fig. 2B). The serum levels of *P. gingivalis* W83-specific IgG were significantly greater ($P<0.01$) in *P. gingivalis*-infected mice compared with sham-infected mice after short-term infection. In sham-infected mice, no production of antibodies against *P. gingivalis* was observed during either short-term or long-term infection periods. However, the infection did induce significantly greater antibody production during short-term infection. Further elevation of antibody levels was observed in response to long-term infection (Fig. 2C). There was no difference in antibody production observed between wild-type and B6.Apoeshl mice.

Deterioration of the serum lipid profile id associated with the infection period

In both mouse strains, oral infection with *P. gingivalis* had no significant effect on the serum lipid profile during short-term infection. In wild-type mice, only HDL cholesterol levels were decreased by long-term infection. In contrast, all cholesterol levels shifted toward atherogenic levels during long-term *P. gingivalis* infection in B6.Apoeshl mice. Total and LDL cholesterol levels were elevated and HDL cholesterol levels were decreased in *P. gingivalis*-infected mice compared with sham-infected mice (Table 1).

An increase in atherosclerosis is associated with *P. gingivalis* infection in B6.Apoeshl mice but not in wild-type mice

Analysis of aortic atherosclerosis demonstrated a significant increase in lesion area during the experimental period in the absence of infection in B6.Apoeshl mice, but not wild-type mice (short-term infection vs. long-term infection in sham-infected mice). *P. gingivalis* infection further increased the lesion size during each infection period, and atherosclerotic plaques comprised >40% of the total vessel area (Fig. 3B). A similar effect on the response to infection was observed in the aortic sinus lesion volume (Fig. 3C). Conversely, no apparent lesions were observed at any point during the experimental period in wild-type mice.

Changes in atherogenicity-related gene expression profiles in aortic tissue are associated with the infection period

Oral infection with *P. gingivalis* significantly increased the expression of Toll-like receptor (TLR) 2 (Fig. 4A) and TLR4 (Fig. 4B) in infected mice compared with sham-infected mice, regardless of whether hyperlipidemia was present. In wild-type mice, a longer bacterial burden induced a further elevation in gene expression, whereas the difference between sham-infected and *P. gingivalis*-infected mice was smaller in long-term infected B6.Apoeshl mice.

Chemokine (C-C motif) ligand 2 (*Ccl2*) and early growth response-1 (*Egr1*), both of which are vascular inflammation-related genes, were also significantly up-regulated in the aortic tissues of *P. gingivalis*-infected mice relative to sham-infected mice (Fig. 4C and 4D). There was no difference in the *Egr1* expression pattern either between short-term infection and long-term infection or between wild-type and B6.Apoeshl mice. The duration of the infection period did not affect *Ccl2* expression in sham-infected mice, and *P. gingivalis* infection consistently induced the up-regulation of gene expression.

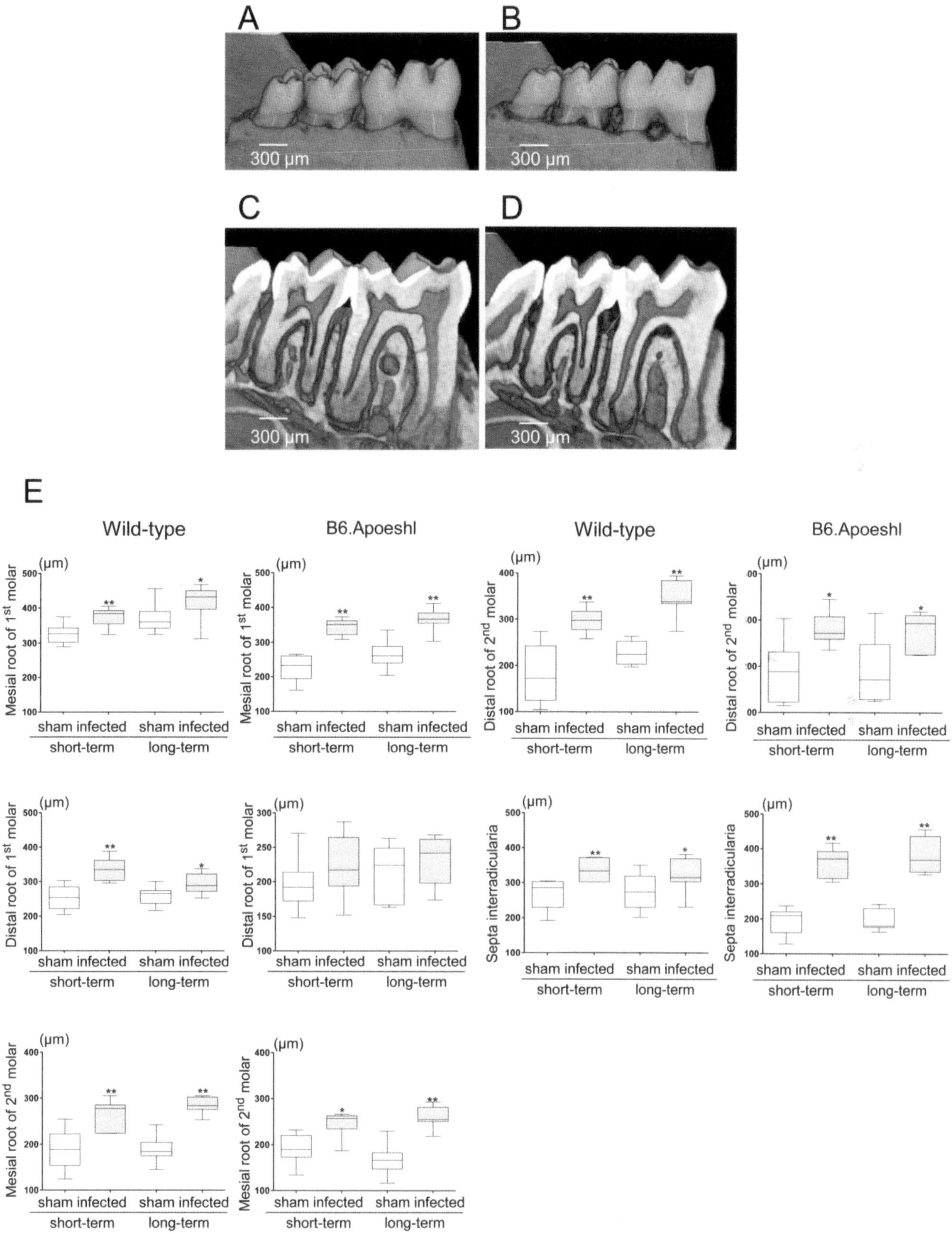

Figure 1. Determination of alveolar bone loss (A–D). Three-dimensional (A and B) and two-dimensional (C and D) microcomputed tomography images of representative samples from sham-infected mice (A and C) and infected mice (B and D) are presented. The infected group (A) showed an increase in the distance from the cement-enamel junction (CEJ) to the alveolar bone crest compared with the sham-infected group (B). Two-dimensional micro-CT sections for the infected group (C) but not the sham-infected group (D) showed alveolar bone loss at the bifurcation.

Numerical analysis of alveolar bone loss between the control group and the infected group (E; N = 10 in each group) was performed. The distance between the cement-enamel junction and alveolar bone crest in each tooth root was determined from three-dimensional micro-CT images using image visualization software. Box plots present medians and the 25th and 75th percentiles as boxes and the 10th and 90th percentiles as whiskers. Significant differences were observed between the infected group and the sham-infected group (* $P<0.01$; ** $P<0.001$, Mann-Whitney U-test).

Because of the importance of lipid metabolism in atherogenesis and the involvement of infection and inflammation in lipid metabolism, the gene expression levels of several cholesterol transport molecules liver X receptors (LXR) α, βand ATP-binding cassette A1 (ABCA1) were examined. Both *Lxrα* and *Lxrβ* were down-regulated during short-term infection, and further down-regulation was observed during long-term infection in wild-type mice (Figs. 4E and 4F). In B6.Apoeshl mice, *Lxrα* showed changes similar to those in wild-type mice, whereas *Lxrβ* did not show any difference following infection. *Abca1* was down-regulated in *P. gingivalis*-infected mice, with a greater reduction being observed during long-term infection. There was no difference in *Abca1* expression between wild-type and B6.Apoeshl mice (Fig. 4G).

Changes in atherogenicity-related gene expression profiles in the liver are associated with the infection period

The expression levels of the inflammation-related markers *Saa1/2* and *Il6* were significantly up-regulated during *P. gingivalis* infection (Figs. 5A and 5B). The expression pattern showed differences between wild-type and B6.Apoeshl mice. Long-term infection tended to produce enhanced up-regulation of *Saa* in wild-type mice, whereas the difference in gene expression was smaller between sham-infected and *P. gingivalis*-infected B6.Apoeshl mice during long-term infection. No such difference was observed for *Il6* expression. The lipid metabolism-related genes *Lxrα* and *Lxrβ*were down-regulated during short-term infection and further down-regulated under long-term infection, regardless of whether hyperlipidemia was present (Figs. 5C and 5D). The gene expression profile of *Abca1* showed a trend similar to that of the *Lxrs*, but a significant reduction was only observed during long-term infection (Fig. 5E). In addition, LDL receptor (*Ldlr*) and inducible degrader of the LDL receptor (*Idol*), another LXR target gene, were analyzed. The expression of *Ldlr* tended to be lower in *P. gingivalis*-infected mice compared with sham-infected mice (Fig. 5F). Consistent with *Lxrs* expressions, *Idol* expression was also decreased in *P. gingivalis*-infected mice compared with sham-infected mice. The change was greater during long-term infection in both wild-type and B6.Apoeshl mice (Fig. 5G).

In contrast to the *Lxrs* and *Abca1*, a marked difference in hydroxymethylglutaryl-coenzyme A reductase (*Hmgcr*) expression was observed between wild-type and B6.Apoeshl mice. Infection with *P. gingivalis* significantly increased the expression of *Hmgcr* as the bacterial burden in wild-type mice increased, while there was no change in the expression levels of this gene in B6.Apoeshl mice (Fig. 5H). A significant down-regulation was also observed in *Adipor2*, which is another antiatherogenic molecule (Fig. 5I).

Because triglyceride levels were significantly down-regulated during *P. gingivalis* infection, particularly during long-term infection, the expression levels of genes critical for the regulation of triglyceride synthesis were analyzed. Both fatty acid synthase (*Fas*) and sterol regulatory element-binding protein 1c (*Srebf1* in mice) expression levels were significantly down-regulated during long-term infection but not during short-term infection in wild-type mice (Figs. 5J and 5K). In B6.Apoeshl mice, *Fas* expression was significantly lower in infected mice compared to sham-infected mice, regardless of the length of the infection period. *Srebf1* expression levels were significantly down-regulated only during long-term infection in this strain of mice.

TLR ligands induce phosphorylation of IRF3 in macrophages

As shown in Fig. 6, the TLR4 ligand *E. coli* LPS and TLR2 ligand Pam3C SK4 clearly induced the phosphorylation of IRF3 in macrophages. *P. gingivalis* LPS, which is known to act as an agonist for both TLR2 and TLR4, also induced IRF3 phosphorylation, although the activity of *P. gingivalis* LPS was much less potent than that of *E. coli* LPS.

Effects of *P. gingivalis* and *E. coli* LPS on cholesterol uptake and efflux from macrophages

Oral infection with *P. gingivalis* down-regulated the expression of the *Lxrs* and *Abca1* in both strains of mice. However, in contrast to the progression of the atherosclerotic lesions in B6.Apoeshl mice, no development of such lesions was observed in wild-type mice. These results suggested that either cholesterol efflux may be much more impaired by the infection in B6.Apoeshl mice than wild-type mice. Alternatively cholesterol efflux may be similar between wild-type and B6.Apoeshl mice, but cholesterol uptake may be higher in B6.Apoeshl mice. This would result in increased cholesterol accumulation and lesion progression. To distinguish between these two hypotheses, the effect of LPS treatment on cholesterol efflux by peritoneal macrophages was quantified in both strains of mice. We found that the apoA1-dependent cholesterol efflux induced by GW3965, a synthetic LXR agonist, was significantly inhibited by LPS treatment. The effect of GW3965 and inhibitory effect of LPS on GW3965-induced apoA1-dependent cholesterol efflux were similar between wild-type mice and B6.Apoeshl mice (Fig. 7A). Basal cholesterol uptake of B6.Apoeshl macrophages was much higher compared to that of wild-type macrophages. LPS treatment in the absence of GW3965 significantly increased cholesterol uptake in both wild-type macrophage and B6.Apoeshl macrophage (Fig. 7B). These results suggested that increased atherosclerotic lesions may be due to the increased uptake of cholesterol into B6.Aoeshl macrophages compared with wild-type macrophages, rather than differences in cholesterol efflux. The differences of these cellular characteristics were further manifested by the LPS stimulation.

Effects of *P. gingivalis* and *E. coli* LPS on LDLR expression in macrophages

The gene expression of LDLR in B6.Apoeshl macrophages was lower than that in wild-type macrophages and stimulation with *P. gingivalis* LPS and *E. coli* LPS increased the gene expression in both strains of mice. Although GW3965 suppressed the *Ldlr* gene expression, either LPS abrogated the effect of GW3965. In contrast to the *Ldlr*, the gene expression of *Idol* was higher in B6.Apoeshl macrophages compared with wild-type macrophages. While GW3965 increased the Idol expression in macrophages of both strains of mice, LPS suppressed the effect of GW3965 (Fig. 8A).

Culture in the sterol-depletion medium strongly induced LDLR protein expression in the macrophage and the addition of GW3965 potently decreased LDLR protein levels in macrophages. P. gingivalis LPS stimulation not only markedly attenuated the suppressive activity of GW3965 on the LDLR expression but also up-regulated the LDLR protein expression in B6.Apoeshl mice.

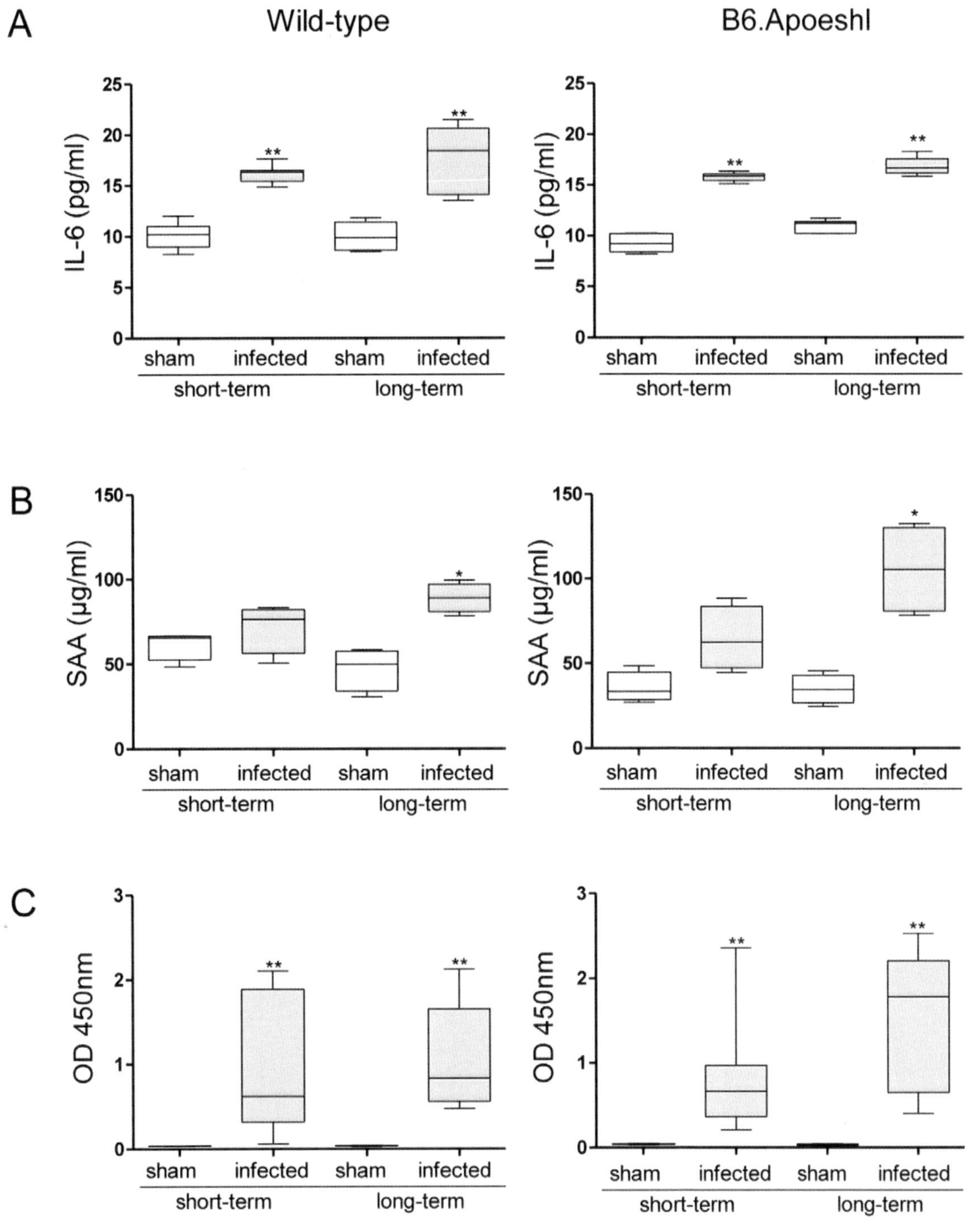

Figure 2. Effects of oral infection with *P. gingivalis* on serum levels of interleukin (IL)-6 (A), serum amyloid A (SAA; B), and anti-*P. gingivalis* antibody (C; N = 5 in each group). All experiments were performed in triplicate wells for each condition and repeated at least twice. Representative data are shown. Box plots present medians and the 25th and 75th percentiles as boxes and the 10th and 90th percentiles as whiskers. Significant differences were observed between the infected group and the sham-infected group (* $P<0.05$; ** $P<0.01$, Mann-Whitney U-test).

Both LPS enhanced LDLR expression in the absence of GW3965 (Fig. 8B).

Discussion

In both wild-type and B6.Apoeshl mice, oral infection with *P. gingivalis* induced alveolar bone resorption, which is a characteristic feature of chronic periodontitis. Both strains of mice also showed elevated levels of serum antibodies against this bacterium, indicating a systemic immune response. Because periodontal tissue destruction is stimulated by inflammatory mediators, rather than by the bacteria themselves [16], the alterations in gene expression levels, the serum lipid profile and serum inflammatory mediators observed in this study could be a consequence of oral infection with *P. gingivalis*. Despite the various systemic effects of oral infection in wild-type mice, the infection did

Table 1. Serum lipid profile associated with infection period in wild-type and B6.Apoeshl mice.

	Short-term			Long-term		
Wild-type						
	Sham-infected	**Infected**	***P*-value**	**Sham-infected**	**Infected**	***P*-value**
Total	102.05±4.73	103.01±4.70	0.841	100.31±6.99	99.06±3.72	0.841
CM	0.58±0.26	0.31±0.17	0.151	0.56±0.23	0.55±0.24	0.917
VLDL	8.09±2.82	6.67±1.08	0.421	8.94±2.12	9.83±3.37	1
LDL	12.72±1.51	11.88±0.97	0.309	11.54±2.37	11.88±2.17	0.548
HDL	80.66±6.12	86.53±5.66	0.222	89.81±1.71	84.88±2.53	0.008
TG	76.79±32.59	47.37±21.04	0.151	20.43±5.21	12.41±3.05	0.016
B6.Apoeshl						
	Short-term			**Long-term**		
	Sham-infected	**Infected**	***P*-value**	**Sham-infected**	**Infected**	***P*-value**
Total	750.26±157.93	775.51±165.26	1	614.29±47.19	756.18±33.93	0.008
CM	43.33±5.11	35.31±2.35	0.056	41.21±3.91	35.67±2.67	0.056
VLDL	458.71±111.32	479.66±143.16	1	398.89±53.60	493.64±45.21	0.032
LDL	249.38±46.71	252.22±34.07	1	179.09±29.93	255.51±27.64	0.016
HDL	34.83±7.73	34.29±8.24	0.841	38.31±4.34	23.35±1.81	0.008
TG	45.21±41.60	59.04±26.80	0.548	67.81±8.30	38.21±10.62	0.008

Values are indicated as mg/dL.
CM indicates chylomicron; VLDL, very low density lipoprotein; LDL, low density lipoprotein; HDL, high density lipoprotein.
N = 5 in each group.

not induce the development of atherosclerotic lesions. The gene expression profiles in the aorta and liver were consistent with proatherogenic profiles. These results are in agreement with the findings related to the effects of other infectious agents, such as *C. pneumonia*, on atherogenesis in mice. However, *C. pneumonia* inoculation in wild-type mice fed a high-fat diet accelerated hypercholesterolemia-induced atherosclerosis [17]. This suggests that infection may play a synergistic role with other preexisting factors, such as hyperlipidemia, to result in the development of atherosclerosis. Therefore, it is important to clarify whether *P. gingivalis* infection has the same effects as *C. pneumonia*. In this context, previous studies have examined the role of periodontal infection using ApoE-deficient mice [9,10]. These studies demonstrated that either oral or intravenous *P. gingivalis* infection accelerated atherosclerosis and raised the levels of systemic inflammatory markers. However, the infection period in these studies was relatively short (3 weeks), and there was no information provided about whether long-term infection mimicked human chronic periodontitis. Furthermore, the ways in which oral infection affects the function of the aorta and liver, which are the organs most relevant to atherogenesis, are unknown.

Our analysis of gene expression levels in the aorta provided new insights into both the mechanisms linking periodontal infection with atherosclerosis and the role of hyperlipidemia in the immune response of B6.Apoeshl mice to *P. gingivalis* infection. During short-term infection, aortic expression of both *Tlr2* and *Tlr4* was significantly up-regulated. However, the stimulatory effect of *P. gingivalis* oral infection was attenuated during long-term infection. Because such attenuation is not seen in wild-type mice, in which the expression of *Tlr2* and *Tlr4* was further elevated after long-term infection compared with short-term infection, the deletion of the *ApoE* gene and/or the resulting hyperlipidemia may have affected the endothelial response. Likewise, the expression of *Egr1* and *Ccl2* was significantly enhanced in B6.Apoeshl mice but this effect was less pronounced than in wild-type mice. Because the expression of both *Egr1* and *Ccl2* is positively regulated by IL-6 in endothelial cells [18], increased serum IL-6 levels in B6.Apoeshl mice compared with wild-type mice would be expected to enhance the transcription of these molecules. Contrary to this assumption, IL-6 did not up-regulate these molecules. These results again suggest that abnormal lipid metabolism may have affected inflammatory responses in endothelial cells. The lipid metabolism–inflammatory response relationship was further highlighted by the observation of alveolar bone resorption. The effect of *P. gingivalis* infection tended to be greater in B6.Apoeshl mice than in wild-type mice. Further studies should be directed at understanding the role of lipid metabolism during the inflammatory response in blood vessels.

Additionally, infection and subsequent inflammation affected lipid metabolism-related gene expression. While the observed changes in *Lxrα* and *Abca1* expression were similar between wild-type and B6.Apoeshl mice with both short-term and long-term infections, *Lxrβ* gene expression was not affected by oral infection with *P. gingivalis* in B6.Apoeshl mice.

LXRs have been identified as central regulators of lipid homeostasis. LXRα is expressed primarily in the liver, intestine, adipose tissue, and macrophages, whereas LXRβ is expressed in many cell types. Endothelial cells also express functional LXRs, and treatment with LXR agonists can up-regulate ABC transporters. This result suggests that LXRs have an antiatherogenic effect in endothelial cells [19,20]. A number of studies have demonstrated that ABCA1 is an efficient exporter of cholesterol from macrophages and other cells, a major determinant of plasma HDL cholesterol levels and a potent cardioprotective factor [21]. The concomitant reduction of *Lxrα* and *Abca1* seen in the livers of infected mice suggests that LXRs are functionally affected by oral

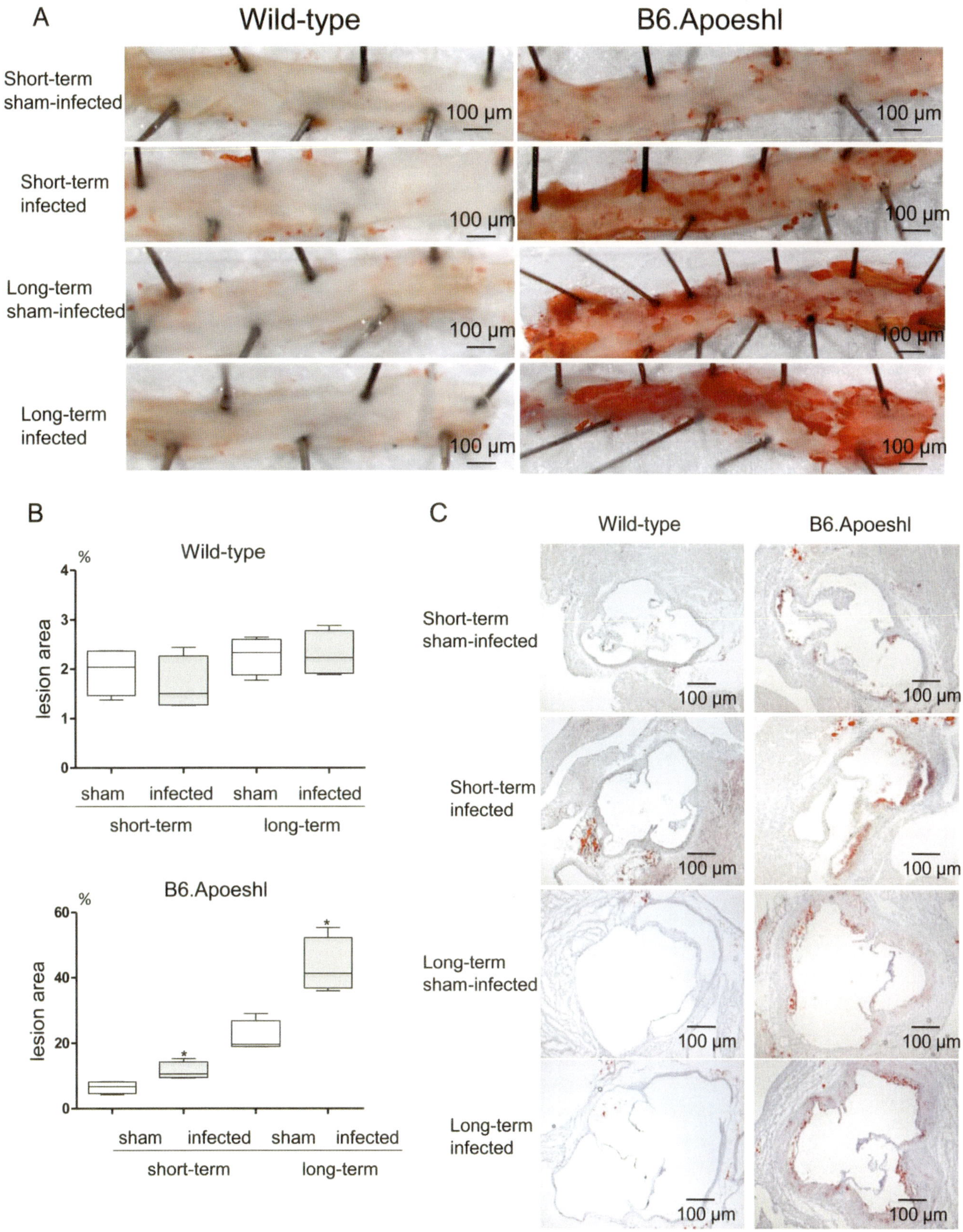

Figure 3. Effects of oral infection with *P. gingivalis* on aortic atherosclerosis in wild-type and B6.Apoeshl mice. (A) Representative aortas from wild-type and B6.Apoeshl mice are depicted. (B) Aortic atherosclerosis expressed as a percentage of the total area (N = 8 in each group). Box plots present medians and the 25th and 75th percentiles as boxes and the 10th and 90th percentiles as whiskers. Significant differences were observed between the infected group and the sham-infected group (* $P<0.01$, Mann-Whitney U-test). (C) Representative aortic sinus cross sections from wild-type and B6.Apoeshl mice. Original magnifications, 40×.

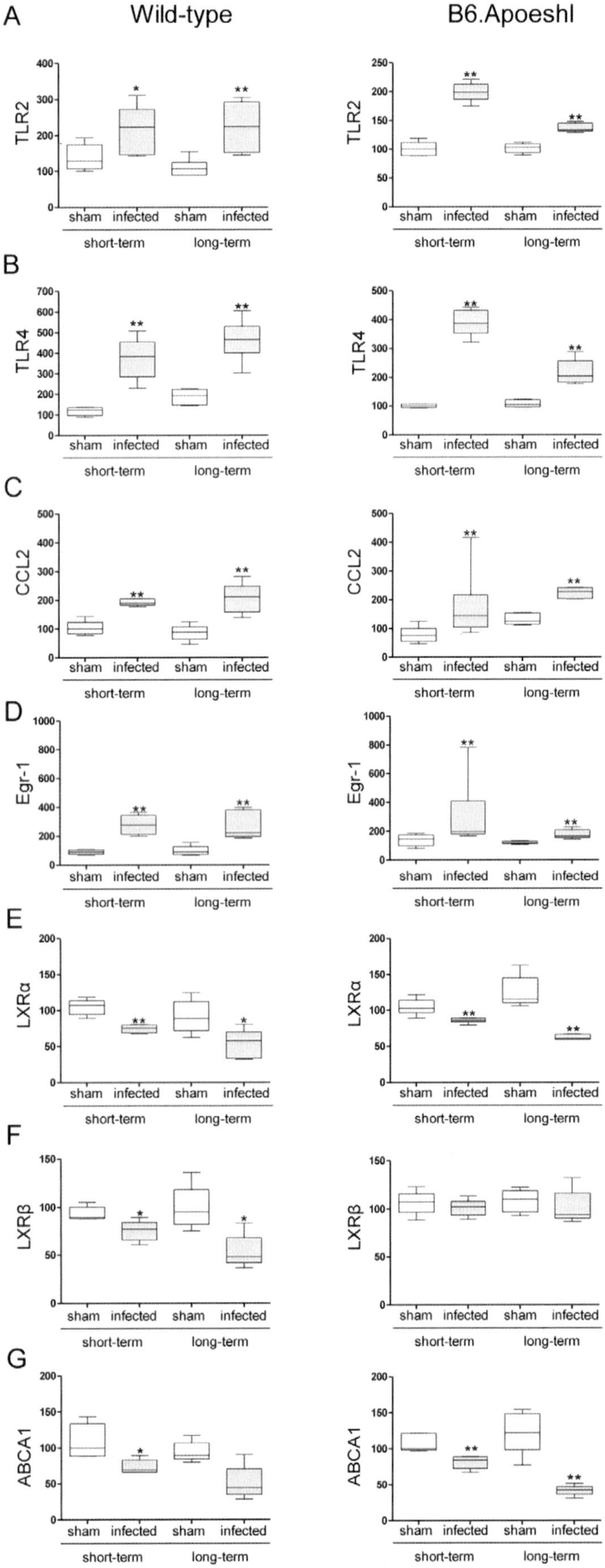
A
Wild-type
B6.Apoeshl
TLR2
sham infected sham infected
short-term long-term
B
TLR4
C
CCL2
D
Egr-1
E
LXRα
F
LXRβ
G
ABCA1

Figure 4. Comparison of relative gene expression levels in the aorta between the control group and the infected group or between the short-term and long-term infected groups (N = 5 in each group). The relative quantity of experimental mRNA was normalized to the relative quantity of glyceraldehyde-3-phosphate dehydrogenase (GAPDH) mRNA. The box plots present medians and the 25th and 75th percentiles as boxes and the 10th and 90th percentiles as whiskers. (* $P<0.01$, Mann-Whitney U-test)

infection with *P. gingivalis*, possibly via crosstalk between LXR and TLR signaling. Castillo et al. [22] demonstrated that activation of TLR3 and TLR4 by microbial ligands blocks the induction of LXR target genes, including *Abca1*, in cultured macrophages and aortic tissues *in vivo*. Crosstalk between LXR and TLR signaling is mediated by interferon regulatory factor 3 (IRF3), a specific effector of TLR3/4 that inhibits the transcriptional activity of LXR. *P. gingivalis* contains diverse TLR ligands, including LPS, lipoproteins, and CpG DNA, which are recognized by TLR4, TLR2, and TLR9, respectively. Although the agonistic activity of *P. gingivalis* LPS is weaker than *E. coli* LPS [23], we found that *P. gingivalis* LPS could also induce phosphorylation of IRF3 in macrophages, albeit to a lesser extent than *E. coli* LPS (Fig. 6). Therefore, TLR signaling-mediated IRF3 activation may be a mechanism for the down-regulation of *Lxr* and *Abca1*.

The functional effect of the change in *Lxrs* and *Abca1* expression levels on the shift in serum lipoproteins (particularly HDL cholesterol) was confirmed by the inhibition of cholesterol efflux by *P. gingivalis* LPS and *E. coli* LPS in peritoneal macrophages. GW3965-induced apoA1-dependent cholesterol efflux was completely abolished by stimulation with LPS. However, the rate of basal and GW3965-induced cholesterol efflux was lower in B6.Apoeshl mice compared with wild-type mice. On the other hand, cholesterol uptake was higher in B6.Apoeshl mice compared to wild-type mice and the uptake was enhanced by the LPS stimulation in both strains of mice.

Plasma cholesterol level is regulated by the LDLR and the expression of the LDLR is regulated at transcriptional and post translational levels. Recently, Zelcer et al. [24] found that LDLR expression is controlled by the LXR-Idol axis where LXR induces Idol, an E3 ubiquitin ligase that triggers LDLR degradation. Given that *Lxrs* are down-regulated in the *P. gingivalis*-infected mice, it is probable that Idol expression is also suppressed in the infected mice compared to sham-infected mice and this change may relate to up-regulation of LDLR. In fact, the expression of the *Idol* gene was significantly lower in the liver of the infected mice and the change was more prominent during the long-term infection in B6.Apoeshl mice. Although the *Ldlr* expression tended to be lower in *P. gingivalis*-infected mice compared to sham-infected mice, the difference was not statistically significant. These changes may have negative effect on Idol-mediated LDLR degradation resulting in the enhanced LDLR expression and subsequent decrease of plasma cholesterol. However, total and LDL cholesterols showed no change in wild-type mice but rather elevation in B6.Apoeshl mice during the long-term infection. *In vitro* stimulation of macrophages with LPS attenuated the GW3965-mediated suppression of the LDLR expression and the effect of *P. gingivalis* LPS was more potent than *E. coli* LPS. The reason for this paradox is unclear. However, Li et al. [25] showed that the acute inflammatory response decrease LDL receptor expression in the liver. In contrast, the same inflammatory stimuli increased the LDLR expression in macrophages. Our results are consistent with these findings. In addition to Idol, the proprotein convertase subtilisin-like kexin type 9 (PCSK9) is also implicated in the regulation of LDLR expression [26]. Although we have not determined whether PCSK9 contributes significantly to LDLR degradation and how its activity is affected by LPS, Feingold et al. [27] showed that inflammation stimulates PCSK9 expression leading to increased LDLR degradation but the underlying mechanisms remain elusive. Nevertheless, oral infection of *P. gingivalis* does affect the expression of the genes that regulate LDLR expression at protein level.

In wild-type mice, genes involved in lipid metabolism, but not the lipid profile itself, were found to be altered by short-term infection with *P. gingivalis*. By contrast, long-term infection reduced HDL cholesterol levels. The exact reasons for the discrepancy between gene expression levels and the lipid profile are not known. However, because the reduction in the expression of the *Abca1* gene, a rate-limiting factor in HDL biogenesis [28], was more pronounced during long-term infection than during short-term infection, it is possible that the suppression of *Abca1* during long-term infection was sufficiently robust to induce a decrease in HDL cholesterol. Few effects of short-term infection with *P. gingivalis* on total cholesterol and the size of the lipoproteins in plasma have been reported [10]. Therefore, it appears that longer-term and chronic infections are necessary to shift the plasma lipid profile toward an atherogenic state, despite the observation of proatherogenic changes in gene expression during short-term infection.

In addition to its effects on HDL cholesterol, *P. gingivalis* infection induced a significant down-regulation of serum triglycerides during long-term infection. *Fas* and *Srebf1*, which are genes involved in the regulation of triglyceride synthesis, were also down-regulated. Enzymes involved in triglyceride synthesis are transcriptionally regulated by SREBP-1c [29] and LXRs [30] in the liver. LXRs are also important regulators of FAS [31]. The conversion of glucose into triglycerides is nutritionally regulated, and both insulin and glucose signaling pathways are involved. Given that LXRs are key regulators of insulin and glucose signaling pathways that were down-regulated in infected mice of both strains, the resulting down-regulation of *Fas* and *Srebf1* and subsequent decrease in serum triglycerides could be due to *P. gingivalis* infection.

Severe periodontitis has been associated with a modest decrease in HDL and LDL cholesterol levels and a more robust increase in plasma triglycerides [32,33]. Although the effects of periodontal infection on the lipid profile of long-term infected B6.Apoeshl mice are slightly different from those seen in human periodontitis, particularly with regard to triglycerides, it is clear that infection does affect lipid metabolism. However, further studies are necessary to clarify the relationship between chronic infection and lipid metabolism. Nevertheless, the systemic inflammation induced by *P. gingivalis* oral infection is associated with a shift to a proatherogenic serum lipid profile that leads to elevated LDL cholesterol and decreased HDL cholesterol levels [34].

In summary, *P. gingivalis* is a representative periodontopathic bacterium that does not have the ability to induce atherosclerosis but can accelerate the progression of atherosclerosis by affecting blood vessel and liver function when hyperlipidemia is present. The results of the present study provide a potential mechanism for this bacterium's contribution to atherogenesis and shed light on the underlying mechanism by which periodontitis affects atherosclerosis and subsequent CHD in humans.

Materials and Methods

Reagents

GW3965 hydrochloride, Sandoz 58-035, Apolipoprotein A-1, simvastatin sodium salt, mevalonic acid and lipoprotein-deficient fetal bovine serum (LPDS) were purchased from Sigma-Aldrich

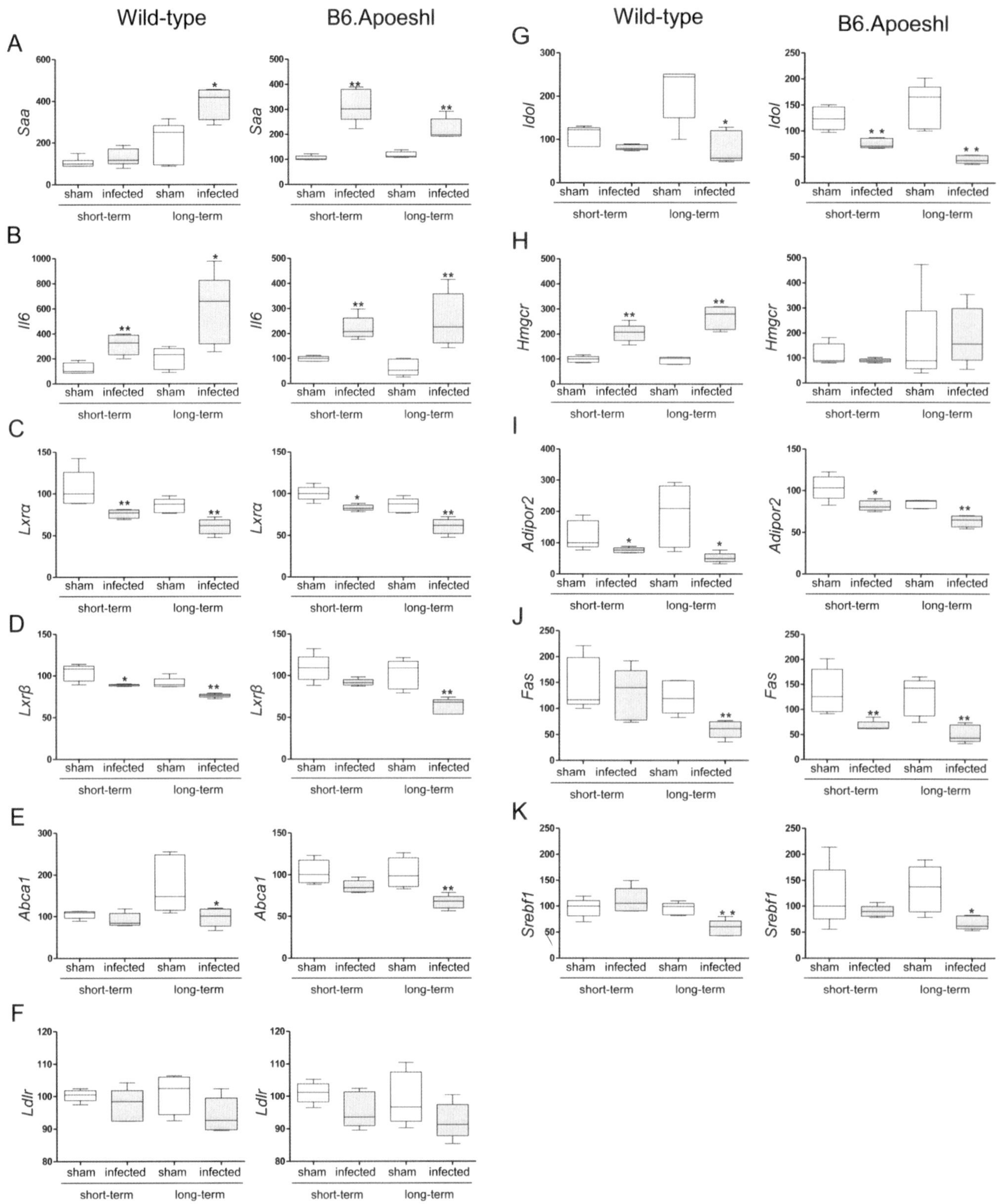

Figure 5. Comparison of the relative gene expression levels in the liver between the control group and the infected groups or between the short-term and long-term infected groups (N = 5 in each group). The relative quantity of mRNA was normalized to the relative quantity of GAPDH mRNA. The box plots present medians and the 25th and 75th percentiles as boxes and the 10th and 90th percentiles as whiskers. (* $P<0.05$; ** $P<0.01$, Mann-Whitney U-test)

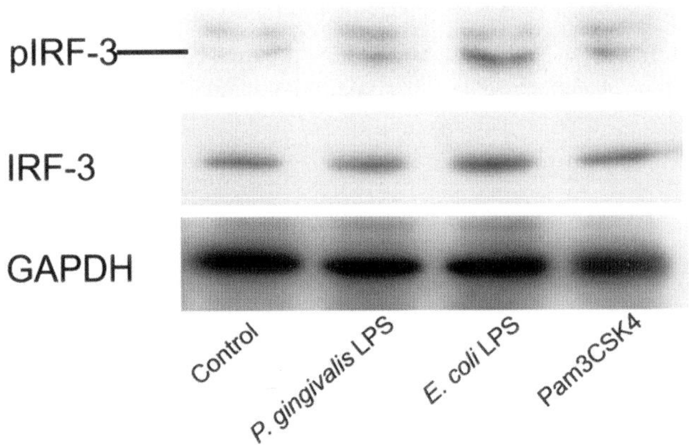

Figure 6. Induction of IRF3 phosphorylation in RAW 264.7 macrophages by TLR2 and TLR4 ligands. Cells were stimulated with 1.0 μg/ml of *P. gingivalis* LPS, 0.1 μg/ml of *E. coli* LPS or 0.1 μg/ml of Pam3CSK4 for 12 hrs. Phosphorylation of IRF3 cellular extracts was analyzed by western blotting. Blot is a representative of three independent experiments.

(St. Louis, MO). BODIPY-cholesterol (23-(dipyrrometheneboron difluoride)-24-norcholesterol was obtained from Avanti Polar Lipids, Inc. (Alabaster, AL). M-PER Mammalian Protein Extraction Reagent and Pierce BCA Protein Assay kit were obtained from Thermo Scientific (Rockford, IL). Pam3Cys-SKKKK x 3HCl (Pam3CSK4) was purchased from EMC microcollections (Tuebingen, Germany). Lipopolysaccharide (LPS) from *Escherichia coli* O111:B4 was purchased from Sigma. LPS from *P. gingivalis* 381 was kindly provided by H. Kumada and T. Umemoto (Department of Microbiology, Kanagawa Dental University, Yokosuka, Japan). Rabbit anti-mouse IRF3 (Santa Cruz Biotechnology, Santa Cruz, CA), rabbit anti-mouse phospho-IRF3 (Cell Signaling Technology, Danvers, MA), rabbit anti-mouse GAPDH (Santa Cruz Biotechnology), peroxidase labeled anti-rabbit antibody (GE Healthcare, Munich, Germany) and ECL Plus Western Blotting Reagent Pack (Amersham Biosciences, Buckinghamshire, UK) were used for western blotting experiments.

Mice

All experiments were performed in accordance with the Regulations and Guidelines on Scientific and Ethical Care and Use of Laboratory Animals of the Science Council of Japan, enforced on June 1, 2006, and approved by the Institutional Animal Care and Use Committee at Niigata University (permit number 39). Six-week-old male C57BL/6 mice and spontaneously hyperlipidemic male C57BL/6.KOR -$Apoe^{shl}$ (B6.Apoeshl) mice [35,36] were obtained from Japan SLC, Inc. (Shizuoka, Japan). The mice were maintained under specific pathogen-free conditions and fed regular chow and sterile water until the commencement of infection at 8 weeks of age.

Bacterial Cultures

P. gingivalis strain W83 was cultured in modified Gifu anaerobic medium (GAM) broth (Nissui, Tokyo, Japan) in an anaerobic jar (Becton Dickinson Microbiology System, Cockeysville, MD) in the presence of an AnaeroPack^{TM} (Mitsubishi Gas Chemical Co. Inc., Tokyo, Japan) for 48 hours at 37°C. Bacterial suspensions were prepared in phosphate-buffered saline (PBS) without Mg^{2+}/Ca^{2+} using established growth curves and spectrophotometric analysis. The number of CFUs was standardized by measuring optical density (600 nm).

Oral Infection

The murine experimental periodontitis model was developed according to Baker et al. [37] with slight modifications. The animals received sulfamethoxazole and trimethoprim at final concentrations of 700 μg/ml and 400 μg/ml, respectively, in water bottles *ad libitum* for 10 days. This treatment was followed by 3 days without antibiotics. The experimental group was then infected. A total of 10^9 CFU of live *P. gingivalis* suspended in 100 μl of PBS with 2% carboxymethyl cellulose (Sigma-Aldrich) was given to each mouse via a feeding needle. This suspension was given either 10 times (short-term infection) or 42 times (long-term infection) at 3-day intervals. The control group received the same pretreatment and was sham infected without the *P. gingivalis*. Two days after the final treatment, the mice were fasted for 16 hours, and oral swabs were obtained and tested for the presence of *P. gingivalis* as previously described [38]. Mice were then euthanized with CO2, and their tissues were removed.

Quantification of Alveolar Bone Loss

For quantitative three-dimensional (3-D) analysis of alveolar bone loss, mandibles were scanned by micro-computerized tomography (micro-CT) (Skyscan 1174; Skyscan, Kontich, Belgium). The micro-CT settings were as follows: pixel size, 1024×1024; slice thickness, 6 μm; magnification, 6×; voltage, 50 kV; and electrical current, 0.08 mA. The 3-D views were constructed with the imaging software program CTan Ver.1.5.0 (SkyScan), and alveolar bone loss was analyzed with the software program CTvol ver.1.9.4 (SkyScan). The sagittal plane of the specimens was set parallel to the x-ray beam axis. The distance from the distal CEJ of the first molar in the middle of the lingual-distal root to the interdental ABC between the first and second molars was measured in the sagittal plane parallel to the lingual-distal root. The measurements of alveolar bone loss in mice were performed by blinded examiners (SM and DY).

Serum Lipoprotein, SAA, IL-6 and IgG Antibody Levels

Sera were obtained prior to euthanasia, and serum cholesterol and triglyceride profiles were analyzed at Skylight Biotech Inc. (Akita, Japan). Serum IL-6 and serum amyloid A (SAA) were measured using commercial ELISA kits (Thermo Scientific and Kamiya Biomedical, Seattle, WA, respectively). *P. gingivalis*-specific IgG antibodies levels were measured by ELISA according to a previously described method [33].

Real-time PCR

Total RNA isolated from aorta, liver tissues and macrophages was extracted using an RNeasy Mini kit and treated with DNase I (Qiagen, Germantown, MD) according to the manufacturer's instructions. Aliquots of RNA were then reverse-transcribed to cDNA using random primers (Takara Bio Inc., Shiga, Japan) and M-MLV reverse transcriptase (Invitrogen, Carlsbad, CA). Primers and probes specific for real-time PCR were purchased from Applied Biosystems (Foster City, CA). Reactions were carried out in a 25- μl mixture in the ABI PRISM 7900HT Sequence Detection System (Applied Biosystems) using TaqMan Gene Expression Assays (Applied Biosystems) containing 900 nM primer and 250 nM probe. The reactions consisted of a 10-minute incubation at 95°C, followed by 40 cycles of a two-step amplification procedure consisting of annealing/extension at

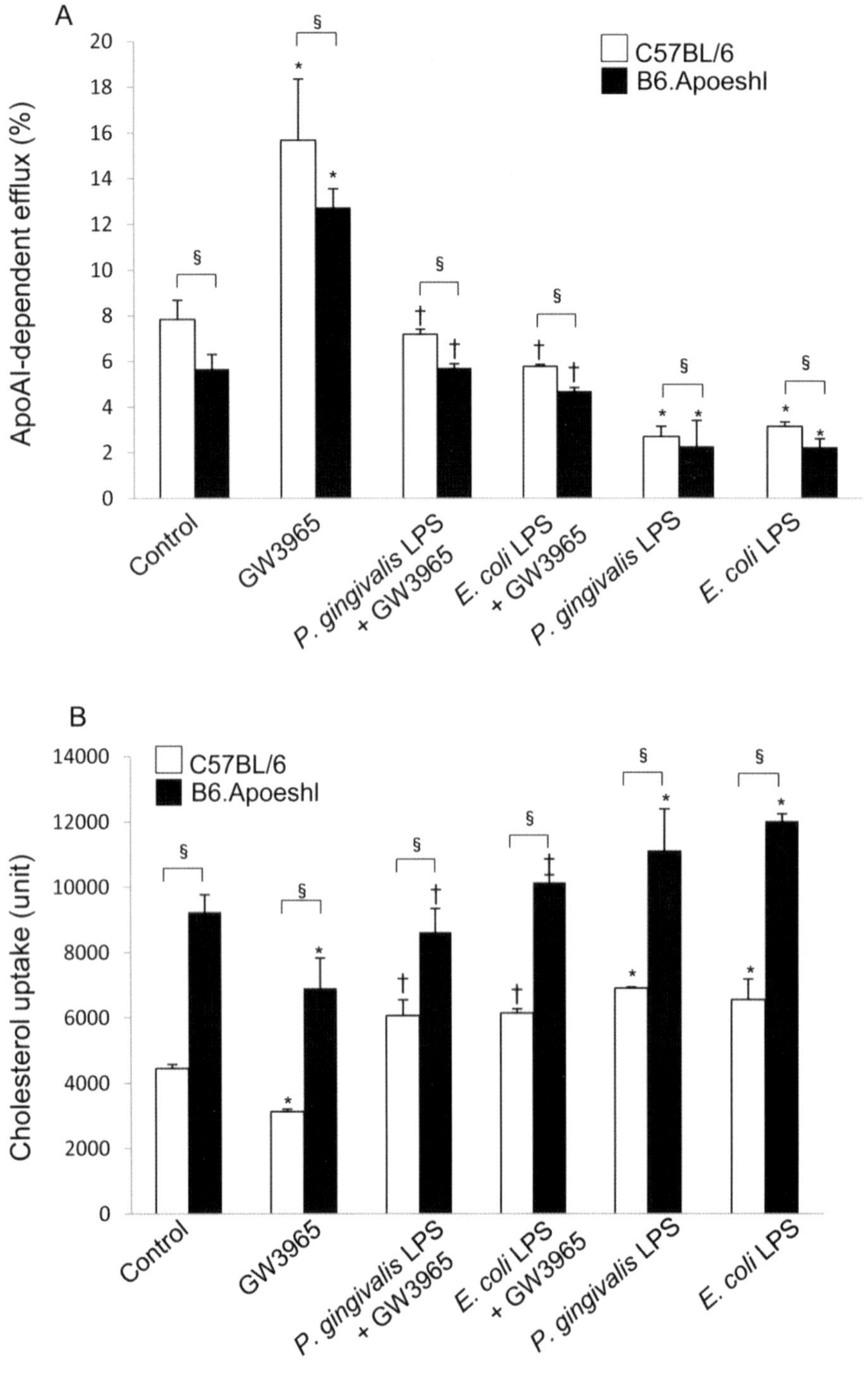

Figure 7. Lipopolysaccharide from *P. gingivalis* and *E. coli* inhibit cholesterol efflux and enhance cholesterol uptake. (A) Peritoneal macrophages from wild-type and B6.Apoeshl mice were loaded with BODIPY-cholesterol and treated with vehicle, 1 µg/ml *P. gingivalis* LPS or 0.1 µg/ml *E. coli* LPS in the presence or absence of 1 µM GW3965. Data are presented as apoA1-dependent cholesterol efflux. (B) Cholesterol uptake was estimated as the total of cellular and effluxed cholesterol. The results are shown as the mean ± S.D. of three independent experiments. There were significant differences found between the wild-type and B6.Apoeshl macrophages (unpaired t-test; § $P<0.05$) and between control and LPS-treated macrophages in the absence (paired t-test; * $P<0.05$) or presence of GW3965 (paired *t*-test; † $P<0.05$).

60°C for 1 minute and denaturation for 15 seconds at 95°C. ABI PRISM SDS 2.0 software (Applied Biosystems) was used to analyze the standards and carry out the quantifications. The relative quantity of each mRNA was normalized to the relative quantity of glyceraldehyde-3-phosphate dehydrogenase (GAPDH) mRNA.

Assessment of the Atherosclerotic Lesion Area

The extent of atherosclerotic lesions in the aortic tree was determined by en face quantification. The aorta was harvested, opened longitudinally, fixed with 4% PFA/PBS and stained with oil red O (Sigma-Aldrich). The stained area was analyzed using ImageJ 1.42 q (Wayne Rasband, National Institutes of Health)

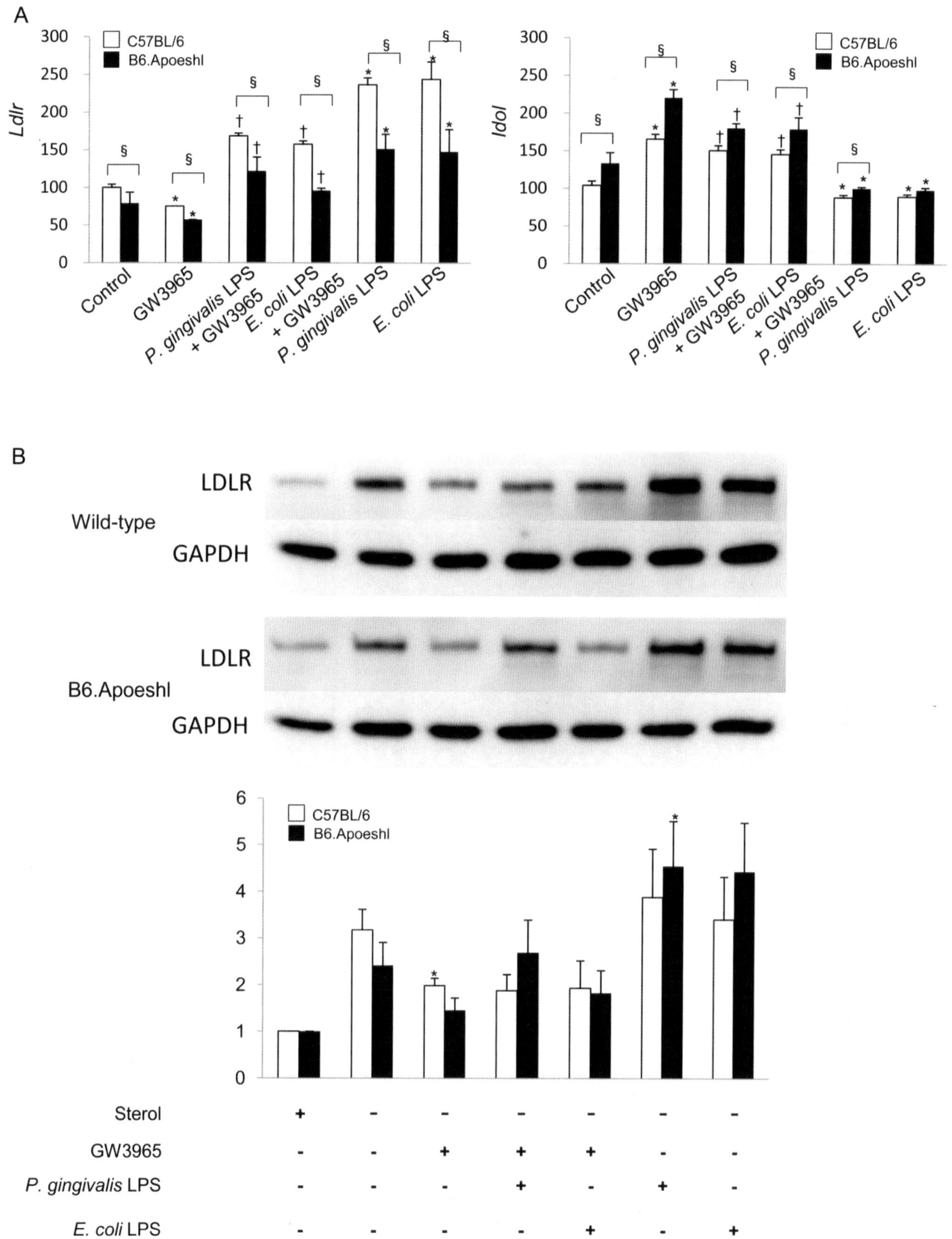

Figure 8. Lipopolysaccharide from *P. gingivalis* and *E. coli* alter the LDLR expression in macrophages. Peritoneal macrophages from wild-type and B6.Apoeshl mice were cultured in the sterol depletion medium for 8 hours and the effect of LPS was evaluated in the presence or absence of GW3965 following 18 hours of incubation. (A) Total RNA was extracted from the cells and gene expression of LDLR and Idol was analyzed by

real-time PCR. Data are expressed as mRNA expression relative to the expression without stimulation. Results are shown as mean ± S.D. of three independent experiments. There were significant differences between the wild-type and B6.Apoeshl macrophages (unpaired t-test; § $P<0.05$) and between control and LPS treated macrophages in the presence (paired t-test; † $P<0.01$) or absence of GW3965 (paired *t*-test; * $P<0.05$). (B) Cell lysates were separated by SDS-PAGE and immunoblotted with anti-LDLR and anti-GAPDH antibodies. Results are representative of those in three independent experiments. The result of densitometric analysis of western blotting shown as mean ± S. E. of three independent experiments. Significant difference between sterol-depletion control and the different LPS stimulations are indicated (paired *t*-test; * $P<0.05$).

and expressed as a proportion of the lesion within the total vessel area. In addition, frozen sections of the proximal aorta were prepared [39]. Briefly, five sections (10 µm thick) per mouse, each separated by 100 µm, were stained with oil red O.

Western blots

For IRF-3 analysis, RAW 264.7 macrophages were seeded in a 24-well culture plate (TPP, Trasadingen, Switzerland) at a concentration of 1×10^6 cells/ml in D-MEM supplemented with 1% penicillin/streptomycin. After 12 hours of incubation, the cells were stimulated for 30 minutes with 1 µg/ml of *P. gingivalis* LPS, 0.1 µg/ml of *E. coli* LPS or 0.1 µg/ml of Pam3CSK4 in medium.

The protein expression of LDLR was evaluated in peritoneal macrophages obtained from wild-type and B6.Apeshl mice. The macrophages were collected 4 days after intraperitoneal injection of aged sterile 3% thioglycollate and cultured in a 12-well culture plate (TPP, Trasadingen, Switzerland) at a concentration of 1×10^6/well in D-MEM supplemented with 10% LPDS, 5 µM simvastatin, and 100 µM mevalonic acid (sterol-depletion medium) for 8 hours and then treated with LPS from *P. gingivalis* (1 µg/ml) and *E. coli* (0.1 µg/ml) in the presence or absence of GW3965 (1 µM) for 18 hours.

The cultured cells were washed twice with ice-cold PBS, and the protein was extracted using M-PER Mammalian Protein Extraction Reagent (Pierce Biotechnology) supplemented with a Halt Protease Inhibitor Cocktail Kit (Thermo Scientific) and Halt Phosphatase Inhibitor Cocktail (Thermo Scientific) according to the manufacturer's instructions. Cell debris was pelleted by centrifugation at 12000 x g for 10 minutes at 4°C. The protein concentration in the supernatant was determined using a Pierce BCA Protein Assay kit (Thermo Scientific) according to the manufacturer's instructions.

Twelve micrograms of each sample was solubilized using SDS sample buffer, separated by SDS-PAGE, transferred to a polyvinylidene difluoride membrane (Immobilon-P; Millipore Co., Bedford, MA), subjected to western blotting with each antibody, and developed with ECL using Lumi Vision PRO 400EX (Aisin, Aichi, Japan). For reprobing of GAPDH, the membranes were washed 3 times with wash buffer (Tris-buffered saline containing 0.1% Tween-20 and 0.5% BSA) and subjected to western blotting with anti-GAPDH antibody, as described above.

Cholesterol influx and efflux in macrophages

Peritoneal macrophages from wild-type and B6.Apoeshl mice were collected 4 days after intraperitoneal injection of aged sterile 3% thioglycollate and plated in a 12-well culture plate (TPP, Trasadingen, Switzerland) at a concentration of 1×10^6/well in D-MEM containing 5% FBS and 1% penicillin/streptomycin, hereafter referred to as medium. Efflux assays were slightly modified from those described by Venkateswaran et al. [40]. Adherent cells were incubated with medium supplemented with ACAT inhibitor (58-035; 2 µg/ml) and BODIPY-cholesterol (10 µg/ml) for 24 hrs. The labeled cells were then treated with *P. gingivalis* LPS (1.0 µg/ml) or *E. coli* LPS (0.1 µg/ml) and/or GW3965 for 4 hrs. After cells were washed with HBSS, ApoA1 (10 µg/ml) was added to the culture and the cells were incubated for and additional12 hrs. Following incubation, the supernatants were removed and the cells were dissolved using M-PER Mammalian Protein Extraction Reagent. The labeled cholesterol in the supernatants and cell fractions was determined using a Versa Fluor Fluorometer (Bio-Rad, Hercules, CA) equipped with the appropriate filters. Uptake of cholesterol in the cells was estimated as the total of released and cellular labeled cholesterol, whereas the ApoA1-dependent efflux of labeled cholesterol from the cells into the medium was determined by calculating the percentage of the total labeled cholesterol in the cells for each condition.

Statistical Analysis

Nonparametric data were evaluated using the Mann-Whitney U test with GraphPad Prism (GraphPad Software, Inc., La Jolla, CA) for two-group comparisons. A probability value (P) <0.05 was considered statistically significant.

Acknowledgments

The authors thank Dr. Yoshibumi Matsushima for kind instruction in the use of C57BL/6.KOR -*Apoe*^{shl} mice.

Author Contributions

Conceived and designed the experiments: KT TN KY. Performed the experiments: TM NT YA H. Miyashita H. Miyazawa SM KT. Analyzed the data: KT TN KY. Contributed reagents/materials/analysis tools: NT YA H. Miyashita SM KT. Wrote the paper: KY.

References

1. O'Connor S, Taylor C, Campbell LA, Epstein S, Libby P (2001) Potential infectious etiologies of atherosclerosis: a multifactorial perspective. Emerg Infect Dis 7: 780–788.
2. Chiu B, Viira E, Tucker W, Fong IW (1997) *Chlamydia pneumoniae*, cytomegalovirus, and herpes simplex virus in atherosclerosis of carotid artery. Circulation 96: 2144–2148.
3. Mendall MA, Goggin PM, Molineaux N, Levy J, Toosy T, et al. (1994) Relation of *Helicobacter pylori* infection and coronary heart disease. Br Heart J 71: 437–439.
4. Bahekar AA, Singh S, Saha S, Molnar J, Arora R (2007) The prevalence and incidence of coronary heart disease is significantly increased in periodontitis: a meta-analysis. Am Heart J 154: 830–837.
5. Humphrey LL, Fu R, Buckley DI, Freeman M, Helfand M (2008) Periodontal disease and coronary heart disease incidence: a systematic review and meta-analysis. J Gen Intern Med 23: 2079–2086.
6. Epstein SE, Zhou YF, Zhu J (1999) Infection and atherosclerosis: emerging mechanistic paradigms. Circulation 100: e20–28.
7. Buhlin K, Hultin M, Norderyd O, Persson L, Pockley AG, et al. (2009) Periodontal treatment influences risk markers for atherosclerosis in patients with severe periodontitis. Atherosclerosis 206: 518–522.
8. Nakajima T, Honda T, Domon H, Okui T, Kajita K, et al. (2010) Periodontitis-associated up-regulation of systemic inflammatory mediator level may increase the risk of coronary heart disease. J Periodont Res 45: 116–122.
9. Gibson FC, 3rd, Hong C, Chou HH, Yumoto H, Chen J, et al. (2004) Innate immune recognition of invasive bacteria accelerates atherosclerosis in apolipoprotein E-deficient mice. Circulation 109: 2801–2806.
10. Lalla E, Lamster IB, Hofmann MA, Bucciarelli L, Jerud AP, et al. (2003) Oral infection with a periodontal pathogen accelerates early atherosclerosis in apolipoprotein E-null mice. Arterioscler Thromb Vasc Biol 23: 1405–1411.

11. Li L, Messas E, Batista EL, Jr., Levine RA, Amar S (2002) *Porphyromonas gingivalis* infection accelerates the progression of atherosclerosis in a heterozygous apolipoprotein E-deficient murine model. Circulation 105: 861–867.
12. Wilson W, Taubert KA, Gewitz M, Lockhart PB, Baddour LM, et al. (2007) Prevention of infective endocarditis: guidelines from the American Heart Association: a guideline from the American Heart Association Rheumatic Fever, Endocarditis, and Kawasaki Disease Committee, Council on Cardiovascular Disease in the Young, and the Council on Clinical Cardiology, Council on Cardiovascular Surgery and Anesthesia, and the Quality of Care and Outcomes Research Interdisciplinary Working Group. Circulation 116: 1736–1754.
13. D'Aiuto F, Parkar M, Nibali L, Suvan J, Lessem J, et al. (2006) Periodontal infections cause changes in traditional and novel cardiovascular risk factors: results from a randomized controlled clinical trial. Am Heart J 151: 977–984.
14. Ramirez-Tortosa MC, Quiles JL, Battino M, Granados S, Morillo JM, et al. (2010) Periodontitis is associated with altered plasma fatty acids and cardiovascular risk markers. Nutr Metab Cardiovasc Dis 20: 133–139.
15. Rufail ML, Schenkein HA, Koertge TE, Best AM, Barbour SE, et al. (2007) Atherogenic lipoprotein parameters in patients with aggressive periodontitis. J Periodont Res 42: 495–502.
16. Seymour GJ, Gemmell E, Reinhardt RA, Eastcott J, Taubman MA (1993) Immunopathogenesis of chronic inflammatory periodontal disease: cellular and molecular mechanisms. J Periodont Res 28: 478–486.
17. Blessing E, Campbell LA, Rosenfeld ME, Chough N, Kuo CC (2001) *Chlamydia pneumoniae* infection accelerates hyperlipidemia induced atherosclerotic lesion development in C57BL/6J mice. Atherosclerosis 158: 13–17.
18. Maekawa T, Takahashi N, Honda T, Yonezawa D, Miyashita H, et al. (2009) *Porphyromonas gingivalis* antigens and interleukin-6 stimulate the production of monocyte chemoattractant protein-1 via the upregulation of early growth response-1 transcription in human coronary artery endothelial cells. J Vasc Res 47: 346–354.
19. Liao H, Langmann T, Schmitz G, Zhu Y (2002) Native LDL upregulation of ATP-binding cassette transporter-1 in human vascular endothelial cells. Arterioscler Thromb Vasc Biol 22: 127–132.
20. Norata GD, Ongari M, Uboldi P, Pellegatta F, Catapano AL (2005) Liver X receptor and retinoic X receptor agonists modulate the expression of genes involved in lipid metabolism in human endothelial cells. Int J Mol Med 16: 717–722.
21. Tang C, Oram JF (2009) The cell cholesterol exporter ABCA1 as a protector from cardiovascular disease and diabetes. Biochim Biophys Acta 1791: 563–572.
22. Castrillo A, Joseph SB, Vaidya SA, Haberland M, Fogelman AM, et al. (2003) Crosstalk between LXR and toll-like receptor signaling mediates bacterial and viral antagonism of cholesterol metabolism. Mol Cell 12: 805–816.
23. Domon H, Honda T, Oda T, Yoshie H, Yamazaki K (2008) Early and preferential induction of IL-1 receptor-associated kinase-M in THP-1 cells by LPS derived from *Porphyromonas gingivalis*. J Leukoc Biol 83: 672–679.
24. Zelcer N, Hong C, Boyadjian R, Tontonoz P (2009) LXR regulates cholesterol uptake through Idol-dependent ubiquitination of the LDL receptor. Science 325: 100–104.
25. Li L, Thompson PA, Kitchens RL (2008) Infection induces a positive acute phase apolipoprotein E response from a negative acute phase gene: role of hepatic LDL receptors. J Lipid Res 49: 1782–1793.
26. Lambert G, Charlton F, Rye KA, Piper DE (2009) Molecular basis of PCSK9 function. Atherosclerosis 203: 1–7.
27. Feingold KR, Moser AH, Shigenaga JK, Patzek SM, Grunfeld C (2008) Inflammation stimulates the expression of PCSK9. Biochemical and biophysical research communications 374: 341–344.
28. Frikke-Schmidt R, Nordestgaard BG, Stene MC, Sethi AA, Remaley AT, et al. (2008) Association of loss-of-function mutations in the ABCA1 gene with high-density lipoprotein cholesterol levels and risk of ischemic heart disease. JAMA 299: 2524–2532.
29. Gonzalez-Baro MR, Lewin TM, Coleman RA (2007) Regulation of triglyceride metabolism. II. Function of mitochondrial GPAT1 in the regulation of triacylglycerol biosynthesis and insulin action. Am J Physiol Gastrointest Liver Physiol 292: G1195–1199.
30. Schultz JR, Tu H, Luk A, Repa JJ, Medina JC, et al. (2000) Role of LXRs in control of lipogenesis. Genes Dev 14: 2831–2838.
31. Chen G, Liang G, Ou J, Goldstein JL, Brown MS (2004) Central role for liver X receptor in insulin-mediated activation of Srebp-1c transcription and stimulation of fatty acid synthesis in liver. Proc Natl Acad Sci U S A 101: 11245–11250.
32. Shimazaki Y, Saito T, Yonemoto K, Kiyohara Y, Iida M, et al. (2007) Relationship of metabolic syndrome to periodontal disease in Japanese women: the Hisayama Study. J Dent Res 86: 271–275.
33. Yamazaki K, Honda T, Domon H, Okui T, Kajita K, et al. (2007) Relationship of periodontal infection to serum antibody levels to periodontopathic bacteria and inflammatory markers in periodontitis patients with coronary heart disease. Clin Exp Immunol 149: 445–452.
34. Khovidhunkit W, Kim MS, Memon RA, Shigenaga JK, Moser AH, et al. (2004) Effects of infection and inflammation on lipid and lipoprotein metabolism: mechanisms and consequences to the host. J Lipid Res 45: 1169–1196.
35. Matsushima Y, Hayashi S, Tachibana M (1999) Spontaneously hyperlipidemic (SHL) mice: Japanese wild mice with apolipoprotein E deficiency. Mamm Genome 10: 352–357.
36. Matsushima Y, Sakurai T, Ohoka A, Ohnuki T, Tada N, et al. (2001) Four strains of spontaneously hyperlipidemic (SHL) mice: phenotypic distinctions determined by genetic backgrounds. J Atheroscler Thromb 8: 71–79.
37. Baker PJ, Evans RT, Roopenian DC (1994) Oral infection with *Porphyromonas gingivalis* and induced alveolar bone loss in immunocompetent and severe combined immunodeficient mice. Arch Oral Biol 39: 1035–1040.
38. Ashimoto A, Chen C, Bakker I, Slots J (1996) Polymerase chain reaction detection of 8 putative periodontal pathogens in subgingival plaque of gingivitis and advanced periodontitis lesions. Oral Microbiol Immunol 11: 266–273.
39. Paigen B, Morrow A, Holmes PA, Mitchell D, Williams RA (1987) Quantitative assessment of atherosclerotic lesions in mice. Atherosclerosis 68: 231–240.
40. Venkateswaran A, Laffitte BA, Joseph SB, Mak PA, Wilpitz DC, et al. (2000) Control of cellular cholesterol efflux by the nuclear oxysterol receptor LXRα. Proc Natl Acad Sci U S A 97: 12097–12102.

14

Bacterial Community Shift in Treated Periodontitis Patients Revealed by Ion Torrent 16S rRNA Gene Amplicon Sequencing

Sebastian Jünemann[1,2]*, Karola Prior[1], Rafael Szczepanowski[1], Inga Harks[1], Benjamin Ehmke[1], Alexander Goesmann[2,3], Jens Stoye[2,4], Dag Harmsen[1]

1 Department for Periodontology, University of Münster, Münster, Germany, **2** Institute for Bioinformatics, Center for Biotechnology, Bielefeld University, Bielefeld, Germany, **3** Bioinformatics Resource Facility, Center for Biotechnology, Bielefeld University, Bielefeld, Germany, **4** Genome Informatics Group, Faculty of Technology, Bielefeld University, Bielefeld, Germany

Abstract

Periodontitis, one of the most common diseases in the world, is caused by a mixture of pathogenic bacteria and inflammatory host responses and often treated by antimicrobials as an adjunct to scaling and root planing (SRP). Our study aims to elucidate explorative and descriptive temporal shifts in bacterial communities between patients treated by SRP alone versus SRP plus antibiotics. This is the first metagenomic study using an Ion Torrent Personal Genome Machine (PGM). Eight subgingival plaque samples from four patients with chronic periodontitis, taken before and two months after intervention were analyzed. Amplicons from the V6 hypervariable region of the 16S rRNA gene were generated and sequenced each on a 314 chip. Sequencing reads were clustered into operational taxonomic units (OTUs, 3% distance), described by community metrics, and taxonomically classified. Reads ranging from 599,933 to 650,416 per sample were clustered into 1,648 to 2,659 non-singleton OTUs, respectively. Increased diversity (Shannon and Simpson) in all samples after therapy was observed regardless of the treatment type whereas richness (ACE) showed no correlation. Taxonomic analysis revealed different microbial shifts between both therapy approaches at all taxonomic levels. Most remarkably, the genera *Porphyromonas*, *Tannerella*, *Treponema*, and *Filifactor* all harboring periodontal pathogenic species were removed almost only in the group treated with SPR and antibiotics. For the species *T. forsythia* and *P. gingivalis* results were corroborated by real-time PCR analysis. In the future, hypothesis free metagenomic analysis could be the key in understanding polymicrobial diseases and be used for therapy monitoring. Therefore, as read length continues to increase and cost to decrease, rapid benchtop sequencers like the PGM might finally be used in routine diagnostic.

Editor: Niyaz Ahmed, University of Hyderabad, India

Funding: SJ was supported by a grant of the German Federal Ministry of Education and Research (BMBF) in the framework of the ParoPhylo project (0313801N). The multi-center study is funded by the German Research Foundation (DFG EH 365/1-1). The funders had no role in study design, data collection and analysis, decision to publish, or preparation of the manuscript.

Competing Interests: The authors have declared that no competing interests exist.

* E-mail: jueneman@cebitec.uni-bielefeld.de

Introduction

Chronic periodontitis has a complex etiology and is an endemic inflammatory disease caused by a mixed bacterial infection with pathogens in intraoral biofilms. It is characterized by severe destruction of teeth supporting periodontal tissues, i.e., the connective tissue attachment apparatus and alveolar bone. Advanced forms of periodontitis may lead to edentulism in adulthood despite therapy and cause high costs for prosthetic rehabilitation. Several bacteria, mainly Gram-negative, are shown to be strongly associated with periodontal infections, e.g. *Porphyromonas gingivalis*, *Tannerella forsythia*, and *Treponema denticola* [1]. Of the about 700 species detected in the oral cavity based on culture and molecular analysis, more than half have not yet been cultivated [2,3]. Approximately 400 of these species have been detected in subgingival pockets, although single patients harbor only a fraction of these species. Recently, next-generation sequencing techniques were used to investigate oral samples from healthy individuals enabling for a deeper coverage of the microbial community [4,5].

Mechanical debridement, i.e. the removal of biofilms from tooth surfaces by scaling and root planing (SRP) is the established gold standard in the treatment of periodontal disease [1] but adjunctive systemic antibiotics are frequently used as supportive therapeutic agents. Two systematic reviews about the impact of various adjunctive antibiotic agents in periodontal therapy conclude that antibiotics may offer a clinical benefit [6,7]. However, it is insufficiently studied which periodontitis patients may profit from antibiotic treatment, what the preferred treatment interval might be, and how antibiotics affect the whole subgingival microflora. Therefore, our study aims to elucidate explorative and descriptive temporal shifts in bacterial communities as analyzed by next-generation sequencing between patients treated by SRP alone versus SRP with adjunctive antibiotics. To explore richness and diversity of subgingival plaque samples the hypervariable region V6 of the 16S rRNA gene was targeted. By using the fast and per experiment rather affordable Ion Torrent's Personal Genome Machine (PGM) a platform was applied that eventually might also be used in routine diagnostics.

Materials and Methods

Patients, Sample Collection and DNA Isolation

In total, samples from four patients were taken before (pre) and two months after (post) intervention. Patients were part of a double-blind, parallel group, randomized, placebo-controlled multi-center efficacy study (ISRCTN64254080). The study was approved by the Medical Ethical Committee of the University Münster (ref: 2006-474-f-A) and a signed written informed consent was obtained from each patient. The four selected patients fulfilled the study's inclusion criteria and were part of one stratum (non-smokers, generalized severe chronic periodontitis, i.e. more than 38% of sites with pocket probing depths of 6 mm or more). The intervention consisted either of mechanical debridement plus 500 mg amoxicillin and 400 mg metronidazole three times daily for 7 days (experimental, Ex; two patients) or mechanical debridement alone (control, Co; two patients). For microbiological analysis, subgingival plaque samples from each patient were pooled. Specimens were taken from four different teeth with at least one site having a pocket probing depth (PPD) of ≥6 mm. Sample teeth were randomly selected before intervention to assure equal distribution throughout the mouth. At the four sample sites supragingival plaque was gently removed, teeth were air-dried and isolated with cotton rolls. One sterile paper point (ISO45, Roeko Dental, Langenau, Germany) was inserted for 10 seconds in each site and all paper points were removed and pooled in one transport tube. Samples were stored at −20°C until further use. Bacterial genomic DNA was isolated and purified with the QiaAmp Mini DNA-Isolation Kit (Qiagen, Hilden, Germany). The protocol followed the manufacturer's instructions with minor modifications, i.e., a pretreatment step with proteinase K (20 mg/ml) at 56°C was carried out overnight. After isolation, the purified DNA was eluted in 200 µl of elution buffer. Quality and purity of the isolated genomic DNA was confirmed by agarose gel-electrophoresis and spectrophotometry on the NanoDrop 2000 device (Fisher Scientific, Schwerte, Germany). DNA concentration was estimated with the Qubit 2.0 instrument applying the Qubit dsDNA HS Assay (Life Technologies, Invitrogen division, Darmstadt, Germany).

16S Primers and Amplicon Library Generation

PCR amplification of the 16S rRNA hypervariable region V6 was performed with a pool of six degenerated forward and six degenerated reverse primers targeting bacteria and archaea as described by Huber at al. [8]. The 5′-ends of the forward primers were fused with the A-Adaptor plus key sequence, whereas the reverse primers were fused with the truncated Pi-adapter sequence (trP1), respectively. The primers were diluted in molecular grade laboratory water and pooled equimolar. For amplicon library preparation 4 ng of each genomic DNA, 1 U Platinum Taq DNA polymerase High Fidelity, 5 mM dNTPs, 2 mM $MgCl_2$ (all Life Technologies), and 10 pmol primer-mix were used per 25 µl amplification reaction. The PCR conditions were as follows: 94°C for 3 min, followed by 36 cycles of 94°C for 15 s, 58°C for 15 s, 68°C for 10 s, and a final elongation step of 68°C for 30 s. Amplicon product purification was performed via gel-electrophoresis on a 1.5% Tris Borat EDTA agarose gel [9] stained with SybrGold (Life Technologies) using the peqGold S gel extraction kit (Peqlab Biotechnologie GmbH, Erlangen, Germany). Control of purification and determination of exact fragment sizes was carried out with the Caliper GX system using the HT DNA High Sensitivity LabChip Kit (Caliper Life Sciences GmbH, Mainz, Germany). Amplicon library concentration was estimated with the Qubit 2.0 instrument using the Qubit dsDNA HS assay (Life Technologies). From the concentration and the average size of each amplicon library, the amount of DNA fragments per micro liter was calculated and libraries were diluted to 2.8×10^8 DNA molecules per micro liter prior to clonal amplification.

Emulsion PCR and Sequencing

The emulsion PCR was carried out applying the Ion XPress Template kit V2.0 (Life Technologies) as described in the appropriate user Guide (Part No. 4469004 Rev. B 07/2011) provided by the manufacturer. Quality and quantity of the enriched spheres were checked on the Guava easyCyte5 system (Millipore GmbH, Schwalbach am Taunus, Germany) as described in the appendix of the Ion Xpress Template Kit User Guide (Part Number 4467389 Rev. B, 05/2011). Sequencing of the amplicon libraries was carried out on the Ion Torrent Personal Genome Machine (PGM) system using the Ion Sequencing 200 kit (all Life Technologies) following the corresponding protocol (Part No. 4471999 Rev B, 13. Oct. 2011) with minor modifications: i) the chip was washed one more time with isopropanol and annealing buffer after chip check and calibration in order to remove possible air bubbles introduced during these procedures; ii) the spheres were loaded twice onto a 314 chip, each loading was followed by four rounds of centrifugation at maximum speed for 15 s (Mini Star, VWR International GmbH, Darmstadt, Germany), shaking on the IKA orbital shaker (IKA-Werke GmbH & Co. KG, Staufen, Germany) equipped with a special chip adapter at 3000 rpm for 10 s, and each loading was finished by a final 15 s centrifugation step; and iii) the complete sample was loaded. For every sample a separate 314 chip (Life Technologies) was used. Raw sequence reads of all samples were deposited at the EBI Short Read Archive (SRA) and can be accessed under the study accession number ERP001440.

Quantification of Selected Periodontal Pathogens

Absolute quantification of *P. gingivalis* and *T. forsythia* in the investigated subgingival plaque samples was achieved by real-time PCR. Genomic DNA of pure cultures of the two species was used to generate standard curves with known amounts of genomic equivalents. Primers and TaqMan probes targeting the 16S rRNA gene were used. Amplification of *P. gingivalis*' 16S rRNA gene was performed in 20 µl reactions composed of 8 µl 2.5× Real Mastermix Probe (5Prime, Hamburg, Germany), 200 nM forward primer (Pg-146f 5′-TGCAACTTGCCTTACAGAGGG-3′), 250 nM reverse primer (Pg-447r 5′-ACTCGTATCGCCCTG-TATTC-3′), and 125 nM TaqMan probe (Pg-195f-FAM 5′-FAM-CGGACTAAAACCGCATACACTTGTATTATTG-BHQ1-3′). Amplification of *T. forsythia's* 16S rRNA gene was done accordingly with 300 nM forward primer (Tf-133f 5′-GGGTGAG-TAACGCGTATGTAACCT-3′), 300 nM reverse primer (Tf-212r 5′-ACCCATCCGCAACCAATAAATC-3′), and 125 nM TaqMan probe (Tf-157f-FAM 5′-FAM-CCCGCAACAGAGG-GATAACCCGG-BHQ1-3′). To each reaction 2 µl of the subgingival plaque DNA was added. All samples were run in duplicates on a MasterCycler realplex^{4}S (Eppendorf, Hamburg, Germany). The PCR conditions were as follows: 95°C for 2 minutes, followed by 40 cycles of denaturation at 95°C for 15 s, and a combined annealing/elongation step at 60°C for 60 s.

Sequence Analysis

Raw sequencing reads were consecutively checked for different quality criteria. Low quality reads were removed as follows: i)

Table 1. Summary of sequence processing.

Sample$	Total reads	High-quality & non-chimeric reads*	De-noised unique reads**
Co-pre-1	613,943	537,150	7,789
Co-post-1	627,905	551,840	5,555
Co-pre-2	620,533	552,247	6,325
Co-post-2	612,292	550,532	8,462
Ex-pre-1	602,209	528,664	5,210
Ex-post-1	599,933	505,452	6,596
Ex-pre-2	565,369	492,048	8,552
Ex-post-2	650,416	566,915	7,144

$Sample abbreviations: Co, control group; Ex, experimental group; pre, before intervention; post, after intervention.
*Number of remaining reads after applying quality criteria as described in the Methods section.
**Unique high quality reads after de-noising the data by Single Linkage Preclustering at 2% edit distance.

reads with no match against the trP1 adapter allowing for up to three errors; ii) reads not matching the degenerated PCR primers with at most two errors; iii) sequences containing ambiguously called bases (N); and iv) reads with an average quality score below the 5th percentile of all reads (95 percent confidence interval). Correctly detected primer sequences were trimmed off during this procedure. Primer matching and trimming were performed by extensions to the Conveyor workflow engine [10] in combination with Cutadapt [11], requiring a minimum primer overlap of 10 bases and penalizing initial gaps in the semi-global alignment. Derived high quality sequences were screened for artificial chimeric formations using the UCHIME algorithm [12]. In order to de-noise sequencing data, reads were further applied to the Single Linkage Preclustering (SLP) method [13] implemented in mothur [14]. In this process, sequences having a pairwise distance less than 2% were clustered using a modified single linkage algorithm and merged while retaining cluster sizes as counts. Following analyses were performed using only high quality reads de-noised by SLP.

Subsequently, operational taxonomic unit (OTU) analysis was done on a clustering basis for each sample individually. Reads were clustered at 97% identity threshold using the complete linkage clustering algorithm implemented in ESPRIT [15]. To meet the known problem of species overestimation [16], reads from singleton OTUs were excluded based on results of another upstream clustering, as recommended [17]. Rarefaction curves and the species richness estimators ACE [18] were calculated by ESPRIT. The abundance accounting Shannon and Simpson diversity indices [19] were computed using the statistical software suite R v 2.9.10 [20] and the vegan R-package [21]. Finally, assignment of taxonomic annotation to high quality reads was achieved using the GAST [22] pipeline with default parameters in combination with the SILVA rRNA database (version 102) [23]. In brief, GAST compares each sequence to a reference database, selects the closest reference(s), and assigns the taxonomy based on the lowest common ancestor for a two-third majority of the references. A schematic overview of the experimental work-flow and applied bioinformatic procedure is given in **Figure S1**.

Results and Discussion

Next-generation sequencing technologies extended our understanding of microbial communities and were applied in a vast number of metagenomic studies. The recently introduced Ion Torrent PGM constitutes a new type of next-generation benchtop sequencing platform. Main advantages of this machine are the small size, low acquisition price, and fast turnaround time. Here, we used the PGM to analyze subgingival plaque samples of four patients for shifts in the microbial community in response to treatment by SRP and SRP with adjunctive antibiotics. Demographic data, baseline and post intervention clinical parameters (pocket probing depth, bleeding on probing (BOP), and plaque index (PI)) are listed in **Table S1**. All clinical parameters improved after intervention in the control and experimental group markedly, i.e. shallow pockets (<=3 mm) increased whereas initially deep sites decreased. No obvious differences between both groups could be observed. Due to limited sample size and short follow-up statistical inference was not performed. However, it is documented in numerous studies and systematic reviews that the administration of adjunctive antibiotics result in further improvements of clinical parameters in comparison to SRP treatment alone e.g. [6,7,24,25].

For the 16S rRNA gene amplicon sequencing we targeted the V6 hypervariable region, corresponding to positions 984–1047 (*Escherichia coli*). Although being a rather short region, it has been shown to enable successful discrimination between different phylotypes [26]. By using the Silva database it was demonstrated in an *in-silico* analysis that more than 97% of V6 tags could be unambiguously mapped at genus level [22]. In addition, V6 was

Table 2. OTU counts, richness and diversity estimates for the bacteria in subgingival plaque samples before and after intervention.

Sample	OTUs*	ACE estimator	Shannon index	Simpson index	Pilous evenness
Co-pre-1	2,365 (5,273)	2,421	4.36	0.05	0.56
Co-post-1	1,710 (3,848)	1,749	4.45	0.02	0.59
Co-pre-2	1,945 (4,377)	1,989	4.42	0.04	0.58
Co-post-2	2,659 (5,705)	2,718	4.91	0.01	0.62
Ex-pre-1	1,648 (3,499)	1,691	3.68	0.11	0.49
Ex-post-1	2,051 (4,449)	2,100	4.03	0.05	0.53
Ex-pre-2	2,412 (6,058)	2,476	4.19	0.05	0.54
Ex-post-2	2,197 (5,051)	2,250	4.38	0.03	0.60

*OTU clusters were generated by complete linkage clustering at 97% identity threshold excluding singleton clusters; numbers in parentheses give OTU counts including singleton clusters.

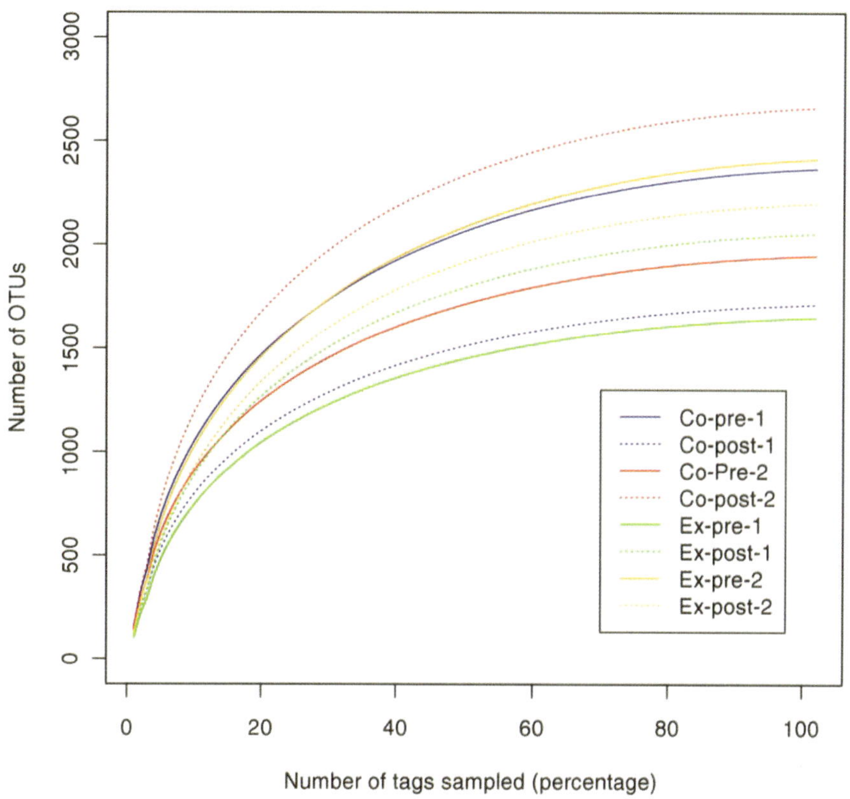

Figure 1. Rarefaction analysis for each sample based on clustering of high quality de-noised reads. In total samples from four patients were analyzed two times, i.e., before (continuous lines) and two months after intervention (dashed lines). Two control group patients (Co) were treated by SRP alone whereas two experimental group patients (Ex) received SRP plus adjunctive antibiotics. Lines are colored according to the sample origin.

not only the hypervariable 16S rRNA gene region used in the first NGS metagenomic amplicon study [27] but is still most frequently applied in environmental and medical microbiology projects e.g. [4,28]. Furthermore, amplicons of single hypervariable regions missing conserved intermediate stretches and short targets in general are less prone to form chimeras, therefore contributing to higher data quality [29]. In total, 4,892,600 sequence reads, ranging from 599,933 to 650,416 per sample and 314 chip were generated on the Ion Torrent PGM machine (**Table 1**). Downstream sequence processing and quality filtering removed about 12.5% of the raw sequencing data. Most sequences were removed from further analysis due to untraceable sequencing or amplification primers (~8%) and significant low quality scores (~4.5%). Chimeric sequences were found only in very small quantities (less than 1% per sample). Sequences of each data set were further de-noised by SLP, by which between 9% and 14% of all reads were compensated for potential sequencing errors resulting in 5,210 to 8,462 unique tag sequences per sample (**Table 1**).

Clustering of de-noised high quality reads at species-level, defined by 3% sequence difference, generated between 3,499 and 6,058 OTUs per specimen (**Table 2**). Exclusion of singleton OTUs prior to computation of community metrics decreased OTU counts to about 50% while affecting only 0.5% of the sequencing data. Non-singleton OTUs ranged from 1,648 to 2,659 counts per sample. ACE species richness estimations were almost identical to the OTU numbers demonstrating a sufficient sampling effort (**Table 2**). This is furthermore supported by rarefaction analysis where all curves almost reached saturated plateau phase (**Figure 1**). No correlation between the number of OTUs and sampling time or treatment type could be observed. Our phylotype estimates were about a log order higher than those determined by cloning and traditional Sanger sequencing [2]. When analyzing pooled supragingival plaque samples from 89 healthy adults by 454 pyrosequencing, Keijser *et al.* reported 10,052 OTUs [4] at 3% difference. The first metagenomic study using Illumina's high-throughput sequencing technology by Lazarevic *et al.* [5] inferred about 8,000 different phylotypes at 3% OTU distance from pooled oral samples of three healthy adults. In contrast, Griffen *et al.* [30] found between 100 and 300 species OTUs in single individuals when analyzing subgingival samples of 29 subjects with chronic periodontitis by 454 pyrosequencing. However, in their study OTUs were not defined by hierarchical clustering but based on similarity to sequences of a curated oral 16S rDNA database [31]. This demonstrates that OTU profiles and metrics based thereupon are highly dependent on data characteristics and applied processing methods. However, community comparisons by species richness and diversity estimates are still meaningful if data were generated and analyzed in the same way. In our study, Shannon and Simpson indices showed a consistent pattern, i.e. increased diversity in all samples after therapy regardless of the treatment type, with sample Ex-Pre-1 representing the least (Shannon: 3.68; Simpson: 0.11) and Co-Post-2 the most diverse (Shannon: 4.91; Simpson: 0.01) community (**Table 2**). As diversity also considers OTU abundances, our results reflect more evenly distributed abundance profiles after treatment, i.e. prevalent organisms of a

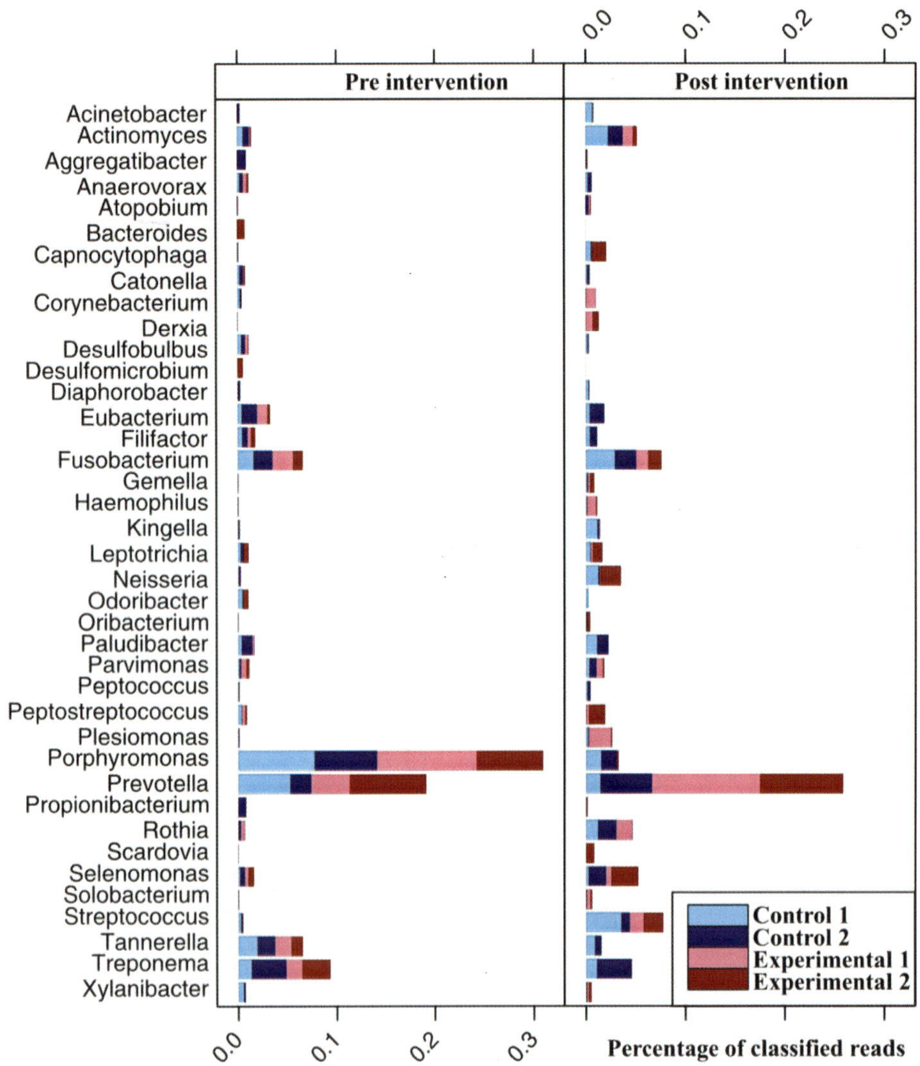

Figure 2. Relative abundance of the most prevalent genera (>= 1% relative abundance within one sample) in subgingival plaque samples before and after intervention. Each bar displays the normalized relative abundance (individual relative abundance divided by the number of analyzed samples at the given time point) of the corresponding genera pre and post intervention. Each bar is further partitioned into four stacked parts for each of the four analyzed patients. The color indicates the type of intervention (blue for control, red for experimental group).

mature biofilm were suppressed by therapy inducing favorable growing conditions for rare and new species. This is also supported by Pielou's evenness values that were indicating more equally distributed OTU abundances among community members in post-treatment samples. It is interesting to note that Kumar at *al.* when comparing subjects with healthy implants and peri-implantitis using 16S pyrosequencing found a significant increase in species diversity in the healthy subgroup [32].

Almost all community members in our samples originated from the bacteria domain. The most prevalent phyla in all samples were: *Bacteroidetes*, *Firmicutes*, *Fusobacteria*, *Proteobacteria*, *Actinobacteria*, *Spirochaetes*, and *Synergistetes* (**Table 1**) comprising together more than 99.8% of all reads. Irrespective of treatment type a shift from Gram-negative *Bacteroidetes* to Gram-positive *Firmicutes* was observed after treatment. At genus level, sequencing reads could be assigned to 330 individual genera, of which 38 were present in all samples with a relative abundance of more than one percent in at least one sample (**Figure 2**). On average, in eight percent of all cases a successful classification at genus level was not possible, resulting in a classification at a higher taxonomic rank (data not shown).

Specimens taken prior to any treatment showed a highly similar community composition by means of taxonomic groups and abundance proportions. *Bacteroidetes*, *Firmicutes*, *Fusobacteria*, and *Spirochaetes* were the most prevalent phyla (**Table 3**), which is in accordance with previous studies [2,4,5]. At genus level the predominant genera were *Porphyromonas*, *Prevotella*, *Treponema*, *Fusobacterium*, and *Tannerella* (**Figure 2**), occupying about 67% of the community sequences. Among these, three genera are of particular interest, as they include the species *Porphyromonas gingivalis*, *Treponema denticola*, and *Tannerella forsythia*, proposed to form the pathogenic 'red complex' consortium in periodontitis [33]. Furthermore, the genus *Prevotella* also includes several known periodontitis associated bacteria (*Prevotella nigrescens*, *Prevotella intermedia*, *Prevotella melaninogenica*) [33,34]. Other genera related to pathogenic organisms could also be identified, but either only in specific samples (e.g. *Aggregatibacter*) or at lower abundances (e.g. *Parvimonas*).

Table 3. Relative abundance of the main phyla identified in subgingival plaque samples.

	Sample							
	Control				Experimental			
	pre		post		pre		post	
Phylum$	1	2	1	2	1	2	1	2
Actinobacteria	3.70	7.15	12.61	13.52	2.44	1.02	12.58	5.57
Bacteroidetes	63.53	44.75	21.43	35.34	63.11	61.45	36.72	40.07
Firmicutes	14.68	14.88	26.36	25.9	16.37	13.22	14.50	30.76
Fusobacteria	6.99	8.19	12.11	8.02	8.27	11.11	4.72	9.08
Proteobacteria	4.65	10.96	22.86	4.05	2.67	2.57	31.36	14.45
Spirochaetes	5.04	13.24	3.98	12.89	6.42	10.11	0.09	0.04
Synergistetes	0.84	0.71	0.25	0.19	0.67	0.42	0.0004	0.0009
Other*	0.32	0.0994	0.2667	0.0705	0.0358	0.0193	0.0255	0.0111
Unclassified**	0.25	0.0147	0.1455	0.0064	0.0013	0.0790	0.0093	0.0089

$Only phyla with a relative abundance of more than half a percent within at least a single sample are shown.
*All remaining phyla with relative abundance lower than half a percent.
**Reads where unambiguous taxonomic classification was not possible.

For post-treatment samples the three most prevalent genera were *Prevotella*, *Streptococcus*, and *Fusobacterium* constituting about 37 percent of the sequences. Specimens of the experimental group showed markedly decreased abundances of the genera *Treponema* and *Filifactor* with frequencies dropping down to complete absence for *Filifactor* in one patient. In the control group these genera remained relatively stable. The genera *Porphyromonas* and *Tannerella* were suppressed in both groups. However, in the experimental group they were virtually absent (**Figure 1**). Due to the limited read length of most next-generation sequencing platforms, taxonomic resolution down to species level is impossible. Therefore, we additionally screened all samples for *P. gingivalis* and *T. forsythia* using species-specific real-time PCR. A positive treatment effect indicated by a reduction of genomic equivalents of both species could be observed irrespectively of the treatment type (**Table 4**). However, in the experimental group *P. gingivalis* and *T. forsythia* were also suppressed to virtual absence, thereby corroborating our NGS data. Our observed bacterial community shifts are in accordance with Valenza *et al.* [35], who did a longitudinal capillary sequencing rDNA cloning study and reported that two months after treatment with SRP plus amoxicillin and metronidazole, disease associated genera were suppressed (e.g. *Treponema*, *Porphyromonas*, *Filifactor*, *Tannerella*). However, these therapy effects were reversible after twelve months. Based on cultivation and on species specific PCR assays the very same effect of systemic adjunctive antibiotics on *P. gingivalis* and *T. forsythia* was previously reported [24,25].

In our study several genera had increased abundance values in the control and experimental group after treatment, i.e. *Prevotella*, *Selenomonas*, *Streptococcus*, *Actinomyces*, and *Rothia*. Of them, *Streptococcus*, *Actinomyces*, and *Rothia* comprise known early colonizer species [36]. The finding that the antibiotic treatment seemed to have selectively eradicated some genera such as *Porphyromonas* while other genera such as *Prevotella* were not affected is difficult to explain. In principle the effects might be due to different recolonization dynamics or antibiotic susceptibility. Since taxonomic resolution down to species-level is impossible we were not able to determine if the sequencing reads counting for the genus *Prevotella* before and after treatment belonged to the same species. *Prevotella loescheii* is known to be an early colonizing partner of receptor-bearing streptococci (first colonizers) [36] therefore a shift from periodontitis associated *Prevotella* species towards the early colonizing species could be conceivable. It is known that the gingival crevicular concentration of metronidazole and amoxicillin is at least ten times the *in-vitro* minimal inhibitory concentration (MIC_{90}) of *P. gingivalis*, *P. intermedia* and *P. nigrescens* [37]. However, some *Prevotella* species might have developed active resistance mechanisms, e.g. Bernal *et al.* reported that about 26% of *P.*

Table 4. Genomic equivalents per microliter of *P. gingivalis* and *T. forsythia* detected by real-time PCR.

	Sample							
	Control				Experimental			
	pre		post		pre		post	
Phylum	1	2	1	2	1	2	1	2
P. gingivalis	338,000	45,499	6,450	2,326	244,000	600,000	n.d.*	n.d.
T. forsythia	98,500	18,601	6,929	10,026	64,500	66,500	1	14

*not detected

intermedia- and *P. nigrescens* isolates are beta-lactamase positive and thereby at least not susceptible to amoxicillin [38]. In addition to the genera *Selenomonas* and *Streptococcus*, Valenza *et al.* [35] also observed for *Prevotella* an increase in abundance early after intervention. In contrast to them we were able to relate effects after treatment either to antibiotic or mechanical debridement therapy by inclusion of a control group.

Whether the detection of selected periodontal pathogens is useful for treatment decision remains questionable. For example, by testing for *A. actinomycetemcomitans*, *Fusobacterium nucleatum spp.*, *P. gingivalis*, *P. intermedia*, *T. denticola*, and *T. forsythia* Cionca *at al.* showed that it was of no predictive value in identifying subjects who would benefit from adjunctive antibiotic treatment [39]. In another recent study the authors suggested a correlation of these species with pocket probing depth rather than periodontal diagnosis [40]. Therefore, analyzing hypothesis free the complete microbial community by NGS might be the key in understanding a chronic disease like periodontitis, as the 'pathogen' might be a disturbed microbial community rather than single organisms [41]. If the in this study observed differences in community profiles and species diversity of periodontitis patients after treatment implies a diagnostic useful prognostic factor for treatment success warrants further experiments with larger sample size, longer follow-up, and a treatment failure subgroup. As performance characteristics like reading length and error rate of the PGM further improves, more specific, e.g. by sequencing longer stretches of adjacent hypervariable regions [31], and less error prone descriptions of the microbial communities will be possible [42].

In conclusion, this translational metagenomic study gives new insights into differences of the subgingival microflora of periodontitis patients for two different treatment regimes. The study results indicate that changes in community profiles and metrics are potentially more diagnostically predictive for treatment success than the detection of selected periodontal pathogens. Monitoring changes in the subgingival microflora with platforms like the PGM might finally pave the way towards routine personalized medicine.

Supporting Information

Figure S1 Schematic overview of the applied experimental and bioinformatic steps throughout the analysis. For a more detailed description of each individual step please see the Methods section.

Table S1 Demographic patient data and clinical parameters at baseline and post intervention.

Acknowledgments

SJ and DH are grateful to Michael Wagner and Matthias Horn (both Department Microbial Ecology, University of Vienna) for giving extensive general advice on how to analyze NGS 16S rRNA gene amplicon data. The authors thank the system administrators of the Bioinformatics Resource Facility at the CeBiTec for technical support and Andreas Schlüter for proof-reading the manuscript.

Author Contributions

Conceived and designed this study: DH. Conceived and designed clinical trial: BE DH. Performed clinical trial: BE IH. Performed Ion Torrent sequencing and real-time PCR: KP RS. Conceived and designed bioinformatic analysis: SJ AG JS. Performed bioinformatic analysis: SJ. First draft of manuscript: SJ DH KP. Contributed and approved the final version of the manuscript: SJ KP RS IH BE AG JS DH.

References

1. Pihlstrom BL, Michalowicz BS, Johnson NW (2005) Periodontal diseases. Lancet 366: 1809–1820.
2. Paster BJ, Olsen I, Aas JA, Dewhirst FE (2006) The breadth of bacterial diversity in the human periodontal pocket and other oral sites. Periodontol 2000 42: 80–87.
3. Dewhirst FE, Chen T, Izard J, Paster BJ, Tanner ACR, et al. (2010) The human oral microbiome. J Bacteriol 192: 5002–5017.
4. Keijser BJF, Zaura E, Huse SM, van der Vossen JMBM, Schuren FHJ, et al. (2008) Pyrosequencing analysis of the oral microflora of healthy adults. J Dent Res 87: 1016–1020.
5. Lazarevic V, Whiteson K, Huse S, Hernandez D, Farinelli L, et al. (2009) Metagenomic study of the oral microbiota by Illumina high-throughput sequencing. J Microbiol Methods 79: 266–271.
6. Herrera D, Sanz M, Jepsen S, Needleman I, Roldán S (2002) A systematic review on the effect of systemic antimicrobials as an adjunct to scaling and root planing in periodontitis patients. J Clin Periodontol 29 Suppl 3: 136–59; discussion 160–2.
7. Haffajee AD, Socransky SS, Gunsolley JC (2003) Systemic anti-infective periodontal therapy: a systematic review. Ann Periodontol 8: 115–181.
8. Huber JA, Welch DBM, Morrison HG, Huse SM, Neal PR, et al. (2007) Microbial population structures in the deep marine biosphere. Science 318: 97–100.
9. Sambrook J, Russell DW (2001) Molecular Cloning: A Laboratory Manual, 3rd edition. Cold Spring Harbor, NY: Cold Spring Harbor Laboratory Press.
10. Linke B, Giegerich R, Goesmann A (2011) Conveyor: a workflow engine for bioinformatic analyses. Bioinformatics 27: 903–911.
11. Martin M (2011) Cutadapt removes adapter sequences from high-throughput sequencing reads. EMBnetjournal 17.1: 10–12.
12. Edgar RC, Haas BJ, Clemente JC, Quince C, Knight R (2011) UCHIME improves sensitivity and speed of chimera detection. Bioinformatics 27: 2194–2200.
13. Huse SM, Welch DM, Morrison HG, Sogin ML (2010) Ironing out the wrinkles in the rare biosphere through improved OTU clustering. Environ Microbiol 12: 1889–1898.
14. Schloss PD, Westcott SL, Ryabin T, Hall JR, Hartmann M, et al. (2009) Introducing mothur: open-source, platform-independent, community-supported software for describing and comparing microbial communities. Appl Environ Microbiol 75: 7537–7541.
15. Sun Y, Cai Y, Liu L, Yu F, Farrell ML, et al. (2009) ESPRIT: estimating species richness using large collections of 16s rRNA pyrosequences. Nucleic Acids Res 37: e76.
16. Kunin V, Engelbrektson A, Ochman H, Hugenholtz P (2010) Wrinkles in the rare biosphere: pyrosequencing errors can lead to artificial inflation of diversity estimates. Environ Microbiol 12: 118–123.
17. Tedersoo L, Nilsson RH, Abarenkov K, Jairus T, Sadam A, et al. (2010) 454 pyrosequencing and sanger sequencing of tropical mycorrhizal fungi provide similar results but reveal substantial methodological biases. New Phytol 188: 291–301.
18. Chao A (1984) Non-parametric estimation of the number of classes in a population. Scandinavian Journal of Statistics 11: 265–270.
19. Magurran AE (2003) Measuring Biological Diversity. Oxford, UK: Blackwell Publishing Limited.
20. Team RDC (2011) R: A Language and Environment for Statistical Computing. R Foundation for Statistical Computing. Vienna, Austria.
21. Dixon P (2003) Vegan, a package of R functions for community ecology. Journal of Vegetation Science 14: 927–930.
22. Huse SM, Dethlefsen L, Huber JA, Welch DM, Relman DA, et al. (2008) Exploring microbial diversity and taxonomy using SSU rRNA hypervariable tag sequencing. PLoS Genet 4: e1000255.
23. Pruesse E, Quast C, Knittel K, Fuchs BM, Ludwig W, et al. (2007) SILVA: a comprehensive online resource for quality checked and aligned ribosomal RNA sequence data compatible with ARB. Nucleic Acids Res 35: 7188–7196.
24. Winkel EG, Van Winkelhoff AJ, Timmerman MF, Van der Velden U, Van der Weijden GA (2001) Amoxicillin plus metronidazole in the treatment of adult periodontitis patients. a double-blind placebo-controlled study. J Clin Periodontol 28: 296–305.
25. Ehmke B, Moter A, Beikler T, Milian E, Flemmig TF (2005) Adjunctive antimicrobial therapy of periodontitis: long-term effects on disease progression and oral colonization. Periodontol 76: 749–759.
26. Liu Z, Lozupone C, Hamady M, Bushman FD, Knight R (2007) Short pyrosequencing reads suffice for accurate microbial community analysis. Nucleic Acids Res 35: e120.
27. Sogin ML, Morrison HG, Huber JA, Welch DM, Huse SM, et al. (2006) Microbial diversity in the deep sea and the underexplored "rare biosphere". Proc Natl Acad Sci U S A 103: 12115–12120.
28. Sundquist A, Bigdeli S, Jalili R, Druzin ML, Waller S, et al. (2007) Bacterial flora-typing with targeted, chip-based pyrosequencing. BMC Microbiol 7: 108.

29. Huber JA, Morrison HG, Huse SM, Neal PR, Sogin ML, et al. (2009) Effect of PCR amplicon size on assessments of clone library microbial diversity and community structure. Environ Microbiol 11: 1292–1302.
30. Griffen AL, Beall CJ, Campbell JH, Firestone ND, Kumar PS, et al. (2012) Distinct and complex bacterial profiles in human periodontitis and health revealed by 16S pyrosequencing. ISME J 6(6): 1176–1185.
31. Griffen AL, Beall CJ, Firestone ND, Gross EL, Difranco JM, et al. (2011) CORE: a phylogenetically-curated 16S rDNA database of the core oral microbiome. PLoS One 6: e19051.
32. Kumar PS, Mason MR, Brooker MR, O'Brein K (2012) Pyrosequencing reveals unique microbial signatures associated with healthy and failing dental implants. J Clin Periodontol 39: 425–433.
33. Socransky SS, Haffajee AD, Cugini MA, Smith C, Kent R Jr (1998) Microbial complexes in subgingival plaque. J Clin Periodontol 25: 134–144.
34. Socransky SS, Haffajee AD (2005) Periodontal microbial ecology. Periodontol 2000 38: 135–187.
35. Valenza G, Veihelmann S, Peplies J, Tichy D, Roldan-Pareja MdC, et al. (2009) Microbial changes in periodontitis successfully treated by mechanical plaque removal and systemic amoxicillin and metronidazole. Int J Med Microbiol 299: 427–438.
36. Kolenbrander PE, Palmer RJ, Rickard AH, Jakubocics NS, Chalmers NI, et al. (2006) Bacterial interactions and successions during plaque development. Periodontol 2000 42: 47–79.
37. Beikler T, Prior K, Ehmke B, Flemming T F (2004) Specific antibiotics in the treatment of periodontitis – a proposed strategy. J Periodontal 75: 169–175.
38. Bernal LA, Guillot E, Paquet C, Mouton C (1998) Beta-lactamase-producing strains in the species *Prevotella intermedia* and *Prevotella nigrescens*. Oral Microbiol Immunol 13: 36–40.
39. Cionca N, Giannopoulou C, Ugolotti G, Mombelli A (2010) Microbiologic testing and outcomes of full-mouth scaling and root planing with or without amoxicillin/metronidazole in chronic periodontitis. J Periodontal 81: 15–23.
40. Riep B, Edesi-Neuss L, Claessen F, Skarabis H, Ehmke B, et al. (2009) Are putative periodontal pathogens reliable diagnostic markers? J Clin Microbiol 47: 1705–1711.
41. Friedrich MJ (2008) Microbiome project seeks to understand human body's microscopic residents. JAMA 300: 777–778.
42. Loman NJ, Misra RV, Dallman TJ, Constantinidou C, Gharbia SE (2012) Performance comparison of benchtop high-throughput sequencing platforms. Nat Biotech 30: 434–439.

15

Education as a Predictor of Chronic Periodontitis

Adrien Boillot[1], Bechara El Halabi[1], George David Batty[4], Hélène Rangé[1], Sébastien Czernichow[2,3], Philippe Bouchard[1]*

1 Department of Periodontology, Service of Odontology, Rothschild Hospital, AP-HP, Paris 7 - Denis Diderot University, U.F.R. of Odontology, Paris, France, **2** Department of Nutrition, Ambroise Paré Hospital, University Versailles St-Quentin, Boulogne-Billancourt, France, **3** INSERM, U1018, Centre for Research in Epidemiology and Population Health, Villejuif, France, **4** Department of Epidemiology and Public Health, University College London, London, United Kingdom

Abstract

Background: The impact of socioeconomic inequalities on health is well-documented. Despite the links of periodontal disease with cardiovascular diseases, adverse pregnancy outcomes and diabetes, no meta-analysis of socioeconomic variations in periodontal disease exists. This meta-analytic review was conducted to determine the extent to which education attainment influences risk of periodontitis in adults aged 35+ years in the general population.

Methods: The authors searched studies published until November 2010 using EMBASE and MEDLINE databases. References listed were then scrutinised, our own files were checked, and, finally, we contacted experts in the field. The authors included only general population-based studies conducted in adults aged 35 years and more. All articles were blind reviewed by two investigators. In the case of disagreement, a third investigator arbitrated. Using PRISMA statement, two reviewers independently extracted papers of interest.

Results: Relative to the higher education group, people with low education attainment experience a greater risk of periodontitis (OR: 1.86 [1.66–2.10]; $p<0.00001$). The association was partially attenuated after adjustment for covariates (OR: 1.55 [1.30–1.86]; $p<0.00001$). Sensitivity analyses showed that methods used to assess periodontitis, definition of cases, study country and categorization of education are largely responsible for the heterogeneity between studies. No significant bias of publication was shown using both the Egger ($p=0.16$) and rank correlation tests ($p=0.35$).

Conclusions: In the studies reviewed, low educational attainment was associated with an increased risk of periodontitis. Although this evidence should be cautiously interpreted due to methodological problems in selected studies, efforts to eliminate educational inequalities in periodontitis should focus on early life interventions.

Editor: Yiqing Song, Brigham & Women's Hospital, Harvard Medical School, United States of America

Funding: The authors have no support or funding to report.

Competing Interests: The authors have declared that no competing interests exist.

* E-mail: phbouch@noos.fr

Introduction

Chronic periodontitis is a bacterially induced inflammatory disease of the soft and hard tissues which support the tooth root [1]. It is caused by an accumulation of dental plaque, organized as a biofilm on the surface of the tooth crown and root [2], which lead to the destruction of periodontal connective tissue and alveolar bone; without treatment this results in tooth loss. Periodontitis may have long term consequences for health by increasing the risk of type 2 diabetes (T2D) [3], obesity [4], metabolic syndrome [5], cardiovascular diseases (CVD) and pulmonary diseases [6–8], adverse pregnancy outcomes [9], and premature mortality [8]. The condition is common, affecting up to 20% of the adult population in industrialised countries [10].

Chronic periodontitis is a multifactorial disease. However, the contribution of the different risk factors/indicators associated with the disease remains unclear. In addition to a role for oral hygiene, age, cigarette smoking [11] and T2D [3] in the aetiology of this disorder, a further risk factor may be poor social circumstances. There are good *prima facie* reasons to anticipate a relationship between low socio-economic status and chronic periodontitis, not least the strong link between socio-economic status and various health behaviours including smoking and diet [12]. Socio-economic adversity is also related to higher rates of a range of other important chronic diseases, including CVD [13] selected cancers [14], and mental illness [15].

Socio-economic status is typically characterised by income, occupational prestige, and educational achievement. Of these, educational attainment is stable across the adult life course [16] and, because it is usually peaks earlier in life than the other socio-economic indicators, it precedes the onset of most major chronic diseases so allowing investigators to separate cause from effect (reverse causality). Identifying socioeconomic at-risk subgroups for chronic periodontitis has the potential to enhance the effectiveness of preventative campaigns by focusing interventions, adopting specific strategies, reducing costs of public health decisions and obtaining active participation of target populations [17]. Given the strong associations described in the literature between chronic periodontitis and various systemic conditions (e.g, cardiovascular disease), such preventive programmes have also a global public health importance.

The most recent systematic review on socioeconomic variations in chronic periodontitis was published five six ago [18]. Accordingly, we undertook an updated systematic review of studies examining the association of educational attainment and chronic periodontitis in adults in the general population. Additionally, we aggregated the results from identified studies by conducting a meta-analysis.

Methods

Identification of Studies

Following the PRISMA statement [19], we performed a systematic review of all published observational studies conducted in individuals aged 35 and older, which investigated the association between level of education and risk of periodontitis. (Table S1)

Two independent reviewers trained in online article searches (AB and BEH) searched English language papers published before November 2010. We used a four-pronged approach to identifying papers. First, the MEDLINE and EMBASE searches were conducted using the MeSH and EMTREE. For MEDLINE, we used the following strategy: ("Periodontal diseases" [MeSH] OR "periodontitis" [MeSH] OR "chronic periodontitis" [MeSH] OR "periodontal attachment loss" [MeSH] OR "periodontal pocket" [MeSH] OR "alveolar bone loss" [MeSH]) AND ("education" [MeSH] OR "educational status" [MeSH] OR "marital status" [MeSH] OR "occupations" [MeSH] OR "income" [MeSH] OR "socioeconomic factors" [MeSH] OR "social class" [MeSH]). Limits: Human, English.. For EMBASE, search strategy was: ("periodontal disease" [EMTREE] OR "periodontitis" [EMTREE] OR "chronic periodontitis" [EMTREE] OR "periodontal pocket" [EMTREE] OR "alveolar bone loss" [EMTREE]) AND ("education" [EMTREE] OR "educational status" [EMTREE] OR "marital status" [EMTREE] OR "occupation" [EMTREE] OR "income" [EMTREE] OR "socioeconomics" [EMTREE] OR "social status" [EMTREE]). Limits: Human, English. Second, references listed in articles of interest were scrutinised. Third, we checked our own files. Fourth, we contacted selected experts in the field.

Inclusion Criteria

We included all observational studies conducted in adults aged 35+ years in the general population with 1) case definition of periodontitis (probing or radiographic assessment, self-reported data) (Text S1), 2) a variable describing the level of education, 3) a quantitative assessment of the relationship between these two variables. Studies conducted in non-representative populations (e.g. samples of attendees in dental settings) were excluded to maximise external validity. When more than one report used the same data, studies resulting in lowest power were excluded except when prospective data were available. In the case of disagreement, the two investigators discussed the article and tried to find agreement. When consensus was not reached, a third investigator (P.B.) was involved until agreement was found.

Data Abstraction

Two investigators (AB, BEH) independently extracted and tabulated basic information on each study: design, country where the study was conducted, sample size, number of cases, age range, definition of chronic periodontitis, partial or full-mouth recording, categories of level of education. Crude odds ratios (OR), or the data to compute them when crude estimates were unavailable, were also identified and extracted. Adjusted effect measures, including the covariates features in the multivariable model, were tabulated.

Data Analysis

We transformed OR by taking their natural logarithms and calculating standard errors and corresponding confidence intervals [20]. Effects measures and their standard errors were pooled using an inverse variance method with random effects to account for statistical heterogeneity between studies. We calculated pooled OR and accompanying 95% confidence interval (95% CI) for the lowest versus the highest categories of education. Heterogeneity was assessed with the I^2 statistic [21]. We carried out sensitivity analyses based on study design (longitudinal versus cross-sectional studies), year of publication (≤2000 versus >2000), region where the study was conducted (US versus non-US countries), sample size (≤1000 versus >1000), age (≥35 versus olders (≥65)), periodontal assessment method (partial-mouth versus full-mouth recording), definition of cases (combined clinical attachment loss (CAL) and periodontal probing depth (PPD) versus single probing measurement), number of categories of education (2 versus >2). Significance was set at $p<0.05$ and 95% CI were quoted throughout [18]. The Kappa statistic was used to assess interrater reliability between the two independent reviewers [22]. Publication bias was assessed by visually examining a funnel plot with asymmetry being formally assessed with both the Egger test [23] and the rank correlation test [24]. The data were analysed using Review Manager (RevMan, version 5.0, The Cochrane Collaboration, 2008). Bias of publication was measured using CMA (Comprehensive Meta Analysis, version 2.2.055, Biostat, 2010).

Results

Study characteristics

The electronic search yielded 6048 publications, including 1288 duplicates. From the 4760 potentially relevant articles identified, 4528 were excluded. Among the 232 remaining papers, hand-searching of references was performed, resulting in 35 additional papers. From the 267 eligible articles, 249 were excluded resulting in 18 studies, which met all the inclusion criteria and were included in the analyses (Figure 1) [25–42]. The kappa coefficient between examiners was 0.78 (0.75–0.80) demonstrating a substantial agreement [43]. Characteristics of the included studies are presented in Table 1–3. The combined population resulted in 40783 participants. Only two studies were longitudinal [31–32]. The included studies were reformed in the following countries (n = 10): Australia, Brazil, Canada, Denmark, Iran, Norway, Sweden, USA, Taiwan, and Thailand. Crude effect estimates were computed in ten studies [27,29–31,33,34,37,39,41–42]. Eight studies met criteria of inclusion, but were excluded because they were conducted in duplicate surveys [44–51].

Four out of 18 studies did not use full-mouth clinical examination [29,35,37,41]. Only six studies, exhibiting a quite different level of adjustment, gave adjusted effect measures [26,29,32,35,38,40]. Two studies were performed on samples of male [28,41]; whereas two other studies were performed on samples of female [30,38]. One study has separated the outcomes

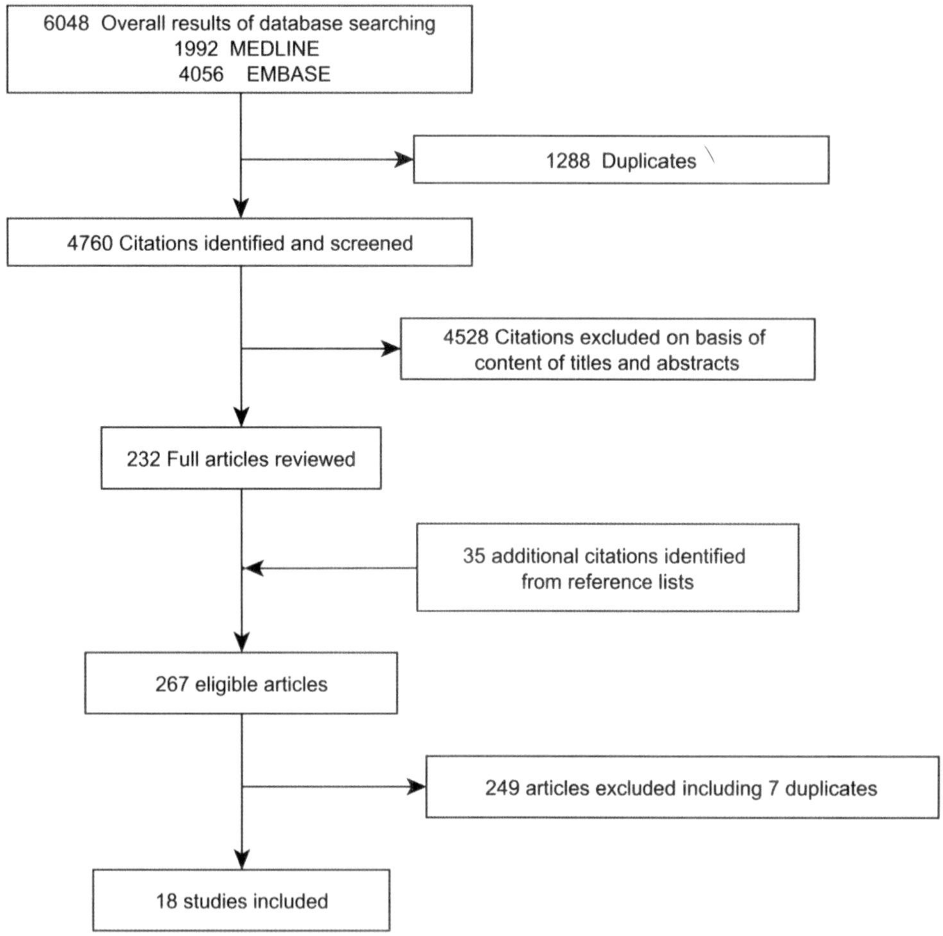

Figure 1. Flow chart for identifying eligible studies.

Table 1. Characteristics of selected US cross-sectional studies in a meta-analysis of education level and chronic periodontitis.

Study name	Study size (of interest/original)	Age (yrs)	Study design	Outcome (No of cases in education groups of interest/Total No of cases)	Comparison groups for education	Variables in multiple adjustment
Beck et al. 1990, USA [25].	689/689	≥65	CS	At least 4 sites with CAL≥5 mm with at least one of those sites with PPD≥4 mm. n = 224/224.	< versus ≥12 years of education.	None.
Borrell et al. 2006, USA [26].	3,240/5,677	≥52	CS	At least two sites with CAL≥6 mm and at least 1 site with PPD≥5 mm. n = 545/963.	<High School versus ≥college.	Age, gender, center, neighbourhood socio-economic score, income.
Dietrich et al. 2006, USA [28].	462/469	47–92	CS	At least one tooth with CAL and PPD≥5 mm. n = 86/86.	≤versus >High School.	None.
Dye et al . 2009, USA [29].	4,014/5,747	≥40	CS	At least one tooth with CAL≥3 mm and PPD≥4 mm. n = 843/1,063.	<High School versus ≥College.	Age, gender, smoking, race, diabetes, periodontal pathogens.
Famili et al. 2005, USA [30].	188/202	≥65	CS	More than 12 teeth with CAL>4 mm. n = 151/163.	≤versus >16 years of education.	None.
Phipps et al. 2009, USA [41].	672/1210	≥65	CS	30% or more of teeth examined with CAL≥5 mm. n = 248/463.	≤High School versus ≥Graduate School	None.

CAL: Clinical Attachment Loss; CPITN: Community Periodontal Index of Treatment Needs; CS: Cross-Sectional; L: Longitudinal; PPD: Periodontal Pocket Depth; t0: Baseline data; Un: Unknown.

Table 2. Characteristics of selected non-US cross-sectional studies in a meta-analysis of education level and chronic periodontitis.

Study name	Study size (of interest/ original)	Age (yrs)	Study design	Outcome (No of cases in education groups of interest/Total No of cases)	Comparison groups for education	Variables in multiple adjustment
Brennan et al. 2007, Australia [27].	709/709	45–54	CS	2 or more sites with CAL≥5 mm and one or more sites with PPD≥4 mm. n = 139/139.	Primary, Secondary, Certificate versus Diploma or degree	None.
Hessari et al. 2007, Iran [33].	2,764/7,949	35–44	CS	At least one sextant with CPITN score 4 (PPD>5.50 mm). Men: n = 136/457. Women: n = 158/360.	Illiterate versus any university education.	None.
Krustrup et al. 2006, Denmark [34].	386/1052	35–44; 65–74	CS	At least one tooth with CAL≥6 mm. n = 22/50.	≤10 versus ≥15 years of education.	None.
Lai et al. 2007, Taiwan [35].	4,347/8,462	35–44	CS	CPITN score 4 (PPD>5,5 mm). n = Un/414.	≤ Junior High School versus ≥ College.	Age, gender, occupation.
Locker et al. 1993, Canada [36].	624/624	≥50	CS	Mean CAL≥3.83. n = Un.	≤ versus >High School.	None.
Mucci et al. 2004, Sweden [37].	14,736/26,690	≥42	CS	Self-reported. Diagnosed by a dentist to have periodontal disease or ever had tooth mobility. n = 2,956/5,527.	Elementary versus University	None.
Nicolau et al. 2007, Brazil [38].	224/224	39,01 (4.70)	CS	More than 42% of teeth with loss of attachment. n = 90/90.	≤ versus >4 years of education.	Age, smoking, plaque, emotionnal support, conditions during childhood.
Paulander et al. 2004, Sweden [39].	549/549	50 ; 55	CS	Highest 20% of the CAL distribution (mean CAL: 2.4–7.1). n = 110/110.	≤ versus >7 years of education.	None.
Peres et al. 2007, Brazil [40].	6,086/11,342	35–44	CS	At least one site with PPD≥4 mm and at least one site with CAL≥4 mm. n = 542/1,018.	≤4 versus ≥12 years of education.	Age, gender, race, income.
Torrungruang et al. 2009, Thailand [42].	453/453	39–59	CS	3 or more sites with PPD≥5 mm. n = 164/164.	≤ versus >High School.	None.

CAL: Clinical Attachment Loss; CPITN: Community Periodontal Index of Treatment Needs; CS: Cross-Sectional; L: Longitudinal; PPD: Periodontal Pocket Depth; t0: Baseline data; Un: unknown.

for each gender [33]. Cases were defined by a combination of CAL and PPD conditions in six studies [25–29,40]; by a single CAL criteria in seven studies [30,31,34,36,38,39,41]; by CPITN score (Community Periodontal Index of Treatment Needs) in two studies [33,35]; and by self-reported assessment in one study (for more informations about periodontal indices, see supplemental material) [36]. No study with radiographic assessment met criteria of inclusion.

Summary estimates

The summary estimates of OR for each study were pooled to give a total estimate of risk (Figure 2). The overall OR (95% CI) for chronic periodontitis was 1.86 (1.66 to 2.10), indicating an increased risk of periodontitis associated with a low level of education when compared with the highest level of education. The effect size among studies showed a moderate to substantial heterogeneity ($I^2 = 55\%$).

Table 3. Characteristics of selected longitudinal studies in a meta-analysis of education level and chronic periodontitis.

Study name	Study size (of interest/ original)	Age (yrs)	Study design	Outcome (No of cases in education groups of interest/Total No of cases)	Comparison groups for education	Variables in multiple adjustment
Gilbert et al. 2005, USA [31].	559/560	≥45	L	At least one site with a 48-month worst attachment level 3 mm or more than the baseline worst attachment level on that same tooth. n = 123/123.	< versus ≥High School.	None.
Hansen et al. 1995, Norway [32].	81/81	35 (t0)	L	Increased in the number of C-scored quadrants (PTNS) from 1973 to 1988 (at least one site with PPD>5 mm). N = 16/16.	≤ versus >10 years of education.	Missing teeth, last dental visit, oral preventive behaviours, socioeconomic proxies, social class.

CAL: Clinical Attachment Loss; CPITN: Community Periodontal Index of Treatment Needs; CS: Cross-Sectional; L: Longitudinal; PPD: Periodontal Pocket Depth; t0: Baseline data; Un: unknown.

Study or Subgroup	log[Odds Ratio]	SE	Weight	Odds Ratio IV, Random, 95% CI
Beck JD 1990 Blacks	1.131	0.332	2.6%	3.10 [1.62, 5.94]
Beck JD 1990 Whites	0.956	0.36	2.3%	2.60 [1.28, 5.27]
Borrell LN 2006 Blacks	0.693	0.186	5.6%	2.00 [1.39, 2.88]
Borrell LN 2006 Whites	0.47	0.122	7.9%	1.60 [1.26, 2.03]
Brennan DS 2007	0.293	0.196	5.3%	1.34 [0.91, 1.97]
Dietrich T 2006	0.086	0.246	4.0%	1.09 [0.67, 1.77]
Dye BA 2009	0.982	0.087	9.5%	2.67 [2.25, 3.17]
Famili P 2005	0.315	0.372	2.2%	1.37 [0.66, 2.84]
Gilbert GH 2005	0.604	0.241	4.1%	1.83 [1.14, 2.93]
Hansen BF 1995	1.29	0.578	1.0%	3.63 [1.17, 11.28]
Hessari H 2007 Females	0.718	0.372	2.2%	2.05 [0.99, 4.25]
Hessari H 2007 Males	0.5	0.206	5.0%	1.65 [1.10, 2.47]
Krustrup 2006	0.531	0.439	1.6%	1.70 [0.72, 4.02]
Lai H 2007	0.315	0.14	7.2%	1.37 [1.04, 1.80]
Locker D 1992	0.788	0.234	4.2%	2.20 [1.39, 3.48]
Mucci LA 2004	0.723	0.043	11.1%	2.06 [1.89, 2.24]
Nicolau B 2007	0.207	0.267	3.6%	1.23 [0.73, 2.08]
Paulander J 2004	0.604	0.22	4.6%	1.83 [1.19, 2.82]
Peres MA 2007	0.788	0.16	6.4%	2.20 [1.61, 3.01]
Phipps KR 2008	0.513	0.176	5.9%	1.67 [1.18, 2.36]
Torrungruand K 2009	0.978	0.248	3.9%	2.66 [1.64, 4.32]
Total (95% CI)			**100.0%**	**1.86 [1.66, 2.10]**

Heterogeneity: $Tau^2 = 0.03$; $Chi^2 = 44.26$, df = 20 (P = 0.001); $I^2 = 55\%$
Test for overall effect: Z = 10.32 (P < 0.00001)

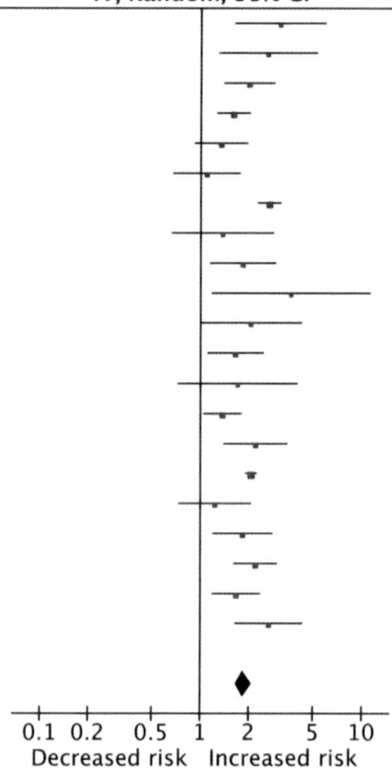

Figure 2. Results of primary meta-analysis: crude risk of periodontitis for individuals with lower education. Legend: Higher level of education as reference. Weights for individual studies calculated with random effects models and inverse variance method. The centre of each black square is placed at the point estimate, the area of the square is proportional to the sample size, and each horizontal line shows the 95% confidence interval for the estimate for each study. Pooled OR (95% CI): 1.86 (1.66–2.10). p<0.00001.

Secondary analyses

Results of the primary analysis were not changed in the sensitivity analysis (Table 4). Two exceptions were the alternative meta-analysis including longitudinal studies and those conducted before year 2000, which enhanced the overall odds ratio (respectively 2.11 (1.22 to 3.63) and 2.57 (1.87 to 3.53)). Within the sensitivity analyses, we examined also various variables as potential sources of heterogeneity. There was evidence of significant heterogeneity across studies that may be explained by geographical differences (Non US: $I^2 = 42\%$ versus US: $I^2 = 68\%$), the extent of the clinical assessment [partial-mouth ($I^2 = 89\%$) versus full-mouth ($I^2 = 22\%$)], and the definition of cases [clinical attachment loss and periodontal probing pocket combined ($I^2 = 74\%$) versus probing pocket depth solely ($I^2 = 0\%$)]. Other sources of heterogeneity have to be interpreted with caution because of the differences in the number of studies in each category. The sensitivity analyses with one by one exclusions showed that one study had a significantly effect on heterogeneity (Data not shown) [29]. When excluded, heterogeneity between studies was nearly non significant ($p = 0.04$, $I^2 = 39\%$).

When pooling studies with adjusted estimates, results were unchanged (OR = 1.55 (1.30 to 1.86); $p<0.00001$) but low heterogeneity between studies was found ($I^2 = 38\%$) (Figure 3). On the contrary, pooling crude estimates for same studies conducted to both an higher heterogeneity ($I^2 = 77\%$) and an higher risk estimate (OR = 1.88 (1.46 to 2.42)) (Data not shown). Funnel plot showed no asymmetry. No significant bias was shown using both the Egger ($p = 0.16$) and rank correlation tests ($p = 0.35$).

Discussion

Principal finding

The present analysis of studies conducted in the general population of adults reveals that individuals with a low level of education have an excess risk of chronic periodontitis when compared with adults with high level of education.

A number of mechanisms may explain this effect. Indirect mechanisms include the link between education and the two main risk factors for chronic periodontitis: smoking [52] and diabetes type 2 [53]. Lower educational attainment, which is a close correlate of IQ, may also directly lead to poorer coping strategies [54], higher BMI [55], lower levels of dental services use [56], low degree of periodontal health awareness [57], and irregular oral self-care practices [58], that in themselves are linked to poor oral hygiene habits may lead to higher levels of dental plaque [59]. Only one study which met our criteria of inclusion showed a significant decrease of the risk to develop chronic periodontitis in the low educated subgroup after adjustment for oral health behaviors [32].

Theories in social epidemiology could also explain such an association. The "pathway model" suggests circumstances in early-life influence social trajectories into and through adulthood, so increasing chronic disease risk [60]. Moreover, low education level is likely to lead to low prestige and low pay occupations, and residing in deprived area. The impact of environmental conditions on periodontal health has been widely described such that individuals living in a neighborhood in the most socially

Table 4. Results of sensitivity analyses to investigate differences between studies included in the meta-analysis (random-effects model).

Included studies	No of studies	OR	95% CI	Residual heterogeneity (I^2)
Study design				
Longitudinal [31,32]	2	2.11*	1.22, 3.63	17%
Cross-sectional [25–30,33–42]	16	1.85***	1.64, 2.09	58%
Baseline data				
≤2000 [25,32,36]	3	2.57***	1.87, 3.53	0%
>2000 [26–31,33–35,37–42]	15	1.79***	1.58, 2.03	61%
Study region				
US [25,26,28–30,41]	6	1.89***	1.51, 2.37	68%
Non US [27,31–40,42]	12	1.83***	1.58, 2.11	42%
Sample size				
≤1000 [25,27,28,30–32,34,36,38,39,41,42]	12	1.78***	1.49, 2.12	31%
>1000 [26,29,33,35,37,40]	6	1.94***	1.65, 2.27	70%
Age (years)				
No limitation [26–29,31–40,42]	15	1.85***	1.62, 2.10	60%
Olders only (≥65) [25,30,41]	3	1.98**	1.41, 2.78	29%
Oral examination				
Partial-mouth [29,35,41]	3	1.85*	1.18, 2.91	89%
Full-mouth [25–28,30–34,36,38–40,42]	14	1.81***	1.59, 2.06	22%
Periodontal assessment				
CAL and PPD [25–29,40]	6	1.93***	1.52, 2.46	74%
CAL or PPD [30–36,38,39,41,42]	11	1.70***	1.49, 1.94	0%
N° of classes for education				
2 [25,27,28,30–32,36,38,39,42]	10	1.81***	1.46, 2.24	42%
2 [26,29,33–35,37,40,41]	8	1.91***	1.66, 2.20	63%

**P*<0.01.
***P*<0.001.
****P*<0.0001.
Higher level of education as reference. Random-effects model and inverse variance method.

Study or Subgroup	log[Odds Ratio]	SE	Weight	Odds Ratio IV, Random, 95% CI
Borrell LN 2006 Blacks	0.693	0.186	14.8%	2.00 [1.39, 2.88]
Borrell LN 2006 Whites	0.182	0.13	21.7%	1.20 [0.93, 1.55]
Dye BA 2009	0.713	0.188	14.6%	2.04 [1.41, 2.95]
Hansen BF 1995	0.723	0.306	7.2%	2.06 [1.13, 3.75]
Lai H 2007	0.336	0.156	18.1%	1.40 [1.03, 1.90]
Nicolau B 2007	0.182	0.327	6.5%	1.20 [0.63, 2.28]
Peres MA 2007	0.405	0.165	17.1%	1.50 [1.09, 2.07]
Total (95% CI)			**100.0%**	**1.55 [1.30, 1.86]**

Heterogeneity: $Tau^2 = 0.02$; $Chi^2 = 9.74$, df = 6 ($P = 0.14$); $I^2 = 38\%$
Test for overall effect: $Z = 4.84$ ($P < 0.00001$)

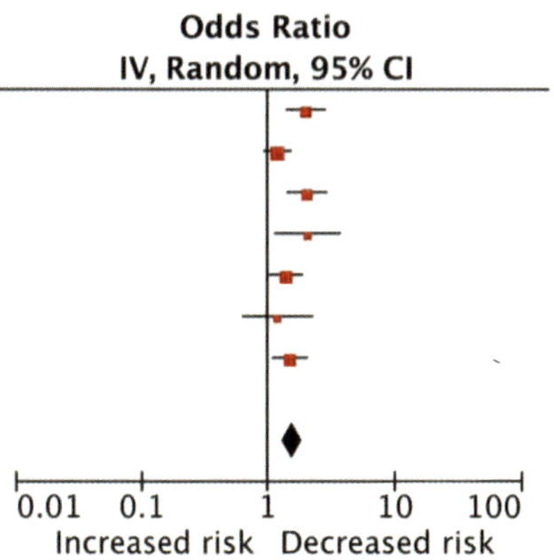

Figure 3. Results of primary meta-analysis: adjusted risk of periodontal diseases for individuals with low education. Legend: Higher level of education as reference. Weights for individual studies calculated with random effects models and inverse variance method. The centre of each black square is placed at the point estimate, the area of the square is proportional to the sample size, and each horizontal line shows the 95% confidence interval for the estimate for each study. Pooled OR (95% CI): 1.55 (1.30–1.86). p<0.00001.

marginalised areas experience twice the risk of periodontitis relative to those in the most affluent [61].

Exploration for heterogeneity

The pooled OR should be interpreted with caution, given the substantial heterogeneity detected between studies. Sensitivity analyses showed that several factors seem to account for this heterogeneity, including the region where the study was conducted, the extent of oral examination, the definition of cases and the number of categories for education level assessment. Taken together these factors might help us to improve our understanding of circumstances under which education interacts with periodontal health. In addition, the heterogeneity indicates that efforts should be made to adopt a standardised methodological approach when studying the association between periodontal diseases and socioeconomic factors.

Partial-mouth examinations may underestimate the prevalence of periodontal diseases [62,63]. Additionally, methods used in partial-mouth examination are numerous. Both result in a lower heterogeneity between studies when excluding studies with partial-mouth examination. For same reasons, exclusion of studies using both CAL and PPD to define periodontitis results in a low heterogeneity between studies. As an illustration, heterogeneity between studies became non-significant when we conducted a one-study removed sensitivity analysis excluding Dye study ($I^2 = 39\%$) [29]. In this cross-sectional study using data from NHANES III survey, cases of periodontitis were defined as a combination of clinical attachment loss and probing pocket depth criteria after a full-mouth examination.

The impact of education on periodontal status does not seem the same according to the geographic area. Heterogeneity was higher for US studies than for studies conducted in other countries. One explanation might be that the US studies were not focused on same spatial units, several using census data, whereas others were conducted in counties or neighbourhoods.

Heterogeneity could also be due to differences in the classification of education attainment. In the sensitivity analyses, we compared studies with two classes of education with other studies. When only studies separating education level into two classes were included in the analysis, a lower heterogeneity was found. This may be due to the method we used. We compared individuals from extreme categories of education attainment. Including studies with more than two classes of education; we excluded all individuals with an intermediate level of education. Further, the classification of education attainment differs between studies. Some authors use corresponding diploma; other authors use years of schooling to categorize the level of education. Both resulted in a higher heterogeneity between studies with more than two classes of education.

Pooling of studies with adjusted estimates showed a decrease in heterogeneity between studies. Confounders such as race, diabetes or smoking are a source of heterogeneity between studies, and no adjustment result in an overestimated association between education and chronic periodontitis [18].

Strengths and limitations

The present study has limitations inherent to meta-analyses. First, the results should be interpreted with caution and should not be considered as causal evidence because all studies were observational and most cross-sectional. Only two prospective studies met our criteria of inclusion [31–32]. Thus, associations are suggestive at best.

Secondly, there was significant heterogeneity between the included studies so overall conclusions must be regarded with caution. When we carried out sensitivity analyses to investigate possible sources of heterogeneity the results highlight a call for standardisation when studying social epidemiology in periodontal health, in particular concerning definition of cases. However, exclusion of only one study [29] resulted in a decrease of heterogeneity between studies, which became non significant ($p = 0.04$). Then, only six studies gave adjusted results for confounders [26,29,32,35,38,40], and two studies were adjusted for smoking [29,38], whereas it was described as a confounding factor [18].

Finally, because the physiopathology mechanisms for aggressive periodontitis differ from those involved in the development of chronic periodontitis [64] *a priori*, we elected not to include studies which captured the former outcome. This may have caused us to misclassify as unaffected some individuals with localized periodontitis. This is likely to have diluted the overall strength of the education-periodontal disease association.

However, our study has several strengths. It is the first, to our knowledge, including such a number of individuals (more than 40000), which quantifies the association between education attainment and periodontal diseases. The analysis is centred on chronic periodontitis, which is the most common form of periodontitis in adults. A previous systematic review has already shown a higher prevalence of periodontitis in a low socioeconomic group but the effect was not quantified [18]. The reason why no meta-analysis was performed in the above study maybe due (1) to the wide range of age (>19 year-old) that may include different diagnosis such as aggressive and chronic periodontitis, (2) to the difficulty to evaluate the socio-economic level in younger populations, and (3) to the low number of studies available when this review was conducted (our Medline search identified a nearly 60% increase in the number of studies from April 2004 to November 2010). Our search was conducted on multiple databases, and references listed in retrieved articles were adequately scrutinised according to the standards guidelines for systematic reviews. Finally, both Egger and rank correlation tests showed no significant bias of publication.

Conclusions and implications

Results from our meta-analysis support the growing body of evidence of a socioeconomic gradient in oral health. The impact is first clinical to identify at-risk patients and adopt preventive attitudes for them, such as motivation to institute healthy behaviours (smoking cessation, oral hygiene instruction, regular dental visits…). This socioeconomic gradient in periodontal health may also have several implications for public health. The association between periodontal disease and other diseases that may compromise health condition emphasises the need to identify at-risk populations. This would permit to target public health actions aiming to prevent periodontal diseases. Identifying socioeconomic at-risk populations for oral diseases enhances the effectiveness of preventive campaigns by focusing interventions, adopting specific strategies and obtaining active participation of target populations. Moreover, because of the associations between education level and various risk factors/indicators for chronic periodontitis, educational attainment appears as a main target in preventing the development of chronic periodontitis. Finally, because of the relationships between chronic periodontitis and numerous systemic conditions, such approaches may lead to the reduction of the morbidity for other chronic diseases and, as a consequence, to decrease the overall healthcare costs.

To conclude, the effect of low education attainment on higher risk of periodontal diseases has a series of potential mechanisms.

This notwithstanding, education may plausibly represent a main target for preventive programmes for periodontal diseases.

Acknowledgments

The authors thank Marco Aurélio Peres, Departamento de Saúde Pública, Universidade Federal de Santa Catarina, Campus Universitário Trindade, Florianópolis, SC 88010-970, Brazil, and Annette Leclerc, Inserm U1018, Epidemiology of occupational and social determinants of health, Center for Research in Epidemiology and Population Health, Inserm, Villejuif, France, for giving additional information, which were necessary to write, respectively, the results and discussion sections.

Author Contributions

Conceived and designed the experiments: AB SC PB. Analyzed the data: AB SC. Wrote the paper: AB BEH GDB HR SC PB. ICMJE criteria for authorship read and met: AB BEH GDB HR SC PB. Agreed with the manuscript's results and conclusions: AB BEH GDB HR SC PB. Collected data: AB BEH HR. Wrote the first draft of the paper: AB GDB SC PB.

References

1. Darveau RP (2010) Periodontitis: a polymicrobial disruption of host homeostasis. Nat Rev Microbiol 8(7): 481–90.
2. Kolenbrander PE, Palmer RJ, Jr., Periasamy S, Jakubovics NS (2010) Oral multispecies biofilm development and the key role of cell-cell distance. Nat Rev Microbiol 8(7): 471–80.
3. Taylor GW (2010) Bidirectional interrelationships between diabetes and periodontal diseases: an epidemiologic perspective. Ann Periodontol 6(1): 99–112.
4. Chaffee B, Weston S (2010) Association Between Chronic Periodontal Disease and Obesity: A Systematic Review and Meta-Analysis. J Periodontol 81(12): 1708–24.
5. D'Aiuto F, Sabbah W, Netuveli G, Donos N, Hingorani AD, et al. (2008) Association of the metabolic syndrome with severe periodontitis in a large U.S. population-based survey. J Clin Endocrinol Metab 93(10): 3989–94.
6. Tonetti MS, D'Aiuto F, Nibali L, Donald A, Storry C, et al. (2007) Treatment of periodontitis and endothelial function. N Engl J Med 356(9): 911–20.
7. Garcia RI, Nunn ME, Vokonas PS (2001) Epidemiologic associations between periodontal disease and chronic obstructive pulmonary disease. Ann Periodontol 6(1): 71–7.
8. Li Q, Chalmers J, Czernichow S, Neal B, Taylor BA, et al. (2010) Oral disease and subsequent cardiovascular disease in people with type 2 diabetes: a prospective cohort study based on the Action in Diabetes and Vascular Disease: Preterax and Diamicron Modified-Release Controlled Evaluation (ADVANCE) trial. Diabetologia 53(11): 2320–7.
9. Wimmer G, Pihlstrom BL (2008) A critical assessment of adverse pregnancy outcome and periodontal disease. J Clin Periodontol 35(8 Suppl): 380–97.
10. Pihlstrom BL, Michalowicz BS, Johnson NW (2005) Periodontal diseases. Lancet 366(9499): 1809–20.
11. Bergstrom J (2006) Periodontitis and smoking: an evidence-based appraisal. J Evid Based Dent Pract 6(1): 33–41.
12. Shankar A, McMunn A, Steptoe A (2010) Health-related behaviors in older adults relationships with socioeconomic status. Am J Prev Med 38(1): 39–46.
13. Kerr GD, Slavin H, Clark D, Coupar F, Langhorne P, et al. (2010) Do Vascular Risk Factors Explain the Association between Socioeconomic Status and Stroke Incidence: A Meta-Analysis. Cerebrovasc Dis 31(1): 57–63.
14. Conway DI, Petticrew M, Marlborough H, Berthiller J, Hashibe M, et al. (2008) Socioeconomic inequalities and oral cancer risk: a systematic review and meta-analysis of case-control studies. Int J Cancer 122(12): 2811–9.
15. Chang-Quan H, Zheng-Rong W, Yong-Hong L, Yi-Zhou X, Qing-Xiu L (2010) Education and risk for late life depression: a meta-analysis of published literature. Int J Psychiatry Med 40(1): 109–24.
16. Ribet C, Melchior M, Lang T, Zins M, Goldberg M, et al. (2007) [Characterisation and measurement of social position in epidemiologic studies]. Rev Epidemiol Sante Publique 55(4): 285–95.
17. Watt RG (2002) Emerging theories into the social determinants of health: implications for oral health promotion. Community Dent Oral Epidemiol 30: 241–47.
18. Klinge B, Norlund (2005) A socio-economic perspective on periodontal diseases: a systematic review. J Clin Periodontol 32 Suppl 6: 314–25.
19. Moher D, Liberati A, Tetzlaff J, Altman DG, The PRISMA Group (2009) Preferred Reporting Items for Systematic Reviews and Meta-Analyses: The PRISMA Statement. PloS Med 6(7).
20. Altman DG, Bland JM (2003) Interaction revisited: the difference between two estimates. BMJ 326(7382): 219.
21. Higgins JP, Thompson SG, Deeks JJ, Altman DG (2003) Measuring inconsistency in meta-analyses. BMJ 327(7414): 557–60.
22. Cohen J (1960) A coefficient of agreement for nominal scales. Educ Psychol Meas 20: 37–46.
23. Egger M, Davey Smith G, Schneider M, Minder C (1997) Bias in meta-analysis detected by a simple, graphical test. BMJ 315(7109): 629–34.
24. Begg CB, Mazumdar M (1994) Operating characteristics of a rank correlation test for publication bias. Biometrics 50(4): 1088–101.
25. Beck JD, Koch GG, Rozier RG, Tudor GE (1990) Prevalence and risk indicators for periodontal attachment loss in a population of older community-dwelling blacks and whites. J Periodontol 61(8): 521–8.
26. Borrell LN, Beck JD, Heiss G (2006) Socioeconomic disadvantage and periodontal disease: The dental atherosclerosis risk in communities study. Am J Public Health 96(2): 332–9.
27. Brennan DS, Spencer AJ, Roberts-Thomson KF (2007) Periodontal disease among 45–54 year olds in Adelaide, South Australia. Aust Dent J 52(1): 55–60.
28. Dietrich T, Krall Kaye E, Nunn ME, Van Dyke T, Garcia RI (2006) Gingivitis susceptibility and its relation to periodontitis in men. J Dent Res 85(12): 1134–7.
29. Dye BA, Herrera-Abreu M, Lerche-Sehm J, Vlachojannis C, Pikdoken L, et al. (2009) Serum antibodies to periodontal bacteria as diagnostic markers of periodontitis. J Periodontol 80(4): 634–47.
30. Famili P, Cauley J, Suzuki JB, Weyant R (2005) Longitudinal study of periodontal disease and edentulism with rates of bone loss in older women. J Periodontol 76(1): 11–5.
31. Gilbert GH, Shelton BJ, Fisher MA (2005) Forty-eight-month periodontal attachment loss incidence in a population-based cohort study: Role of baseline status, incident tooth loss, and specific behavioral factors. J Periodontol 76(7): 1161–70.
32. Hansen BF, Bjertness E, Gronnesby JK, Eriksen HM (1995) Changes in periodontal treatment needs. A follow-up study of Oslo citizens from the ages of 35 to 50 years. J Periodontal Res 30(6): 410–7.
33. Hessari H, Vehkalahti MM, Eghbal MJ, Murtomaa HT (2007) Oral health among 35- to 44-year-old Iranians. Med Princ Pract 16(4): 280–5.
34. Krustrup U, Erik Petersen P (2006) Periodontal conditions in 35–44 and 65–74-year-old adults in Denmark. Acta Odontol Scand 64(2): 65–73.
35. Lai H, Lo MT, Wang PE, Wang TT, Chen TH, et al. (2007) A community-based epidemiological study of periodontal disease in Keelung, Taiwan: a model from Keelung community-based integrated screening programme (KCIS No. 18). J Clin Periodontol 34(10): 851–9.
36. Locker D, Leake JL (1993) Risk indicators and risk markers for periodontal disease experience in older adults living independently in Ontario, Canada. J Dent Res 72(1): 9–17.
37. Mucci LA, Hsieh CC, Williams PL, Dickman PW, Bjorkman L, et al. (2004) Birth order, sibship size, and housing density in relation to tooth loss and periodontal disease: a cohort study among Swedish twins. Am J Epidemiol 159(5): 499–506.
38. Nicolau B, Netuveli G, Kim JW, Sheiham A, Marcenes W (2007) A life-course approach to assess psychosocial factors and periodontal disease. J Clin Periodontol 34(10): 844–50.
39. Paulander J, Axelsson P, Lindhe J, Wennstrom JL (2004) Some characteristics of 50/55-year-old individuals with various experience of destructive periodontal disease: A cross-sectional study. Acta Odontol Scand 62(4): 199–206.
40. Peres MA, Antunes JLF, Boing AF, Peres KG, Bastos JLD (2007) Skin colour is associated with periodontal disease in Brazilian adults: A population-based oral health survey. J Clin Periodontol 34(3): 196–201.
41. Phipps KR, Chan BK, Jennings-Holt M, Geurs NC, Reddy MS, et al. (2009) Periodontal health of older men: the MrOS dental study. Gerodontology 26(2): 122–29.
42. Torrungruang K, Bandhaya P, Likittanasombat K, Grittayaphong C, Torrungruang K, et al. (2009) Relationship between the presence of certain bacterial pathogens and periodontal status of urban Thai adults. J Periodontol 80: 122–29.
43. Landis JR, Koch GG (1977) The measurement of observer agreement for categorical data. Biometrics 33(1): 159–74.
44. Brown LF, Beck JD, Rozier RG (1994) Incidence of attachment loss in community-dwelling older adults. J Periodontol 65(4): 316–23.
45. Cascaes AM, Peres KG, Peres MA (2009) Periodontal disease is associated with poor self-rated oral health among Brazilian adults. J Clin Periodontol 36(1): 25–33.
46. Dolan TA, Gilbert GH, Ringelberg ML, Legler DW, Antonson DE, et al. (1997) Behavioral risk indicators of attachment loss in adult Floridians. J Clin Periodontol 24(4): 223–32.

47. Hansen BF, Bjertness E, Gjermo P (1990) Changes in periodontal disease indicators in 35-year-old Oslo citizens from 1973 to 1984. J Clin Periodontol 17(4): 249–54.
48. Hansen BF, Bjertness E, Gronnesby JK (1993) A socio-ecologic model for periodontal diseases. J Clin Periodontol 20(8): 584–90.
49. Hessari H, Vehkalahti M, Eghbal M, Murtomaa H, Hessari H, et al. (2009) Lifelong exposure to smoking and oral health among 35- to 44-year-old Iranians. Oral Health Prev Dent 7(1): 61–8.
50. Torrungruang K, Tamsailom S, Rojanasomsith K, Sutdhibhisal S, Nisapakultorn K, et al. (2005) Risk indicators of periodontal disease in older Thai adults. J Periodontol 76(4): 558–65.
51. Tsai C, Hayes C, Taylor GW (2002) Glycemic control of type 2 diabetes and severe periodontal disease in the US adult population. Community Dent Oral Epidemiol 30(3): 182–92.
52. Huisman M, Van Lenthe FJ, Giskes K, Kamphuis CB, Brug J, et al. (2011) Explaining socio-economic inequalities in daily smoking: a social-ecological approach. Eur J Public Health. In press.
53. Kavanagh A, Bentley RJ, Turrell G, Shaw J, Dunstan D, et al. (2010) Socioeconomic position, gender, health behaviours and biomarkers of cardiovascular disease and diabetes. Soc sci Med 71: 1150–60.
54. Christensen U, Schmidt L, Kriegbaum M, Hougaard CO, Holstein BE (2006) Coping with unemployment: does educational attainment make any difference? Scand J Public Health 34: 363–70.
55. Molarius A, Seidell JC, Sans S, Tuomilehto J, Kuulasmaa K (2000) Educational level, relative body weight, and changes in their association over 10 years: an international perspective from the WHO MONICA Project. Am J Public Health 90: 1260–68.
56. Lang IA, Gibbs SJ, Steel N, Melzer D (2008) Neighbourhood deprivation and dental service use: a cross-sectional analysis of older people in England. J Public Health 30: 472–78.
57. Alwaeli HA, Al-Jundi SH (2005) Periodontal disease awareness among pregnant women and its relationship with socio-demographic variables. Int J Dent Hyg 3: 74–82.
58. Petersen PE, Aleksejuniene J, Christensen LB, Eriksen HM, Kalo I (2000) Oral health behavior and attitudes of adults in Lithuania. Acta Odontol Scand 58: 243–48.
59. Zini A, Sgan-Cohen HD, Marcenes W (2011) Socio-economic position, smoking, and plaque: a pathway to severe chronic periodontitis. J Clin Periodontol 38: 229–35.
60. Graham H (2002) Building an inter-disciplinary science of health inequalities: the example of lifecourse research. Soc Sci Med 55: 2005–16.
61. Borrell LN, Burt BA, Warren RC, Neighbors HW (2006) The role of individual and neighborhood social factors on periodontitis: the third National Health and Nutrition Examination Survey. J Periodontol 77: 444–53.
62. Eaton KA, Duffy S, Griffiths GS, Gilthorpe MS, Johnson NW (2001) The influence of partial and full-mouth recordings on estimates of prevalence and extent of lifetime cumulative attachment loss: a study in a population of young male military recruits. J Periodontol 72(2): 140–5.
63. Borges-Yanez SA, Maupome G, Jimenez-Garcia G (2004) Validity and reliability of partial examination to assess severe periodontitis. J Clin Periodontol 31(2): 112–8.
64. Lang N, Bartold PM, Cullinan M, Jeffcoat M, Mombelli A, et al. (1999) Consensus Report: Aggressive Periodontitis. Ann Periodontol 4: 53.

16

Investigation of the Effect of Type 2 Diabetes Mellitus on Subgingival Plaque Microbiota by High-Throughput 16S rDNA Pyrosequencing

Mi Zhou[1]¶, Ruichen Rong[2]¶, Daniel Munro[2], Chunxia Zhu[1], Xiang Gao[2], Qi Zhang[1,3]*, Qunfeng Dong[2,4]*

1 State Key Laboratory Breeding Base of Basic Science of Stomatology, Key Laboratory of Oral Biomedicine Ministry of Education, School and Hospital of Stomatology, Wuhan University, Wuhan, Hubei, China, **2** Department of Biological Sciences, University of North Texas, Denton, Texas, United States of America, **3** Department of Endodontics, School of Stomatology, Tongji University, Shanghai, China, **4** Department of Computer Science and Engineering, University of North Texas, Denton, Texas, United States of America

Abstract

Diabetes mellitus is a major risk factor for chronic periodontitis. We investigated the effects of type 2 diabetes on the subgingival plaque bacterial composition by applying culture-independent 16S rDNA sequencing to periodontal bacteria isolated from four groups of volunteers: non-diabetic subjects without periodontitis, non-diabetic subjects with periodontitis, type 2 diabetic patients without periodontitis, and type 2 diabetic patients with periodontitis. A total of 71,373 high-quality sequences were produced from the V1-V3 region of 16S rDNA genes by 454 pyrosequencing. Those 16S rDNA sequences were classified into 16 phyla, 27 classes, 48 orders, 85 families, 126 genera, and 1141 species-level OTUs. Comparing periodontally healthy samples with periodontitis samples identified 20 health-associated and 15 periodontitis-associated OTUs. In the subjects with healthy periodontium, the abundances of three genera (*Prevotella*, *Pseudomonas*, and *Tannerella*) and nine OTUs were significantly different between diabetic patients and their non-diabetic counterparts. In the subjects carrying periodontitis, the abundances of three phyla (*Actinobacteria*, *Proteobacteria*, and *Bacteriodetes*), two genera (*Actinomyces* and *Aggregatibacter*), and six OTUs were also significantly different between diabetics and non-diabetics. Our results show that type 2 diabetes mellitus could alter the bacterial composition in the subgingival plaque.

Editor: Michael Tunney, Queens University Belfast, Ireland

Funding: Funding for this study was provided by the National Natural Science Foundation of China (Grant No. 81070824), the Fundamental Research Funds for the Central Universities, and the PhD Candidates Self-research (Including 1+4) Program of Wuhan University (No. 201001304275580), the Research Initiation Grant at University of North Texas, and the undergraduate student research training grant to the University of North Texas from the Howard Hughes Medical Institute through the Precollege and Undergraduate Science Education Program. The funders had no role in study design, data collection and analysis, decision to publish, or preparation of the manuscript.

Competing Interests: The authors have declared that no competing interests exist.

* E-mail: qizhang@tongji.edu.cn (QZ); Qunfeng.Dong@unt.edu (QD)

¶ These authors contributed equally to this work.

Introduction

Periodontitis is an inflammatory disorder, in which dental plaque bacteria induce exacerbated host immune response that destroys the gingival epithelium and alveolar bone, eventually leading to loss of teeth [1]. It is well established that the bacterial composition in periodontitis is different than that associated with healthy periodontium ([2], [3]). For example, periodontitis bacterial communities are more diverse than those in healthy tissue [4], and the disease microbiome harbors significantly enriched metabolic pathways adapted for oxygen-poor environments as well as lipid degradation pathways associated with known virulence-related activities [5].

Chronic periodontitis is often associated with diabetic patients with poor glycemic control ([6], [7], [8], [9], [10]). Diabetes mellitus significantly contributes to the severity, prevalence, and progression of periodontal disease ([11], [12], [13], [14]). Elevated oxidative stress responses, inflammatory cytokines, and receptor for advanced glycation end products (RAGE)-mediated damages have been observed under diabetic conditions in response to periodontal pathogens ([15], [16], [17], [18], [19], [20], [21] [22], [23], [24]), illustrating that diabetes mellitus significantly increases the host hyper-inflammatory response to periodontitis [14].

Besides affecting host immune response, diabetes mellitus also changes the oral environment, which may result in a different periodontal bacteria community than that in non-diabetic conditions. For example, increased gingival crevicular fluid glucose levels in diabetic patients [25] could provide an altered source of nutrition affecting the growth of certain bacterial species [26]. However, the extent of such effects on the subgingival microbiota composition still remains unclear ([14], [26]). Previous studies were mainly based on traditional methods such as checkerboard DNA-DNA hybridization and PCR to investigate the differences of the selected subgingival bacteria in diabetics compared with non-diabetics (*e.g.*, [27], [28], [29], [30], [31], [32], [33], [34], [35]). Instead of surveying the entire bacterial community, such traditional methods mainly suffered from limited detection of a small number of selected species [3]. For example, Field *et al.* [35] recently compared subgingival plaque microbiota in different backgrounds of periodontitis and diabetes mellitus, but their study was limited by the scope of quantitative PCR. They were only able to evaluate three bacterial species (*Aggregatibacter actinomycetemcomitans*, *Fusobacterium nucleatum*, and *Porphyromonas gingivalis*) in subgingival plaque and found no significant differences of these bacteria between type 2 diabetes mellitus patients and non-diabetic controls.

The aim of the present study was to examine whether diabetes mellitus might affect subgingival bacterial composition by high-throughput 16S rDNA sequencing with the 454 pyrosequencing technology [36], which has been widely adopted by numerous human microbiome projects including several studies characterizing the oral microbiome (e.g., [37], [38], [39], [40], [41], [42], [43]). Our study design included non-diabetic subjects without periodontitis (P−D−), non-diabetic subjects with periodontitis (P+D−), type 2 diabetic patients without periodontitis (P−D+), and type 2 diabetic patients with periodontitis (P+D+). The comparisons of the P−D− vs. P+D− and P−D+ vs. P+D+ groups were critical for discovering health-associated and periodontitis-associated bacteria in both diabetes-negative and diabetes-positive backgrounds, which were essential for understanding the interactions between periodontitis and diabetes mellitus. Based on our knowledge, our study is the first to apply 454 pyrosequencing to the above four groups of subjects.

While this manuscript was being prepared, Casarin *et al.* [44] reported a survey on the subgingival biodiversity in type 2 diabetic subjects by 16S rDNA sequencing using the traditional cloning-based Sanger sequencing method. Three important differences exist between our study and that of Casarin *et al.* [44]. First, Casarin *et al.* only included P+D+ and P+D− in their study. Second, Casarin *et al.* used paper points to collect subgingival biofilm, whereas we used a curette as the sample collection instrument. Paper points are generally limited to sampling the flowing or loosely adherent plaque, while a curette can also collect the more tightly-attached tooth or epithelium plaque ([45], [46]). Third, we were able to achieve much deeper sequencing depth with 454 pyrosequencing than that of the traditional Sanger sequencing used by Casarin *et al.* Overall, our study presents a distinct examination of the effects of diabetes mellitus on the subgingival bacterial community.

Materials and Methods

Ethics statement

Human subjects participated in the study after they signed the written informed consent in accordance with the study protocol approved by the Ethics Committee of the Faculty of Medicine for Human Studies, School & Hospital of Stomatology, Wuhan University (protocol number 2011029).

Sample collection

Thirty-one Chinese subjects satisfied the inclusion criteria, which required no usage of antibiotics or non-steroidal anti-inflammatory drugs and no smoking in the three months prior to the sampling. Those selected participants, between 30 and 65 years old, had at least 20 teeth without any clinical signs of oral mucosal disease or root caries. None of them were either pregnant or HIV positive. They had also not been previously treated with any periodontal therapy or surgery. Table S1 shows all the clinical parameters of the 31 participating subjects. Fisher's exact test (p-value = 0.88) and ANOVA test (p-value = 0.11) confirmed that no gender or age bias, respectively, existed among the four subject groups in this study. The sampling procedure was similar to what was used in Paster *et al.* [47], as briefly described below. Subjects with type 2 diabetes had been diagnosed for at least one year with HbA1c ≥6.5%, fasting plasma glucose test ≥7.0 mmol/L, or OGTT 2 hour glucose test ≥11.1 mmol/L. Periodontitis was defined by the following criteria: at least 30% of sites with probing depth and attachment loss, and more than four with probing depth ≥4 mm and clinical attachment loss ≥2 mm. Subgingival plaque samples were extracted from the four deepest sites of the molars in the participants using sterile Gracey curettes and transferred into 200 μL of phosphate-buffered saline (PBS) buffer for immediate freezing at −70°C.

DNA extraction and sequencing

Total DNA was isolated with a Qiagen DNA MiniAmp kit (Qiagen, Valencia, CA, USA) following the manufacturer's instruction on the tissue protocol. The universal primers targeting the 16S rDNA V1–V3 hypervariable region were used for PCR amplification: forward primer (8F, 5′-AGAGTTTGATCCTGGCTCAG-3′) and reverse primer (533R, 5′-TTACCGCGGCTGCTGGCAC-3′). The V1–V3 region was chosen because it could provide good detection of the oral microbiome [48]. The PCR primers were also tagged by unique barcodes for multiplex sequencing. PCR amplification was performed in the 20 μL reactions with 2.5 mM dNTPs, 5 μM forward and reverse primers, 20–50 ng template DNA, 1× polymerase buffer, and Platinum Taq DNA Polymerase High-Fidelity enzyme 0.4 U (Life Technologies, USA). After initial denaturation at 95°C for 4 minutes, 25 cycles of PCR were performed (denaturation at 95°C for 30 s, annealing at 55°C for 30 s, and extension at 72°C for 30 s). PCR amplicons were purified using AxyPrep DNA Gel Extraction kit (Axygen Biosciences, USA) according to the manufacturer's protocol,and visualized by electrophoresis in 1% agarose gels. Purified DNA samples were diluted in 30 uL 1× TE; an equal volume 2× PicoGreen working solution was added for a total reaction volume of 60 μL in a minicell cuvette. Fluorescence was measured on a Turner Biosystems TBS-380 Fluorometer using the 465–485/515–575-nm excitation/emission filter pair. Following quantification, purified amplicons were combined in equimolar ratios into a single tube. After preparing amplicons using the emPCR Kit II (according to the manufacturer's protocol), pyrosequencing was carried out on a 454 Life Sciences Genome Sequencer FLX Titanium instrument (Roche, USA). All of the sequences and associated metadata were deposited to the NCBI Sequence Read Archive [49] under the accession number SRA062091.

Sequence analysis

The Mothur software (version 1.23.0, [50]) was applied to process the sequence reads as previously described [51]. Briefly, sequence reads were deconvoluted into individual samples based on perfect match to the barcode sequences. Primers and barcodes were trimmed from each read and the trimmed sequences shorter than 200 bp were discarded. Low-quality and chimeric sequences were removed with default Mothur parameters. The remaining high-quality sequences were binned into species-level operational taxonomic units (OTUs), which is commonly defined by the level of 16S rDNA sequence similarity (i.e., ≥97% for a 'species'-level phylotype, [52]) based on the average neighbor algorithm in the Mothur package. As reported previously, the resulting number of OTUs may represent an inflated number of true species ([53], [54]). Therefore, during our manual process of species-level classification, we also merged some OTUs of interest that matched to the same reference database sequences with high confidence (e.g., ≥97% identity), which is similar to other published species-level classification methods (e.g., [55]). To avoid bias caused by the different sequencing depths of samples, we followed the normalization procedure previously published in Hawlena *et al* [51]. Briefly, 1000 sequences were randomly selected without replacement from each sample. This step of random sampling was repeated 1000 times and averaged to get the mean size of each OTU per normalized sample for statistical comparison. Taxonomic classification (from phylum to genus level) of the sequence reads was performed by the RDP Classifier (version 2.4, [56]) with the default 0.8 confidence threshold. Classification of the selected OTUs to the species level was achieved by BLASTing the OTU sequences against the NCBI 16S rDNA collection [57], SILVA database version 114 [58], and HOMD database version 12 [59] with manual inspection of the alignment results (minimum percentage of identity and coverage in the alignments as 97% and 95%, respectively). UniFrac analysis and non-metric multidimensional scaling (NMDS) were performed using the R packages *phyloseq* [60] and *vegan* [61], respectively. Both Wilcoxon rank-sum test and Fisher's exact test were performed with customized scripts that were implemented with the freely available R software environment (http://www.r-project.org). Relative abundance of each OTU was used in the statistical tests. In order to exclude rare OTUs that might be associated with large random sampling errors, only the OTUs with at least 0.5% relative abundance in one or more of the sample groups (*i.e.*, P−D−, P−D+, P+D−, and P+D+) were tested for their differential abundance or prevalence by the Wilcoxon rank-sum test and Fisher's exact test, respectively.

Results and Discussion

Taxonomic classification of 16S rDNA sequences

From 31 participating subjects, 71,393 high-quality 16S rDNA sequences were obtained after filtering out low-quality, chimeric, and non-bacterial sequences. The sequencing depth was similar among different sample groups although a slightly smaller amount of sequences were generated from the P+D− group (2504±357 in P−D+, 2611±216 in P−D−, 2361±470 in P+D+, and 1662±323 in P+D−). Compared to the 16S study by Casarin *et al.* [44] in which 87.4 sequences per subject were generated using Sanger sequencing, we achieved a much deeper sequencing depth with the 454 pyrosequencing technology (*i.e.*, 2,302 sequences per subject on average). Of those high-quality sequences, 87.22% could be classified into 126 genera, which belong to 16 phyla, 27 classes, 48 orders, and 85 families. The average percentage of classified sequences at the genus level is 91.01%±3.07% for P−D+, 91.68%±5.47% for P−D−, 87.32%±7.31% for P+D+, and 87.52%±7.72% for P+D−. No obvious bias in the proportion of unclassifiable sequences among different sample groups was observed (p = 0.40 based on the ANOVA test). All the sequences were clustered into 1,141 species-level OTUs based on their shared sequence similarity.

Effects of periodontitis on subgingival plaque microbiota compositions

The bacterial compositions at the community level in the different periodontitis groups were compared by unweighted UniFrac distance, which is commonly used in microbial ecology for quantitatively measuring compositional differences among microbial communities by calculating the length proportion of unique branches to each sample-specific taxon in a phylogenetic tree constructed from 16S rDNA sequences [62]. Figure 1 shows that the samples in the periodontitis-positive groups (*i.e.*, P+D− or P+D+) are well separated from those in the periodontitis-negative groups (*i.e.*, P−D− or P−D+) based on the unweighted UniFrac distances measured at the OTU level (Figures 1A and 1B), reflecting that the bacterial compositions in periodontitis and healthy samples were distinct. The significantly different bacterial communities between the periodontitis-negative and periodontitis-positive groups could also be confirmed by PERMANOVA test (p<0.01). Similar to our results, several other high-throughput 16S rDNA surveys also showed different subgingival bacterial compositions in non-diabetic subjects with periodontitis and healthy controls ([4], [5], [47], [63], [64]). Additionally, our results further show that compositional shifts in the subgingival plaque bacterial community associated with periodontitis also exist in diabetic patients.

Standard statistical methods (*i.e.*, Wilcoxon rank-sum test for relative abundance and Fisher's exact test for prevalence) were applied to pinpoint signature bacteria that were significantly different between the periodontitis-positive and periodontitis-negative samples. If the prevalence or relative abundances of the signature OTUs were significantly higher in the periodontitis-positive groups, the bacteria were designated as periodontitis-associated. Otherwise, the bacteria were designated as health-associated if they were significantly more abundant in periodontitis-negative groups. In total, 20 and 15 signature OTUs were designated as health-associated and periodontitis-associated bacteria, respectively (Tables 1 and S2). Many of our designations were consistent with previous studies ([47], [63], [64],[65], [66], [67], [68], [69], [70], [71], [72]), such as periodontitis-associated OTU0001 (*Porphyromonas gingivalis*), OTU0004 (genus of *Leptotrichia*), OTU0010 (*Tannerella forsythia*), OTU0011 (*Treponema denticola*), OTU2003 (*Treponema medium*), and OTU2006 (*Prevotella intermedia*), as well as heath-associated OTU0003 (*Corynebacterium matruchotii*), OTU0019 (*Neisseria elongate*), OTU0052 (*Streptococcus infantis*), and OTU0161 (*Capnocytophaga sputigena*) ([47], [63], [69], [70], [71], [73]). The reported roles of some other bacteria in periodontitis are often unclear. In addition, 13 signature OTUs were not classifiable at species or higher taxonomic levels (Table 1); therefore we were unable to validate their designated associations based on literature search. Such unclassified species might represent novel bacteria previously unknown to be involved in periodontitis.

From the diabetes-negative group, 20 species-level OTUs were identified as signature bacteria differentiating the P+D− from the P−D− samples. Similarly from the diabetes-positive group, 21 OTUs were identified as signature bacteria differentiating the P+D+ from the P−D+ samples (Tables 1 and S2). Out of all the signature OTUs, only six OTUs were shared in the above diabetes-positive and diabetes-negative groups, 14 OTUs were unique to the diabetes-negative group, and 15 OTUs were unique to the diabetes-positive group. The six shared OTUs were OTU0011 (*Treponema denticola*), OTU0052 (*Streptococcus infantis*), OTU0343 (family of *Prevotellaceae*), OTU2002 (*Streptococcus gordonii*), OTU2005 (*Actinomyces naeslundii*), and OTU2006 (*Prevotella intermedia*). Except for OTU0343, all the shared OTUs were reported previously as being associated with either periodontitis or healthy periodontium ([5], [47], [63], [64], [65], [66], [67]). For example, *T. denticola* is part of the "red complex" associated with periodontitis ([64], [67]). OTU0343 could only be classified as *Prevotellaceae* at the family level with high confidence. This OTU was designated as periodontitis-associated bacteria since its relative abundance was 3.15% in P+D− compared to 0.069% in P−D− samples (p-value = 0.028), and 0.99% in P+D+ compared to 0% in P−D+ samples (p-value = 0.025). The six shared OTUs may represent the core periodontal bacterial community that is commonly involved in pathogenesis or prevention of periodontitis regardless of diabetes status. The other 29 OTUs were identified as health- or periodontitis-associated bacteria only in either the

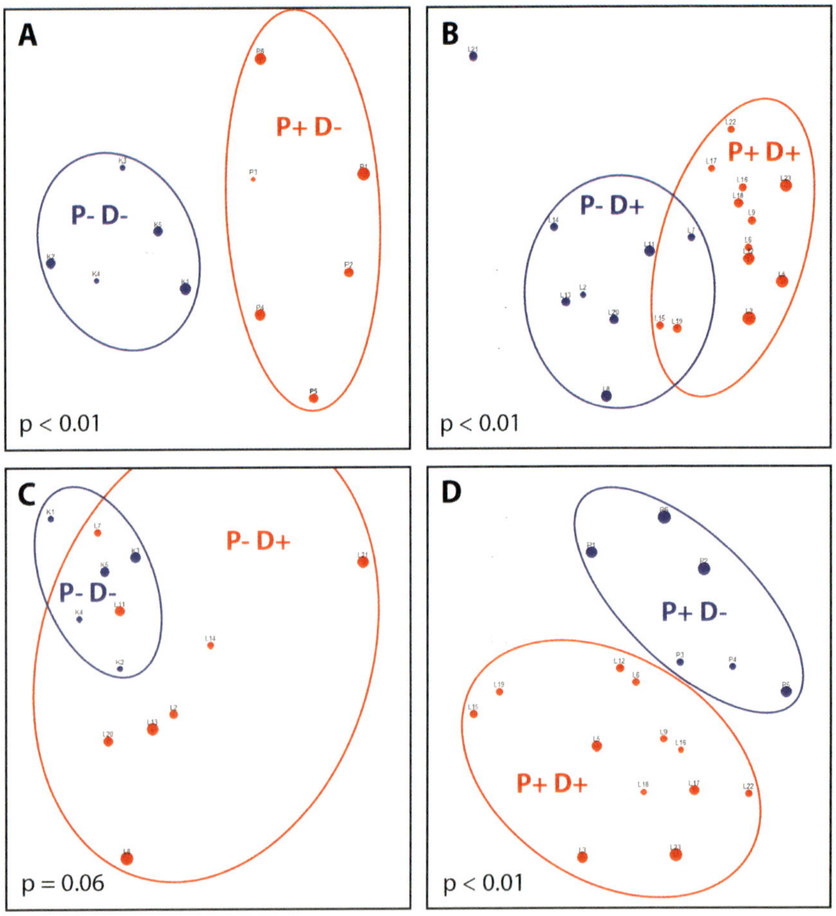

Figure 1. Subgingival plaque bacterial community composition comparison. The figure shows the results of non-metric multidimensional scaling (NMDS) applied to the unweighted UniFrac distances between different subsets of samples. The X- and Y-axes represent the first and second NMDS dimensions, respectively. The label next to each data point indicates the sample name. (A) Among diabetes-negative samples, a PERMANOVA test indicates significant ($p<0.01$) differences in the UniFrac distances according to the presence or absence of periodontitis. (B) A similar comparison among diabetes-positive samples is also significant ($p<0.01$). (C) Among periodontitis-negative samples, there is no clear separation based on diabetes status ($p=0.06$). (D) In periodontitis-positive samples, however, significant differences do exist based on diabetes status ($p<0.01$).

Table 1. Health-associated and periodontitis-associated OTUs.

	Health-associated bacteria OTUs	Periodontitis-associated bacteria OTUs
Significance uniquely identified in the diabetes-negative background	OTU0003 *Corynebacterium matruchotii* OTU0016 family of *Propionibacteriaceae* OTU0020 *Prevotella loescheii* OTU0025 genus of *Aggregatibacter* OTU0026 *Selenomonas noxia* OTU0088 *Cardiobacterium hominis* OTU0094 *Neisseria flavescens* OTU0096 *Cardiobacterium valvarum* OTU0102 family of *Leptotrichiaceae* OTU0127 genus of *Leptotrichia* OTU0161 *Capnocytophaga sputigena* OTU2004 *Porphyromonas sp.*	OTU2001 *Selenomonas sputigena* OTU0507 family of *Prevotellaceae*
Significance identified in the both diabetes-positive and diabetes-negative backgrounds	OTU0052 *Streptococcus infantis* OTU2002 *Streptococcus gordonii* OTU2005 *Actinomyces naeslundii*	OTU0011 *Treponema denticola* OTU2006 *Prevotella intermedia* OTU0343 family of *Prevotellaceae*
Significance uniquely identified in the diabetes-positive background	OTU0019 *Neisseria elongate* OTU0028 *Rothia dentocariosa* OTU0194 genus of *Veillonella* OTU0214 *Haemophilus parainfluenzae* OTU0280 genus of *Neisseria*	OTU0001 *Porphyromonas gingivalis* OTU0004 genus of *Leptotrichia* OTU2003 *Treponema medium* OTU0009 order of *Bacteroidales* OTU0010 *Tannerella forsythia* OTU0017 family of *Synergistaceae* OTU0044 *Porphyromonas endodontalis* OTU0056 unclassified OTU0058 *Filifactor alocis* OTU0101 genus of *Leptotrichia*

All OTUs listed had significantly different abundances or prevalence between the healthy and periodontitis samples within the diabetes-negative group, diabetes-positive group, or in both groups, as indicated by the three rows. The two columns indicate whether each OTU was more abundant or prevalent in periodontitis-negative or periodontitis-positive samples.

diabetes-negative or the diabetes-positive group based on their small p-values in the statistical tests. However, 24 of those 29 OTUs displayed consistently higher (or lower) prevalence or abundance in periodontitis-negative samples compared to periodontitis-positive samples in both diabetes-positive and diabetes-negative groups, despite non-significant p-values in one of the groups. If larger sample sizes were obtained, statistically significant p-values could have potentially been achieved for those "unique" OTUs, leading to more observations of "shared" signature OTUs. For example, OTU2003 (*Treponema medium*) was only identified as periodontitis-associated in the diabetes-positive background. In the diabetes-negative background, the p-value of this species was not significant in the two-tailed Wilcoxon rank-sum test, but its relative abundance was clearly higher in the P+D− samples (3.21%) than in the P−D− samples (0.92%), indicating its association with periodontitis (one-tailed test does show significance, $p = 0.04$). On the contrary, five of those 29 signature OTUs did not follow the same trend, prompting the possibility that "health-associated" or "periodontitis-associated" bacteria might need to be defined in the context of diabetes. For example, the relative abundance of OTU0020 (*Prevotella loescheii*) in P+D− and P−D− samples was 0.33% and 5.05%, respectively, highly enriched in the healthy periodontium samples in the diabetes-negative background ($p = 0.004$). However, its relative abundance in P+D+ and P−D+ samples was 1.16% and 0.33%, respectively, displaying a trend of enrichment in the periodontitis samples in the diabetes-positive background.

Effects of diabetes mellitus on subgingival plaque microbiota compositions

We also compared P−D− with P−D+ as well as P+D− with P+D+ to investigate the effects of diabetes mellitus on the subgingival plaque microbiota in subjects with or without periodontitis. Although the P−D− samples could not be easily separated from the P−D+ samples based on unweighted UniFrac distances (Figure 1C; PERMANOVA test, $p = 0.06$), three genera and nine OTUs had significantly different abundance between the P−D− and P−D+ samples (Tables 2 and S2). At the genus level, *Prevotella* ($p = 0.019$) and *Tannerella* ($p = 0.042$) were enriched in the P−D− samples while *Pseudomonas* ($p = 0.045$) was more associated with the P−D+ samples. At the OTU level, we were not able to designate OTU0125 (the order of *Actinomycetales*, unclassifiable at family level or below) or OTU0193 (the genus of *Prevotella*, unclassifiable at species level) as either health-associated or periodontitis-associated bacteria. All of the remaining seven OTUs could be considered as putative health-associated bacteria based on the above comparisons of their relative abundances in periodontitis-positive and periodontitis-negative groups. Only one of those seven health-associated OTUs, OTU0280 (genus of *Neisseria*), was enriched in the P−D+ samples. The other six health-associated OTUs significantly decreased their abundances in the P−D+ samples ($p < 0.05$): OTU0003 (*Corynebacterium matruchotii*), OTU0020 (*Prevotella loescheii*), OTU0094 (*Neisseria flavescens*), OTU0096 (*Cardiobacterium valvarum*), OTU0102 (family of *Leptotrichiaceae*, unclassifiable at the genus level or below), and OTU0187 (*Capnocytophaga ochracea*; although the relative abundance of this OTU was not significantly different in the comparison of the periodontitis-negative and the periodontitis-positive groups, its association with healthy periodontium has been reported in previous studies (*e.g.*, [73])). The tendency of reduced abundance of health-associated bacteria in the P−D+ samples might predispose the diabetic patients to greater risk of periodontitis.

In the periodontitis-positive group, the P+D+ samples could be separated from the P+D− samples based on unweighted UniFrac distances (Figure 1D; PERMANOVA test, $p < 0.01$). At the phylum level, both *Actinobacteria* ($p = 0.0013$) and *Proteobacteria* ($p = 0.041$) had significantly higher abundance in P+D+, while *Bacteroidetes* was more abundant in P+D− ($p = 0.018$). Casarin *et al.* [44] also detected the same trend for the above three phyla in diabetic subjects. At the genus level, *Actinomyces* ($p = 0.0057$) and *Aggregatibacter* ($p = 0.00037$) were more abundant or prevalent in the P+D+ samples. Both *Actinomyces* and *Aggregatibacter* were also observed by Casarin *et al.* [44] to be more associated with their P+D+ subjects. At the OTU level, six significantly different OTUs were detected between the P+D+ and P+D− samples in our study (Tables 2 and S2): OTU0015 (classified as *Burkholderiales* at the order level), OTU0046 (*P. tannerae*), OTU0016 (classified as *Propionibacteriaceae* at the family level), OTU0161 (*Capnocytophaga sputigena*), OTU0010 (*T. forsythia*) and OTU0343 (classified as *Prevotellaceae* at the family level). OTU0161 (*C. sputigena*) was designated as putative health-associated bacteria in our data set, which is also consistent with its reported association with healthy periodontal sites ([69], [70]). We observed that this species was more abundant in the P+D+ than in the P+D− samples. The increase of *Capnocytophaga* species in P+D+ subjects was also reported by Casarin *et al.* [44]. *C. sputigena* is a known glucose-fermenting species ([74], [73], [70]), which might explain its higher abundance in diabetic patients. Besides the species of *C. sputigena*, the relative abundance of OTU0016 (classified as *Propionibacteriaceae* at the family level) was also higher in the P+D+ samples. OTU0016 was designated as health-associated bacteria based on the above comparisons of its relative abundances in periodontitis-positive and periodontitis-negative groups, although it is difficult to verify the role of the unclassified species of *Propionibacteriaceae* in the literature. The physiological impacts of the higher abundance of such health-associated subgingival bacteria on periodontitis in diabetic patients are unclear.

In our data set, OTU0010 (*Tannerella forsythia*) was more likely to be detected in the P+D+ samples than in the P+D− samples. This OTU was detected in all 12 samples in the P+D+ group, while it was present in only three out of six total P+D− samples (Fisher's exact test, $p = 0.025$). Contradictory to our observations, the PCR results by Sardi *et al.* [34] and Campus *et al.* [75] (both using a curette) and 16S rDNA sequencing by Casarin *et al.* (using paper points) [44] indicated that *T. forsythia* is more prevalent in P+D− subjects. On the other hand, Li *et al.* (using paper points) [76] also detected higher prevalence and abundance of *T. forsythia* by PCR in P+D+ subjects, which is in agreement with our results. *T. forsythia* is a major component of the "red complex" associated with periodontitis ([64], [67]). Our result indicates that the higher prevalence of this well-known periopathogen in diabetic patients could contribute to their severity of periodontitis.

It is noteworthy to mention that we did not detect any significant difference for the other two components of the "red complex", *P. gingivalis* and *T. denticola*, when comparing the P+D+ samples with the P+D− samples, although both species were identified as periodontitis-associated bacteria in our data set. *P. gingivalis* was the most abundant species in our periodontitis-positive samples. Its average relative abundance in the P+D− and P+D+ samples was 17.85% and 12.48%, respectively ($p > 0.05$ in both Wilcoxon rank-sum test and Fisher's exact test). Our observation of *P. gingivalis* is supported by Yuan *et al.* [33], Sardi *et al.* [34], Field *et al.* [35], and Li *et al.* [76] (all of their results were based on PCR), although Campus *et al.* [75] and Casarin *et al.* [44] reported higher prevalence or abundance of this species in their P+D− subjects. The average relative abundance of *T. denticola* in

Table 2. Signature OTUs associated with diabetic and non-diabetic samples.

		Health-associated OTUs	Periodontitis-associated OTUs	Other OTUs
Periodontitis negative	↑ in Diabetes	OTU0280 genus of *Neisseria*		OTU0125 order of *Actinomycetales*
	↓ in Diabetes	OTU0003 *Corynebacterium matruchotii* OTU0020 *Prevotella loescheii* OTU0096 *Cardiobacterium valvarum* OTU0094 *Neisseria flavescens* OTU0102 family of *Leptotrichiaceae* OTU0187 *Capnocytophaga ochracea*		OTU0193 genus of *Prevotella*
Periodontitis positive	↑ in Diabetes	OTU0016 family of *Propionibacteriaceae* OTU0161 *Capnocytophaga sputigena*	OTU0010 *Tannerella forsythia*	OTU0015 order of *Burkholderiales*
	↓ in Diabetes		OTU0343 family of *Prevotellaceae*	OTU0046 *Prevotella tannerae*

Within the periodontitis-negative and periodontitis-positive sample groups, the listed OTUs were significantly either more or less abundant in diabetes-positive samples than in diabetes-negative samples, as indicated by the rows. The three columns indicate whether each OTU was significantly enriched in periodontitis-negative samples, periodontitis-positive samples, or neither, as found in the comparisons shown in Table 1.

our P+D− and P+D+ samples was 2.41% and 2.38%, respectively. Consistent with our results, Hintao *et al.* [30] (based on checkerboard DNA-DNA hybridization) and Yuan *et al.* [33] (based on PCR) also did not detect any significant difference for this species between their P+D− and P+D+ subgingival samples. In addition, we noticed that Casarin *et al.* [44] (based on 16S rDNA Sanger sequencing) did not find *T. denticola* to be significantly different in their study either, although Li *et al.* [76] observed a higher abundance and prevalence of this species in their P+D+ subjects. The source of such discrepancies in results is unclear, although it has been reported that subgingival microbiota could differ by geographic location, possibly due to lifestyle differences ([77], [78]).

Potential limitation

Our relatively small sample size is largely due to our rigorous criteria for subject recruitment in China. We excluded cigarette smokers and subjects with other systemic illness. We also excluded subjects with root caries since it is well known that the pathogenic bacteria of caries are highly different from those associated with periodontitis ([79], [80]). Despite our relatively small sample size, we could still detect differences among subject groups at both the bacterial community level and the individual bacteria level. However, small sample size inevitably limits the statistical power. We might have missed some bacteria that exist at different abundances in the different sample groups.

Another limitation is the relatively short read length (i.e., around 500 bp) associated with the 454 pyrosequencing technology. The BLAST-based species-level classification of short reads can be very challenging because multiple reference sequences in the database may match equally well to the query sequence. In our study, we manually examined the BLAST alignments and classified OTUs at species level only if the annotated top hit matched better than the other database hits. Nevertheless, manual assignment is subjective by nature as in many other aspects of bioinformatics inferences where it is difficult to deploy any automatic cutoff. We have decided to provide all the OTU sequences (File S1) for other researchers to verify our species classification of their OTUs of interest and compare with the latest database records in the future.

Conclusions

We have conducted the first high-throughput 16S rDNA pryosequencing to compare the subgingival plaque microbiota in non-diabetic subjects without periodontitis, non-diabetic subjects with periodontitis, type 2 diabetic patients without periodontitis, and type 2 diabetic patients with periodontitis. Based on the comparisons, a number of health-associated and periodontitis-associated bacteria were detected in both diabetic and non-diabetic backgrounds. In both periodontitis-negative and periodontitis-positive groups, we also detected that diabetic and non-diabetic subjects harbored bacteria at several taxonomic levels with significantly different prevalence or abundance.

Supporting Information

Figure S1 Distribution of all signature OTUs among four subject groups. The bar-plot shows the distribution of all signature OTUs among the four subject groups. The bar heights correspond to relative abundance percentage, and are log-scaled. The error bar indicates one unit of standard error.

Table S1 Clinical parameters of the participant subjects. Each subject was given an ID (column 1) and assigned a group according to periodontitis and diabetes statuses. Gender and age were recorded. Probing depth (PD) indicates the average depth in millimeters of the four deepest periodontal pockets. Attachment loss (AL) indicates the average tooth support tissue loss in millimeters of the same four sites. For subjects with diabetes, fasting blood sugar (FBS), two-hour postprandial blood sugar (PBS), and glycosylated hemoglobin, the three-month average glucose level (HbA1c), were recorded.

Table S2 Classification of all signature OTUs. These signature OTUs had significantly different abundances or prevalence in at least one of the following sample group comparisons: P−D− vs. P+D−, P−D+ vs. P+D+, P−D− vs. P−D+, or P+D− vs. P+D+ (see figure S1 for the distribution of the signature OTUs). Any significant ($p<0.05$) Wilcoxon rank-sum test or Fisher's exact test p-values are stated in the corresponding column. For the two comparisons of periodontal health, the "Association with periodontal health of subjects" column indicates whether the OTU is enriched in the periodontitis-negative or periodontitis-positive samples of that comparison. Similarly for the two comparisons of diabetes status, the "Association with diabetes status of subjects" column indicates the sample group with the higher abundances for that OTU.

File S1 FASTA-format sequences for all the OTUs. Sequences for each OTU are provided in a FASTA-format file.

Acknowledgments

We thank Drs. Feng Lu and Guangda Xiang for their guidance in working with the diabetic patients in this project. Their expertise in diabetes mellitus also helped us with experimental design and data analysis. We also thank Kashi Revanna for his assistance in the data management. The two anonymous reviewers also provided very constructive suggestions to improve the manuscript.

Author Contributions

Conceived and designed the experiments: QZ QD. Performed the experiments: MZ CZ. Analyzed the data: RR MZ DM XG QD. Contributed reagents/materials/analysis tools: MZ RR DM CZ. Wrote the paper: QD MZ RR DM XG QZ.

References

1. Graves DT, Li J, Cochran DL (2011) Inflammation and uncoupling as mechanisms of periodontal bone loss. J Dent Res 90: 143–153.
2. Pihlstrom BL, Michalowicz BS, Johnson NW (2005) Periodontal diseases. Lancet 366: 1809–1820.
3. Socransky SS, Haffajee AD (2005) Periodontal microbial ecology. Periodontol 2000 38: 135–187.
4. Griffen AL, Beall CJ, Campbell JH, Firestone ND, Kumar PS, et al. (2012) Distinct and complex bacterial profiles in human periodontitis and health revealed by 16S pyrosequencing. ISME J 6: 1176–1185.
5. Liu B, Faller LL, Klitgord N, Mazumdar V, Ghodsi M, et al. (2012) Deep sequencing of the oral microbiome reveals signatures of periodontal disease. PLoS One 7: e37919.
6. Taylor GW (2001) Bidirectional interrelationships between diabetes and periodontal diseases: an epidemiologic perspective. Ann Periodontol 6: 99–112.
7. Nelson RG, Shlossman M, Budding LM, Pettitt DJ, Saad MF, et al. (1990) Periodontal disease and NIDDM in Pima Indians. Diabetes Care 13: 836–840.
8. Shlossman M, Knowler WC, Pettitt DJ, Genco RJ (1990) Type 2 diabetes mellitus and periodontal disease. J Am Dent Assoc 121: 532–536.
9. Loe H (1993) Periodontal disease. The sixth complication of diabetes mellitus. Diabetes Care 16: 329–334.
10. Lakschevitz F, Aboodi G, Tenenbaum H, Glogauer M (2011) Diabetes and periodontal diseases: interplay and links. Curr Diabetes Rev 7: 433–439.
11. Taylor GW, Borgnakke WS (2008) Periodontal disease: associations with diabetes, glycemic control and complications. Oral Dis 14: 191–203.
12. Mealey BL, Oates TW (2006) Diabetes mellitus and periodontal diseases. J Periodontol 77: 1289–1303.
13. Taylor GW, Burt BA, Becker MP, Genco RJ, Shlossman M, et al. (1996) Severe periodontitis and risk for poor glycemic control in patients with non-insulin-dependent diabetes mellitus. J Periodontol 67: 1085–1093.
14. Lalla E, Papapanou PN (2011) Diabetes mellitus and periodontitis: a tale of two common interrelated diseases. Nat Rev Endocrinol 7: 738–748.
15. Salvi GE, Collins JG, Yalda B, Arnold RR, Lang NP, et al. (1997) Monocytic TNF alpha secretion patterns in IDDM patients with periodontal diseases. J Clin Periodontol 24: 8–16.
16. Salvi GE, Yalda B, Collins JG, Jones BH, Smith FW, et al. (1997) Inflammatory mediator response as a potential risk marker for periodontal diseases in insulin-dependent diabetes mellitus patients. J Periodontol 68: 127–135.
17. Karima M, Kantarci A, Ohira T, Hasturk H, Jones VL, et al. (2005) Enhanced superoxide release and elevated protein kinase C activity in neutrophils from diabetic patients: association with periodontitis. J Leukoc Biol 78: 862–870.
18. Ohnishi T, Bandow K, Kakimoto K, Machigashira M, Matsuyama T, et al. (2009) Oxidative stress causes alveolar bone loss in metabolic syndrome model mice with type 2 diabetes. J Periodontal Res 44: 43–51.
19. Lalla E, Lamster IB, Drury S, Fu C, Schmidt AM (2000) Hyperglycemia, glycoxidation and receptor for advanced glycation endproducts: potential mechanisms underlying diabetic complications, including diabetes-associated periodontitis. Periodontol 2000 23: 50–62.
20. Marette A (2004) Pathogenic role of inflammatory cytokines in obesity: from insulin resistance to diabetes mellitus. Nestle Nutr Workshop Ser Clin Perform Programme 9: 141–150; discussion 151–143.
21. Alexandraki K, Piperi C, Kalofoutis C, Singh J, Alaveras A, et al. (2006) Inflammatory process in type 2 diabetes: The role of cytokines. Ann N Y Acad Sci 1084: 89–117.
22. Kardesler L, Buduneli N, Cetinkalp S, Lappin D, Kinane DF (2011) Gingival crevicular fluid IL-6, tPA, PAI-2, albumin levels following initial periodontal treatment in chronic periodontitis patients with or without type 2 diabetes. Inflamm Res 60: 143–151.
23. King GL (2008) The role of inflammatory cytokines in diabetes and its complications. J Periodontol 79: 1527–1534.
24. Preshaw PM, Alba AL, Herrera D, Jepsen S, Konstantinidis A, et al. (2012) Periodontitis and diabetes: a two-way relationship. Diabetologia 55: 21–31.
25. Ficara AJ, Levin MP, Grower MF, Kramer GD (1975) A comparison of the glucose and protein content of gingival fluid from diabetics and nondiabetics. J Periodontal Res 10: 171–175.
26. Ohlrich EJ, Cullinan MP, Leichter JW (2010) Diabetes, periodontitis, and the subgingival microbiota. J Oral Microbiol 2.
27. Mashimo PA, Yamamoto Y, Slots J, Park BH, Genco RJ (1983) The periodontal microflora of juvenile diabetics. Culture, immunofluorescence, and serum antibody studies. J Periodontol 54: 420–430.
28. Thorstensson H, Dahlen G, Hugoson A (1995) Some suspected periodontopathogens and serum antibody response in adult long-duration insulin-dependent diabetics. J Clin Periodontol 22: 449–458.
29. Sbordone L, Ramaglia L, Barone A, Ciaglia RN, Iacono VJ (1998) Periodontal status and subgingival microbiota of insulin-dependent juvenile diabetics: a 3-year longitudinal study. J Periodontol 69: 120–128.
30. Hintao J, Teanpaisan R, Chongsuvivatwong V, Ratarasan C, Dahlen G (2007) The microbiological profiles of saliva, supragingival and subgingival plaque and dental caries in adults with and without type 2 diabetes mellitus. Oral Microbiol Immunol 22: 175–181.
31. Lalla E, Kaplan S, Chang SM, Roth GA, Celenti R, et al. (2006) Periodontal infection profiles in type 1 diabetes. J Clin Periodontol 33: 855–862.
32. Ebersole JL, Holt SC, Hansard R, Novak MJ (2008) Microbiologic and immunologic characteristics of periodontal disease in Hispanic americans with type 2 diabetes. J Periodontol 79: 637–646.
33. Yuan K, Chang CJ, Hsu PC, Sun HS, Tseng CC, et al. (2001) Detection of putative periodontal pathogens in non-insulin-dependent diabetes mellitus and non-diabetes mellitus by polymerase chain reaction. J Periodontal Res 36: 18–24.
34. Sardi JC, Duque C, Camargo GA, Hofling JF, Goncalves RB (2011) Periodontal conditions and prevalence of putative periodontopathogens and Candida spp. in insulin-dependent type 2 diabetic and non-diabetic patients with chronic periodontitis–a pilot study. Arch Oral Biol 56: 1098–1105.
35. Field CA, Gidley MD, Preshaw PM, Jakubovics N (2012) Investigation and quantification of key periodontal pathogens in patients with type 2 diabetes. J Periodontal Res 47: 470–478.
36. Margulies M, Egholm M, Altman WE, Attiya S, Bader JS, et al. (2005) Genome sequencing in microfabricated high-density picolitre reactors. Nature 437: 376–380.
37. Human Microbiome Consortium (2012) Structure, function and diversity of the healthy human microbiome. Nature 486: 207–214.
38. Lazarevic V, Whiteson K, Hernandez D, Francois P, Schrenzel J (2010) Study of inter- and intra-individual variations in the salivary microbiota. BMC Genomics 11: 523.
39. Dong Q, Nelson DE, Toh E, Diao L, Gao X, et al. (2011) The microbial communities in male first catch urine are highly similar to those in paired urethral swab specimens. PLoS One 6: e19709.
40. Dong Q, Brulc JM, Iovieno A, Bates B, Garoutte A, et al. (2011) Diversity of bacteria at healthy human conjunctiva. Invest Ophthalmol Vis Sci.
41. Wolfe AJ, Toh E, Shibata N, Rong R, Kenton K, et al. (2012) Evidence of uncultivated bacteria in the adult female bladder. J Clin Microbiol 50: 1376–1383.
42. Ahn J, Yang L, Paster BJ, Ganly I, Morris L, et al. (2011) Oral microbiome profiles: 16S rRNA pyrosequencing and microarray assay comparison. PLoS One 6: e22788.
43. Hooda S, Boler BM, Serao MC, Brulc JM, Staeger MA, et al. (2012) 454 pyrosequencing reveals a shift in fecal microbiota of healthy adult men consuming polydextrose or soluble corn fiber. J Nutr 142: 1259–1265.
44. Casarin RC, Barbagallo A, Meulman T, Santos VR, Sallum EA, et al. (2012) Subgingival biodiversity in subjects with uncontrolled type-2 diabetes and chronic periodontitis. J Periodontal Res.
45. Hartroth B, Seyfahrt I, Conrads G (1999) Sampling of periodontal pathogens by paper points: evaluation of basic parameters. Oral Microbiol Immunol 14: 326–330.
46. Tanner AC, Goodson JM (1986) Sampling of microorganisms associated with periodontal disease. Oral Microbiol Immunol 1: 15–22.
47. Paster BJ, Boches SK, Galvin JL, Ericson RE, Lau CN, et al. (2001) Bacterial diversity in human subgingival plaque. J Bacteriol 183: 3770–3783.

48. Kumar PS, Brooker MR, Dowd SE, Camerlengo T (2011) Target region selection is a critical determinant of community fingerprints generated by 16S pyrosequencing. PLoS One 6: e20956.
49. Shumway M, Cochrane G, Sugawara H (2010) Archiving next generation sequencing data. Nucleic Acids Res 38: D870–871.
50. Schloss PD, Westcott SL, Ryabin T, Hall JR, Hartmann M, et al. (2009) Introducing mothur: open-source, platform-independent, community-supported software for describing and comparing microbial communities. Appl Environ Microbiol 75: 7537–7541.
51. Hawlena H, Rynkiewicz E, Toh E, Alfred A, Durden LA, et al. (2012) The arthropod, but not the vertebrate host or its environment, dictates bacterial community composition of fleas and ticks. ISME J.
52. Stackebrandt E, Goebel BM (1994) A place for DNA-DNA reassociation and 16S rRNA sequence analysis in the present species definition in bacteriology. Int J Syst Bacteriol 44: 846–849.
53. Quince C, Lanzen A, Curtis TP, Davenport RJ, Hall N, et al. (2009) Accurate determination of microbial diversity from 454 pyrosequencing data. Nat Methods 6: 639–641.
54. Kunin V, Engelbrektson A, Ochman H, Hugenholtz P (2010) Wrinkles in the rare biosphere: pyrosequencing errors can lead to artificial inflation of diversity estimates. Environ Microbiol 12: 118–123.
55. Fettweis JM, Serrano MG, Sheth NU, Mayer CM, Glascock AL, et al. (2012) Species-level classification of the vaginal microbiome. BMC Genomics 13 Suppl 8: S17.
56. Wang Q, Garrity GM, Tiedje JM, Cole JR (2007) Naive Bayesian classifier for rapid assignment of rRNA sequences into the new bacterial taxonomy. Appl Environ Microbiol 73: 5261–5267.
57. Johnson M, Zaretskaya I, Raytselis Y, Merezhuk Y, McGinnis S, et al. (2008) NCBI BLAST: a better web interface. Nucleic Acids Res 36: W5–9.
58. Quast C, Pruesse E, Yilmaz P, Gerken J, Schweer T, et al. (2013) The SILVA ribosomal RNA gene database project: improved data processing and web-based tools. Nucleic Acids Res 41: D590–596.
59. Chen T, Yu WH, Izard J, Baranova OV, Lakshmanan A, et al. (2010) The Human Oral Microbiome Database: a web accessible resource for investigating oral microbe taxonomic and genomic information. Database (Oxford) 2010: baq013.
60. McMurdie PJ, Holmes S (2012) Phyloseq: a bioconductor package for handling and analysis of high-throughput phylogenetic sequence data. Pac Symp Biocomput: 235–246.
61. Oksanen J, Kindt R, Legendre P, O'Hara RB, Simpson GL, et al. (2012) vegan: Community Ecology Package. R package version 20-5.
62. Lozupone C, Lladser ME, Knights D, Stombaugh J, Knight R (2011) UniFrac: an effective distance metric for microbial community comparison. ISME J 5: 169–172.
63. Kumar PS, Griffen AL, Barton JA, Paster BJ, Moeschberger ML, et al. (2003) New bacterial species associated with chronic periodontitis. J Dent Res 82: 338–344.
64. Kumar PS, Griffen AL, Moeschberger ML, Leys EJ (2005) Identification of candidate periodontal pathogens and beneficial species by quantitative 16S clonal analysis. J Clin Microbiol 43: 3944–3955.
65. Ashimoto A, Chen C, Bakker I, Slots J (1996) Polymerase chain reaction detection of 8 putative periodontal pathogens in subgingival plaque of gingivitis and advanced periodontitis lesions. Oral Microbiol Immunol 11: 266–273.
66. Socransky SS, Haffajee AD, Cugini MA, Smith C, Kent RL, Jr. (1998) Microbial complexes in subgingival plaque. J Clin Periodontol 25: 134–144.
67. Holt SC, Ebersole JL (2005) Porphyromonas gingivalis, Treponema denticola, and Tannerella forsythia: the "red complex", a prototype polybacterial pathogenic consortium in periodontitis. Periodontol 2000 38: 72–122.
68. Moter A, Hoenig C, Choi BK, Riep B, Gobel UB (1998) Molecular epidemiology of oral treponemes associated with periodontal disease. J Clin Microbiol 36: 1399–1403.
69. Colombo AP, Boches SK, Cotton SL, Goodson JM, Kent R, et al. (2009) Comparisons of subgingival microbial profiles of refractory periodontitis, severe periodontitis, and periodontal health using the human oral microbe identification microarray. J Periodontol 80: 1421–1432.
70. Colombo AP, Bennet S, Cotton SL, Goodson JM, Kent R, et al. (2012) Impact of periodontal therapy on the subgingival microbiota of severe periodontitis: comparison between good responders and individuals with refractory periodontitis using the human oral microbe identification microarray. J Periodontol 83: 1279–1287.
71. Shaddox LM, Huang H, Lin T, Hou W, Harrison PL, et al. (2012) Microbiological characterization in children with aggressive periodontitis. J Dent Res 91: 927–933.
72. Nadkarni MA, Browne GV, Chhour KL, Byun R, Nguyen KA, et al. (2012) Pattern of distribution of Prevotella species/phylotypes associated with healthy gingiva and periodontal disease. Eur J Clin Microbiol Infect Dis 31: 2989–2999.
73. Holdeman LV, Moore WE, Cato EP, Burmeister JA, Palcanis KG, et al. (1985) Distribution of capnocytophaga in periodontal microfloras. J Periodontal Res 20: 475–483.
74. Socransky SS, Holt SC, Leadbetter ER, Tanner AC, Savitt E, et al. (1979) Capnocytophaga: new genus of gram-negative gliding bacteria. III. Physiological characterization. Arch Microbiol 122: 29–33.
75. Campus G, Salem A, Uzzau S, Baldoni E, Tonolo G (2005) Diabetes and periodontal disease: a case-control study. J Periodontol 76: 418–425.
76. Li C, Liu J, Tan L, Yu N, Lin L, et al. (2012) The Sociodemographic Characteristics, Periodontal Health Status, and Subgingival Microbiota of Chronic Periodontitis Patients With Type 2 Diabetes Mellitus: A Case Control Study in a Chinese Population. J Periodontol.
77. Haffajee AD, Bogren A, Hasturk H, Feres M, Lopez NJ, et al. (2004) Subgingival microbiota of chronic periodontitis subjects from different geographic locations. J Clin Periodontol 31: 996–1002.
78. Kim TS, Kang NW, Lee SB, Eickholz P, Pretzl B, et al. (2009) Differences in subgingival microflora of Korean and German periodontal patients. Arch Oral Biol 54: 223–229.
79. Liljemark WF, Bloomquist C (1996) Human oral microbial ecology and dental caries and periodontal diseases. Crit Rev Oral Biol Med 7: 180–198.
80. Paster BJ, Olsen I, Aas JA, Dewhirst FE (2006) The breadth of bacterial diversity in the human periodontal pocket and other oral sites. Periodontol 2000 42: 80–87.

17

Neutrophil Mobilization by Surface-Glycan Altered Th17-Skewing Bacteria Mitigates Periodontal Pathogen Persistence and Associated Alveolar Bone Loss

Rajendra P. Settem, Kiyonobu Honma, Ashu Sharma*

Department of Oral Biology, School of Dental Medicine, University at Buffalo, State University of New York, Buffalo, New York, United States of America

Abstract

Alveolar bone (tooth-supporting bone) erosion is a hallmark of periodontitis, an inflammatory disease that often leads to tooth loss. Periodontitis is caused by a select group of pathogens that form biofilms in subgingival crevices between the gums and teeth. It is well-recognized that the periodontal pathogen *Porphyromonas gingivalis* in these biofilms is responsible for modeling a microbial dysbiotic state, which then initiates an inflammatory response destructive to the periodontal tissues and bone. Eradication of this pathogen is thus critical for the treatment of periodontitis. Previous studies have shown that oral inoculation in mice with an attenuated strain of the periodontal pathogen *Tannerella forsythia* altered in O-glycan surface composition induces a Th17-linked mobilization of neutrophils to the gingival tissues. In this study, we sought to determine if immune priming with such a Th17-biasing strain would elicit a productive neutrophil response against *P. gingivalis*. Our data show that inoculation with a Th17-biasing *T. forsythia* strain is effective in blocking *P. gingivalis*-persistence and associated alveolar bone loss in mice. This work demonstrates the potential of O-glycan modified *Tannerella* strains or their O-glycan components for harnessing Th17-mediated immunity against periodontal and other mucosal pathogens.

Editor: Özlem Yilmaz, University of Florida, United States of America

Funding: This work was supported by U.S. Public Health R01 grants DE14749 and DE19424. The funder had no role in study design, data collection and analysis, decision to publish, or preparation of the manuscript.

Competing Interests: The authors have declared that no competing interests exist.

* Email: sharmaa@buffalo.edu

Introduction

The oral pathogen *Tannerella forsythia* and its cohabiting partner *Porphyromonas gingivalis* have been implicated in periodontitis, a polymicrobial disease that often leads to tooth loss in adults. These bacteria form biofilms in subgingival crevices (spaces between the gums and teeth) and instigate inflammatory responses destructive to the tooth supporting structures. In order to colonize and persist in the host environment, pathogens have constantly evolved strategies to modulate the innate as well as the adaptive immunity of the host. In this regard, the periodontal pathogen *T. forsythia* induce the development of Th2 responses, resulting in inflammatory alveolar bone loss [6]. This bacterium expresses a uniquely glycosylated surface envelope, known as the surface (S)-layer, which plays an immunomodulatory role in influencing the immunity [1]. The *T. forsythia* S-layer has recently been shown to be important in delaying the cytokine responses of the monocyte and macrophage cells *in vitro* [2]. More recently, we have shown that an O-glycan structural core linked to the bacterium's S-layer proteins is critical in shaping the cytokine responses of antigen-presenting cells and adaptive T cell immunity *in vivo* [3]. Furthermore, in a mouse model of periodontitis we demonstrated that a terminal pseudaminic acid and N-acetylmannosaminuronic containing tri-saccharide branch on an O-glycan core linked to the *Tannerella* surface proteins plays a role in dampening Th17 differentiation and mitigating neutrophil infiltration to the gingival tissue [3]. Likewise, *P. gingivalis*, has its own specific mechanisms proficient for evading and paralyzing the innate and adaptive immunity, and is considered a keystone pathogen whose colonization results in oral microbial dysbiosis [4]. The dysbiotic flora resulting from *P. gingivalis* colonization is thought to induce an exaggerated and dysfunctional immune response culminating in alveolar bone loss and other pathologies characteristic of periodontitis [4]. Targeting *P. gingivalis* is thus an attractive strategy to block disease pathogenesis. In this study we tested whether oral inoculation with an O-glycan altered *T. forsythia* strain ED1 [3], capable of inducing Th17-dependent neutrophil responses, would be efficacious in eradicating *P. gingivalis* in a mouse model. Our results demonstrate that oral inoculation with a Th17-biasing *T. forsythia* strain is able to confer protection against *P. gingivalis* colonization and associated alveolar bone loss.

Materials and Methods

Bacterial strains and culture conditions

P. gingivalis ATCC 33277, *T. forsythia* ATCC 43037 and *T. forsythia* ED1 inactivated in the gene encoding UDP-*N*-acetylmannosaminuronic dehydrogenase were grown in broth or agar plates containing 1.5% agar under anaerobic conditions as described previously [3,5].

Mice and bacterial inoculation

Specific-pathogen-free BALB/cJ mice (Jackson Laboratory, Bar Harbor, ME, USA), 5–6 weeks old (female) at the start of the experiment were maintained in the Laboratory Animal Facility of the University at Buffalo. Mice were maintained and handled in strict accordance with the recommendations in the Guide for the Care and Use of Laboratory Animals of the National Institutes of Health. The study protocol was approved by the Institutional Animal Care and Use Committee (IACUC) of the University at Buffalo (IACUC Approval # ORB05072Y). All efforts were made to minimize suffering and tissues were harvested after euthanizing animals with carbon dioxide inhalation. After 1-week quarantine period, mice were given kanamycin (1 mg/mL) in drinking water *ad libitum* for 5 days followed by a two-day antibiotic-free period to suppress the resident bacteria. Mice were divided into four groups (16 mice per group). The experimental protocol has been schematically summarized in Fig, 1. The control group received six doses of 200 μL of vehicle 1% carboxymethyl cellulose (CMC) without bacteria at 48 h intervals via oral gavage (group 1, sham-infected). Group 2 (control) received three doses of 10^8 cfu *P. gingivalis* cells in 200 μL 1% CMC at 48 h intervals three days after priming with six doses of vehicle. Groups 3 and 4 were subjected to infection priming by oral gavage with six doses of 10^8 cfu *T. forsythia* cells in 200 μL 1% CMC at 48 h intervals with either the live wild-type ATCC 43037 (groups 3) or trisaccharide O-glycan deficient *T. forsythia* ED1 strain (group 4). Three days after the last dose, *T. forsythia*-primed groups 3 and 4 were challenged with three doses of 10^8 cfu *P. gingivalis* cells in 200 μL of 1% CMC at 48 h intervals as above.

Specific IgG response by ELISA

T. forsythia wild-type, ED1 and *P. gingivalis* strain specific IgG antibody responses were measured by ELISA as described previously [6]. Briefly, 96-well Immuno-Maxisorp plates (Nalgene Nunc International, Rochester, NY) coated with formalin-fixed bacteria (10^9 cells/mL and 100 μL/well) were incubated with serial dilutions of mouse sera, followed by HRP-conjugated goat anti-mouse IgG (Bethyl Laboratories, TX). ELISA wells were color developed with TMB Micro well enzyme substrate (Kirkegaards and Perry, MD) and plates were read at 495 nm. Titers were defined as the $\log^2$ of the highest dilution with a signal that was 0.1 optical density units above the background level.

Assessment of alveolar bone loss

Horizontal bone loss around the maxillary molars was assessed by a morphometric method. After 6 weeks following the first infection mice were scarified, skulls were autoclaved, de-fleshed and immersed overnight in 3% hydrogen peroxide and then stained with 1% methylene blue as described previously [6]. The distances between the alveolar bone crest (ABC) and cement-enamel junction (CEJ) considered as alveolar bone loss were measured by two independent evaluators in blinded fashion at 7 buccal sites on each side with the help of a dissecting microscope attached to an imaging system with a software (Aquinto imaging system, a4i America, Brook-Anco, Rochester, NY).

Intracellular staining and FACS analysis

The following Abs and isotype controls were purchased from e-Biosciences: PE-conjugated anti–IFN-γ and rat IgG2a; PE-conjugated anti–IL-5; PECy5-labeled anti-CD4; anti-CD80 (16-10A**1**) and anti-CD83 (Michel-17); rat IgG1, IgG2a, and IgG2b; PE-conjugated anti-CD11c (N418); hamster IgG; PE-conjugated anti–IL-17A (eBio17B7); and rat IgG2a. For intracellular staining, cell suspensions from cervical lymph nodes (cLNs) were stimulated with anti-CD3 and anti-CD28 Abs (eBioscience) for 48 h, followed by PMA (50 ng/ml), ionomycin (1 μg/ml), and brefeldin A (10 μg/ml) for 6 h. Cells were washed, incubated with FcR block (1 μg/ml; eBiosciences), and stained for CD4. Cells were fixed with 2% paraformaldehyde, permeabilized with 0.1% saponin (Sigma), and stained for IL-5, IL-17 and IFN-γ. Cells were analyzed on a FACS Calibur (BD Biosciences) with FCS Express software (DeNovo Software).

Quantification of osteoclasts by TRAP staining

Mouse maxillary and mandibular bones ($n = 4$–6) were fixed in 10% phosphate-buffered formalin and decalcified in 10% EDTA. The samples were then embedded in paraffin, and sections at 4 μm were prepared and stained for tartrate-resistant acid phosphatase (TRAP; Sigma). TRAP-stained whole slides were digitally scanned immediately with a Scan Scope CS system (Aperio) to minimize color fading. The scanned slides were viewed with Image Scope viewing software (Aperio). The right maxillary and mandibular inter dental areas (average of 10 higher power fields per slide) of the crestal alveolar bone from the first molar to third molar were used to quantify osteoclasts.

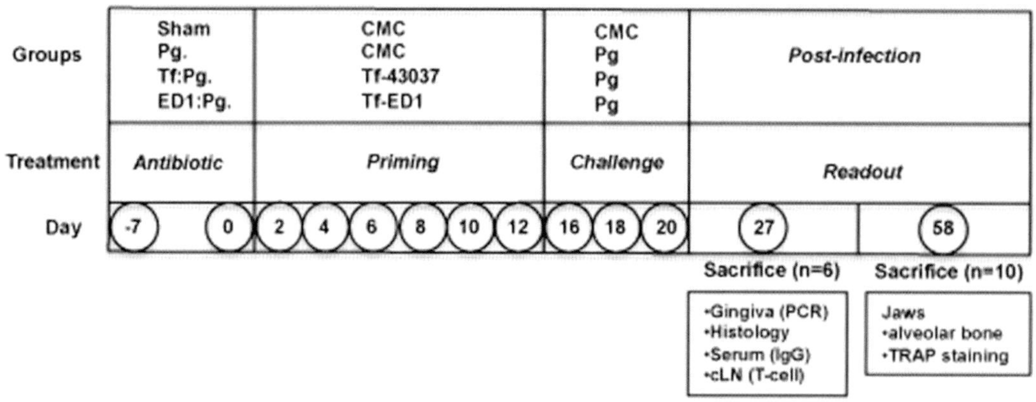

Figure 1. Schematic representation of infection and tissue harvesting schedules.

Quantification of CD45$^+$ cells and infiltrated neutrophils

The right and left halves of the maxillary and mandibular bones with soft tissues were recovered and processed as follows. The left maxillary and mandibular tissues were used for DNA extraction (see below) and the right maxillary and mandibular tissues were used for histology after embedding in paraffin. Briefly, 4 µm sections were cut from the embedded tissues, deparafinized in xylene and hydrated in graded ethanol prior to antibody staining as follows. Specimens were first incubated at 90°C for 10 min with BD Retrievagen A (BD PharMingen) for antigen retrieval and then sequentially incubated in: (i) blocking solution containing 0.1% Triton X-100 in 0.1 M PBS (PBST) for 1 h at room temperature; (ii) monoclonal rat anti-mouse CD45 (BD PharMingen) antibody diluted 1:30 in PBST or anti-neutrophil marker antibody (NIMP-R14, Santa Cruz Biotechnology, CA, USA) for 1 h at room temperature. The slides were incubated with a biotinylated secondary antibody (goat anti-rat IgG) followed by an avidin-biotin complex developed with 3, 3-diaminobenzidine (DAB) (Vector Labs, Burlingame, CA). The slides were counter stained with haematoxylin. After each step, slides were rinsed in PBST (3×10 min). Slides were scanned at an absolute magnification of 400× using the Aperio Scan Scope CS system (Aperio Technologies, Vista, CA). Slides (six slides per mouse) were viewed and analyzed using desktop personal computers employing the virtual image viewer software (Aperio). Antibody positive cells (stained brown) were enumerated manually in the inter-dental areas from the first to third molar at randomly selected locations in each slide (6 per slide). The areas associated with these locations were then obtained from the software to calculate the average cell densities per square millimeter.

Assessment of bacterial colonization levels by real-time PCR

DNA was isolated from left maxillary and mandibular tissues (soft gingival and hard tissue) of each mouse a tissue DNA isolation kit (DNAeasy from Qiagen, Valencia, CA). *P. gingivalis* and *T. forsythia* levels in the tissues were determined by quantitative real-time PCR as described previously [3]. Briefly, *T. forsythia* or *P. gingivalis* specific 16S rDNA amplicons from tissue samples were amplified in a real-time PCR reaction with specific primer sets (*Tf*: 5′-GCGTATGTAACCTGCCCGCA-3′ and 5′-TGCTTCAG-TTCAGTTATACCT-3′; *Pg*: 5′-CTTGACTTCAGTGGCGG-CAG-3′ and 5′-AGGGAAGACGGTTTTCACCA-3′) and SYBR green master mix using MyiCycler (Bio-Rad laboratories). In addition, mouse glyceraldehyde-3-phosphate dehydrogenase (*gapdh*) gene amplified (primers 5-GCACAGTCAAGGCCGA-GAAT-3 and 5-GCCTTCTCCATGGTGGTGAA-3) from the same sample was used to normalize bacterial loads in extracted tissues as per previously described method [3]; bacterial loads were expressed as the number of $\log_{10}$ bacterial genomes per 10^9 copies of *gapdh*. Ct values were converted to weights of DNA by interpolation from DNA weights versus a Ct standard curve. For calculating the number of bacterial genomes from the quantities of DNA, the genome size of 3.4 Mb and 2.35 Mb for *T. forsythia* and *P. gingivalis* respectively (http://www.homd.org) were used.

Data analysis

Data were analyzed with Graph Pad Prism software (Graph Pad, San Diego, CA). Comparisons between groups were made using a Student's *t* test (between two groups) or ANOVA (multiple group comparisons) as appropriate. Statistical significance was defined as $p<0.05$.

Results

Neutrophil mobilization to gingivae is enhanced and *P. gingivalis* persistence is moderately reduced in O-glycan-deficient ED1-primed mice

Previous studies from our laboratory showed that the O-glycans linked to the proteinaceous surface (S) - layer in the periodontal pathogen *T. forsythia* plays an immunomodulatory role in mice [3,6]. Specifically, a *Tannerella* strain ED1 lacking the terminal trisaccharide motif comprising a modified pseudaminic acid and two *N*-acetylmannosaminuronic residues on a protein linked O-glycan core induces a Th17- response [3]. We tested whether a Th17-driven neutrophil response orchestrated by the ED1 strain would be productive in clearing *P. gingivalis*. Briefly, mice were inoculated with either the vehicle, wild-type *T. forsythia* or ED1 strains and then challenged with *P. gingivalis* as described (summarized in Fig. 1). Serum IgG titers against bacteria were also determined 1-week after the last infection dose to confirm that mice were productively infected. *T. forsythia* or *P. gingivalis*-specific IgG titers were significantly elevated in groups infected with the corresponding species over the sham-infected group (Fig. 2). Background antibody titers against *T. forsythia* or *P. gingivalis* in sham-infected groups were also observed, this likely reflects the presence of cross-reacting common antigens between these bacteria and the resident oral flora. Antibody titers against *T. forsythia* and *P. gingivalis* were also elevated in groups receiving both *T. forsythia* and *P. gingivalis* (Fig. 2). Th- cell response were evaluated by intracellular staining followed by flow cytometry on T cell populations from draining lymph nodes; single cell suspensions from cervical lymph nodes (cLNs) stimulated with anti-CD3, -CD28 antibodies and ionomycin were surface stained for cell surface marker CD4 and intracellularly for subset effector cytokines IL-5 (Th2), IFN-γ (Th1) and IL-17 (Th17). The results showed that the ED1-primed group (ED1: Pg) exhibited significantly higher levels of Th17 cells in cLNs compared to all other groups (Fig. 3). Mice infected with the wild-type *T. forsythia* and *P. gingivalis* (Tf:Pg) or *P. gingivalis* alone (Pg) showed an increase in the numbers of Th2 cells compared to the sham or ED1 infected mice (Fig. 3). To evaluate the inflammatory activity locally in the periodontal area, the left maxillae were collected, sectioned and stained with mouse specific CD45 and neutrophil (Gro$^+$) antibodies as described previously [3]. The results showed that CD45$^+$ inflammatory cells were elevated in all groups infected with bacteria compared to the control group (sham-infected). Moreover, the numbers of CD45$^+$ cells were highest in the groups primed with ED1 (Fig. 4A). A similar trend was observed with neutrophils (Fig. 4B). ED1 primed and *P. gingivalis* challenged mice showed an increase in the numbers of Gro$^+$ cells compared to all other groups (Fig. 4B). In addition, the level of neutrophil infiltration in each group paralleled the Th17 responses in the bacterial infected groups. Together these results indicated that mice primed with ED1 develop a sustained Th17-mediated neutrophil response which is not perturbed by *P. gingivalis* challenge (ED1:Pg). To evaluate if neutrophil infiltration due to ED1 was effective in clearing *P. gingivalis*, bacteria were quantified by quantitative PCR as described previously [3]. The results showed that the *P. gingivalis* colonization was significantly reduced in ED1- primed compared to the *T. forsythia* wild-type - primed mice ($P<0.05$). A trend toward reduced *P. gingivalis* colonization in the ED1-primed (ED1:Pg) group compared to the sham-primed (Pg) group was observed. However, this reduction in colonization did not reach the statistical significance ($P=0.067$) (Fig. 5). With respect to *Tannerella*, the numbers of genomes recovered from the Tf:Pg group were approximately100-fold

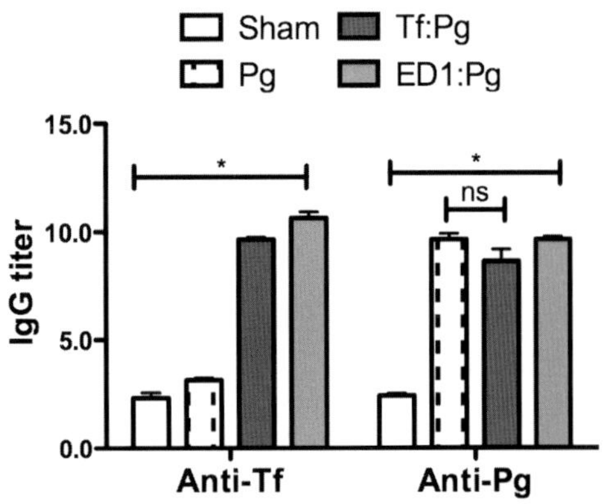

Figure 2. Antibody titers against *T. forsythia* and *P. gingivalis* after infection. Sera from mice 1-week after the last infection were analyzed by ELISA for *T. forsythia* and *P. gingivalis* specific IgG. Antibody levels are presented as $\log_2$ titers. Data are from one of two independent experiments with similar results (mean ± s.d, of 6 mice per group; *, $p<0.05$).

higher than the ED1:Pg group. This is likely due to the fact that ED1 is significantly more prone to capture and killing by antigen-presenting cells than the wild-type strain [3], No *P. gingivalis* or *T, forsythia* were detected in sham-infected animals; Ct values higher than the cutoff set at 40 cycles and similar to template absent water control (Fig. 5).

The O-glycan deficient ED1 strain protects mice from *P. gingivalis*-induced alveolar bone loss

To assess whether *P. gingivalis* clearance reciprocally reduces alveolar bone loss, mice jaws were harvested 6-weeks after the first *P. gingivalis* infection dose and the alveolar bone loss in each group was assessed as the average total distance between ABC-CEJ per mouse. The data showed that ED1 primed and *P. gingivalis* challenged mice (ED1:Pg) exhibited reduced alveolar bone loss as compared to the *T. forsythia* wild-type primed–*P. gingivalis* challenged (Tf:Pg) or the *P. gingivalis* alone challenged (Pg) mice (Fig. 6 A). The net bone loss calculated as the total mean bone loss in the sham infected group subtracted from the bacteria infected group was significantly less in the ED1:Pg group compared to the Pg alone or Tf:Pg groups. As an additional measure of alveolar bone loss, osteoclastic activity in the interdental region was evaluated for each group for tartrate-resistant alkaline phosphatase (TRAP) staining. The results showed that the TRAP activity in each group correlated with the alveolar bone loss of the corresponding group; ED1-primed mice exhibited lower osteoclastic activity compared to *T. forsythia* wild-type or *P. gingivalis* infected groups (Fig. 6 C&D).

Discussion

It is well established that periodontal disease is a polymicrobial infection with the black-pigmented anaerobe *P. gingivalis* playing a key role alongside *T. forsythia* in periodontal disease and that *P. gingivalis* is adept in immune subversion strategies that allow the

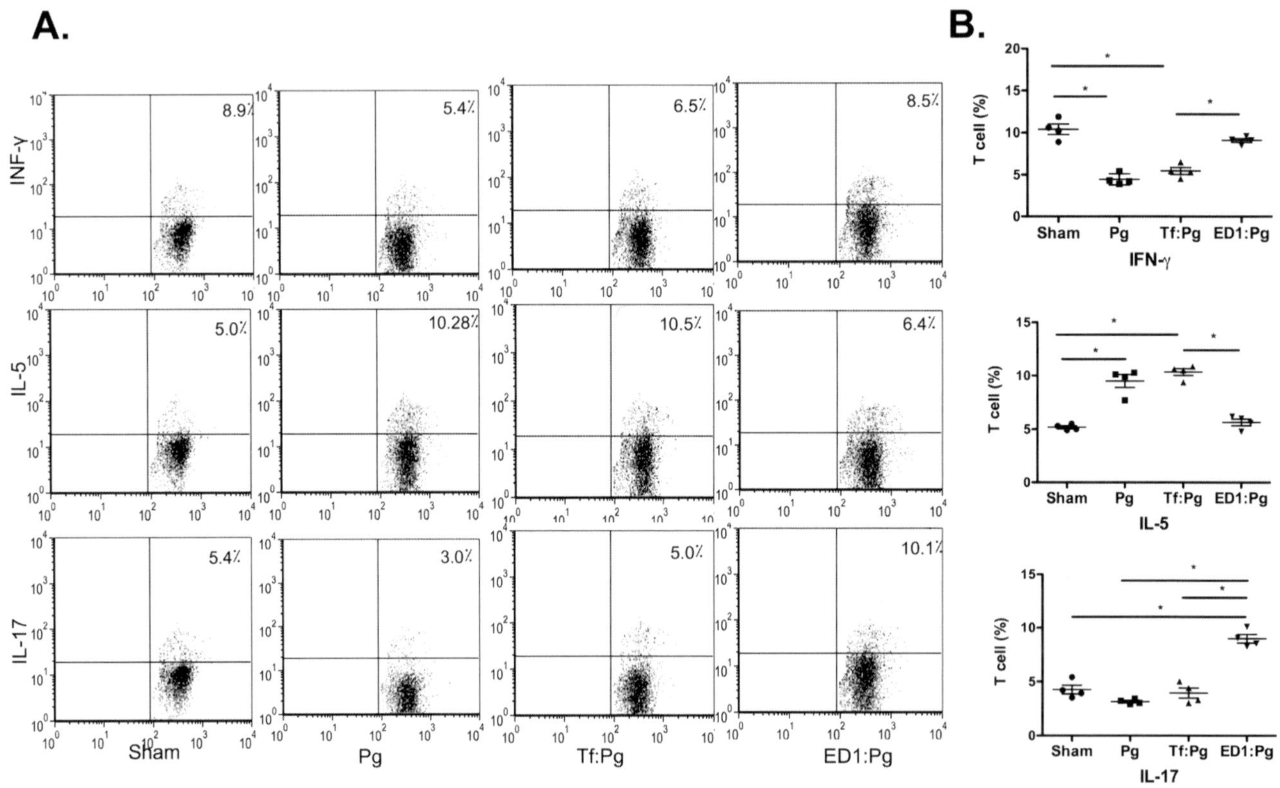

Figure 3. Flow cytometric analysis of cytokine production in CD4⁺ T cells from mice after infection. Draining lymph node cells from all groups were stimulated *in vitro* with anti-CD3 and anti-CD28 Abs for 48 h. Cells were then stimulated with PMA and ionomycin for 4–6 h prior to intracellular staining for IL-5, IFN-γ or IL-17 (A) Representative flow cytometry dot plots of CD4⁺ T cells from sham- and bacteria- infected mice intracellularly stained for IL-5, IFN-γ or IL-17. (B) Bar graphs showing percentages of specific cytokine positive T cells for each group. Data are from one of two independent experiments with similar results (mean ± s.d of 6 mice per group; *, $p<0.05$, n.s, not significant).

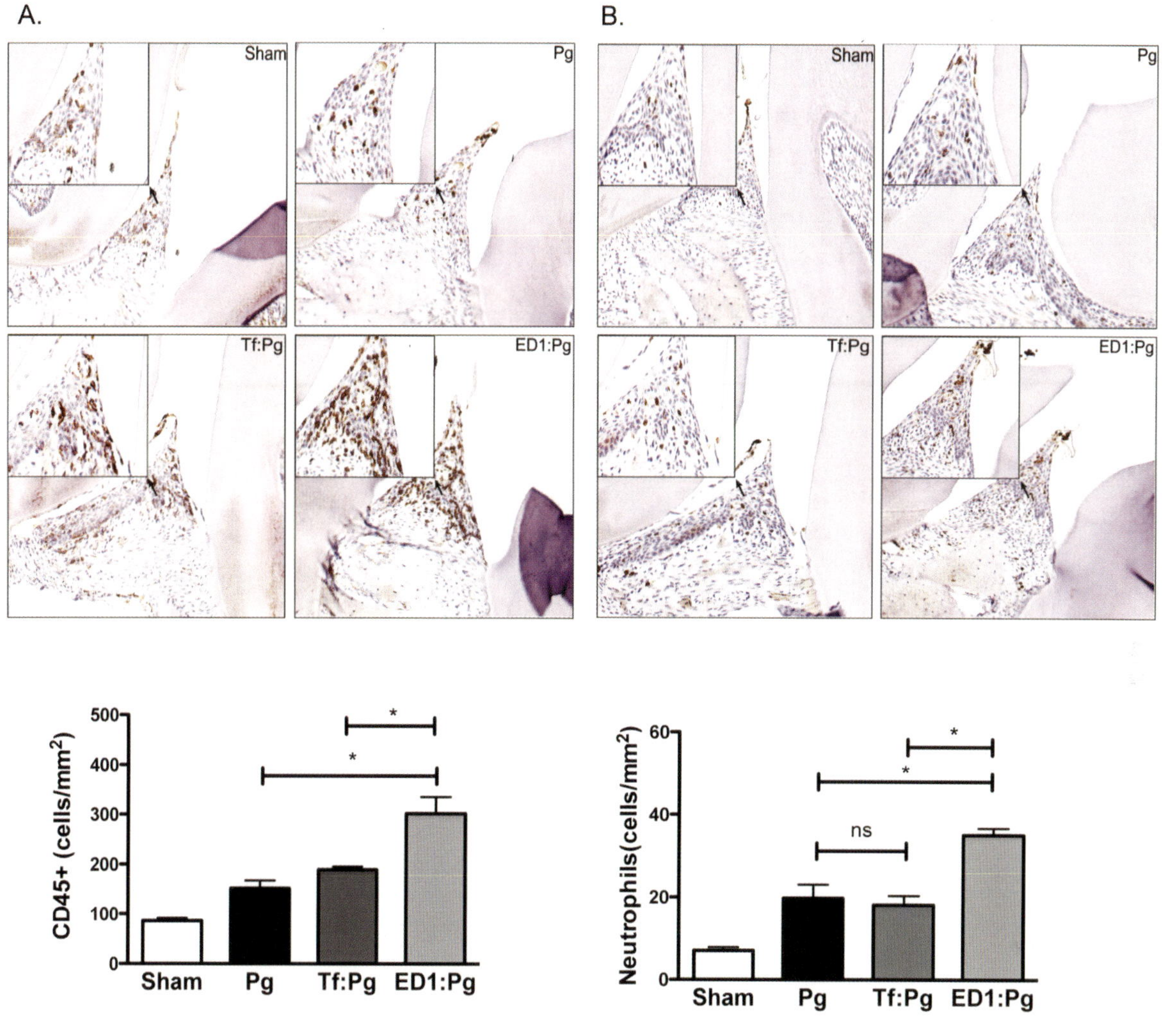

Figure 4. Lymphocyte/neutrophil infiltration in gingival tissues of mice primed with ED1 and infected with *P. gingivalis*. Immunohistochemical staining for total CD45 positive inflammatory cells (A) and neutrophils (B) in gingival tissue. All images are representative of 400× magnification. Slide images were viewed with Aperio Image Scope viewing software and the inter-dental areas from the first to third molar were used to quantify inflammatory cells. Bar graphs below each image show numbers of CD45 positive or neutrophil antibody positive cells (brown color). Data are from one of two independent experiments with similar results (mean ± s.d. of 6 mice per group; *, $p<0.05$).

bacterium to persist in the host [7]. We sought to explore whether neutrophil mobilization to gingival tissue through oral inoculation with Th17-biasing strains of *T. forsythia* could impair *P. gingivalis* persistence in the oral cavity. *P. gingivalis* is a keystone pathogen whose presence results in the development of a dysbiotic subgingival microbial community [4], triggering a dysregulated immune response culminating in inflammatory alveolar bone destruction, a hallmark of periodontitis. *P. gingivalis* utilizes a plethora of strategies to weaken the host innate and adaptive immunity that allow the bacterium to increase its colonization potential and existence in the oral cavity [7]. We reasoned that approaches by which neutrophil recruitment to the gingival tissues could be enhanced would be beneficial in clearing *P. gingivalis*, and thus in mitigating inflammatory alveolar bone loss. Our results demonstrated that by priming with Th17-biasing *T. forsythia* ED1 strain a productive neutrophil response able to block *P. gingivalis* colonization and associated alveolar bone loss was achieved in a mouse model. As shown, increased Th17-linked neutrophil infiltration into the gingival epithelium was observed in mice primed with the O-glycan altered *T. forsythia* ED1 strain, which

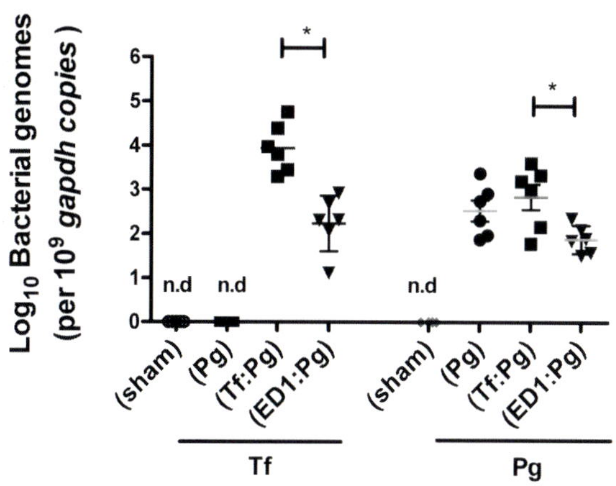

Figure 5. *P. gingivalis* persistence in the gingival tissues following priming with ED1. Bacterial loads in gingival tissues from mice were determined by quantitative PCR. Data are from one of two independent experiments with similar results (mean ± s.d. of 6 mice/group; *, $p<0.05$).

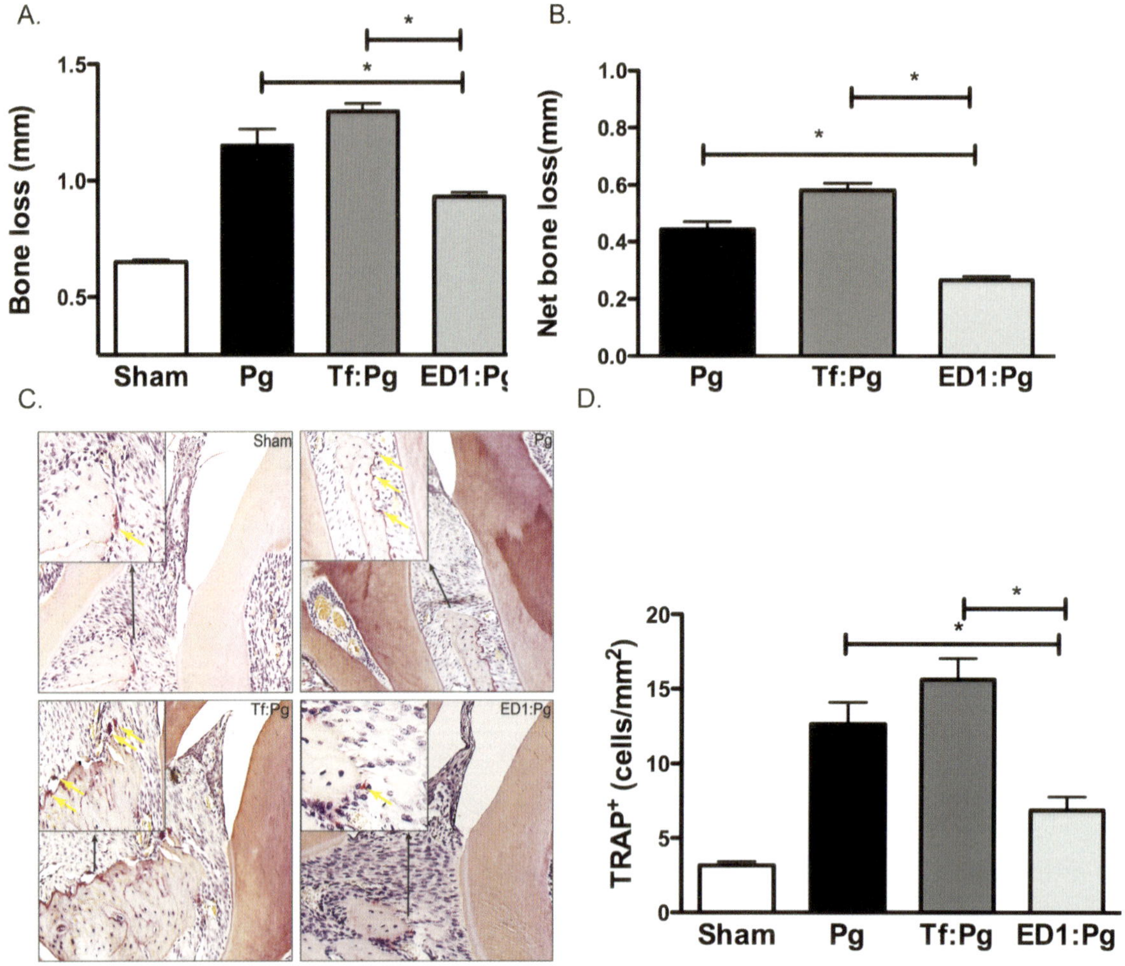

Figure 6. *P. gingivalis*-induced alveolar bone loss in mice primed with ED1. *A & B, alveolar bone levels.* A, Alveolar bone loss was assessed after 6 weeks by measuring the distance from the ABC to the CEJ at 14 maxillary buccal sites (7 sites on each side) per mouse and the total alveolar mean bone loss per group was plotted. B, Net bone loss induced by *P. gingivalis* in wild-type or ED1 primed groups was calculated as mean total ABC-CEJ distance of bacterially infected group minus mean total ABC-CEJ distance of the sham-infected group. *C & D,* osteoclastic activity measured as numbers of TRAP positive cells. C, Representative histological sections showing TRAP$^+$ cells (indicated with yellow arrows) lining the bone crest in each group. (D) Average number of TRAP$^+$ cells in 10 high power magnification fields/slide (4 mice/group). Data are from one of two independent experiments with similar results (mean $\pm$ s.d, of six mice in A & B or four mice in C & D; *, $p<0.05$).

also led to *P. gingivalis* clearance from the gingival tissues and reduced alveolar bone loss.

Here we utilized an attenuated strain of *T. forsythia* ED1 to induce a Th17 dependent neutrophil response able to clear *P. gingivalis*. ED1 lacks a trisaccharide motif consisting of a pseudaminic acid with two mannosaminuronic residues at the terminal end of an O-glycan core linked to the bacterial surface-layer proteins via serine threonine residues [8]. While the exact mechanism by which the O-glycan trisaccharide motif in *T. forsythia* modulates T cell immunity is not yet known, we envision that these O-glycans differentially regulate C-type lectin receptor(s) signaling to orchestrate the expression of T cell differentiation cytokines in dendritic cells and macrophages [1]. In general, a clear mechanistic understanding of how bacterial polysaccharides regulate T cell polarization is currently lacking because polysaccharide antigens are thought to be T cell independent antigens. However, the orchestration of T cell immunity via microbe associated glycans has been observed in other settings as well. For example surface capsular polysaccharide modified with methyl phosphoramidate in *Campylobacter jejuni* has been shown to modulate Th17 immunity against the pathogen and its persistence in the host [9]. The polysaccharide antigen (PSA) expressed by the ubiquitous human gut commensal and opportunistic pathogen *Bacteroides fragilis* down regulates Th17 differentiation and promotes IL-10-producing FoxP3$^{(+)}$ Treg cells in the gut mucosa [10–12]. Similarly, polysaccharides with immunomodulatory roles have also been identified in bacteria such as *Streptococcus pneumoniae* and *Staphylococcus aureus* type-5 and 8 [13,14].

In the gingival sulcus, neutrophils and Th17 responses play protective roles by clearing *P. gingivalis*. Neutrophils are sentinel cells of the innate immune system that keep the gingival surface free of pathogenic bacteria by forming a protective 'wall' [15,16]. At the same time, a heightened neutrophil infiltration could be detrimental to the host due to the toxic effects of neutrophil components [16,17]. Thus, the regulation of neutrophil function is critical in determining the severity and extent of periodontal inflammation. Likewise, IL-17 producing Th17 cells have been associated with both immune pathology and protection against infectious diseases. Th17 cells play an essential role in protective immunity against pathogens by coordinating early neutrophil recruitment into local sites of infection [18]. IL-17, in addition to orchestrating the chemokine cascades required for neutrophil mobilization, may also augment the killing activity of neutrophils even in the absence of pathogen opsonization with antibody or complement [19]. IL-17 driven neutrophil mobilization has been demonstrated to be critical in protection against *P. gingivalis* induced alveolar bone loss in a mouse model [20]. On the other hand, IL-17 produced byTh17 cells themselves can drive periodontal bone loss in chronic *P. gingivalis* infections [21]. In chronic settings neutrophils themselves can also become a source of IL-17, leading to IL-17-dependent inflammatory bone loss [22]. However, the complex role of IL-17 (Th17) in periodontitis remains to be determined [23]. A number of strategies that focus on exploiting host responses for the treatment of periodontitis are currently being explored. These include, but are not limited to, vaccine strategies to block *P. gingivalis* colonization [24] and targeted therapeutics modulating inflammatory cascades regulated by complement [25], glycogen synthase kinase 3β signaling [26] and T regulatory cells [27]. Bacterial S-layer proteins self-assemble *in vitro* to form nanoaggregates [28], which have been proposed as vehicles for vaccine antigen or therapeutic delivery. We envision that S-layer nanoaggregates from the ED1 strain could be directly delivered to gingival mucosa for the induction of local Th17 immunity for the eradication of *P. gingivalis*. We caution that all of the strategies described aimed at modulating host inflammatory responses require a careful analysis to weigh their associated advantages and risks. For instance anti-inflammatory therapies might lead to the colonization of pathogens such as *Candida* sp. whose colonization and virulence are kept in check via Th17 responses.

Acknowledgments

We thank Dr. Graham Stafford for critical reading of the manuscript.

Author Contributions

Conceived and designed the experiments: AS. Performed the experiments: RPS KH. Analyzed the data: RPS KH AS. Contributed to the writing of the manuscript: RPS AS.

References

1. Settem RP, Honma K, Stafford GP, Sharma A (2013) Protein-linked glycans in periodontal bacteria: prevalence and role at the immune interface. Front Microbiol 4: PMID: 24146665 (open access).
2. Sekot G, Posch G, Messner P, Matejka M, Rausch-Fan X, et al. (2011) Potential of the Tannerella forsythia S-layer to delay the immune response. J Dent Res 90: 109–114.
3. Settem RP, Honma K, Nakajima T, Phansopa C, Roy S, et al. (2012) A bacterial glycan core linked to surface (S)-layer proteins modulates host immunity through Th17 suppression. Mucosal Immunol 6: 415–426.
4. Hajishengallis G, Darveau RP, Curtis MA (2012) The keystone-pathogen hypothesis. Nat Rev Microbiol.
5. Honma K, Mishima E, Inagaki S, Sharma A (2009) The OxyR homologue in *Tannerella forsythia* regulates expression of oxidative stress responses and biofilm formation. Microbiology 155: 1912–1922.
6. Myneni SR, Settem RP, Connell TD, Keegan AD, Gaffen SL, et al. (2011) TLR2 signaling and Th2 responses drive *Tannerella forsythia*-induced periodontal bone loss. Journal of Immunology 187: 501–509.
7. Hajishengallis G, Lamont RJ (2014) Breaking bad: Manipulation of the host response by *Porphyromonas gingivalis*. Eur J Immunol 44: 328–338.
8. Posch G, Pabst M, Brecker L, Altmann F, Messner P, et al. (2011) Characterization and scope of S-layer protein O-glycosylation in *Tannerella forsythia*. J Biol Chem 286: 38714–38724.
9. Maue AC, Mohawk KL, Giles DK, Poly F, Ewing CP, et al. (2012) The polysaccharide capsule of Campylobacter jejuni 81–176 modulates the host immune response. Infect Immun.
10. Surana NK, Kasper DL (2012) The yin yang of bacterial polysaccharides: lessons learned from B. fragilis PSA. Immunol Rev 245: 13–26.
11. Ochoa-Reparaz J, Mielcarz DW, Wang Y, Begum-Haque S, Dasgupta S, et al. (2010) A polysaccharide from the human commensal Bacteroides fragilis protects against CNS demyelinating disease. Mucosal Immunol 3: 487–495.
12. Mazmanian SK, Round JL, Kasper DL (2008) A microbial symbiosis factor prevents intestinal inflammatory disease. Nature 453: 620–625.
13. Gonzalez-Fernandez A, Faro J, Fernandez C (2008) Immune responses to polysaccharides: lessons from humans and mice. Vaccine 26: 292–300.
14. Tzianabos AO, Finberg RW, Wang Y, Chan M, Onderdonk AB, et al. (2000) T cells activated by zwitterionic molecules prevent abscesses induced by pathogenic bacteria. J Biol Chem 275: 6733–6740.
15. Darveau RP (2010) Periodontitis: a polymicrobial disruption of host homeostasis. Nat Rev Microbiol 8: 481–490.
16. Scott DA, Krauss J (2012) Neutrophils in periodontal inflammation. Front Oral Biol 15: 56–83.
17. Nussbaum G, Shapira L (2011) How has neutrophil research improved our understanding of periodontal pathogenesis? Journal of Clinical Periodontology 38 Suppl 11: 49–59.
18. Curtis MM, Way SS (2009) Interleukin-17 in host defence against bacterial, mycobacterial and fungal pathogens. Immunology 126: 177–185.
19. Lu YJ, Gross J, Bogaert D, Finn A, Bagrade L, et al. (2008) Interleukin-17A mediates acquired immunity to pneumococcal colonization. PLoS Pathog 4: e1000159.
20. Yu JJ, Ruddy MJ, Wong GC, Sfintescu C, Baker PJ, et al. (2007) An essential role for IL-17 in preventing pathogen-initiated bone destruction: recruitment of neutrophils to inflamed bone requires IL-17 receptor-dependent signals. Blood 109: 3794–3802.
21. Moutsopoulos NM, Kling HM, Angelov N, Jin W, Palmer RJ, et al. (2012) *Porphyromonas gingivalis* promotes Th17 inducing pathways in chronic periodontitis. J Autoimmun 39: 294–303.
22. Hajishengallis E, Hajishengallis G (2013) Neutrophil Homeostasis and Periodontal Health in Children and Adults. J Dent Res.
23. Cheng WC, Hughes FJ, Taams LS (2014) The presence, function and regulation of IL-17 and Th17 cells in periodontitis. J Clin Periodontol.
24. Choi JI, Seymour GJ (2010) Vaccines against periodontitis: a forward-looking review. J Periodontal Implant Sci 40: 153–163.
25. Hajishengallis G, Lambris JD (2013) Complement-targeted therapeutics in periodontitis. Adv Exp Med Biol 734a: 197–206.
26. Adamowicz K, Wang H, Jotwani R, Zeller I, Potempa J, et al. (2012) Inhibition of GSK3 abolishes bacterial-induced periodontal bone loss in mice. Mol Med 18: 1190–1196.
27. Glowacki AJ, Yoshizawa S, Jhunjhunwala S, Vieira AE, Garlet GP, et al. (2013) Prevention of inflammation-mediated bone loss in murine and canine periodontal disease via recruitment of regulatory lymphocytes. Proc Natl Acad Sci U S A 110: 18525–18530.
28. Ilk N, Egelseer EM, Sleytr UB (2011) S-layer fusion proteins–construction principles and applications. Curr Opin Biotechnol 22: 824–831.

18

Artificial Neural Networks for the Diagnosis of Aggressive Periodontitis Trained by Immunologic Parameters

Georgios Papantonopoulos[1]*, Keiso Takahashi[2], Tasos Bountis[3], Bruno G. Loos[4]

1 Center for Research and Applications of Nonlinear Systems, Department of Mathematics, University of Patras, Patras, Greece, **2** Department of Conservative Dentistry, School of Dentistry, Ohu University, Fukushima, Japan, **3** Laboratory of Nonlinear Systems and Applied Analysis, Department of Mathematics, University of Patras, Patras, Greece, **4** Department of Periodontology, Academic Center for Dentistry Amsterdam (ACTA), University of Amsterdam and VU University, Amsterdam, The Netherlands

Abstract

There is neither a single clinical, microbiological, histopathological or genetic test, nor combinations of them, to discriminate aggressive periodontitis (AgP) from chronic periodontitis (CP) patients. We aimed to estimate probability density functions of clinical and immunologic datasets derived from periodontitis patients and construct artificial neural networks (ANNs) to correctly classify patients into AgP or CP class. The fit of probability distributions on the datasets was tested by the Akaike information criterion (*AIC*). ANNs were trained by cross entropy (*CE*) values estimated between probabilities of showing certain levels of immunologic parameters and a reference mode probability proposed by kernel density estimation (KDE). The weight decay regularization parameter of the ANNs was determined by 10-fold cross-validation. Possible evidence for 2 clusters of patients on cross-sectional and longitudinal bone loss measurements were revealed by KDE. Two to 7 clusters were shown on datasets of CD4/CD8 ratio, CD3, monocyte, eosinophil, neutrophil and lymphocyte counts, IL-1, IL-2, IL-4, INF-γ and TNF-α level from monocytes, antibody levels against A. *actinomycetemcomitans* (*A.a.*) and *P.gingivalis* (*P.g.*). ANNs gave 90%–98% accuracy in classifying patients into either AgP or CP. The best overall prediction was given by an ANN with *CE* of monocyte, eosinophil, neutrophil counts and CD4/CD8 ratio as inputs. ANNs can be powerful in classifying periodontitis patients into AgP or CP, when fed by *CE* values based on KDE. Therefore ANNs can be employed for accurate diagnosis of AgP or CP by using relatively simple and conveniently obtained parameters, like leukocyte counts in peripheral blood. This will allow clinicians to better adapt specific treatment protocols for their AgP and CP patients.

Editor: Ali Al-Ahmad, University Hospital of the Albert-Ludwigs-University Freiburg, Germany

Funding: The Academic Center for Dentistry Amsterdam (ACTA) (author B.G.L.) is supported in part by a grant from the University of Amsterdam for research into the focal point "Oral infections and Inflammation". This research has been co-financed by the European Union (European Social Fund, ESF) and Greek national funds through the Operational Program "Education and Lifelong Learning" of the National Strategic Reference Framework (NSRF) – Research Funding Program: THALES: Investing in knowledge society through the European Social Fund. The funders had no role in study design, data collection and analysis, decision to publish, or preparation of the manuscript.

Competing Interests: The authors have declared that no competing interests exist.

* E-mail: ppntnpls@otenet.gr

Introduction

Periodontitis is a bacterial-driven chronic inflammatory destructive disease of the tissues surrounding and supporting the dental root [1]. Severe periodontitis affects around 8.5% of the general population, while a moderate form of the disease is present in 30% and a mild form in 9% of adults aged 30 and older [2].

Periodontitis is a complex disease, where multiple causal factors simultaneously and interactively play a role. There are four main causal risk factors, i.e. the subgingival microbiota (the bacterial biofilm), individual genetic variations, life style and systemic factors [3]. It is a well-known fact that the behavior of a complex system cannot be explained by isolating its components [4]. Currently two clinical types of periodontitis are recognized; the aggressive (AgP) and the chronic (CP) form [5]. Due to the complexity of the pathogenesis of the disease, there is no single clinical, microbiological, histopathological, genetic test or combinations of them to discriminate AgP from CP patients [6].

Clinical identification of AgP cases is based on rapid attachment loss and bone destruction, the absence of systemic factors to explain this progression rate and familial aggregation [7]. Any age upper limit in discriminating AgP from CP is arbitrary. Nevertheless, given the same amount of periodontal destruction individuals with AgP are found considerably younger than CP patients. The age of 35 has been used as a cut-off point to discriminate between AgP and CP [8]. It is realized that is difficult to distinguish between the two phenotypes at the initial stages of periodontitis, thus preventing proper early clinical management of AgP, which is generally found more demanding.

Complexity is understood through modeling and simulation [4]. In a recent study [9] using cellular automata experiments, periodontitis was described as a system out of equilibrium with the level of the host immune response determining its entropy rate. In a subsequent study [10] a chaotic map was analyzed, expressed by a particular equation, which accurately models periodontitis progression in connection to the variation of the host immune response level. By renormalization arguments, two zones of disease activity were identified, a fast and a slow progressing zone, corresponding to AgP and CP respectively. Based on the above, we may now pose the hypothesis that different entropy rates might indeed reflect the presence of distinct patient clusters in immunologic and clinical datasets.

Histograms are the oldest probability density estimators [11], but suffer from certain important drawbacks; they are discontinuous and hardly appropriate for representing bivariate or trivariate data. Nonparametric kernel density estimation (KDE) methods on the other hand, reveal structure in datasets, such as skewness and multimodality that might be missed by classical parametric methods [12]. KDE is an unsupervised learning procedure that can be used for nonparametric classification tasks [13]. In general, when a desired outcome is known, a learning process is called supervised, otherwise it is unsupervised learning.

Artificial neural networks (ANNs) are considered powerful nonlinear statistical tools to model complex relationships between inputs and outputs. Therefore, they appear appropriate in searching for parameters that could achieve an accurate diagnosis of AgP or CP. ANNs consist of a set of simple units called neurons by analogy with the biological neurons [14]. Neurons are linked to each other by a weighted connection which is called synapsis, and are organized in layers: Information is fed to neurons of the input layer, and then processed in the hidden layer and finally exits to the neurons of the output layer. ANNs can be adaptive to external or internal changes and "learn" from the data entered into them. For instance, one type of ANN is the multilayer perceptron (MLP); this is a feedforward ANN trained by the backwards propagation of the error found in the outcome layer. It can be used for supervised learning classification procedures.

The first aim of this study was to estimate the probability density functions of a set of observed clinical and immunologic data in periodontitis patients. Secondly we investigated the fit of the data to various probability distribution models. Based on these findings we developed ANNs able to classify periodontitis patients belonging to either one of the two different clinical forms, aggressive or chronic form.

Materials and Methods

Study population

Data were retrieved from previous studies that provided 4 distinct patient samples. From one study [15], we obtained 29 periodontitis patients with severely advanced disease as evidenced by clinical and radiographic examination, which were clinically followed and maintained for 5 to 8 years (we designate this as sample-1). At baseline examination, they had ≥14 teeth present and at least 50% of their teeth showed bone loss of ≥50% of their root length. We used data on baseline radiographic mean bone loss and on longitudinal mean radiographic bone loss level change. From Loos et al. [16,17] studies from 76 periodontitis patients (the same group for both studies to which we will refer as sample-2) we derived datasets of total number of monocytes, lymphocytes, basophils, neutrophils and eosinophils in peripheral blood, as well as the total number of CD3, CD4, CD19 cells and the CD4/CD8 ratio. For sample-2 radiographic bone loss measurements were also available (% of teeth with bone loss of ≥50% of the tooth root length). From Graswinckel et al. [18] we used the datasets for IgA, IgM and IgG from 80 periodontitis patients (sample-3). From Takahashi et al. [19] (sample-4) we derived data of serum antibody levels in 162 periodontitis patients against *Aggregatibacter actinomycetemcomitans* (*A.a.*) (Y4 antigen), *A.a.* (ATCC 29523), *A.a.* (SUNY67), *Porphyromonas gingivalis* (*P.g.*) (FDC381), *P.g.* (SU63), *Eikenella corrodens* (*E.c.*) (ATCC 23834), *Prevotella intermedia* (*P.i.*) (ATCC 25611), *Prevotella nigrescens* (*P.i.*) (ATCC 33563), *Capnocytophaga ochracea* (*C.o.*) (S3), *Wolinella succinogens* (ATCC 29543), *Treponema Denticola* (*T.d.*) (ATCC 35405) and *Fusobacterium nucleatum* (*F.n.*) (ATCC 25586). In addition we derived data of IL-1, IL-2, IL-4, IL-6, TNF-α and INF-γ levels produced by mononuclear cells from peripheral blood.

The undefined periodontitis patients, those with adult periodontitis (AP) or those with localized (L) or generalized (G) early onset periodontitis (EOP) from the studies from which data were retrieved [16–19] were reclassified as previously described [9]. Those with an age at the time of diagnosis >35 years or originally having AP, were reclassified as CP; patients ≤35 years were classified as AgP; those with L- or G-EOP were all classified as AgP. EOP (a term used in the 1989 world workshop in clinical periodontics, preserved in the 1996 modification and changed to AgP in 1999) is considered to have its onset from puberty until 35 years [20].

Therefore from sample-2 we derived 23 AgP and 53 CP cases; from sample-3 18 AgP and 62 CP cases. For these two samples we had an exclusion of 20% of the initially recruited patients for various reasons that could affect their immunologic profile (like chronic medical disorder, pregnancy, trauma, recent tooth extraction, etc). From sample-4 we obtained 68 AgP and 43 CP cases. A group of 51 patients "suspected for EOP", was declared suspected for AgP with no definitive criteria for a final diagnosis; they had severe periodontitis and a disease history that suggested EOP, but were >35 years at the first examination and with no family members diagnosed with EOP. Patients in sample-4 were recruited as they presented at the Okayama University Dental Hospital over a period of 10 years.

Kernel density estimation

For the estimation of univariate or bivariate probability densities of the data distribution of the various parameters, an appropriate kernel function is needed [21]. The process of choosing a kernel function is described in Text S1 in File S1.

Fit of the data distributions to probability models

The fit of the available data distributions was tested in five well known probability models for continuous variables: the Normal, the Exponential, the Weibull, the Pareto and the Gamma models. They all have been extensively used and applied on biological systems [22]. A first visual appreciation of the fit was judged by quantile to quantile (Q-Q) plots. Subsequently, comparisons between models were based on the Akaike information criterion (*AIC*) [23,24], which safe-guards against overfitted models [25].

Construction of artificial neural networks

We built MLP ANNs to classify periodontitis patients. A diagram of the MLP ANN applied in this study is presented in Figure 1. It depicts the three types of layers, the input, the hidden and the output layer along with the interweaving of their neurons. We trained ANNs using cross entropy values (*CE*) [26] of immunological parameters of periodontitis patients in reference to a target probability value revealed by KDE.

The first step in the construction process was to calculate the probability $p(x)$ of demonstrating a certain level of an immunological parameter (x) in an individual patient. We used for that the cumulative probability function (cpf) of the corresponding probability model. At a second step, we computed cross entropy (*CE*) values [26] for each patient between the previously described probability $p(x)$ for selected immunologic parameters and a reference probability value, the target probability $t_{i(CP)}$. We used the formula

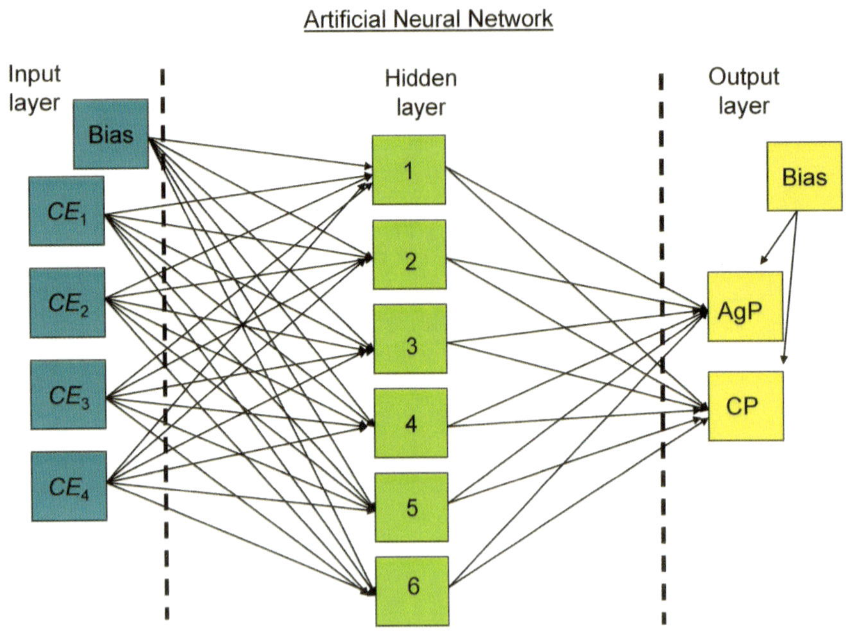

Figure 1. Multilayer perceptron feedforward neural network with error backpropagation. The information (cross entropy values of immunological parameters for each patient) is inserted in the input neurons. At the hidden layer, here with 6 neurons, we sum the information and transfer it (through the sigmoid function) to the outcome layer, where the sigmoid function exits an AgP or CP verdict. Bias neurons have a constant value and help the network to learn patterns. They are independent from other neurons and can shift the curve of the sigmoid function to the left or to the right. The classification error found at the outcome layer backpropagates in the network and synaptic weights are adapted accordingly as the network learns from its error and tries to minimize it.

$$CE_i = -\left(t_{i(CP)} \ln p(x_i)\right)$$

where i = 1, 2, ...N and N is the number of the immunological parameters (x) inserted into the ANN. CE is a nonsymmetric measure of the difference between two probability distributions. The target probability distribution $t_{i(CP)}$ was estimated by direct application of the appropriate cpf; we used the mode value of x with the highest density probability of the immunologic data distribution (indicated by KDE) as the reference point. We assumed that the highest density modes represent clusters inhabited mostly by the CP patients.

Our pruning strategy in feature selection at the input layer was based on automatic relevance determination (ARD) [27]. According to the method, features whose posterior weight distributions show low variance are discarded. The weight decay regularization parameter was determined by a 10-fold cross-validation process [28] (see text S1). If 10-fold cross validation is used for the determination of the weight decay regularization parameter, usually there is no need to use cross validation to determine the number of the hidden units [28]. We determined the number of hidden units and the maximum number of epochs by experimentation (we stopped increasing iterations when the sum of squares error stopped improving) [27,28]. Finally, since the results of the networks are sensitive to the initial weight values, we tried 10 random initial weight configurations and we computed the mean prediction rates [28]. We report the technical features of the ANNs, such as maximum number of epochs (iterations) and learning methods applied, as well as sensitivity, specificity and overall accuracy of the ANNs against the original clinical diagnosis.

Results

From 4 distinct samples we derived clinical and immunologic data and performed KDE. From sample-1 on baseline and longitudinal bone loss data KDE revealed possible evidence of two clusters of patients (Figure 2A, B). On sample-2 for the dataset of % of teeth with bone loss ≥50% of their root length, possible evidence of two main clusters was also found (Figure 2C). KDE on sample-2 revealed three to seven clusters for monocytes, basophils, neutrophils, eosinophils and lymphocytes counts (Figure 2Q, R, S, T & X) and two clusters for CD3 (Figure 2L). From sample-3, IgA and IgM data showed one mode (Figure 2V & W) while IgG data (Figure 2U) showed two clusters. From sample-4, KDE gave possible evidence of two main clusters for IL-2, IL-4, IL-6, TNF-α, INF-γ, (Figure 2D, E, F, H, J & K), and of 2 to 3 modes for antibody IgG titers against the 12 examined bacteria (graphs are shown for three of them) (Figure 2M, N & O).

Some bivariate KDE were generated. Using longitudinal bone loss data in relation to age (sample-1), we identified two clusters of patients (Figure 3A). The majority of patients clustered around the mode of 0.2 mm of longitudinal bone loss over the follow up period, while a small cluster of patients showed a mode with an almost 5 times higher value for this parameter. In the bivariate KDE of the CD4/CD8 ratio in relation to age (sample-2) (Figure 3B) or in relation to % of teeth with bone loss ≥50% of their root length (Figure 3C), two clusters at modes $x = 1.5$ and $x = 1.9$ are found.

We found the baseline and longitudinal bone loss measurements to fit to the Normal model (Table S1 in File S1). Most of the immunologic data fitted to the Gamma model (Figure S1, Table S1 in File S1). We built three ANNs with three kinds of immunologic parameters as inputs: leukocytes (ANN_1) (from sample-2), interleukins (ANN_2) and IgG antibody titers (ANN_3)

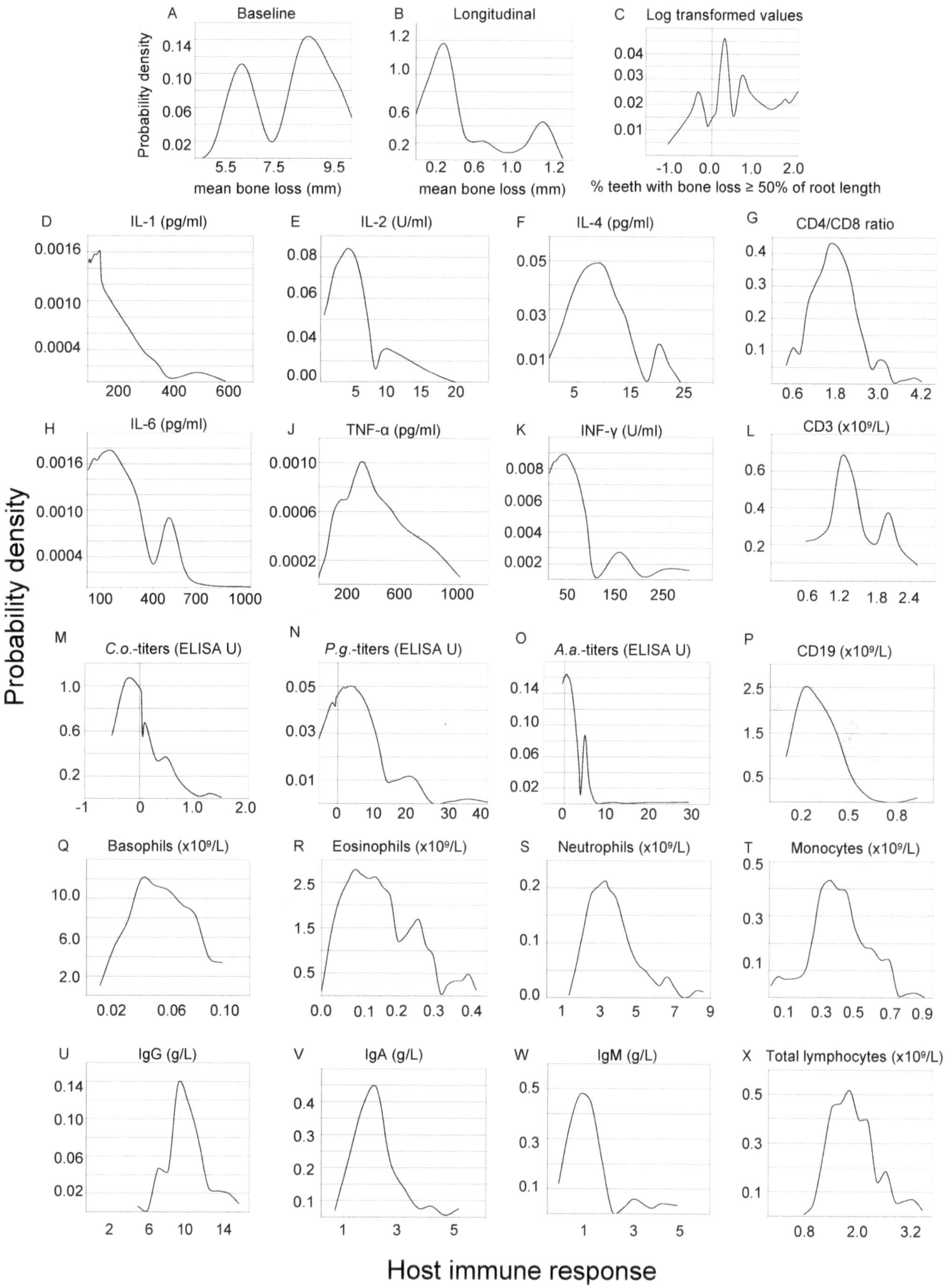
A Baseline
B Longitudinal
C Log transformed values
Probability density
mean bone loss (mm)
mean bone loss (mm)
% teeth with bone loss ≥ 50% of root length
D IL-1 (pg/ml)
E IL-2 (U/ml)
F IL-4 (pg/ml)
G CD4/CD8 ratio
H IL-6 (pg/ml)
J TNF-α (pg/ml)
K INF-γ (U/ml)
L CD3 (x10⁹/L)
M C.o.-titers (ELISA U)
N P.g.-titers (ELISA U)
O A.a.-titers (ELISA U)
P CD19 (x10⁹/L)
Q Basophils (x10⁹/L)
R Eosinophils (x10⁹/L)
S Neutrophils (x10⁹/L)
T Monocytes (x10⁹/L)
U IgG (g/L)
V IgA (g/L)
W IgM (g/L)
X Total lymphocytes (x10⁹/L)
Probability density
Host immune response

Figure 2. Univariate kernel density estimation (KDE) graphs. Graphs A to C. Univariate KDE for radiographic bone loss measurements: modes (single, bimodal or multimodal) are defined as the values that appear more frequent. Graphs A & B from sample-1. In graph C (sample-2) we log transformed the confined data to find support in the interval ($-\infty$, $+\infty$) (see text S1). Graphs D to X. Univariate KDE for immunologic data: possible evidence of multimodality for the CD4/CD8 ratio, CD3, lymphocytes, monocytes, eosinophils, basophils and neutrophils counts (sample-2), IgG levels (sample-3), IL-2, IL-4, IL-6, INF-γ, TNF-α, IgG *A.a.* titers and IgG *C.o.* titers (sample-4). Mini clusters close to each other are detected for IL-1 and IgG *P.g* titers (sample-4).

(from sample-4). We didn't mix parameters from the two samples. The results of ARD on feature selection are presented in Table S2 in File S1. ANN_1 showed high accuracy (98.1%) followed close by ANN_2 (95.6%), while ANN_3 was left behind in overall accuracy (90%) (Table 1). For comparison to the ANNs performance, we conducted canonical discriminant analysis and binary logistic regression using the above selected inputs. They both displayed inferior results compared to the ANNs (Table S3 in File S1).

Discussion

We found by KDE techniques possible evidence of two modes in radiographic bone loss and selected immunologic data. We also fitted probability models to our datasets. In training ANNs we used *CE* values instead of original data. This might seem an unnecessary complication, but the ANNs were trained far better providing higher prediction accuracy. We can only speculate on the reason for that. It might have been that the smoothing parameter in KDE fine-tuned the complexity of ANNs via a shrinking effect on weights; increasing complexity directly relates to an increasing variance of ANNs test error and poorer prediction outcome [28,29]. The nonsymmetric nature of *CE* might also have facilitated the learning process.

ANNs have been used in monitoring medical conditions, where a complex combination of changes in multiple variables is associated with the onset of a disease [30]. ANNs simulate the *tabula rasa* or clean-slate learning we find associated with biological processes [14]. ANNs using the softmax transfer function and the *CE* error function are equivalent to linear logistic regression in the hidden units [28]. However, a growing number of studies in various scientific fields indicate that ANNs provide higher prediction accuracy than multiple regression models in solving classification problems [31]. This was also shown by our results (Table S3 in File S1). We must note however, that the performance of an ANN is variable, depending on the learning method used. In fact, ANNs in supervised machine learning methodology are found to approximate any function with arbitrary accuracy. However, they are susceptible to the overfitting problem [29]. Our results indicate that ANNs can be helpful in the diagnosis of AgP in a periodontal practice, while they appear unsuitable for monitoring the general population where a test with almost 100% specificity is required.

Clustering periodontal patients to gain insight into the pathogenesis of periodontitis is not a new idea. Among the vast literature, we can distinguish a study that analysed differences among 5 groups of patients [32]; grouping was based on pocket depth (PD) and bleeding on probing scores (BOP). Using logistic regression *C. rectus* antibody titers was the best single predictor among all IgG titers of one of the 5 phenotypes and *P. gingivalis* titers found the best single predictor of other three phenotypes. The study supported the microbial specificity of periodontitis pathogenesis. However, the discontinuity of the grouping method used in the study, like in the use of histograms, translates into inefficient use of the data and causes huge difficulties when derivatives of the estimates are required. The situation can be perplexed by the combination of two parameters (PD and BOP). In contrast, KDE when used as intermediate component of another method, like in the current study, is particularly justified as an alternative to histograms.

The main body of the periodontal literature relevant to cluster analysis is based on similarities of subgingival microbiota, followed by investigation of clinical and immunologic differences among clusters. For example, hierarchical cluster analysis identified 5 groups of AgP patients of similar subgingival microbiota [33]; IL-1β/IL-10 ratio in gingival crevicular fluid (GCF) was significantly different among groups. A recent review underscored the fact that although bacteria initiate periodontitis, disease progression is multidimensional and poorly understood [34]. Our unsupervised grouping method on immunologic parameters from peripheral blood determined clusters by local maxima of the overall density function. However, one can question the validity of the *in vitro* interleukin evaluation tests. Using parameters from GCF or saliva [35] is an alternative that may enhance the prediction or generalization ability of ANNs. Our hypothesis that the host immune response level is the determinant of periodontitis disease rate [8], agrees with the recently proposed paradigm for periodontitis pathogenesis [36]; it is suggested that even the immune response level mounted at the early stage of gingivitis is the determinant factor of periodontitis progression and not the presence of specific bacteria known for their virulent properties. On this basis it becomes meaningful to use immunologic parameters by nonlinear methods to discriminate AgP from CP.

It is currently understood that for the behavior of a complex disease many components intricately and dynamically interact; the emergence of the behavior of a complex system cannot be explained by considering its contributing parts separately (the whole does not equal the sum of the parts) [4]. The biological relevance of our results can be evaluated through the above realization. A complex system is not static: it undergoes continuous scale transformations. At one scale some factors compete to each other and at another scale below or above they act in synergy. That makes it difficult to find significant differences between AgP and CP when simple comparisons are made, for example by mean values of immunologic parameters. On the other hand, ANNs start nearly linear (with weights near zero) and become nonlinear as the weights increase [28]. As they grow they learn the nonlinear patterns of the data through the backpropagation of their misclassification error. However, the problem with ANNs remains their generalization ability and overfitting is always a concern [28,29].

The limitations of the methodology used in this study should be addressed. First of all, there are no rules for determining how large a sample should be for justifying the application of ANNs. However, having larger samples would allow us to leave a portion of the patients entirely out of the training process to finally evaluate upon this portion the general performance of the models. This seems to be an objective way to test the generalization ability of the models. Secondly, regarding the ANNs design, it is better to have too many hidden units than too few. The number of hidden units varies in relation to the number of inputs and the size of the training sample, usually being in the range of 5 to 100 [28]. With too few hidden units, the model might not have enough flexibility to capture the nonlinearities in the data; with too many hidden

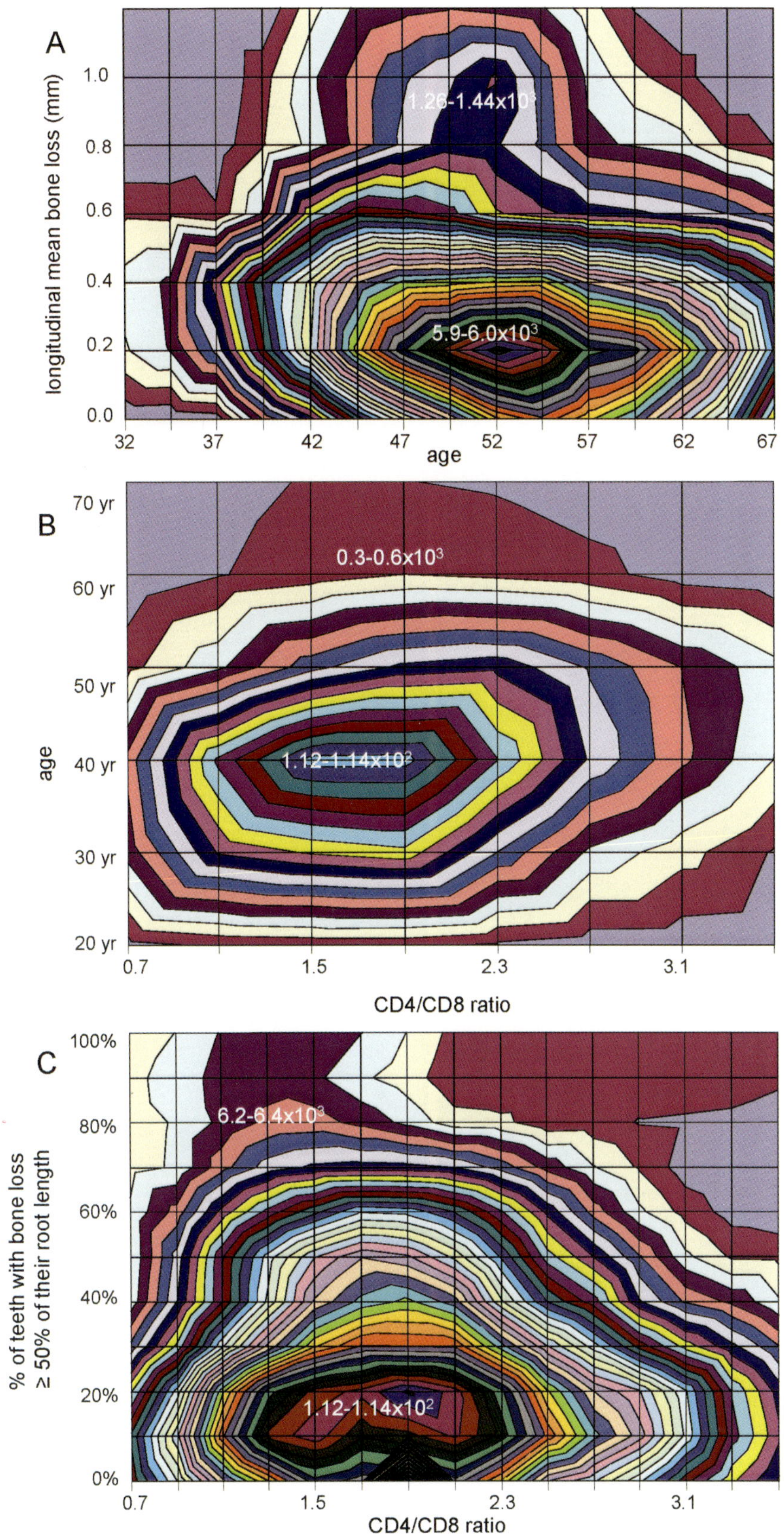

Figure 3. Bivariate kernel density estimation (KDE) for some selected parameters. (A) Contour plot for bivariate KDE of longitudinal radiographic bone loss level (sample-1) in relation to age: this topographical-like plot shows a main cluster with 0.2 mm longitudinal bone loss and a small cluster with almost five times greater bone loss. (B) Contour plot for bivariate KDE: By estimating probability density for CD4/CD8 ratio by age (sample-2), we see two clusters although not separated distinctly, at modes of 1.5 and 1.9. (C) Contour plot for bivariate KDE: By estimating

probability density for CD4/CD8 ratio (sample-2) by disease severity (% of teeth with bone loss ≥ of 50% of their root length), we reveal two distinct clusters of patients, with modes at *x* values of 1.5 and 1.9.

units the model will suffer from overfitting. Overfitting is avoided by early stopping or regularization. A common technique of regularization is to add a penalty in the error function, as we actually did (see text S1). By early stopping or by regularization we want to stop training well before we approach the global minimum, where neural networks with too many weights generally overfit the data. Third, not removing irrelevant input features would affect the classification accuracy of the network. Feature pruning typically increases the generalization ability of classifiers [29]. It is realized, however, that a variable, even though useless by itself, can be useful in combination with others [37]. Therefore, a limited set of candidate features may miss a potent combination of features. On the other hand, the variance-bias trade-off problem calls for our attention when we increase the complexity of the model. Too many features will decrease the training error by overfitting and at the same time will increase the test (generalization) error [28].

The diagnostic criteria for AgP and CP were different among the 4 patient groups used for this study. One sample [15] was selected on the basis of the presence of severe periodontitis with no discrimination of AgP or CP. The sole criterion of disease severity was obviously inadequate to predict the future behaviour of all patients. A small subgroup of patients showed a 5 times higher rate of longitudinal bone loss than the main cluster of patients (Figure 3A). This is definitely a group of patients with aggressive disease behavior. Takahashi's group [19] used the current classification scheme [5]; however, discrimination of AgP and CP was as much as possible precise, resulting in a group of "suspected" for AgP patients, which contributed to KDE but was not used in ANNs. The other two samples used in this study suffered of a crude method in designating patients into the AgP or CP group. Obviously one can argue why we should concern ourselves for a complicated method while by taking the age of 35 as a cutoff point, one has a classification [38]. However we demonstrated that even in "noisy" samples (some AgP cases are declared CP and vice versa) a host immune classifier can work with arbitrary accuracy. We assume this kind of noise is present even with the established criteria for AgP diagnosis [5]. Recently a

Table 1. Characteristics of three artificial neural networks (ANN) built on immunological parameters.

Input neurons	Network's description	Results[f]
ANN_1		
CE[a] values of	#[o] of hidden layers = 1,	Sensitivity = 98,6%,
1. CD4/CD8[b]	# of neurons in hidden layer = 9,	Specificity = 97.9%
2. Neutrophils	max. # of epochs[c] = 900,	Accuracy = 98.1%
3. Monocytes	weight decay regularization parameter[d] = 0.0001,	
4. Eosinophils	learning method = batch[e], gradient descent.	
ANN_2		
CE values of	# of hidden layers = 1,	Sensitivity = 92.3%,
1. IL-1[g]	# of neurons in hidden layer = 10,	Specificity = 96.9%
2. IL-4	max. # of epochs = 800,	Accuracy = 95.6%
3. IFN-γ[h]	weight decay regularization parameter = 0.0005,	
4. TNF-α[i]	learning method = batch, gradient descent.	
ANN_3		
CE values of	# of hidden layers = 1,	Sensitivity = 91.1%,
1. *A.a.*[k] titers	# of neurons in hidden layer = 10,	Specificity = 89.4%
2. *P.g.*[l] titers	max. # of epochs = 1000,	Accuracy = 90.0%
3. *C.o.*[m] titers	weight decay regularization parameter = 0.005,	
4. *F.n.*[n] titers	learning method = batch, gradient descent.	

[a]CE = Cross entropy. Feature selection by automatic relevance determination.
[b]CD = cluster of differentiation.
[c]epoch = iteration.
[d]Determined by 10-fold cross validation.
[e]Batch training passes all input data before updating the synaptic weights.
[f]The mean values of 10 random configurations of initial weights are reported (mean values of sensitivity, specificity and overall accuracy of the ANNs against the original clinical diagnosis).
[g]IL = interleukin.
[h]INF = interferon.
[i]TNF = tumor necrosis factor.
[k]*A.a.* = *Aggregatibacter actinomycetemcomitans*(Y4 antigen).
[l]*P.g.* = *Porphyromonas gingivalis*(FDC381 antigen).
[m]*C.o.* = *Capnocytophaga ochracea.*
[n]*F.n.* = *Fusobacterium nucleatum.*
[o]# = Number.

study using a transcriptome classifier with four supervised learning methods reported good prediction results by one of the four; AgP or CP diagnosis was strictly made by the established criteria [39]. The authors suggested possible heterogeneity within the AgP and CP classes based on the variability of the results of the four methods. The combined use of unsupervised with supervised learning methods can be an attempt to reduce true misclassification error [28]. We realize that the AgP diagnostic criteria for the patients of sample-2 limit the generalization ability of the ANN results based on it.

In conclusion, we demonstrated by KDE methods possible evidence of two clusters on clinical and most immunological data from periodontitis patients. By the use of ANNs we can effectively classify periodontitis patients by their immune response profile into the AgP or CP class. We anticipate that future work on bigger samples extending the results of the present study and employing a wider array of parameters can turn personalized treatment of periodontitis from concept to reality.

Supporting Information

File S1 This file includes the following: Text S1. Selection of a kernel function; Fitting clinical datasets to probability models; Constructing multilayer perceptron neural networks. **Table S1.** The fit of probability distribution models to clinical and immunological data. **Table S2.** Input feature selection by automatic relevance determination. **Table S3.** Comparison of two multivariate analyses to artificial neural networks.

Figure S1 An example of quantile to quantile plots.

Author Contributions

Conceived and designed the experiments: GP BGL. Performed the experiments: GP BGL KT. Analyzed the data: GP TB. Contributed reagents/materials/analysis tools: BGL KT. Wrote the paper: GP BGL TB.

References

1. Kinane DF, Berglund T, Lindhe J (2008) Pathogenesis of periodontitis. In: Lindhe J, Karring T, Lang NP, editors. Clinical Periodontology and Implant Dentistry. Blackwell Munksgaard: Oxford. pp. 285–306.
2. Eke PI, Dye BA, Wei L, Thornton-Evans GO, Genco RJ (2012) Prevalence of periodontitis in adults in the United States: 2009 and 2010. J Dent Res 91:914–920.
3. Laine ML, Crielaard W, Loos BG (2012) Genetic susceptibility to periodontitis. Periodontol 2000 58:37–68.
4. Nicolis G, Nicolis C (2012) Foundations of complex systems: emergence, information and prediction. World Scientific: Singapore. 12 p.
5. Armitage GC (1999) Developement of a classification system for periodontal diseases and conditions. Ann Periodontol 4:1–6.
6. Armitage GC (2013) Learned and unlearned concepts in periodontal diagnostics: a 50-year perspective. Periodontol 2000 62:20–36.
7. Tonetti MS, Mombelli A (2008) Aggressive periodontitis. In: Lindhe J, Karring T, Lang NP, editors. Clinical Periodontology and Implant Dentistry. Blackwell Munksgaard: Oxford. pp. 428–458.
8. Armitage GC, Cullinan MP (2010) Comparison of the clinical features of chronic and aggressive periodontitis. Periodontol 2000 53:12–27.
9. Papantonopoulos G, Takahashi K, Bountis T, Loos BG (2013a) Using cellular automata experiments to model periodontitis: A first step towards understanding the nonlinear dynamics of the disease. Int J Bifurcation Chaos 23:1350056.
10. Papantonopoulos G, Takahashi K, Bountis T, Loos BG (2013b) Mathematical modeling suggests periodontitis behaves as a nonlinear chaotic dynamical process. J Periodontol 84(10):e29–e39.
11. Silverman BW (1986) Density estimation for statistics and data analysis. Chapman and Hall: London. 6 p.
12. Simonoff JS (1996) Smoothing methods in statistics. New York: Springer-Verlag: New York. 13 p.
13. Sheather SJ (2004) Density estimation. Stat Science 19:588–597.
14. Abdi H (2003) Neural networks. In: Lewis-Beck M, Bryman A, Futing T, editors. Encyclopaedia of Social Sciences Research Methods. Sage: Thousand Oaks (CA). pp. 725–729.
15. Papantonopoulos G (2004) Effect of periodontal therapy in smokers and nonsmokers with advanced periodontal disease: Results after maintenance therapy for a minimum of 5 years. J Periodontol 75:839–843.
16. Loos BG, Craandijk J, Hoek FJ, Wertheim-van Dillen PME, van der Velden U (2000) Elevation of systemic markers related to cardiovascular diseases in the peripheral blood of periodontitis patients. J Periodontol 71:1528–1534.
17. Loos BG, Roos MT, Schellekens PT, van der Velden U, Miedema F (2004) Lymphocyte number and function in relation to periodontitis and smoking. J Periodontol 75:557–564.
18. Graswinckel JEM, van der Velden U,van Winkelhoff AJ, Hoek FJ, Loos BG (2004) Plasma antibody levels in periodontitis patients and controls. J Clin Periodontol 31:562–568.
19. Takahashi K, Ohyama H, Kitanaka M, Sawa T, Mineshiba J, et al. (2001) Heterogeneity of host immunological risk factors in patients with aggressive periodontitis. J Periodontol 72:425–437.
20. Kinane DF (2001) Periodontal disease in children and adolescents: introduction and classification. Periodontol 2000 26:7–15.
21. Hall P, Kang KH (2005) Bandwidth choice for nonparametric classification. Ann Statist 33:284–306.
22. Vose D (2008) Risk analysis: A quantitative guide. West Sussex: John Wiley & Sons. 115 p.
23. Sakamoto Y, Ishikuro M, Kitaqawa G (1986) Akaike information criterion statistics. Springer-Verlag: New York. 56 p.
24. Myung J (2003) Tutorial on maximum likelihood estimation. J Math Psychol 47:90–100.
25. Burnham KP, Anderson DR (2004) Multimodel inference: understanding AIC and BIC in model selection. Sociol Methods Res 33:261–304.
26. de Boer PT, Kroese DP, Mannor S, Rubinstein RY (2005) A tutorial on the cross-entropy method. Ann Oper Res 134:18–67.
27. Neal R, Zhang J (2006) High dimensional classification with bayesian neural networks and dirichlet diffusion trees. In: Guyon I, Gunn S, Nikravesh M, Zadeh L, editors. Feature Extraction, Foundations and Applications. Springer: New York. pp. 265–296.
28. Hastie T, Tibshirani R, Friedman J (2009) The elements of statistical learning: Data mining, inference, and prediction. Springer: New York. 389 p.
29. Zhang GP (2000) Neural networks for classification: A survey. IEEE Trans Syst Man Cybern 30:451–462.
30. Mazurowski MA, Habas PA, Zurada JM, Lo JY, Baker JA, et al. (2008) Training neural network classifiers for medical decision making; The effects of imbalanced datasets on classification performance. Neural Netw 21:427–436.
31. Shi H-Y, Lee K-T, Lee H-H, Ho W-H, Sun D-P, et al. (2012) Comparison of artificial neural network and logistic regression models for predicting in-hospital mortality after primary liver cancer surgery. PLOS ONE 7(4):e35781.
32. Offenbacher S, Barros SP, Singer RE, Moss K, Williams RC, et al. (2007) Periodontal disease at the biofilm-gingival interface. J Periodontol 78:1911–1925.
33. Teles RP, Gursky LC, Faveri M, Rosa EA, Teles FRF, et al. (2010) Relationships between subgingival microbiota and GCF biomarkers in generalized aggressive periodontitis. J Clin Periodontol 37: 313–323.
34. Razzouk S, Termechi O (2013) Host genome, epigenome, and oral microbiome interactions: towards personalized periodontal therapy. J Periodontol 84:1266–1271.
35. Loos BG, Tjoa S (2005) Host-derived diagnostic markers for periodontitis: do they exist in gingival crevicular fluid? Periodontol 2000 39:53–72.
36. Bartold PM, Van Dyke E (2013) Periodontitis: a host-mediated disruption of microbial homeostasis. Unlearning learned concepts. Periodontol 2000 62:203–217.
37. Guyon I, Elisseeff A (2003) An introduction to variable and feature selection. J Mach Learn Res 3:1157–1182.
38. Van der Velden U (2005) Purpose and problems of periodontal disease classification. Periodontol 2000 39:13–21.
39. Kebschull M, Guarnieri P, Demmer RT, Boulesteix AL, Pavlidis P, et al. (2013) Molecular Differences between Chronic and Aggressive Periodontitis. J Dent Res 92:1081–1088.

Global Metabolomic Analysis of Human Saliva and Plasma from Healthy and Diabetic Subjects, with and without Periodontal Disease

Virginia M. Barnes[1], Adam D. Kennedy[3], Fotinos Panagakos[1], William Devizio[1], Harsh M. Trivedi[1], Thomas Jönsson[3], Lining Guo[3], Shannon Cervi[2], Frank A. Scannapieco[2]*

1 Colgate Palmolive Technology Center, Piscataway, NJ, United States of America, **2** Metabolon, Durham, NC, United States of America, **3** Department of Oral Biology, School of Dental Medicine, University at Buffalo, State University of New York, Buffalo, NY, United States of America

Abstract

Recent studies suggest that periodontal disease and type 2 diabetes mellitus are bi-directionally associated. Identification of a molecular signature for periodontitis using unbiased metabolic profiling could allow identification of biomarkers to assist in the diagnosis and monitoring of both diabetes and periodontal disease. This cross-sectional study identified plasma and salivary metabolic products associated with periodontitis and/or diabetes in order to discover biomarkers that may differentiate or demonstrate an interaction of these diseases. Saliva and plasma samples were analyzed from 161 diabetic and non-diabetic human subjects with a healthy periodontium, gingivitis and periodontitis. Metabolite profiling was performed using Metabolon's platform technology. A total of 772 metabolites were found in plasma and 475 in saliva. Diabetics had significantly higher levels of glucose and α-hydroxybutyrate, the established markers of diabetes, for all periodontal groups of subjects. Comparison of healthy, gingivitis and periodontitis saliva samples within the non-diabetic group confirmed findings from previous studies that included increased levels of markers of cellular energetic stress, increased purine degradation and glutathione metabolism through increased levels of oxidized glutathione and cysteine-glutathione disulfide, markers of oxidative stress, including increased purine degradation metabolites (e.g. guanosine and inosine), increased amino acid levels suggesting protein degradation, and increased ω-3 (docosapentaenoate) and ω-6 fatty acid (linoleate and arachidonate) signatures. Differences in saliva between diabetic and non-diabetic cohorts showed altered signatures of carbohydrate, lipid and oxidative stress exist in the diabetic samples. Global untargeted metabolic profiling of human saliva in diabetics replicated the metabolite signature of periodontal disease progression in non-diabetic patients and revealed unique metabolic signatures associated with periodontal disease in diabetics. The metabolites identified in this study that discriminated the periodontal groups may be useful for developing diagnostics and therapeutics tailored to the diabetic population.

Editor: Özlem Yilmaz, University of Florida, United States of America

Funding: This study was funded by a grant from Colgate Palmolive Co. The funder and Metabolon provided support in the form of salaries for authors VMB, FP, WD, HMT, and TJ, LG, ADK respectively, but did not have any additional role in the study design, data collection and analysis, decision to publish, or preparation of the manuscript. The specific roles of these authors are articulated in the "author contributions" section.

Competing Interests: This research was supported by Colgate Palmolive Co. VMB, FP, WD, and HMT are employed by Colgate. Other authors (TJ, LG, and ADK) are employed by Metabolon, a commercial company specializing in metabolomic analysis. Both Metabolon and the University at Buffalo (FAS and SC) received funding from Colgate Palmolive to complete these studies. There are no patents, products in development, or marketed products to declare.

* Email: fas1@buffalo.edu

Introduction

Periodontal disease is a chronic bacterial infection causing persistent gingival inflammation, and in some cases connective tissue destruction and bone resorption around the teeth. It is also characterized by pocket formation and recession. Although advances in dental care has resulted in improved periodontal status in certain populations, disparities persist as severe periodontitis is often found to be exaggerated in certain segments of the population, for example those from a low socio-economic background [1]. It is well known that bacteria colonize the teeth to form a biofilm, called dental plaque, which initiates gingivitis, and sometimes progresses to periodontitis. Release of bacterial products from the biofilm induces local inflammation. Without treatment, periodontal tissue destruction, bone resorption and tooth loss may ensue [1]. Periodontal disease also has been associated with several systemic diseases, including cardiovascular disease, diabetes mellitus, respiratory disease, rheumatoid arthritis, chronic kidney disease, and adverse pregnancy outcomes [2–6].

The gingival epithelium forms a crevice around each tooth that provides a protected space for bacterial colonization and proliferation [7–10]. Analysis of gingival crevicular fluid (GCF) [11] and saliva [12–14] from periodontal patients has identified a variety of inflammatory mediators and tissue-destructive molecules, including metalloproteinases [15–23] and metabolic signatures associated with host-bacterial interactions to be elevated when compared to periodontally health patients.

Diabetic patients have a high prevalence of gingivitis, periodontitis, oral candidiasis, and xerostomia, and the severity of these diseases are correlated with the duration of diabetes and degree of glycemic control [24,25]. Poor glycemic control has been shown to be associated with poor periodontal health, of which the molecular signatures may be monitored using modern "omics" -based methods [26–30].

Saliva is a complex secretory fluid that contains trace metals, metabolites, biochemicals, proteins, glycoproteins, lipds, etc., that serve a spectrum of physiological needs. Saliva is a critical source of tissue lubricants, tooth mineralizing factors, acid buffers, toxin neutralizers, and antimicrobial components [31–35]. The ability to use saliva to evaluate physiological conditions, follow disease progression, and monitor post-treatment therapeutic results through noninvasive methods is an important objective for healthcare in general and periodontology in particular. We have previously performed a series of untargeted global metabolomic profiling tests of GCF and saliva samples from subjects with healthy gingiva, gingivitis, and periodontitis that have suggested a rigorous set of potential biomarkers for monitoring periodontal disease status and examining the effectiveness of oral care treatment that resolves the metabolic signature of inflammation [11,12,36,37]. Many metabolites associated with inflammation, oxidative stress, tissue degradation, and bacterial metabolism were found to be significantly elevated in periodontal disease and reduced by treatment [37]. Validation of such biomarkers will provide an objective phenotype to allow practitioners to diagnose disease, monitor patient disease activity and determine the effectiveness of treatment.

Metabolomic profiling is a rapidly evolving technology that has been increasingly used to discover early markers of disease [11,12,37–40]. Whole saliva can be easily collected through noninvasive means and has considerable potential to monitor general health and disease status. With the advancement of technological means such as metabolomics, saliva can be leveraged as a clinical and diagnostic tool because of its potential to mirror oral and systemic health conditions [41–45]. To this end, metabolomic signatures were determined in saliva and compared to those in plasma from orally healthy subjects and periodontal subjects, with and without type 2 diabetes, in an effort to identify unique metabolomic profiles and biomarkers of periodontal disease in both systemic health and diabetes. Based on our previous results from biomarker identification of periodontal disease progression [11,12,37], we performed a discovery study to identify biomarkers of decreased periodontal health as monitored by biochemical profiling of saliva and plasma collected from orally healthy subjects and those with gingivitis and periodontitis using an unbiased metabolomic profiling approach based on liquid and gas chromatography/mass spectrometry (LC/MS and GC/MS).

Materials, Participants, and Methods

Experimental Design and Participants

This cross-sectional clinical study enrolled adult male and female subjects from the Buffalo, New York area and was conducted in accordance with the Helsinki Declaration. The Institutional Review Board at the University at Buffalo approved the protocol (ORB0650111E), including the clinical examination, collection of saliva and plasma samples. All subjects read and signed a written informed consent before their enrollment into the study. The inclusion criteria were: age between 18 and 65 years, in good general health (n = 81), or subjects diagnosed with diabetes (n = 80); and a minimum of 20 natural teeth (excluding third molars) present. Exclusion criteria included: inability or unwillingness to sign the informed consent form, diagnosis of a medical condition which required pre-medication prior to dental visits/procedures, 5 or more decayed untreated teeth at screening (cavities), diagnosis of other diseases of the hard or soft oral tissues, impaired salivary function, use of antibiotics or antimicrobial drugs within 30 days prior to the first study visit, a history of uncharacterized systemic disease, pregnant or nursing women, participation in any other clinical study within 1 week prior to enrollment into this study, present use of tobacco products, subjects who required dental treatment during the duration of the study, immune compromised individuals (e.g. those diagnosed with HIV, AIDS, or taking immunosuppressive drug therapy), or subjects who received periodontal treatment within the previous 30 days.

Subjects were evaluated by a single dental examiner (SC) for inclusion/exclusion criteria. At the first visit, participants received a tube of standard, non-anti-microbial fluoridated toothpaste with instructions for use, in order to minimize variations in results that might be driven by the use of different toothpastes. A fasting blood sample was then collected from subjects self-identifying as diabetic to confirm diabetic status. During the second visit, subjects gave an update on their medical and medication history, contributed saliva and blood samples, had an assessment of their oral tissues to assess periodontal status, to monitor adverse events since the first visit and answer questions regarding their compliance as to the use of the standard toothpaste. A minimum of 0.5 ml of unstimulated saliva and 10 ml of blood was collected. Subjects were asked to refrain from eating or drinking (excluding water) from 11:00 PM the previous night; to brush their teeth and entire mouth the evening before the saliva donation, but not the morning of collection. Blood samples were obtained after collection of the saliva. Saliva was collected into sterile polypropylene tubes and immediately frozen in a dry ice bath and stored at −80 degrees C until shipped to Metabolon. No preservatives were added to the saliva samples

Definition of oral status groups

Within the diabetic or non-diabetic cohorts, three sub-groups were established: periodontal health, gingivitis and periodontitis. Subjects were stratified according to the gingivitis index: Healthy: These subjects had an average full mouth Modified Gingival Index (MGI) [46] score below 1.0, with fewer than 3 bleeding on probing (BOP) sites and minimal dental plaque present as scored by the method of Sillness and Lõe [47]. Gingivitis: These subjects had an average full mouth MGI score between 1 and 2 with multiple BOP sites and periodontal pockets <4 mm. Periodontitis: These subjects had an average full mouth MGI of 2.0 or greater with multiple BOP sites, and 2 or more periodontal pockets with probing depths of 5 mm or more in at least two quadrants. Plaque at any level was present. Measurement of oral indices was performed as per Lobene et al. [46] as follows: 0 = normal, 1 = mild inflammation of the gingival unit (slight change in color, little change in texture of any portion of the gingival unit), 2 = mild inflammation of the entire gingival unit, 3 = moderate inflammation (moderate change in texture, redness, edema and hypertrophy of the gingival unit, 4 = severe inflammation (marked redness and edema/hypertrophy, spontaneous bleeding or ulceration) of the gingival unit. Plaque indices were assessed for 6 surfaces on each tooth and the plaque index score was the average of the scores obtained from all teeth. The amount of plaque observed on each tooth was scored 0 to 3 as follows: 0 = no plaque notes; 1 = plaque seen only on the tip of an explorer passed over the tooth surface;

Table 1. Sample Size of Study Groups.

	Healthy	Gingivitis	Periodontal	Totals
Diabetic	28	27	26	**81**
Non-Diabetic	25	26	29	**80**
Totals	**53**	**53**	**55**	**161**

2 – plaque obvious with the naked eye; 3 = gross deposits of plaque present over the entire tooth.

Systemic Health Selection Criteria/Assessment for Diabetes Status

For this study, diabetes status was established by self-reported history. Subjects who reported a history of diabetes were asked to confirm diabetic status by providing blood samples to measure HbA1c values. An individual was defined with Type 2 diabetes if hemoglobin A1C≥6.5%. Due to financial limitations, HbA1c levels were not assessed for those not reporting a history of diabetes. As a recent study suggested, the prevalence of diabetes (as measured by HbA1c>6.4) is likely low (extrapolated to be 5.0% with diabetes and 9.5% with pre-diabetes) in dental patients unaware of their diabetes status [48], we assumed that the prevalence of diabetes in the non-diabetes subject in this study would be similar and therefore not compromise the analysis.

Saliva and Plasma Sample Collection

Saliva was collected in 50 mL polypropylene tubes and plasma was collected in Vacutainer tubes and anti-coagulated with EDTA. Samples were immediately frozen in a dry ice bath and stored at −80°C.

Metabolomic Profiling Technology

Metabolomic profiling was performed as described previously [12,49]. In summary, after the extraction of metabolites from each sample, the extracts were analyzed by GC/MS and LC/MS. We carried out chromatographic separation, followed by full-scan mass spectroscopy, to record and quantify all detectable ions presented in the samples [50]. We identified metabolites with

Table 2. Demographics of Study Subjects.

Healthy n = 53		
	Non DM	**DM**
Total	**28**	**25**
Male	9	14
Female	19	11
Mean Age	37.5 (15.2)	50.2 (11.0)
Mean BMI	26.1 (4.2)	33.6 (9.9)
Mean HbA1C*	no data	7.1 (1.1)
Gingivitis n = 53		
	Non DM	**DM**
Total	**27**	**26**
Male	11	10
Female	16	16
Mean Age	35.9 (12.0)	53.8 (7.5)
Mean BMI	26.9 (5.7)	33.1 (7.6)
Mean HbA1C	no data	7.2 (1.5)
Periodontal n = 55		
	Non DM	**DM**
Total	**26**	**29**
Male	11	19
Female	15	10
Mean Age	49.7 (10.8)	54.5 (6.8)
Mean BMI	30.3 (6.0)	32.8 (7.9)
Mean HbA1C	no data	7.7 (1.9)

*HbA1c testing was done on purported diabetic subjects only.

Table 3. Overall statistical analysis of saliva and plasma samples from the healthy periodontal cohorts.

Summary of Altered Metabolites	*t*-Test Saliva (Diabetic vs. Non-diabetic)	*t*-Test Plasma (Diabetic vs. Non-diabetic)
Total number of comparisons $p \leq 0.05$	69	174
Biochemical direction of change	66 ↑/3 ↓*	115 ↑/59 ↓**

*66 metabolites were increased in saliva from subjects with diabetes, 3 metabolites were increased in saliva from non-diabetic subjects.
**115 metabolites were increased in plasma from subjects with diabetes, 59 metabolites were increased in plasma from non-diabetic subjects.

known chemical structure by matching the ions' chromatographic retention index and mass spectral fragmentation signatures with reference library entries created from authentic standard metabolites under the identical analytical procedure as the experimental samples [51]. For ions that were not covered by the standards, additional library entries were added based on their unique ion signatures (chromatographic and mass spectral). After this, these ions could be routinely detected and quantified.

Statistical Analysis

After normalization and imputation, the data were log-transformed. We then performed ANOVA and *t* tests to compare data obtained from the healthy, gingivitis, and periodontitis samples. Multiple comparisons were accounted for with the false discovery (FDR) rate method, and each FDR was estimated by *q*-values.

Results

A total of 174 subjects were enrolled in this study (Table 1). The mean age of the non-diabetic subjects tended to be younger than the diabetic subjects (Table 2). Diabetic subjects had a higher BMI for all groups (Table 2). HbA1C testing confirmed diabetic status of the subjects self-reporting as diabetic.

An untargeted metabolomic profiling approach was used to assess the chemical milieu of saliva and plasma. In total, 161 individual saliva samples were collected, 80 from subjects with diabetes and 81 from subjects without diabetes. We detected 475 and 772 metabolites in saliva and plasma, respectively, of which 370 and 430 could be mapped to known chemical structures (Tables S1 and S2).

Characterization of Diabetic and Non-Diabetic Samples

Welch's two sample *t* tests and ANOVA identified statistically significant differences in these saliva samples between non-diabetic subjects and those with diabetes. Approximately 14% of the detected metabolites (69 of 475) in saliva showed altered levels ($p \leq 0.05$) among the healthy samples when compared to the diabetic cohort, suggesting that these may be markers of diabetic status in humans (Table 3). Alternatively, comparison of the plasma from the same subjects resulted in 174 statistically significant changes. ANOVA analysis with either matrix did not produce a list of metabolites largely different from the *t* tests (data not shown).

Glycemic control can be monitored by changes in 1,5-anhydroglucitol (1,5-AG). 1,5-AG is reabsorbed in the renal tubules, a process competitively inhibited by glucosuria, which leads to a reduction in its level in plasma. Thus, the greater the degree of glucosuria, the lower the amount of 1,5-AG present in the plasma [52–54]. The correlation between this reduction and the amount of glucose present in urine is so close that 1,5-AG represents a sensitive, real-time marker of glycemic control [55]. Thus, elevations of 1,5-AG in plasma are highly indicative of reduced glucosuria as a consequence of improved glycemic control. Not surprisingly, subjects with diabetes had significantly lower 1,5-AG and significantly higher levels of glucose in their plasma (Table 4). Additionally, diabetic subjects had significantly lower 1,5-AG in their saliva for all periodontal disease groups and higher levels of glucose in their saliva (Table 4). These observations lend confidence to the appropriateness of the control group, which was based on self-report of diabetes. None of the non-diabetic subjects had metformin in their plasma or saliva (data not shown).

α-hydroxybutyrate (AHB) is an early marker for insulin resistance in humans [52] as it arises from states of lactic and ketoacidosis or disrupted energy metabolism [56–61]. AHB levels were increased significantly in the diabetic cohort in plasma (Table 4) and were increased significantly in saliva in the healthy and gingivitis cohorts (data not shown). This may be a reflection of the increased energetic stress induced by the infection during the development of periodontitis or a translation of insulin resistance markers to saliva.

High-Level Characterization of Diabetic and Non-Diabetic Periodontal Cohorts

The analysis of each periodontal cohort (diabetic and non-diabetic) separately resulted in the identification of several

Table 4. Relative levels of biochemicals linked to diabetic status in saliva and plasma*.

Matrix	Biochemical Name	Fold Change (Diabetc/Non-diabetic)	P value	Q value
Saliva	1-5 anhydroglucitol (1,5-AG)	0.93	0.0417	0.3041
	Glucose	2.66	0.0074	0.2228
	α-hydroxybutyrate (AHB)	2.14	0.0009	0.0958
Plasma	1-5 anhydroglucitol (1,5-AG)	0.61	0.0007	0.0168
	Glucose	1.35	9.46×10^{-6}	0.0009
	α-hydroxybutyrate (AHB)	1.59	0.0012	0.0255

*Metformin was not detected in any of the non-diabetic samples.

Table 5. Overall statistical analysis of saliva samples comparing periodontal cohorts from diabetics and non-diabetics.

Summary of Altered Biochemicals	*t*-Test Saliva (Diabetic Gingivitis vs. Diabetic Healthy)	*t*-Test Saliva (Diabetic Periodontitis vs. Diabetic Healthy)	*t*-Test Saliva (Non-diabetic gingivitis vs. Non-diabetic Healthy)	*t*-Test Saliva (Non-diabetic periodontitis vs. Non-diabetic Healthy)
Total number of comparisons $p \leq 0.05$	35	54	20	64
Biochemical direction of change	25 ↑/10 ↓*	12 ↑/42 ↓**	17 ↑/3 ↓***	62 ↑/2 ↓****

*25 metabolites were increased in saliva from subjects with gingivitis, 10 metabolites were increased in saliva from diabetic, non-gingivitis subjects.
**12 metabolites were increased in saliva from diabetic subjects with periodontitis, 42 metabolites were increased in saliva from diabetic, periodontally healthy subjects.
***17 metabolites were increased in saliva from non-diabetic gingivitis subjects without diabetes, 3 metabolites were increased in saliva from non-diabetic, periodontally healthy subjects.
****62 metabolites were increased in saliva from non-diabetic periodontitis subjects, 2 metabolites were increased in saliva from non-diabetic, periodontally healthy subjects.

metabolites that were associated with the progression of gingival status (Table 5). The most striking find in the study was the direction of change in the periodontitis samples in the diabetic cohort. In the non-diabetic cohort, metabolites increased in abundance through disease progression, whereas many biochemicals increased in abundance when comparing the healthy to gingivitis groups, but then decreased in abundance in the diabetic subjects with periodontal disease suggesting an interaction between the diabetes signature and the periodontal signature.

Both periodontal status and diabetes status of the subjects were major driving factors in the biochemical changes observed. For the majority of metabolites with altered concentrations in the non-diabetic cohort, the levels at gingivitis samples were found to be intermediate between those levels found in healthy and periodontitis samples (Table S1). This suggests that the metabolic changes induced by gingivitis are a continuum of those of periodontitis.

Analysis of the Non-Diabetic Saliva Samples

Barnes et al. found differences in the biochemical signatures in saliva between non-diabetic subjects with healthy gingiva or periodontitis [12]. This report showed increased levels of metabolites in the saliva of the periodontal population reflecting enhanced degradation of macromolecules, including proteins, lipids, nucleotides and polysaccharides. Comparison of the non-diabetic cohort from the current study with these previous studies showed similar results (Table 6). This metabolic signature, which includes elevated levels of ω-6 fatty acids, is indicative of a hyper-inflammatory environment resulting from chronic bacterial infection and further support for increased macromolecular degradation of the periodontal tissues resulting from inflammation. Several metabolic signatures supported the notion that a more diverse and active microbial flora accompanied the inflammatory response resulting in gingivitis and periodontitis. Aromatic amino acid metabolites likely derived from bacteria were increased in periodontitis samples (Table 6). Moreover, carnitine, which is often the sole source of carbon and nitrogen for bacteria, was also elevated. Periodontal saliva samples also contained elevated levels of 3-dehydrocarnitine, a bacterial degradation product of carnitine, further supporting the utilization of carnitine in oral bacterial metabolism.

Table 6. Comparison of biochemical changes to previously published results.

Biochemical Pathway/Name	Barnes et al., J. Dent. Res. [12] Saliva Periodontitis vs. Healthy	Current Study Saliva (Non-diabetic subjects only) Periodontitis vs. Healthy
Purine Degradation (Link to Oxidative Stress)	Increased*	Increased
Dipeptides (Macromolecular degradation of proteins)	Increased	Increased
Amino Acid Metabolites (p-cresol sulfate, Bacterial)	Increased	Increased
Carbohydrates (monosaccharides indicative of amylase activity)	Increased	Increased
Energy Metabolites (TCA cycle, indicative of energetic stress)	Unchanged	Increased
Uridine (DNA/RNA Degradation)	Increased	Increasing trend**
Allantoin	Increased	Increasing trend
ω-6 fatty acids (link to inflammation)	Increased	Increased
Fatty Acids	Increased	Increased
Acetylcarnitine	Increased	Increased
Carnitine	Increased	Unchanged
3-dehydrocarnitine	Increased	Increased

*Increased with statistically significant differences ($p \leq 0.05$) in biochemicals from those pathways. I
**Increasing trend reflects differences ($0.05 < p \leq 0.10$) in biochemicals from those pathways.

Table 7. Relative levels of biochemicals linked to purine degradation and anti-oxidant status in saliva samples from diabetics.

Biochemical Name	Fold Change (Diabetic -Gingivitis/Diabetic - Healthy)	P value	Q value
Adenosine	1.37	0.0943	0.6881
Inosine	1.70	0.0294	0.629
Guanine	2.40	0.0673	0.6546
Guanosine	2.06	0.0343	0.629
Xanthine	1.49	0.0434	0.629
Glutathione, oxidized (GSSG)	1.40	0.07	0.6546
Cysteine-glutathione disulfide	1.57	0.061	0.6444

Comparison of Biochemical Signatures in Saliva Samples from Diabetics vs Non-Diabetic subjects

Oxidative Stress and Anti-Oxidant Capacity. Purine degradation is regulated, in part, by oxidative stress [62], and increased purine degradation serves as an indication of an increased inflammatory response. Specifically, the conversion of hypoxanthine to xanthine and the subsequent conversion of xanthine to uric acid require O_2 to activate xanthine oxidase [63,64] and these reactions are coupled with a reduction of oxygen to generate superoxides in the form of O_2^- and H_2O_2. Urate is known to function in redox balance as a radical scavenger or antioxidant under conditions of oxidative stress and in the process converted to other products (e.g. allantoin). In the context of gingival disease, increased oxidative stress would result in higher levels of purine degradation metabolites, reflected in increased levels of hypoxanthine and xanthine. The results of this study are consistent with the results from previous studies [11,37]. Metabolites in the purine degradation pathway were statistically elevated in the diabetic cohort compared to the non-diabetic cohort (Table 7).

The levels of cysteine-glutathione disulfide and oxidized glutathione increased with gingival disease in non-diabetics and diabetics (Table 7). Glutathione plays a central role in the cellular defense against free radicals and xenobiotics. The increased levels of these oxidized glutathione species in saliva indicated increased oxidative stress.

Lipid and Sphingolipid Metabolism. Several lipid inflammatory mediators increased significantly in saliva from both the non-diabetic and diabetic groups during periodontal disease progression (Table 8). In this state of oxidative stress, lipoxygenase enzymes oxidize fatty acids to generate lipid signaling molecules such as 12-HETE. In saliva, arachidonate and 12-HETE increased in the non-diabetic cohort with periodontal disease and also increased in the diabetic gingivitis cohort compared to the healthy group, but was reduced in periodontitis (Table 8). Sphingomyelin, ceramides and glycosphingolipids are molecules that reside in the plasma membrane and participate in intracellular signaling cascades. Palmitoyl sphingomyelin was elevated in saliva of diabetic and non-diabetic subjects periodontitis (Table 8).

Discussion

We used metabolomic profiling technology to analyze saliva from subjects with and without diabetes who had a healthy gingiva, gingivitis, or periodontitis. In addition to verifying previously published observations in saliva [12] and GCF [11,37], we also identified in the present study salivary biochemical changes associated with diabetes, as well as changes associated with periodontal disease. The results from this analysis show that human diabetic subjects with periodontal disease have an increased purine degradation signature, a decreased redox balance capacity (Table 7) and altered ω-3/ω-6 fatty acid profiles (Table 8) in saliva.

Redox balance is vital for maintaining cellular homeostasis. Oxidative stress, caused by over production of reactive oxygen species and insufficient cellular anti-oxidant capabilities, can lead to cell damage. Glutathione and other anti-oxidant molecules serve to protect cellular proteins and structures from oxidative stress caused by reactive oxygen species. Glutathione is a thiol-containing tripeptide that plays a central role in cellular defense against free radicals and xenobiotics [65–68] and is the major intracellular redox mediator and it is pivotal for controlling the electrical or redox gradient across the mitochondrial inner-membrane [69,70]. Glutathione in the mitochondrial intermembrane space plays a intricate role in the mechanism of redox balance in living cells through its linkage to the redox milieu in the cytosol [71]. Oral interventions that enhance redox balance have been shown to be effective at relieving oral symptoms. For

Table 8. Fatty acids and sphingomyelins inreased in saliva from subjects with diabetes and periodontal disease.

Biochemical Name	Fold Change (Diabetic - Gingivitis/Diabetic - Healthy)	P value	Q value
12-HETE	2.41	0.0127	0.629
Linoleate (18:2n6)	3.22	0.0269	0.629
Linolenate [α or γ; (18:3n3 or 6)]	4.52	0.0476	0.629
Docosapentaenoate (n3 DPA; 22:5n3)	1.63	0.0483	0.629
Arachidonate (20:4n6)	2.00	0.0631	0.6517
Palmitoyl sphingomyelin	1.65	0.0422	0.629

example, Hansen and Grunnet showed that taurine plays a significant role in mitochondria in pH buffering that not only affects the status of glutathione, but also the NADH/NAD+ redox pair [72]. These molecules were all found to be elevated in saliva from the diabetic subjects.

Several lipid compounds are important for the initiation and propagation of inflammatory signaling in cells and tissues. Linoleic acid and arachidonic acid give rise to many of these metabolites. These lipid signaling inflammatory mediators are liberated from the plasma membrane phospholipids by phospholipase A_2 enzymes ultimately resulting in the production of linoleic and arachidonic acid-derived eicosanoids which help to mediate the inflammatory response [73]. Arachidonic acid release can also be initiated by collagen, thrombin, bradykinin, serotonin, and adrenaline, which increase in tissues during tissue damage and the early stages in inflammation and oxidative stress. Immune cells such as macrophages and neutrophils produce reactive oxygen species and reactive nitrogen species during cell activation that have the potential to damage lipids, proteins, and other molecules. Interestingly, these compounds were found to be elevated in the saliva of diabetic subjects with gingivitis.

Mobilization of lipid signaling pathways results in the synthesis of ceramides or the liberation of ceramides from intracellular stores. The activity of ceramidases results in the formation of sphingosine and sphingomyelin molecules that function in an array of intracellular signaling or maintenance of cell membrane architecture including apoptosis [74,75]. Depending on the specific cellular type and mechanism of activation, sphingomyelins and ceramides can serve activation or inhibitory purposes [76]. The formation of ceramides and sphingomyelins has been linked to cell death through nutrient starvation [74–76] as well as an important signaling molecule for cell differentiation and polarity [77]. *Porphyromonas gingivalis* is known to induce and alter sphingomyelin and ceramide signaling during infection [78].

Prediction of risk and accurate diagnosis of current disease activity may facilitate effective prevention and treatment of gingival diseases. GCF and saliva have been extensively examined in attempts to assess the oral disease status. The markers identified in this study may be leveraged to monitor the effectiveness of interventions as well as identify the mechanisms of action for these interventions. Several different approaches have confirmed that identifying a single marker characteristic of a disease is unlikely; rather, a combination of biomarkers would likely constitute an effective clinical test. For example, insulin resistance is a feature if the pre-diabetes stage in humans prior to the development of diabetes. Untargeted biochemical profiling to identify biomarkers of insulin resistance following the development of targeted assays and validation of the targeted assays in a clinical cohort resulted in the development of a diagnostic that monitors insulin sensitivity status in humans [52,79]. By monitoring selected metabolites representing the diverse biochemical pathways, it is therefore possible to identify unique biomarkers and to monitor during the course of periodontal treatment in diabetics. In conclusion, this study demonstrated that biochemical profiling technology is a powerful tool for dental research and the results provide new mechanistic insights and treatment strategies that could be specific for oral health of diabetics. Additionally, the biochemicals identified in this study that segregated the individuals by periodontal status could be leveraged or developed into a rapid diagnostic to monitor periodontal disease activity.

Supporting Information

Table S1 Saliva Metabolic Profiling and Pathway Analysis. Statistical analyses for each biochemical detected in saliva between each of the gingival and diabetic cohorts.

Table S2 Plasma Metabolic Profiling and Pathway Analysis. Statistical analyses for each biochemical detected in plasma between each of the gingival and diabetic cohorts.

Author Contributions

Conceived and designed the experiments: VMB FP WD HMT TJ LG FAS. Performed the experiments: TJ LG ADK SC FAS. Analyzed the data: VMB LG ADK FAS. Contributed reagents/materials/analysis tools: LG ADK. Contributed to the writing of the manuscript: ADK FAS VMB FP LG.

References

1. Leyden JJ, Thiboutot D, Shalita A (2004) Photographic review of results from a clinical study comparing benzoyl peroxide 5%/clindamycin 1% topical gel with vehicle in the treatment of rosacea. Cutis 73: 11–17.
2. Gutman DA, Cooper LA, Hwang SN, Holder CA, Gao J, et al. (2013) MR imaging predictors of molecular profile and survival: multi-institutional study of the TCGA glioblastoma data set. Radiology 267: 560–569.
3. Demmer RT, Desvarieux M (2006) Periodontal infections and cardiovascular disease: the heart of the matter. J Am Dent Assoc 137 Suppl: 14S–20S; quiz 38S.
4. Tonetti MS, D'Aiuto F, Nibali L, Donald A, Storry C, et al. (2007) Treatment of periodontitis and endothelial function. N Engl J Med 356: 911–920.
5. Pussinen PJ, Tuomisto K, Jousilahti P, Havulinna AS, Sundvall J, et al. (2007) Endotoxemia, immune response to periodontal pathogens, and systemic inflammation associate with incident cardiovascular disease events. Arterioscler Thromb Vasc Biol 27: 1433–1439.
6. Pussinen PJ, Paju S, Mantyla P, Sorsa T (2007) Serum microbial- and host-derived markers of periodontal diseases: a review. Curr Med Chem 14: 2402–2412.
7. Nieman DC, Shanely RA, Gillitt ND, Pappan KL, Lila MA (2013) Serum metabolic signatures induced by a three-day intensified exercise period persist after 14 h of recovery in runners. J Proteome Res 12: 4577–4584.
8. Scannapieco FA (1994) Saliva-bacterium interactions in oral microbial ecology. Crit Rev Oral Biol Med 5: 203–248.
9. Scannapieco FA, Bergey EJ, Reddy MS, Levine MJ (1989) Characterization of salivary alpha-amylase binding to Streptococcus sanguis. Infect Immun 57: 2853–2863.
10. Scannapieco FA, Solomon L, Wadenya RO (1994) Emergence in human dental plaque and host distribution of amylase-binding streptococci. J Dent Res 73: 1627–1635.
11. Barnes VM, Teles R, Trivedi HM, Devizio W, Xu T, et al. (2009) Acceleration of purine degradation by periodontal diseases. J Dent Res 88: 851–855.
12. Barnes VM, Ciancio SG, Shibly O, Xu T, Devizio W, et al. (2011) Metabolomics reveals elevated macromolecular degradation in periodontal disease. J Dent Res 90: 1293–1297.
13. Christodoulides N, Floriano PN, Miller CS, Ebersole JL, Mohanty S, et al. (2007) Lab-on-a-chip methods for point-of-care measurements of salivary biomarkers of periodontitis. Ann N Y Acad Sci 1098: 411–428.
14. Miller CS, King CP Jr, Langub MC, Kryscio RJ, Thomas MV (2006) Salivary biomarkers of existing periodontal disease: a cross-sectional study. J Am Dent Assoc 137: 322–329.
15. Akalin FA, Baltacioglu E, Alver A, Karabulut E (2007) Lipid peroxidation levels and total oxidant status in serum, saliva and gingival crevicular fluid in patients with chronic periodontitis. J Clin Periodontol 34: 558–565.
16. Akalin FA, Isiksal E, Baltacioglu E, Renda N, Karabulut E (2008) Superoxide dismutase activity in gingiva in type-2 diabetes mellitus patients with chronic periodontitis. Arch Oral Biol 53: 44–52.
17. Pradeep AR, Kumar MS, Ramachandraprasad MV, Shikha C (2007) Gingival crevicular fluid levels of neopterin in healthy subjects and in patients with different periodontal diseases. J Periodontol 78: 1962–1967.
18. Pradeep AR, Manjunath SG, Swati PP, Shikha C, Sujatha PB (2007) Gingival crevicular fluid levels of leukotriene B4 in periodontal health and disease. J Periodontol 78: 2325–2330.
19. Waddington RJ, Embery G, Samuels RH (1994) Characterization of proteoglycan metabolites in human gingival crevicular fluid during orthodontic tooth movement. Arch Oral Biol 39: 361–368.
20. Embery G, Waddington R (1994) Gingival crevicular fluid: biomarkers of periodontal tissue activity. Adv Dent Res 8: 329–336.

21. Alpagot T, Bell C, Lundergan W, Chambers DW, Rudin R (2001) Longitudinal evaluation of GCF MMP-3 and TIMP-1 levels as prognostic factors for progression of periodontitis. J Clin Periodontol 28: 353–359.
22. Alpagot T, Silverman S, Lundergan W, Bell C, Chambers DW (2001) Crevicular fluid elastase levels in relation to periodontitis and metabolic control of diabetes. J Periodontal Res 36: 169–174.
23. Kardesler L, Buduneli N, Cetinkalp S, Lappin D, Kinane DF (2011) Gingival crevicular fluid IL-6, tPA, PAI-2, albumin levels following initial periodontal treatment in chronic periodontitis patients with or without type 2 diabetes. Inflamm Res 60: 143–151.
24. Acker-Hewitt TL, Shafer BM, Saunders MJ, Goh Q, Luden ND (2012) Independent and combined effects of carbohydrate and caffeine ingestion on aerobic cycling performance in the fed state. Appl Physiol Nutr Metab 37: 276–283.
25. Garcia-German D, Viloria F, Menendez P, Canillas F (2012) [Letter in reference to the article "surgery on the wrong side: implication for the patient and the professional. Experience in a major ambulatory surgery of the foot unit"]. Rev Esp Cir Ortop Traumatol 56: 421; author reply 422.
26. Keles GC, Cetinkaya BO, Eroglu C, Simsek SB, Kahraman H (2010) Vascular endothelial growth factor expression levels of gingiva in gingivitis and periodontitis patients with/without diabetes mellitus. Inflamm Res 59: 543–549.
27. Salvi GE, Franco LM, Braun TM, Lee A, Rutger Persson G, et al. (2010) Pro-inflammatory biomarkers during experimental gingivitis in patients with type 1 diabetes mellitus: a proof-of-concept study. J Clin Periodontol 37: 9–16.
28. Sima C, Rhourida K, Van Dyke TE, Gyurko R (2010) Type 1 diabetes predisposes to enhanced gingival leukocyte margination and macromolecule extravasation in vivo. J Periodontal Res 45: 748–756.
29. Xiang X, Duarte PM, Lima JA, Santos VR, Goncalves TD, et al. (2013) Diabetes-Associated Periodontitis Molecular Features in Infrared Spectra of Gingival Crevicular Fluid. J Periodontol.
30. Yoon AJ, Cheng B, Philipone E, Turner R, Lamster IB (2012) Inflammatory biomarkers in saliva: assessing the strength of association of diabetes mellitus and periodontal status with the oral inflammatory burden. J Clin Periodontol 39: 434–440.
31. Mandel ID (1989) The role of saliva in maintaining oral homeostasis. J Am Dent Assoc 119: 298-304.
32. Stuchell RN, Blitzer A, Mandel ID (1984) Medical management of non-neoplastic salivary gland disease. Otolaryngol Clin North Am 17: 697–703.
33. Tabak LA, Levine MJ, Mandel ID, Ellison SA (1982) Role of salivary mucins in the protection of the oral cavity. J Oral Pathol 11: 1–17.
34. Dunn W, Griffith JW, Morrison MT, Tanquary J, Sabata D, et al. (2013) Somatosensation assessment using the NIH Toolbox. Neurology 80: S41–44.
35. Hargreaves CE, Grasso M, Hampe CS, Stenkova A, Atkinson S, et al. (2013) Yersinia enterocolitica provides the link between thyroid-stimulating antibodies and their germline counterparts in Graves' disease. J Immunol 190: 5373–5381.
36. Barnes VM, Arvanitidou E, Szewczyk G, Richter R, DeVizio W, et al. (2011) Evaluation of the antiplaque efficacy of two cetylpyridinium chloride-containing mouthwashes. J Clin Dent 22: 200–203.
37. Barnes VM, Teles R, Trivedi HM, Devizio W, Xu T, et al. (2010) Assessment of the effects of dentifrice on periodontal disease biomarkers in gingival crevicular fluid. J Periodontal 81: 1273–1279.
38. Ganti S, Weiss RH (2011) Urine metabolomics for kidney cancer detection and biomarker discovery. Urol Oncol 29: 551–557.
39. Lobene RR, Kashket S, Soparkar PM, Shloss J, Sabine ZM (1979) The effect of cetylpridinium chloride on human plaque bacteria and gingivitis. Pharmacol Ther Dent 4: 33–47.
40. Fredericks MA, Lobene RR, Mundy P (1971) A model for teaching social concepts to dental auxiliaries. J Dent Educ 35: 232–235.
41. Bessonneau V, Bojko B, Pawliszyn J (2013) Analysis of human saliva metabolome by direct immersion solid-phase microextraction LC and benchtop orbitrap MS. Bioanalysis 5: 783–792.
42. Zhang A, Sun H, Wang X (2012) Saliva metabolomics opens door to biomarker discovery, disease diagnosis, and treatment. Appl Biochem Biotechnol 168: 1718–1727.
43. Al-Tarawneh SK, Border MB, Dibble CF, Bencharit S (2011) Defining salivary biomarkers using mass spectrometry-based proteomics: a systematic review. OMICS 15: 353–361.
44. Rathnayake N, Akerman S, Klinge B, Lundegren N, Jansson H, et al. (2013) Salivary biomarkers for detection of systemic diseases. PLoS ONE 8: e61356.
45. Rathnayake N, Akerman S, Klinge B, Lundegren N, Jansson H, et al. (2013) Salivary biomarkers of oral health: a cross-sectional study. J Clin Periodontol 40: 140–147.
46. Lobene RR, Weatherford T, Ross NM, Lamm RA, Menaker L (1986) A modified gingival index for use in clinical trials. Clin Prev Dent 8: 3–6.
47. Silness J, Loe H (1964) Periodontal Disease in Pregnancy. Ii. Correlation between Oral Hygiene and Periodontal Condtion. Acta Odontol Scand 22: 121–135.
48. Genco RJ, Schifferle RE, Dunford RG, Falkner KL, Hsu WC, et al. (2014) Screening for diabetes mellitus in dental practices: A field trial. J Am Dent Assoc 145: 57–64.
49. Judice PB, Matias CN, Santos DA, Magalhaes JP, Hamilton MT, et al. (2013) Caffeine intake, short bouts of physical activity, and energy expenditure: a double-blind randomized crossover trial. PLoS ONE 8: e68936.
50. Evans A, DeHaven CD, Barrett T, Mitchell M, Milgram E (2009) Integrated, nontargeted ultrahigh performance liquid chromatography/electrospray ionization tandem mass spectrometry platform for the identification and relative quantificationof the small-molecule complement of biological systems. Anal Chem 81: 6656–6667.
51. DeHaven CD, Evans AM, Dai H, Lawton KA (2010) Organization of GC/MS and LC/MS metabolomics data into chemical libraries. J Cheminformatics 2: 9–21.
52. Gall WE, Beebe K, Lawton KA, Adam KP, Mitchell MW, et al. (2010) Alpha-hydroxybutyrate is an early biomarker of insulin resistance and glucose tolerance in a nondiabetic population. PLoS ONE 5: 1–10.
53. Nerby CL, FStickle DF (2009) 1,5-anhydroglucitol monitoring in diabetes: A mass balance perspective. Clin Biochem 42: 158–167.
54. Toth BI, Geczy T, Griger Z, Dozsa A, Seltmann H, et al. (2009) Transient receptor potential vanilloid-1 signaling as a regulator of human sebocyte biology. J Invest Dermatol 129: 329–339.
55. Buse JB, Freeman JL, Edelman SV, Jovanovic L, McGill JB (2003) Serum 1,5-anhydroglucitol (GlycoMark): a short-term glycemic marker. Diabetes Technol Ther 5: 355–363.
56. Brass EP (1986) Effect of alpha-ketobutyrate on palmitic acid and pyruvate metabolism in isolated rat hepatocytes. Biochim Biophys Acta 888: 18–24.
57. Landaas S (1975) The formation of 2-hydroxybutyric acid in experimental animals. Clin Chim Acta 58: 23–32.
58. Landaas S, Pettersen JE (1975) Clinical conditions associated with urinary excretion of 2-hydroxybutyric acid. Scand J Clin Lab Invest 35: 259–266.
59. Pettersen JE, Landaas S, Eldjarn L (1973) The occurrence of 2-hydroxybutyric acid in urine from patients with lactic acidosis. Clin Chim Acta 48: 213–219.
60. Silva AR, Ruschel C, Helegda C, Wyse AT, Wannmacher CM, et al. (2001) Inhibition of in vitro CO2 production and lipid synthesis by 2-hydroxybutyric acid in rat brain. Braz J Med Biol Res 34: 627–631.
61. Yang W, Roth KS (1985) Defect in alpha-ketobutyrate metabolism: a new inborn error. Clin Chim Acta 145: 173–182.
62. Quinlan GJ, Lamb NJ, Tilley R, Evans TW, Gutteridge JM (1997) Plasma hypoxanthine levels in ARDS: implications for oxidative stress, morbidity, and mortality. Am J Respir Crit Care Med 155: 479–484.
63. Quick KL, Hardt JI, Dugan LL (2000) Rapid microplate assay for superoxide scavenging efficiency. J Neurosci Methods 97: 139–144.
64. Becker BF (1993) Towards the physiological function of uric acid. Free Radic Biol Med 14: 615–631.
65. Forman HJ, Dickinson DA (2003) Oxidative signaling and glutathione synthesis. Biofactors 17: 1–12.
66. Pastore A, Federici G, Bertini E, Piemonte F (2003) Analysis of glutathione: implication in redox and detoxification. Clin Chim Acta 333: 19–39.
67. Wu G, Fang YZ, Yang S, Lupton JR, Turner ND (2004) Glutathione metabolism and its implications for health. J Nutr 134: 489–492.
68. Townsend DM, Tew KD, Tapiero H (2003) The importance of glutathione in human disease. Biomed Pharmacother 57: 145–155.
69. Garcia-Ruiz C, Colell A, Morales A, Kaplowitz N, Fernandez-Checa JC (1995) Role of oxidative stress generated from the mitochondrial electron transport chain and mitochondrial glutathione status in loss of mitochondrial function and activation of transcription factor nuclear factor-kappa B: studies with isolated mitochondria and rat hepatocytes. Mol Pharmacol 48: 825–834.
70. Garcia-Ruiz C, Morales A, Colell A, Ballesta A, Rodes J, et al. (1995) Feeding S-adenosyl-L-methionine attenuates both ethanol-induced depletion of mitochondrial glutathione and mitochondrial dysfunction in periportal and perivenous rat hepatocytes. Hepatology 21: 207–214.
71. Kojer K, Bien M, Gangel H, Morgan B, Dick TP, et al. (2012) Glutathione redox potential in the mitochondrial intermembrane space is linked to the cytosol and impacts the Mia40 redox state. Embo J 31: 3169–3182.
72. Hansen SH, Grunnet N (2013) Taurine, glutathione and bioenergetics. Adv Exp Med Biol 776: 3–12.
73. Calder PC (2006) n-3 polyunsaturated fatty acids, inflammation, and inflammatory diseases. Am J Clin Nutr 83: 1505S–1519S.
74. Guenther G, Peralta E, Rosales K, Wong S, Siskind L, et al. (2008) Ceramide starves cells to death by downregulating nutrient transporter proteins. Proc Natl Acad Sci U S A 105: 17402–17407.
75. Peralta E, Edinger A (2009) Ceramide-induced starvation triggers homeostatic autophagy. Autophagy 5: 407–409.
76. Mao C, Obeid LM (2008) Ceramidases: regulators of cellular responses mediated by ceramide, sphingosine, and sphingosine-1-phosphate. Biochim Biophys Acta 1781: 424–434.
77. Bieberich E (2011) Ceramide in stem cell differentiation and embryo development: novel functions of a topological cell-signaling lipid and the concept of ceramide compartments. J Lipids In Press.
78. Nichols FC, Rojanasomsith K (2006) Porphyromonas gingivalis lipids and diseased dental tissues. Oral Microbiol Immunol 21: 84–92.
79. Cobb J, Gall W, Adam KP, Nakhle P, Button E, et al. (2013) A novel fasting blood test for insulin resistance and prediabetes. J Diabetes Sci Technol 7: 100–110.

Chair-Side Quantitative Oral-Microflora Screening for Assessing Familial Correlation of Periodontal Status and Caries Prevalence

Yung-Kai Huang[1], Wei-Fang Lee[2], Meng-Jiy Wang[3], Yus-Han Sophie Chang[4], Wen-Shiun Tchaou[4], Wei-Jen Chang[5], Sheng-Yang Lee[5,6], Joen-Rong Sheu[7,8], Nai-Chia Teng[4,5]*

1 School of Oral Hygiene, College of Oral Medicine, Taipei Medical University, Taipei, Taiwan, **2** School of Dental Technology, College of Oral Medicine, Taipei Medical University, Taipei, Taiwan, **3** Department of Chemical Engineering, National Taiwan University of Science and Technology, Taipei, Taiwan, **4** Division of Oral Rehabilitation and Center of Pediatric Dentistry, Department of Dentistry, Taipei Medical University Hospital, Taipei, Taiwan, **5** School of Dentistry, College of Oral Medicine, Taipei Medical University, Taipei, Taiwan, **6** Dental Department of Wan-Fang Hospital, Taipei Medical University, Taipei, Taiwan, **7** Department of Pharmacology, School of Medicine, College of Medicine, Taipei Medical University, Taipei, Taiwan, **8** Graduate Institute of Medical Sciences, College of Medicine, Taipei Medical University, Taipei, Taiwan

Abstract

Aim: Our goal was to investigate the relationship between clinical status and the presence of carious or periodontal pathogens among parent-child familial pairs. Clinical practices of risk assessment with consideration of familial pathogen interaction might reduce the need for therapy, improve patient outcomes, and ultimately reduce oral disease burden. Materials and Methods: In this study, we enrolled 30 parent-child pairs, with the children exhibiting complete deciduous dentition or mixed dentition with only permanent first molars. Clinical statuses were evaluated using caries and periodontal disease indicators, including the sum of decay and the number of missing or filled teeth (DMFT) for adults, decay, extraction caused by dental disease, and filled teeth (deft), for children, probing depth, and plaque control record (PCR). Supra- and sub-gingival bacteria were determined based on semi-quantitative measurements of microbial infection by using data from the Dentocult® SM test (caries-related organisms) and the PerioCheck® test (periodontal disease-related organisms). Results: No statistically significant relationship was detected between the prevalence of periodontal pathogens and that of cariogenic pathogens in the oral cavity. However, the clinical status of caries (DMFT) was negatively correlated with the clinical status of periodontal disease (pocket depth) in parents who were infected with dominant periodontal pathogens ($r = -0.59$, $p<0.01$). Parents' DMFT scores were positively correlated with children's deft and PCR scores. PCR and deft scores of children appeared to decrease significantly with the parent's pocket depth. Conclusion: The study showed that the quantity of caries pathogens were not significant related to periodontal pathogens, but the caries clinical outcome is negative related with periodontal clinical outcome between familial pairs.

Editor: Michael Glogauer, University of Toronto, Canada

Funding: This study was supported by a research grant from the Taipei Medical University -National Taiwan University of Science and Technology Joint Research Program (TMU-NTUST-100-01).The funders had no role in study design, data collection and analysis, decision to publish, or preparation of the manuscript.

Competing Interests: The authors have declared that no competing interests exist.

* E-mail: dianaten@tmu.edu.tw

Introduction

Dental caries and periodontitis are the most widespread oral diseases in populations of all ages. Recent epidemiological surveys have revealed that 60% of the U.S. population present with mild forms of periodontal disease and that 64% of seniors (adults aged 65 y and older) exhibit either moderate or severe periodontitis [1]. Various factors including nutritional status, tobacco and alcohol use, hygiene, and stress have been linked to a wide range of oral diseases, forming the foundation of the commonly used risk-factor approach for preventing oral diseases [2,3]. Among these, oral hygiene is one of the most critical factors for preventing oral diseases, particularly caries and periodontal disease [4]. The relationship between oral hygiene and intra-oral pathogenesis has been defined, and the advanced relationship between pathogenesis and dental caries or periodontal disease has also been investigated [4,5]. The core of traditional dentistry is based on the treatment of oral diseases. For dental caries, treatment is typically initiated when lesions are clinically detectable and tissue damage is irreversible; a similar approach can be applied in treating periodontal disease. Remarkable advances have now been made in the field of oral microbiology, particularly with regards to adjunct diagnosis.

Streptococcus mutans is the principal cariogenic pathogen [6,7]. The early acquisition of *S. mutans* has been reported to be due to mother-to-child transmission: children whose mothers have high levels of salivary *S. mutans* acquire caries earlier and also have higher counts of *S. mutans* than have children whose mothers have low levels of *S. mutans* [8]. *Actinobacillus actinomycetemcomitans*, *Porphyromonas gingivalis*, *Prevotella intermedius*, and *Bacterioids forsythus* are the strongest putative pathogens in periodontitis [9]. Moreover, the occurrence of intrafamilial transmission of periodontal pathogens has been suggested by previous studies. Parents are the first people who interact with their children and are thus a potential source of infection, and the detection of periodontal pathogens in children at an early age may indicate endogenous infection [10,11].

People with salivary bacterial counts of *S. mutans* and *P. gingivalis* in excess of 1×10^5, and 4×10^6 colony forming units (CFU)/mL are regarded to have a high risk of developing dental caries and periodontitis, respectively. However, little research supports a relationship between streptococci (*S. mitis* and *S. sanguis*) and periodontal pathogens. Previous in vitro studies have suggested that the growth of *S. mutans* is related to *P. gingivalis* [12,13], but no direct evidence has been presented of this relationship in the human oral cavity. Microbial tests, such as Dentocult® SM Strip and PerioCheck®, have been developed that are easy to use at the chair-side. The Dentocult test is a simple and clinically acceptable method that might facilitate the procedure of determining the amount of bacteria present in dental plaques and mobilized into the saliva. PerioCheck® is a rapid chair-side test used to detect the presence of neutral proteases [14]. The presence of neutral proteases has been implicated in collagen breakdown, which is a key feature of periodontal disease [15]. The PerioCheck® method has been demonstrated to exhibit a high sensitivity (88%) when diagnosing periodontitis [16]. These diagnostic tests can detect the presence of active disease, predict future disease progression, and evaluate the response to clinical therapy, thereby improving the clinical management of patients. However, thus far, a comprehensive understanding of the pathogenesis of dental caries and periodontal disease, particularly the transmission between child and parent or caregiver, has been lacking. In this study, we investigated the relationship between clinical status and the presence of carious or periodontal pathogens among child-parent pairs. Clinical practices of risk assessment with a consideration of familial pathogen interaction might reduce the need for therapy, improve patient outcomes, and ultimately reduce the burden of oral disease.

Materials and Methods

Participants

Thirty parent-child pairs were recruited for this study. Children aged 3–7 years exhibiting complete deciduous dentition or mixed dentition with only permanent first molars were considered eligible for enrollment. The parents of all enrolled children had no chronic or systemic diseases, were not pregnant, and had no history of dental disease beside caries. The study was approved by the Taipei Medical University Joint Institutional Review Board. Before conducting interviews and collecting specimens, written informed consent was obtained from the parents of all children who participated in the study. The study complied with the World Medical Association Declaration of Helsinki.

Caries Examination and Oral Hygiene Evaluation

A questionnaire was completed by parents to provide information on their socioeconomic status and their child's oral health habits (infant feeding history, current diet, oral hygiene practices) and systemic health and medication. All children were examined by a dentist who was trained and assessed in relation to an experienced oral epidemiologist. The dentist demonstrated >90% reliability before the training session was completed. Dental examination for caries was conducted in fully equipped dental units, using an illuminated mouth mirror and a CPI probe (CP-11.5B6, Hu-Friedy, Chicago, IL, US). The tooth status was assessed through visual inspection, aided by tactile inspection if necessary. The World Health Organization (WHO) criteria for the diagnosing and coding of dental caries were used. Dental caries were scored using the sum of decay and the number of missing or filled teeth (DMFT) for adults and decay, extraction caused by dental disease, and filled teeth (deft) for children. The plaque control record (PCR) developed by O'Leary was used to examine the dental hygiene status of parents and children [17].

Periodontal Status and Classification

To evaluate periodontal health, periodontal examinations were performed on adults, which included full mouth periodontal charting that was conducted using a periodontal probe and the gingival index. The American Dental Association periodontal classification was used to identify or categorize each patient's periodontal status. After clinical and radiographic data were gathered, the patients were classified into one of the 4 case types: Type I, for gingivitis; Type II, for early periodontitis; Type III, for moderate periodontitis; and Type IV, for advanced periodontitis. A similar assessment was not performed on the children because most children do not exhibit severe periodontal disease.

Oral Bacteria Tests

Study participants were asked to refrain from using oral hygiene procedures the night before the day of the study. Saliva collection was scheduled at the beginning of the day. Participants were first asked to swallow preexisting saliva. Subsequently they were to chew a standard piece of paraffin wax (Orion Diagnostics kit). The saliva that was produced was collected in a sterile plastic recipient. A minimum of 2 mL of saliva had to be collected. The plaque sample was collected from every quadrant by using sterile mini-brushes. The collection was from the interproximal area between the primary first molar and primary second molar. Immediately after collection, both the saliva and the plaque *S. mutans* samples were assessed using the Dentocult SM® dip strip (Orion Diagnostica, Espoo, Finland). The growth density on the strips was classified according to the manufacturer's instructions and expressed as scores of 0, 1, 2, and 3, which correspond to *S. mutans* growth levels of $\leq$104, $\leq 10^5$, 10^5–10^6, and $\geq 10^6$ CFU/mL.

PerioCheck® (CollaGenex Pharmaceuticals, Newtown, PA, USA) is a quick and simple periodontal diagnostic tool that is used to detect peptidase activity specifically attributed to *Treponema denticola*, *P. gingivalis*, and *B. forsythus*. Periodontal pathogens residing in the periodontal pocket react specifically to the peptidase. A composite score ranging from 0 to 2, assigned based on comparing the blue color of the test result with a standard color chart, was used to determine the amount of bacteria in samples.

Statistical Analyses

Data were analyzed using SAS 9.2 software (Cary, NC, USA). Student's t test was used to test for significant differences in DMFT, deft or PCR scores of samples in relation to demography strata, oral hygiene strata, or a pathogen level of 0 or above. Analysis of variance (ANOVA) was used to test the PCR and deft scores of children among the children's age groups and main caregiver categories. Fisher's exact test was used to evaluate differences in the categorical variables of periodontal status and caries indices. The strength of the association between periodontal indices (PCR, gingival index, and depth) and the caries index (DMFT) was noted using a correlation coefficient. Linear regression was used to elucidate the relationship between parent DMFT and child deft or PCR scores. A probability level (alpha) of less than 0.05 was used as the criterion for significance.

Table 1. Mean PCR and deft scores of children according to demography and oral hygiene habits in children and caregivers.

		PCR	p- value	deft	p- value
	N	Mean ± SE		Mean ± SE	
Gender			0.08[a]		0.39[a]
Girls	19	78.35±7.38		9.47±1.04	
Boys	11	92.40±2.47		7.82±1.76	
Age (y)			0.10[b]		0.81[b]
3–4	12	86.80±4.45		9.58±1.45	
5	10	69.76±12.80		8.20±1.65	
6–7	8	95.73±1.39		8.63±1.37	
Single child			0.08[a]		0.28[a]
No	21	89.08±4.37		9.52±1.06	
Yes	9	70.50±12.06		7.33±1.80	
Eat/drink before bedtime			0.08[a]		<0.01[a]
No	18	77.70±7.79		6.44±1.01	
Yes	12	92.20±2.12		12.50±1.08	
Snack consumption			0.44[a]		0.73[a]
Rare	7	73.19±15.87		8.29±2.49	
Yes	23	86.64±4.25		9.04±0.96	
Frequency of brushing			<0.01[a]		0.54[a]
Less than daily	2	100.00±0.00		11.00±1.00	
Once or more per day	28	82.32±5.16		8.71±0.98	
Floss used			0.30[a]		0.44[a]
No	18	87.69±5.46		9.00±1.19	
Yes	12	77.22±9.03		8.67±1.49	
Main caregiver			0.59[b]		0.44[b]
Mother	15	80.61±9.89		9.60±0.89	
Mother and father	9	81.55±9.48		9.22±2.90	
Others	6	93.65±3.37		6.50±2.20	
Main caregiver's education			0.09[a]		0.40[a]
High school	7	92.85±3.60		10.29±1.04	
University and above	23	80.66±6.18		8.43±1.15	
Main Caregiver's occupation			0.02[b]		0.36[b]
Employer/professional	6	94.13±2.59		11.67±1.2	
Employee/professional	8	59.67±14.56		6.75±2.42	
Employee/non-professional	10	87.97±4.64		9.00±1.53	
Unemployed	6	97.22±1.96		8.67±1.48	
Floss used frequency of main caregiver			0.48[b]		0.73[b]
Occasion	18	88.31±5.20		9.39±1.20	
Once/day	7	75.07±12.07		8.57±1.76	
Twice/day	5	78.00±6.17		7.40±2.71	
Dental care utilization of main caregiver			0.78[b]		0.70[b]
Once/half year	4	92.2±4.34		8.25±2.46	
Once/one year	14	83.07±8.1		9.71±1.52	
Once/more than one year	12	81.11±7.85		8.08±1.29	

[a]p value for student t test.
[b]p value for ANOVA test.
Abbreviations: deft, decay, extraction, and filled teeth; PCR, plaque control records; SE, standard error.

Table 2. Association between the results of chair-side semi-quantitative microbial infection measurements and caries index or periodontal clinical status in parent and child.

Microbial results - parents		**DMFT**	**PCR**	**Pocket depth**	**Gingival index**
	N	Mean ± SE			
Plaque SM					
0	8	10.13±1.93	75.02±7.65	2.22±0.25	1.26±0.08
1–3	22	13.91±0.85	86.65±2.86	2.07±0.15	1.61±0.09
p value[a]		0.04	0.18	0.62	0.04
Saliva SM					
0	6	9.33±2.41	71.89±10.05	2.37±0.32	1.37±0.13
1–3	24	13.79±0.81	86.46±2.63	2.05±0.13	1.55±0.09
p value[a]		0.03	0.05	0.31	0.36
PerioCheck®					
0	8	10.00±1.33	82.68±5.37	1.92±0.23	1.26±0.09
1–2	22	13.95±0.93	83.86±3.67	2.18±0.15	1.61±0.09
p value[a]		0.04	0.86	0.37	0.04
Microbial results - children	**N**	**deft**	**PCR**		
Plaque SM					
0	9	7.44±2.14	66.45±13.79		
1–3	21	9.48±0.95	90.81±2.78		
p value[a]		0.31	0.11		
Saliva SM					
0	13	8.08±1.61	75.93±10.24		
1–3	17	9.47±1.07	89.29±3.32		
p value[a]		0.46	0.23		
PerioCheck®					
0	9	7.66±1.38	84.77±9.57		
1–2	21	9.38±1.17	82.96±5.78		
p value[a]		0.40	0.73		

[a]p value for student t test.
Abbreviations: DMFT, decay and the number of missing or filled teeth; deft, decay, extraction, and filled teeth; PCR, plaque control records; SE, standard error; SM, *Streptococcus mutans*.

Results

Table 1 presents the PCR and deft scores in relation to demography and oral hygiene habits of children. The deft scores of children who routinely ate or drank before bedtime were significantly higher than those of children who did not have the habit of eating or drinking before bedtime. The PCR scores of children who brushed their teeth less frequently than daily were significantly higher than those of children whose brushing frequency was once or more per day. The PCR scores of children whose caregivers' occupation were professional employee were significantly lower than those of children whose caregivers' occupation were other three categories.

The results in Table 2 reveal the association between the use of the chair-side semi-quantitative assays to measure microbial infection and the caries index or periodontal clinical status in the parent and child. The mean scores of DMFT and deft were 12.90 and 8.87 in parents and children, respectively. The mean DMFT score of parents who tested positive for plaque *S. mutans* was higher than that of parents who tested negative ($p = 0.03$, student *t*-test). Parents identified to carry microbial infections (based on the *S. mutans* Dentocult SM® and PerioCheck® results) had a significantly higher DMFT score than parents who tested negative for microbial infection. Periodontal clinical status was only assessed on parents and the mean periodontal pocket depth and gingival index were 2.11 mm and 1.37, respectively. Plaque *S. mutans*-positive parents had a higher gingival index than parents who tested negative for plaque *S. mutans* ($p = 0.04$). Parents who tested positive on the PerioCheck® test had higher a gingival index than those who tested negative ($p = 0.04$).

The results in Table 3 indicate the association between periodontal and cariogenic pathogens. Relative to parents who tested negative for plaque *S. mutans*, the parents who tested positive showed higher rates of periodontal pathogens, but the difference was not statistically significant (50.00% vs. 81.82%, $p = 0.16$). The parents' status of periodontal pathogens (determined using PerioCheck®) was not associated with the children's *S. mutans* or pathogen status. These results suggest that no statistically significant relationship exists between the prevalence of periodontal pathogens and that of cariogenic pathogens in the oral cavity.

To explore the relationship between the periodontal clinical status or periodontal pathogens and caries indices, we compared

Table 3. Association between periodontal and cariogenic pathogens.

	Parent PerioCheck®			Child PerioCheck®	
	0	1+		0	1+
	N (%)			N (%)	
Parent plaque SM			Child plaque SM		
0	4 (50.00)	4 (18.18)	0	4 (44.44)	5 (23.81)
1+	4 (50.00)	18 (81.82)	1+	5 (55.56)	16 (76.19)
p value[a]	0.16		p value[a]	0.39	
Parent saliva SM			Child saliva SM		
0	3 (37.50)	3 (13.64)	0	6 (66.67)	7 (33.33)
1+	5 (62.50)	19 (86.36)	1+	3 (33.33)	14 (66.67)
p value[a]	0.30		p value[a]	0.12	
Child plaque SM			Parent plaque SM		
0	4 (50.00)	5 (22.73)	0	2 (22.22)	6 (28.57)
1+	4 (50.00)	17 (77.27)	1+	7 (77.78)	15 (71.43)
p value[a]	0.20		p value[a]	1.00	
Child saliva SM			Parent saliva SM		
0	5 (62.50)	8 (36.36)	0	2 (33.33)	7 (29.17)
1+	3 (37.50)	14 (63.64)	1+	4 (66.67)	17 (70.83)
p value[a]	0.24		p value[a]	1.00	
Child PerioCheck®			Parent PerioCheck®		
0	2 (22.22)	6 (28.57)	0	4 (50.00)	5 (22.73)
1+	7 (77.78)	15 (71.43)	1+	4 (50.00)	17 (77.27)
p value[a]	1.00		p value[a]	0.20	

[a]p value for Fishers exact test.
SM: *Streptococcus mutans.*

the DMFT and PCR scores and the periodontal status in parents (Fig. 1). The DMFT scores of parents who exhibited moderate periodontitis (Type III) or advanced periodontitis (Type IV) were significantly lower than those of parents who had gingivitis (Type I) or early periodontitis (Type II) (Fig. 1A). The DMFT scores of patients without any detectable dominant periodontal pathogens (PerioCheck® = 0) were lower than those of patients in whom the dominant periodontal pathogens were present (PerioCheck® ≥ 0). The rates of testing negative for periodontal pathogens (PerioCheck® = 0) in the periodontal classification Types I, II, and III/IV were 75%, 12.5%, and 12.5%, respectively, and the PerioCheck® test results were not significantly associated with the periodontal classifications (p = 0.58 in the χ^2 test). By contrast, the status of cariogenic pathogens (plaque or saliva *S. mutans*) was associated with DMFT scores, but not with pocket depth (data not shown).

Table 4 presents the correlation coefficients for caries indices and periodontal status in parents. The DMFT score was negatively correlated with pocket depth ($r = -0.49$, $P<0.01$), but the correlation was not observed in patients in whom the dominant periodontal pathogens were not detected (PerioCheck® = 0). The negative correlation was stronger ($r = -0.59$, $P<0.01$) in patients with dominant periodontal pathogens when compared with all patients. These results indicate that DMFT scores and pocket depth are correlated in an oral environment containing periodontal dominant pathogens.

We examined the relationship between the dental caries index of children (PCR and deft) and the parents' caries clinical status or periodontal clinical status (Fig. 2). The PCR and deft scores of children appeared to increase significantly with the parents' DMFT scores increasing (Figs. 2A and 2B) and appeared to decrease with the parent's pocket depth increasing (Figs. 2C and 2D).

Discussion

The results in Table 1 indicate that the children's deft score was influenced by the habit of eating or drinking before bedtime. The children's PCR score was influenced by the frequency of brushing. We used the habit of eating or drinking before bedtime as a factor in a multivariate model in which children's deft score was used as a dependent variable. The association between children's deft score and parents' DMFT score or parents' pocket depth was statistically significant ($\beta = 0.45$, $p<0.01$ for parents' DMFT; $\beta = -0.38$, $p<0.01$ for parents' pocket depth). We used the frequency of brushing as a factor in a multivariate model in which children's PCR score was used as a dependent variable. The association between children's PCR score and parents' DMFT score or parents' pocket depth was statistically significant ($\beta = 2.94$, $p<0.01$ for parents' DMFT; $\beta = -14.4$, $p = 0.03$ for parents' pocket depth).

Dental caries and periodontal disease are the most common diseases of the oral cavity. Both diseases are known to be associated with microorganisms that colonize the tooth surface. The influence of the family in the establishment of pathogenic microorganisms in children has been documented [18,19]. However, even when an oral disease is present, a microbial

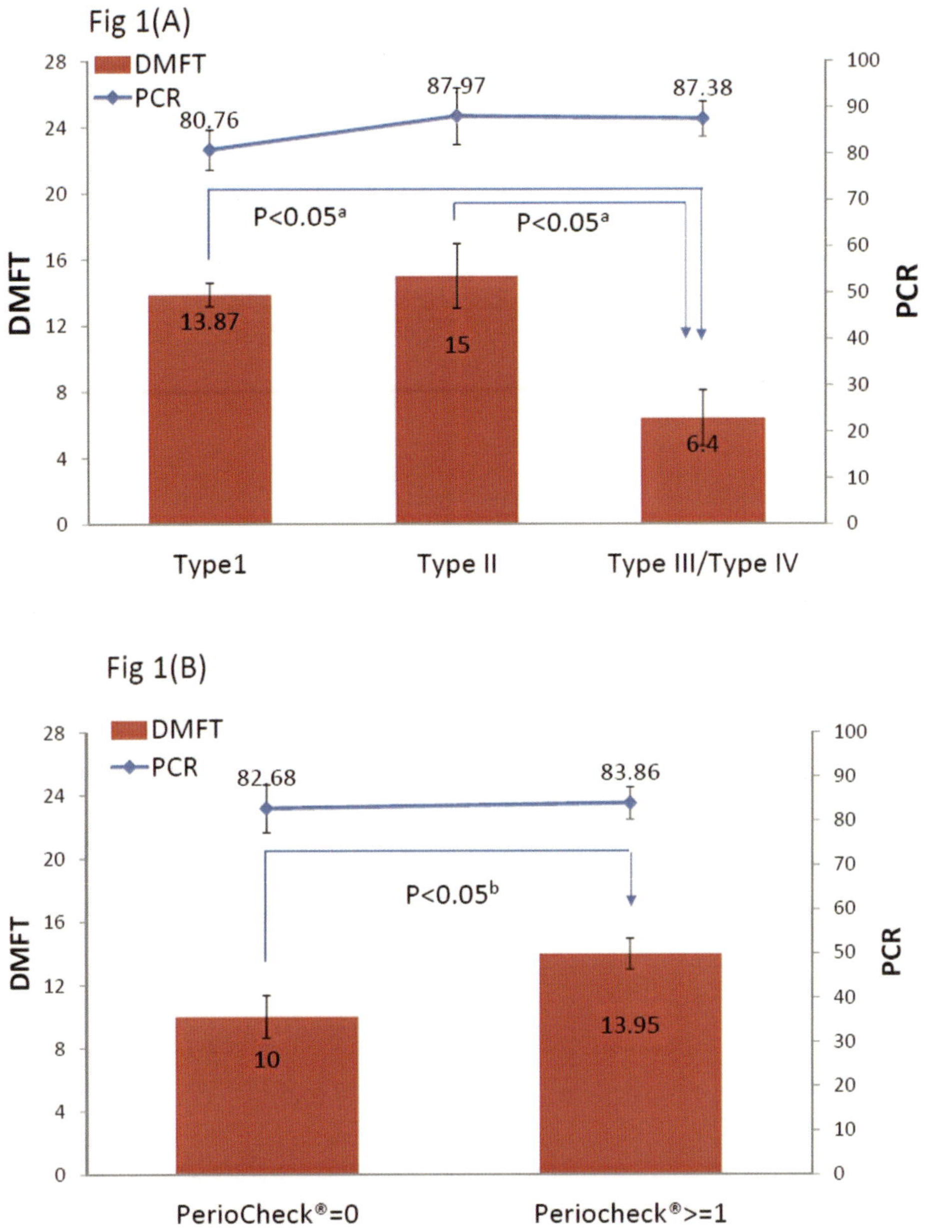

Figure 1. Comparison of DMFT and PCR scores in relation to periodontal status in parents. (A): Distribution of DMFT and PCR scores among periodontal classification types. (B): DMFT and PCR score distribution in relation to PerioCheck® status. [a]Significantly different ($p<0.05$) from periodontal classification Type I based on analysis of variance and Scheffe's test. [b]Significantly different ($p<0.05$) based on Student's *t* test. Abbreviations: DMFT, decay and the number of missing or filled teeth; PCR, plaque control records.

sample is rarely taken and tested to confirm the presence of microorganisms [20]. Because dental caries and periodontal disease have been reported to have a genetic basis [21], certain people may be predisposed to or have a greater likelihood of hosting these bacteria and might thus suffer from poor oral health. Knowledge of the underlying familial microbial infection could be used in assessing the risk of disease development and progression, which would facilitate dental counseling and the use of preventive protocols.

It is very interesting that the positive detection of *S. mutans* in parents by using the Dentocult® SM strip test was highly correlated with positive detection in their children. When parents exhibited *S. mutans*-positive plaques, their children carried the plaque *S. mutans* at a rate that was significantly higher than in children of parents who tested negative for plaque *S. mutans* (90.48% vs. 33.33%). A strong association was also detected between the presence of plaque *S. mutans* in parents and the presence of saliva *S. mutans* in their children (data not show). Microbial monitoring has been considered as an alternative method for evaluating current caries activity and future caries risk. Chair-side evaluation of salivary and plaque *S. mutans* levels (e.g., Dentocult-SM) has been used in numerous studies [22]. The practicality of the test in children has been evaluated and the test has been demonstrated to be accurate [23]. Moreover, the microbial counts on the strip have been determined to be an accurate indicator of infection [24]. A systematic review has

Table 4. Correlation coefficients of caries indices and periodontal status in parent.

	PCR	Gingival index	Pocket depth
DMFT	−0.02	0.20	−0.49**
PCR	1.00	0.24	0.19
Gingival index		1.00	0.15
Pocket depth			1.00
PerioCheck® = 0, N = 8			
	PCR	**Gingival index**	**Pocket depth**
DMFT	0.45	−0.14	−0.63
PCR	1.00	0.24	0.19
Gingival index		1.00	0.15
Pocket depth			1.00
PerioCheck® ≥ 1, N = 22			
	PCR	**Gingival index**	**Pocket depth**
DMFT	−0.16	0.11	−0.59**
PCR	1.00	0.34	0.25
Gingival index		1.00	0.15
Pocket depth			1.00

Abbreviations: DMFT, decay and the number of missing or filled teeth; PCR, plaque control records.
**p<0.01.

confirmed that the presence of *S. mutans* in both the plaque and the saliva of young caries-free children was associated with a considerable increase in the risk of early childhood caries (ECC) [25].

In this study, we determined that the chair-side Dentocult® SM score may be an indicator of the present clinical status only for parents (Table 2): the Dentocult SM score was not significantly related to deft status. The paired child-deft and parent-DMFT scores were positive correlated (Fig. 2A), indicating that genetic factors might play a key role in the clinical status of dental caries. The levels of *S. mutans* in saliva and plaque were shown to predict caries activity, but the clinical status of the children was more closely related to their parents' clinical status in this cross-sectional study.

In this study, the parents' scores on both the Periocheck® and the Dentocult SM tests were correlated with the gingival index (Table 2). The presence of high numbers of pathogens at the site of the tooth may induce gingival inflammation, but the quantity of pathogen was related neither to the pocket depth nor to the PCR. A previous cross-sectional analysis indicated that *P. gingivalis* from tongue and subgingival samples and *B. forsythus* from subgingival samples were associated with early periodontitis in adults [26]. Watson et al. (1991) reported that young children are colonized by *P. gingivalis*, *T. denticola*, and *T. forsythensis*. Children whose parents were colonized by bacteria that test positively with benzoyl-DL-arginine-naphthylamide (BANA) were significantly more likely to exhibit a positive BANA reaction than children of parents who were not colonized by BANA test-positive bacteria. Furthermore, children displaying BANA-positive plaques were more likely than children without such plaques to have parents, caregivers, or other family members who were older and had a history of periodontal disease [27,28]. In this study, we noted that parents who were PerioCheck® positive were more likely have children who tested positive in PerioCheck® than parents who were PerioCheck® negative, but the difference was not statistically significant (Table 4). Our results agree with the previous studies in which the BANA test was used.

Our results indicated that the PerioCheck® score was not correlated with saliva *S. mutans* (Table 3). Moreover, the DMFT scores of patients with moderate or advanced periodontitis were lower than those of gingivitis patients (Fig. 1). Based on the results, we conclude that plaque *S. mutans* and PerioCheck® scores were correlated with gingival status. These data suggest that PerioCheck® can serve as a chair-side indicator of clinical severity, but gingivitis is more related to supragingival pathogens. Recently, periodontal therapy has been reported to lead to a change in microbial flora, from a predominantly periodontal pathogenic organism to one that is more cariogenic [29,30]. Patients whose periodontal disease had been treated were found to exhibit high microorganism recovery during follow-up [31,32], and, similarly, patients who had been treated for periodontal disease showed higher *S. mutans* levels than untreated patients did [29]. Periodontitis patients who were not treated displayed high recovery rates of *S. mutans* in saliva, tongue dorsum, buccal mucosa, and supra- and sub-gingival plaque [33].

The salivary levels of *P. gingivalis* and *S. mutans* have been assessed using the polymerase chain reaction method to compare periodontal disease and dental caries [34]. The results suggested that the salivary levels of *S. mutans* were significantly higher in the healthy group than in periodontitis patients, and that salivary levels of *P. gingivalis* were significantly higher in the caries-free group than in the periodontally healthy group with caries. Data obtained using semi-quantitative detection tools in this study did not reveal an inverse correlation between *S. mutans* and periodontic pathogens. Furthermore, patients exhibiting poor oral hygiene had both higher saliva *S. mutans* levels and Periocheck® scores, both in parent and child groups (Fig. 2).

Although antagonistic interactions between *S. sanguis* and *Porphyromonas* species in vivo have been reported, these interactions might be related to the resistance to colonization after infection with gram-positive streptococci [13,35]. In these studies, polymerase chain reaction was used to detect the pathogens, and some of the samples were collected from gingival sulcus. Despite the changes in the proportion of *S. mutans* in the subgingival sample before and after therapy, the bacterium persisted in the oral cavity of patients treated for periodontitis. The subgingival area is an ecological niche, and the high proportions of *S. mutans* in this niche after periodontal therapy indicate a shift from gram-negative bacteria to gram-positive bacteria including *S. mutans*. In this study, we did not use polymerase chain reaction to detect oral pathogens, but instead used a method that is more practical for the clinician. Dentocult SM was used to detect the presence of *S. mutans* in supragingival plaques and saliva, and PerioCheck® was used to detect the organism in the subgingival plaque. The periodontal and caries pathogens, which resided in the oral cavity but not in the same ecological niche, showed no antagonistic interactions.

In this study, we did not detect an inverse correlation between the scores of PerioCheck® and DMFT, but parents with severe periodontitis had significantly lower DMFT scores (Fig. 1A), which suggests high rates of familial transmission and habitation of the pathogens. Because the periodontitis status of children cannot be detected, PerioCheck® serves as a crucial indicator of the early acquisition of these organisms by children. The periodontitis risk-assessment model should include a pathogen score and the clinical

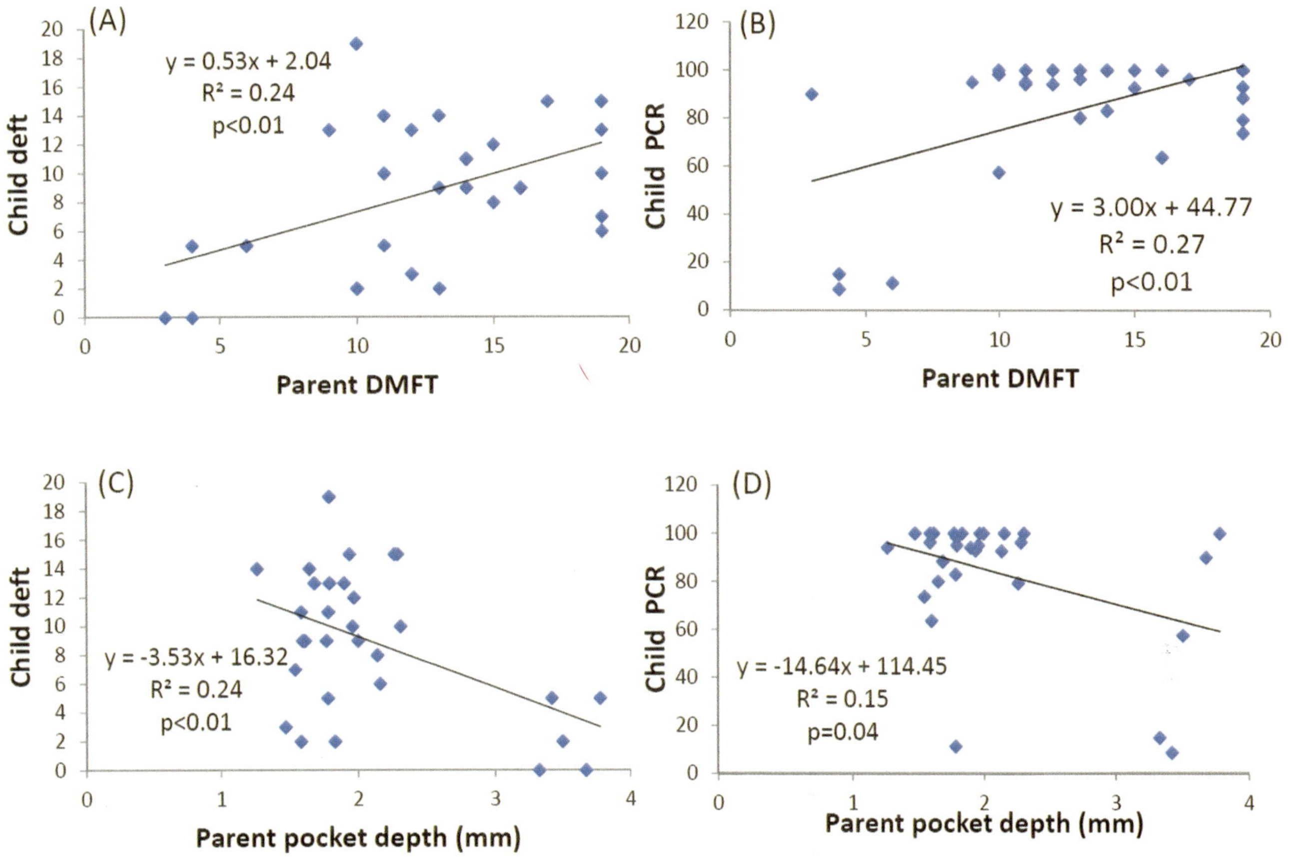

Figure 2. Scatterplots indicating the relationships between child caries index and parent caries index or clinical periodontal outcome. Scatterplots of (A) child deft and parent DMFT scores; (B) child PCR and parent DMFT scores; (C) child deft scores and parent pocket depth; and (D) child PCR scores and parent pocket depth. Abbreviations: deft, decay, extraction, and filled teeth; DMFT, decay and the number of missing or filled teeth; PCR, plaque control records.

status (DMFT and periodontal status) of the caregiver or parent; the use of such a model could help identify children who face a high risk of periodontal disease and exclude those whose risk of developing the disease is low. An understanding of the risk factors involved in initial periodontitis and the use of an appropriate diagnostic sampling protocol will be invaluable not only in identifying people who face the risk of suffering from periodontitis, but also in developing effective disease intervention measures [36].

Another key result obtained in this study was the correlation detected between the pocket depth and the caries index. Our data indicate that parents exhibiting greater pocket depth developed fewer dental caries (Table 4), and, moreover, that their children had fewer dental caries (Fig. 2C). The clinical severity of the periodontal status appeared to be inversely correlated with dental caries, particularly when the pathogen could be isolated. Therefore, both pathogen detection and genetic factors should be considered in risk assessment when evaluating periodontal and dental caries clinical status in children.

This cross-sectional study was conducted to elucidate the familial correlation of microbial levels with periodontal status and caries development. The 30 parent-child pairs were recruited from dental clinics, and the caries- and periodontal-related microbial levels were measured using semi-quantitative microbial commercial kits. This study should be extended using a larger sample size.

People who are at risk of suffering from periodontal disease or dental caries could be identified and targeted for intervention. Moreover, understanding the interaction between genetic and environmental factors is critical: evidence indicates that dental caries and periodontitis are multifactorial infectious diseases caused by numerous contributory environmental factors and that a strong genetic component is involved in the etiology of these diseases. Additional studies on twins, families, and animal models should be conducted to broaden the current understanding of the genetic component of dental caries and periodontitis.

Author Contributions

Conceived and designed the experiments: WFL YHSC WST JRS. Performed the experiments: YHSC WST NCT. Analyzed the data: YKH MJW SYL. Contributed reagents/materials/analysis tools: WFL WJC NCT. Wrote the paper: WFL YKH MJW NCT. Partly contributed to the conception and design of the work, and recruited the study subjects: YHSC WST SYL.

References

1. Eke PI, Dye BA, Wei L, Thornton-Evans GO, Genco RJ (2012) Prevalence of periodontitis in adults in the United States: 2009 and 2010. J Dent Res 91: 914–920.
2. Sheiham A, Watt RG (2000) The common risk factor approach: a rational basis for promoting oral health. Community Dent Oral Epidemiol 28: 399–406.
3. WHO (1997) Oral Health Surveys - Basic Methods. 4th Ed.

4. Selwitz RH, Ismail AI, Pitts NB (2007) Dental caries. The Lancet 369: 51–59.
5. Tomas I, Diz P, Tobias A, Scully C, Donos N (2012) Periodontal health status and bacteraemia from daily oral activities: systematic review/meta-analysis. Journal of Clinical Periodontology 39: 213–228.
6. Bowen WH (2002) Do we need to be concerned about dental caries in the coming millennium? Crit Rev Oral Biol Med 13: 126–131.
7. Kuramitsu HK (2003) Molecular genetic analysis of the virulence of oral bacterial pathogens: an historical perspective. Crit Rev Oral Biol Med 14: 331–344.
8. van Loveren C, Buijs JF, ten Cate JM (2000) Similarity of bacteriocin activity profiles of mutans streptococci within the family when the children acquire the strains after the age of 5. Caries Res 34: 481–485.
9. Ezzo PJ, Cutler CW (2003) Microorganisms as risk indicators for periodontal disease. Periodontol 2000 32: 24–35.
10. Asikainen S, Chen C, Slots J (1996) Likelihood of transmitting Actinobacillus actinomycetemcomitans and Porphyromonas gingivalis in families with periodontitis. Oral Microbiol Immunol 11: 387–394.
11. Dogan B, Kipalev AS, Okte E, Sultan N, Asikainen SE (2008) Consistent intrafamilial transmission of Actinobacillus actinomycetemcomitans despite clonal diversity. J Periodontol 79: 307–315.
12. Dalwai F, Spratt DA, Pratten J (2007) Use of quantitative PCR and culture methods to characterize ecological flux in bacterial biofilms. J Clin Microbiol 45: 3072–3076.
13. Hillman JD, Socransky SS, Shivers M (1985) The relationships between streptococcal species and periodontopathic bacteria in human dental plaque. Arch Oral Biol 30: 791–795.
14. Bowers JE, Zahradnik RT (1989) Evaluation of a chairside gingival protease test for use in periodontal diagnosis. J Clin Dent 1: 106–109.
15. Eley BM, Cox SW (1995) Bacterial proteases in gingival crevicular fluid before and after periodontal treatment. Br Dent J 178: 133–139.
16. Hemmings KW, Griffiths GS, Bulman JS (1997) Detection of neutral protease (Periocheck) and BANA hydrolase (Perioscan) compared with traditional clinical methods of diagnosis and monitoring of chronic inflammatory periodontal disease. J Clin Periodontol 24: 110–114.
17. O'Leary TJ, Drake RB, Naylor JE (1972) The plaque control record. J Periodontol 43: 38.
18. Kononen E, Saarela M, Karjalainen J, Jousimies-Somer H, Alaluusua S et al(1994) Transmission of oral Prevotella melaninogenica between a mother and her young child. Oral Microbiol Immunol 9: 310–314.
19. Morinushi T, Lopatin DE, Van PN, Ueda Y (2000) The relationship between gingivitis and colonization by Porphyromonas gingivalis and Actinobacillus actinomycetemcomitans in children. J Periodontol 71: 403–409.
20. Loesche W (2007) Dental caries and periodontitis: contrasting two infections that have medical implications. Infect Dis Clin North Am 21: 471–502.
21. Hassell TM, Harris EL (1995) Genetic influences in caries and periodontal diseases. Crit Rev Oral Biol Med 6: 319–342.
22. Olak J, Mandar R, Karjalainen S, Soderling E, Saag M (2007) Dental health and oral mutans streptococci in 2–4-year-old Estonian children. Int J Paediatr Dent 17: 92–97.
23. Karjalainen S, Soderling E, Pienihakkinen K (2004) Validation and inter-examiner agreement of mutans streptococci levels in plaque and saliva of 10-year-old children using simple chair-side tests. Acta Odontol Scand 62: 153–157.
24. Pienihakkinen K, Jokela J (1995) A simple method for monitoring mutans streptococci in young children. Eur J Oral Sci 103: 61–62.
25. Thenisch NL, Bachmann LM, Imfeld T, Leisebach MT, Steurer J (2006) Are mutans streptococci detected in preschool children a reliable predictive factor for dental caries risk? A systematic review. Caries Res 40: 366–374.
26. Tanner AC, Paster BJ, Lu SC, Kanasi E, Kent R, et al(2006) Subgingival and tongue microbiota during early periodontitis. J Dent Res 85: 318–323.
27. Watson MR, Lopatin DE, Bretz WA, Ertel IJ, Loesche WJ (1991) Detection of two anaerobic periodontopathogens in children by means of the BANA and ELISA assays. J Dent Res 70: 1052–1056.
28. Lee Y, Straffon LH, Welch KB, Loesche WJ (2006) The transmission of anaerobic periodontopathic organisms. J Dent Res 85: 182–186.
29. Quirynen M, Gizani S, Mongardini C, Declerck D, Vinckier F et al (1999) The effect of periodontal therapy on the number of cariogenic bacteria in different intra-oral niches. J Clin Periodontol 26: 322–327.
30. Haffajee AD, Socransky SS (1994) Microbial etiological agents of destructive periodontal diseases. Periodontol 2000 5: 78–111.
31. Loesche WJ (1986) Role of Streptococcus mutans in human dental decay. Microbiol Rev 50: 353–380.
32. Van der Reijden WA, Dellemijn-Kippuw N, Stijne-van Nes AM, de Soet JJ, van Winkelhoff AJ (2001) Mutans streptococci in subgingival plaque of treated and untreated patients with periodontitis. J Clin Periodontol 28: 686–691.
33. Loesche WJ, Syed SA, Schmidt E, Morrison EC (1985) Bacterial profiles of subgingival plaques in periodontitis. J Periodontol 56: 447–456.
34. Iwano Y, Sugano N, Matsumoto K, Nishihara R, Iizuka T et al(2010) Salivary microbial levels in relation to periodontal status and caries development. J Periodontal Res 45: 165–169.
35. Fiehn NE, Klausen B, Evans RT (1992) Periodontal bone loss in Porphyromonas gingivalis-infected specific pathogen-free rats after preinoculation with endogenous Streptococcus sanguis. J Periodontal Res 27: 609–614.
36. Rudney JD, Michalowicz BS, Krig MA, Kane PK, Pihlstrom BL (1994) Genetic contributions to saliva protein concentrations in adult human twins. Arch Oral Biol 39: 513–517.

Dental Follicle Cells Rescue the Regenerative Capacity of Periodontal Ligament Stem Cells in an Inflammatory Microenvironment

Jia Liu[1,2]ᵠ, Liying Wang[1,2]ᵠ, Wenjia Liu[2,3]ᵠ, Qiang Li[4], Zuolin Jin[1]*, Yan Jin[2,3]*

1 State Key Laboratory of Military Stomatology, Department of Orthodontics, School of Stomatology, The Fourth Military Medical University, Xi'an, Shaanxi, China, **2** State Key Laboratory of Military Stomatology, Center for Tissue Engineering, School of Stomatology, The Fourth Military Medical University, Xi'an, Shaanxi, China, **3** Research and Development Center for Tissue Engineering, Fourth Military Medical University, Xi'an, Shaanxi, China, **4** State Key Laboratory of Military Stomatology, Department of General Dentistry & Emergency, School of Stomatology, The Fourth Military Medical University, Xi'an, Shaanxi, China

Abstract

Aims: Periodontal ligament stem cells (PDLSCs) are one of the best candidates for periodontal regeneration. Their function could be impaired in periodontitis microenvironment. Dental follicle cells (DFCs), serving as precursor cells and mesenchymal stem cells, have intimate connection with PDLSCs. However, it is still unknown whether DFCs could provide a favorable microenvironment to improve the proliferation and differentiation capacity of PDLSCs from healthy subjects (HPDLSCs) and patients diagnosed with periodontitis (PPDLSCs).

Methods: HPDLSCs, PPDLSCs and DFCs were harvested and identified using microscopic and flow cytometric analysis. Then, the coculture systems of DFCs/HPDLSCs and DFCs/PPDLSCs were established with 0.4 μm transwell, in which all the detection indexs were obtained from HPDLSCs and PPDLSCs. The expression of stemness-associated genes was detected by real-time PCR, and the proliferation ability was assessed using colony formation and cell cycle assays. The osteogenic differentiation capacity was evaluated by real-time PCR, western blot, ALP activity, Alizarin Red S staining and calcium level analysis, while the adipogenic differentiation capacity was determined by real-time PCR and Oil Red O staining. The cell sheet formation in vitro was observed by HE staining and SEM, and the implantation effect in vivo was evaluated using HE staining and Masson's trichrome staining.

Results: PPDLSCs had a greater proliferation capability but lower osteogenic and adipogenic potential than HPDLSCs. DFCs enhanced the proliferation and osteogenic/adipogenic differentiation of HPDLSCs and PPDLSCs to different degrees. Moreover, coculture with DFCs increased cell layers and extracellular matrix of HPDLSCs/PPDLSCs cell sheets in vitro and improved periodontal regeneration by HPDLSCs/PPDLSCs in vivo.

Conclusions: Our data suggest that the function of PPDLSCs could be damaged in the periodontitis microenvironment. DFCs appear to enhance the self-renewal and multi-differentiation capacity of both HPDLSCs and PPDLSCs, which indicates that DFCs could provide a beneficial microenvironment for periodontal regeneration using PDLSCs.

Editor: Irina Kerkis, Instituto Butantan, Brazil

Funding: This work was supported by grants from the Nature Science Foundation of China (31030033 and 81271176) and the National Basic Research Program (973 Program) (2010CB944800 and 2011CB964700). The funders had no role in study design, data collection and analysis, decision to publish, or preparation of the manuscript.

Competing Interests: The authors have declared that no competing interests exist.

* Email: zuolinj@fmmu.edu.cn (ZJ); yanjin@fmmu.edu.cn (YJ)

ᵠ These authors contributed equally to this work.

Introduction

Periodontitis is a chronic infectious disease that can lead to the destruction of periodontal tissues and even tooth loss [1,2]. Therapeutic strategies for the treatment of periodontitis include not only the control of local inflammation but also the regeneration of new periodontal tissues attached to the surface of the tooth root. Although stem cell biology and guided tissue regeneration (GTR) have provided advances in inflammation control, they still have limitations for the recovery of a functional periodontium [3].

Tissue engineering has recently been shown to be a promising approach for periodontal regeneration [4–6], and strategies using mesenchymal stem cells (MSCs) are especially promising [7]. Periodontal ligament stem cells (PDLSCs) have been identified as a type of MSCs present in periodontal tissues and are capable of differentiating into cementum-forming cells, bone-forming cells, adipocytes and collagen-forming cells. After transplantation into immunocompromised mice, PDLSCs are able to generate cementum/PDL-like structures [8–11]. Compared with MSCs from other tissue sources, PDLSCs are more similar to the native periodontal tissues with regard to morphology, structure and characteristics, making them the best candidate for periodontal regeneration [12–14]. Therefore, optimizing the characteristics and function of PDLSCs to regenerate periodontal tissues (including fibrous tissues and bones) is an important topic in this field.

The extracellular microenvironment is known to affect the proliferation and differentiation of MSCs [15–17]. It has previously been demonstrated that the periodontitic microenvironment can decrease the osteogenic ability of PDLSCs [18]. In contrast, a favorable microenvironment, such as that provided by conditioned medium from young periodontal ligament cells, can enhance the proliferation and differentiation of PDLSCs from aged donors [19].

Dental follicle cells (DFCs), which are a type of MSCs found in periodontal tissues, are young precursor cells present during tooth development [20]. DFCs are intimately associated with PDLSCs, both structurally and functionally, during tooth development. In this study, we established a co-culture system for DFCs and PDLSCs using transwell to simulate the natural microenvironment present during tooth development. PDLSCs were obtained from healthy subjects (HPDLSCs) and patients diagnosed with periodontitis (PPDLSCs). We postulated that DFCs, as a homologous precursor cell type, could provide a beneficial microenvironment to optimize the characteristics of PDLSCs (both HPDLSCs and PPDLSCs) through cell-to-cell interactions.

Materials and Methods

Study Subjects and Ethics Statement

HPDLSCs for primary culture (n = 15) were obtained from healthy periodontal tissues of 10 orthodontic patients (25–43 years old) undergoing premolar and third molar extractions. PPDLSCs for primary culture (n = 10) were obtained from 6 periodontitis patients (28–52 years old) who were diagnosed by the same periodontics specialist based on the clinical manifestation of alveolar bone loss (≥1/3) and more than one periodontal pocket (depth≥5 mm). DFCs for primary culture (n = 8) were obtained by culturing tissue explants from healthy subjects whose third molars were being extracted for orthodontic reasons during the phase of tooth germ development. The subjects included in this study did not have a history of systemic disease, smoking or special medication. All samples were collected at the Department of Oral and Maxillofacial Surgery of the School of Stomatology at the Fourth Military Medical University. All participants provided written informed consent, and the study was approved by the Ethics Committee of School of Stomatology, Fourth Military Medical University (Xi'an, China).

Cell Culture

For cell isolation, the teeth were first washed in sterile phosphate-buffered saline (PBS). The periodontal ligament (PDL) was then gently separated from the middle part of the root surface and cut into small pieces (1 mm^3) under a microscope. Colonies were established from single cells using the limiting dilution technique to obtain homogeneous populations of HPDLSCs and PPDLSCs, as previously described [21,22]. The culture medium was changed every 2 days. After 2–3 weeks of culture, the single cell-derived clones were harvested and mixed together. Multiple colony-derived HPDLSCs and PPDLSCs at passage 2–4 were used in our experiments. For each experiment, PDLSCs at the same passage were used.

Flow Cytometric Analysis

For identification of the MSC phenotype, approximately 5×10^5 PDLSCs were incubated with PE-conjugated monoclonal antibodies against human Stro-1, CD29, CD45, CD90, CD105 and CD146 (BD Bioscience, San Jose, CA, USA). The cells were incubated with the specified antibodies for 1 hour in a 4°C lucifugal environment. After washing three times with PBS containing 30 ml/L fetal bovine serum (FBS), the cells were subjected to flow cytometric analysis using a Beckman CoulterE-

Table 1. Primer sequences.

Gene	Primer sequence
β-actin	Forward 5′-TGG CAC CCA GCA CAA TGA A-3′
	Reverse 5′-CTA AGT CAT AGT CCG CCT AGA AGC A-3′
Klf4	Forward 5′-GAG CCC AAG CCA AAG AGG-3′
	Reverse 5′-ATC CAC AGC CGT CCC AGT C-3′
Sox2	Forward 5′-ATG GGT TCG GTG GTC AAC TC-3′
	Reverse 5′-CGC TCT GGT AGT GCT GGG A-3′
Oct4	Forward 5′-CCT GTC TCC GTC ACC ACT CTG-3′
	Reverse 5′-AAC CCT GGC ACA AAC TCC-3′
Runx2	Forward 5′-CCC GTG GCC TTC AAG GT-3′
	Reverse 5′-CGT TAC CCG CCA TGA CAG TA-3′
ALP	Forward 5′-GGA CCA TTC CCA CGT CTT CAC-3′
	Reverse 5′-CCT TGT AGC CAG GCC CAT TG-3′
OCN	Forward 5′-CCC AGG CGC TAC CTG TAT CAA-3′
	Reverse 5′-GGT CAG CCA ACT CGT CAC AGT C-3′
PPARγ	Forward 5′-CCA CTT TGA TTG CAC TTT GGT ACT CTT G-3′
	Reverse 5′-CTT CAC TAC TGT TGA CTT CTC CAG CAT TTC-3′

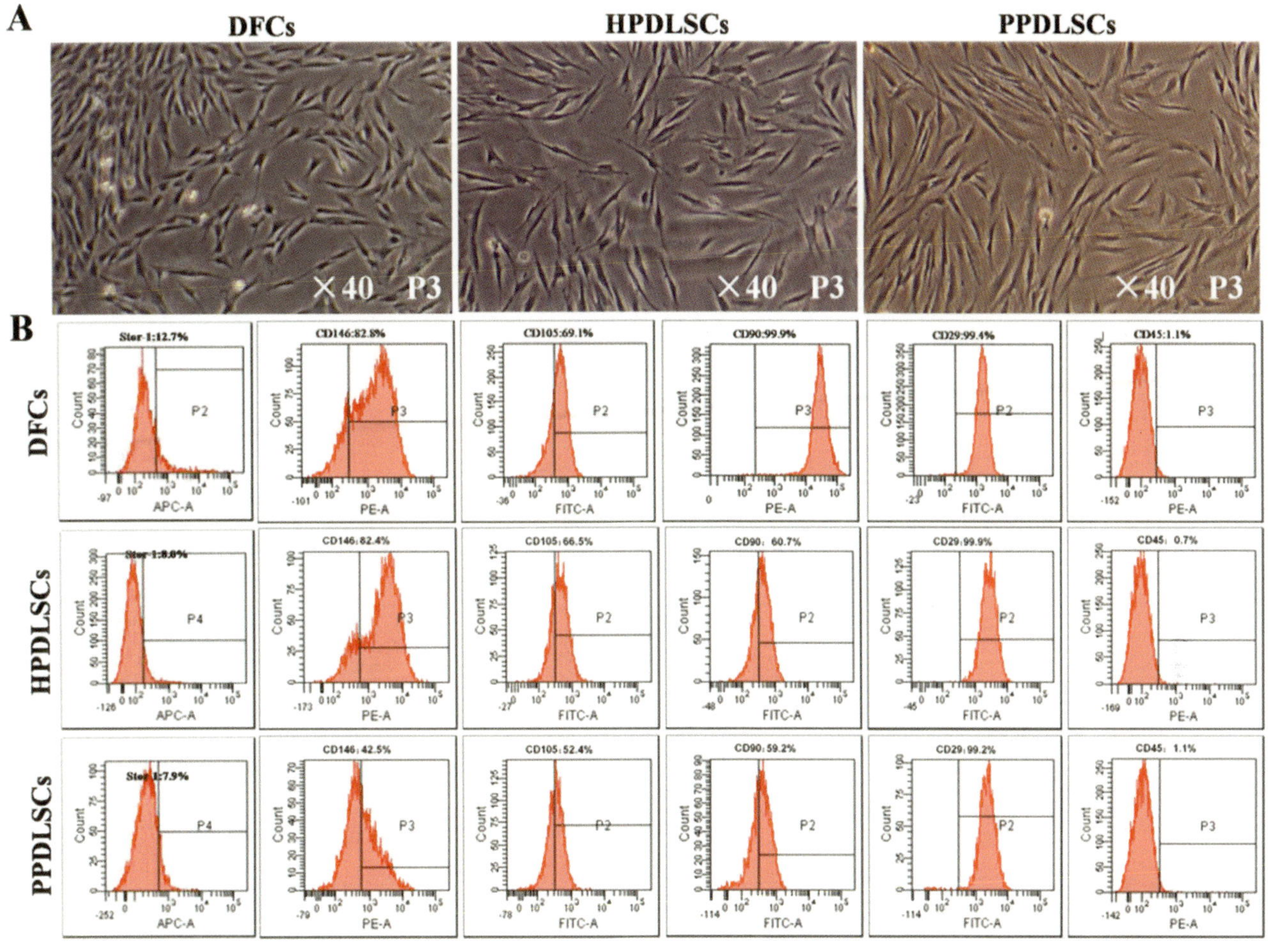

Figure 1. Isolation and identification of HPDLSCs, PPDLSCs, and DFCs. A: Morphologies of DFCs, HPDLSCs, and PPDLSCs observed by microscopy. **B:** Mesenchymal stem cell phenotype examination by flow cytometric analysis.

pics XL instrument (Beckman Coulter, Fullerton, CA, USA) for cell phenotype characterization.

For cell cycle analysis, HPDLSCs and PPDLSCs (approximately 2×10^4 cells) were cultured in 6-well plates with serum-free α-MEM, and DFCs (5×10^4) were seeded in transwell chambers with 0.4 μm pores (Millicell, Millipore, MA, USA). After culturing for 24 hours, the transwell was placed into the 6-well plates to establish the DFC/HPDLSC and DFC/PPDLSC co-culture systems. The control groups consisted of monocultured HPDLSCs or PPDLSCs in the plates, with no cells in the transwell chambers. The monocultured and co-cultured HPDLSCs and PPDLSCs were maintained separately in their own systems for 5 days. Then, single-cell suspensions (5×10^5 HPDLSCs and PPDLSCs each) were washed with PBS containing 30 ml/L FBS, fixed with 75% ethanol and subjected to cell cycle analysis by flow cytometry. The fractions of cells in the G_1, S and G_2 phases of the cell cycle were measured, and the proliferation index (PI, the percentage of cells in G_2+S phases) was analyzed.

Colony-Forming Assays

Single-cell suspensions (50 cells) of HPDLSCs and PPDLSCs in α-MEM (10% FBS) were seeded in 6-well plates (Corning, Lowell, MA, USA), and DFCs (5×10^4) were seeded in the transwell chambers (Millipore, Billerica, MA, USA). After 6 hours, the co-culture and monoculture systems were established, as described above. The HPDLSCs and PPDLSCs cultures were fixed in 4% paraformaldehyde and stained with 0.1% toluidine blue at day 10. The stained cultures were analyzed by microscopy, and aggregates containing 50 or more cells were counted as colonies. The number of colonies per well was counted, and the colony-forming rate was calculated.

Real-time PCR

Total RNA was isolated from the HPDLSCs and PPDLSCs using Trizol reagent (Invitrogen, Carlsbad, CA, USA), and reverse transcription was performed using the PrimeScript RT reagent kit (Takara, Bio, Otsu, Japan). The primer sequences used in the experiment are listed in Table 1. Real-time PCR reactions were performed using the SYBR Premix Ex Taq II kit (Takara, Bio, Otsu, Japan) and an applied Bio-systems CFX96TM Real-Time sequence detection system (Applied Biosystems, Darmstadt, Germany).

Osteogenic and Adipogenic Differentiation

For osteogenesis, HPDLSCs and PPDLSCs were plated at a density of 5×10^4 cells per well in 6-well plates, and DFCs were plated in transwell chambers (Millipore, Billerica, MA, USA) at the same density to establish co-culture and monoculture systems. After reaching 80% confluence, HPDLSCs and PPDLSCs were cultured in osteogenic medium (α-MEM supplemented with 5%

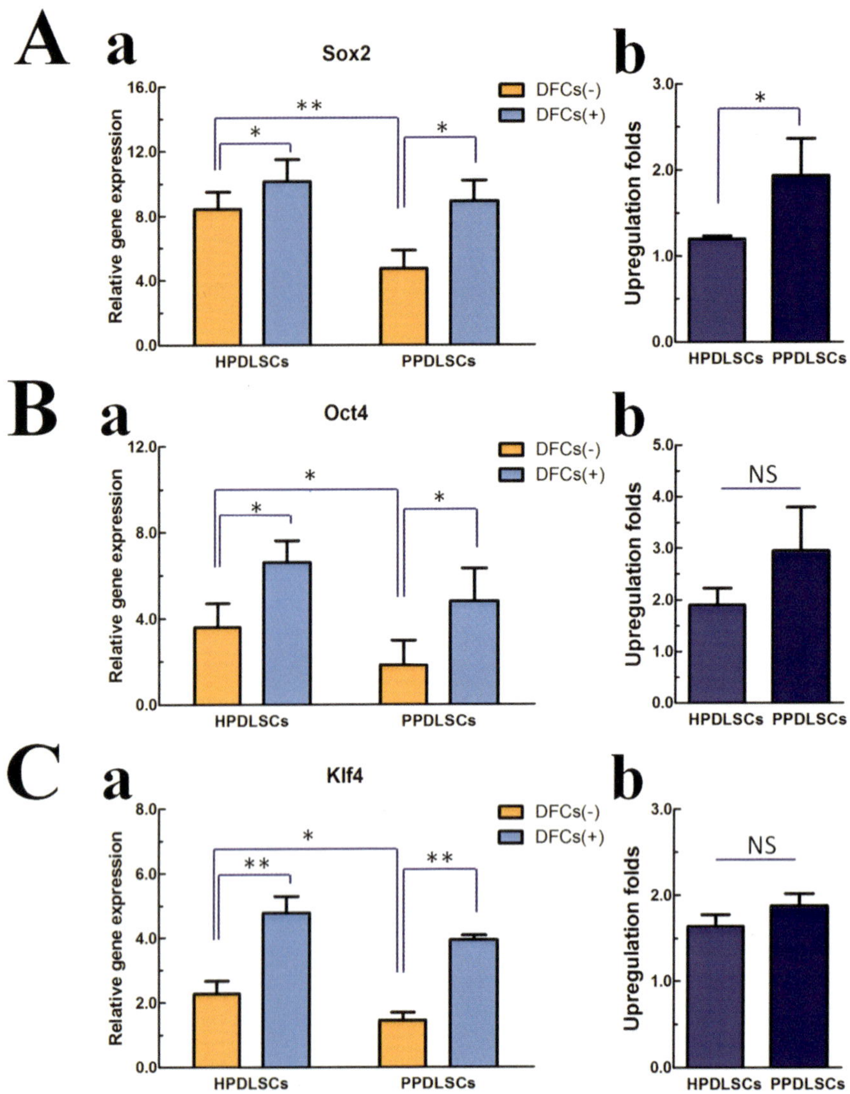

Figure 2. Effects of DFCs on the stemness of HPDLSCs and PPDLSCs. Expression levels of the stemness-related genes Sox2 (**Aa**), Oct4 (**Ba**), and Klf4 (**Ca**) were examined by real time RT-PCR after 14 days of culture with osteogenic supplements. Upregulation folds of Sox2 (**Ab**), Oct4 (**Bb**), and Klf4 (**Cb**) gene levels by coculture with DFCs were quantitatively analyzed in HPDLSCs and PPDLSCs. Notes: DFCs (–), monocultured PDLSCs that were cultured with transwell containing no DFCs; DFCs (+), co-cultured PDLSCs that were cultured with transwell seeded with a specific number of DFCs. Bars represent the mean ± S.D. (n = 3). *$p<0.05$, **$p<0.01$, ***$p<0.001$.

FBS, 100 nM dexamethasone (Sigma, Santa Clara, CA, USA), 50 pg/ml ascorbic acid (Sigma, Santa Clara, CA, USA) and 5 mM β-glycerophosphate (Sigma, Santa Clara, CA, USA)) for 7–28 days. The media were changed every 3 days. For the differentiation analysis, the cells were washed twice in PBS and fixed in 4% paraformaldehyde for 30 min. Subsequently, alkaline phosphatase (ALP) staining was performed using the BCIP/NBT Alkaline Phosphatase Color Development Kit (Beyotime, Shanghai, China), and ALP activity was measured using the Alkaline Phosphatase (AKP/ALP) Detection Kit (Jiancheng Bioengineering, Nanjing, China). Mineralized nodules were stained with Alizarin Red S (pH 4.2) (Kermel, Tianjin, China) for 15 min at room temperature. Calcium levels were measured using a calcium colorimetric assay kit (BioVision, San Francisco, CA, USA).

For adipogenesis, HPDLSCs and PPDLSCs were plated at a density of 5×10^4 cells per well in 6-well plates and co-cultured with DFCs at the same density. After reaching 80% confluence, the HPDLSCs/PPDLSCs were cultured in adipogenic medium (α-MEM supplemented with 5% FBS, 0.5 mM methylisobutylxanthine (Sigma, Santa Clara, CA, USA), 0.5 μM hydrocortisone (Sigma, Santa Clara, CA, USA), and 60 μM indomethacin (Sigma, Santa Clara, CA, USA) for 7–21 days. For analysis, the adipogenic cultures were fixed in 4% paraformaldehyde for 30 min and stained with fresh Oil Red O solution (Sigma, Santa Clara, CA, USA) for 15 min. To quantify the amount of Oil Red O-stained lipids, the stain was solubilized in isopropanol for 5 minutes at room temperature. The solubilized stain (150 μL) was then transferred to the wells of a 96-well plate, and the absorbance was measured at 520 nm.

Protein Isolation and Western Blot Analysis

Total protein was extracted from the cells by lysis in RIPA buffer (10 mM Tris-HCl, 1 mM EDTA, 1% sodium dodecyl sulfate, 1% Nonidet P-40, 1:100 proteinase inhibitor cocktail,

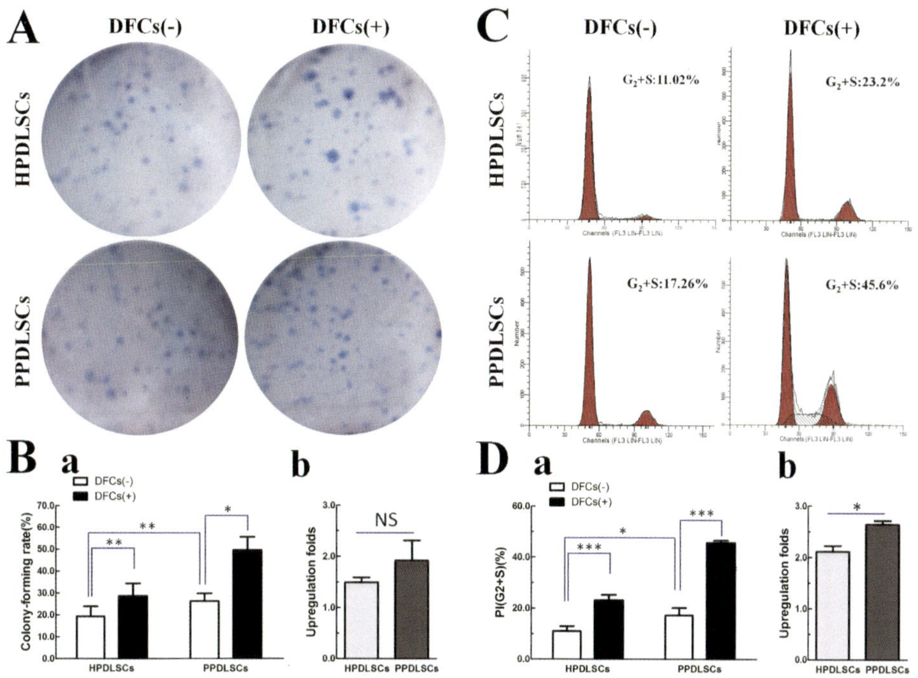

Figure 3. Effects of DFCs on proliferation of HPDLSCs and PPDLSCs. A: The colony forming rate was determined using colony-forming assays at day 10. **B:** Quantitative data for the colony-forming assays, **a:** Colony-forming rate of monocultured and cocultured HPDLSCs/PPDLSCs; **b:** Upregulation folds of colony-forming rate by coculture with DFCs in HPDLSCs and PPDLSCs. **C:** The percentage of cells in G2+S phases was measured by flow cytometry at day 5. **D:** Quantitative data of the cell cycle analysis, **a:** PI of HPDLSCs and PPDLSCs in monocultured and cocultured systems; **b:** Upregulation folds of PI in HPDLSCs and PPDLSCs by cocultured with DFCs. Notes: DFCs (–), monocultured PDLSCs that were cultured with transwell containing no DFCs; DFCs (+), co-cultured PDLSCs that were cultured with transwell seeded with a specific number of DFCs. Bars represent the mean ± S.D. (n = 3). $^*p<0.05$, $^{**}p<0.01$, $^{***}p<0.001$.

50 mM b-glycerophosphate and 50 mM sodium fluoride). The protein concentration in the extracted lysates was determined using a protein assay solution based on the absorbance at 595 nm (Bio-Rad, Hercules, CA, USA). Additionally, 20 to 50 mg of the cell lysate samples were separated by 10% SDS-PAGE and then transferred to a polyvinylidene fluoride (PVDF) membrane (Bio-Rad, Hercules, CA, USA). The membranes were blocked with 5% milk for 2 hours and then incubated with anti-Runx2 (Abcam, Cambridge, UK) and anti-β-actin (Cell Signaling Technology, Beverly, MA, USA) primary antibodies. The immune complexes were then incubated with horseradish peroxidase-conjugated anti-rabbit or anti-mouse IgG antibodies (Boshide, Beijing, China). Immunodetection was performed using the Western-Light Chemiluminescent Detection System (Peiqing, Shanghai, China).

Culture of Cell Sheets

HPDLSCs and PPDLSCs were seeded in 6-well plates at a density of 2×10^5 cells per well, and DFCs were seeded in transwell chambers at the same density. Co-culture and monoculture systems were set up after 24 hours. After 8–9 days of culture in normal α-MEM medium containing 5% FBS and ascorbate (50 μg/ml), cell-matrix sheets of HPDLSCs and PPDLSCs had formed and could be easily detached from the bottom of the culture plates using a cell scraper.

H&E Staining

The sheets were fixed in 4% phosphate-buffered paraformaldehyde for 24 h, embedded in paraffin, sectioned longitudinally and stained with hematoxylin and eosin (H&E). The H&E staining results were evaluated using an Olympus BX50 compound microscope (Olympus Optical, Tokyo, Japan).

Scanning Electron Microscopy (SEM)

To evaluate matrix secretion by the co-cultured and monocultured HPDLSCs and PPDLSCs, specimens were serially dehydrated with 70%, 75%, 80%, 90%, 95%, and 100% alcohol for 5 min each. The specimens were then sputter-coated with gold using a standard protocol and observed by SEM using a scanning electron microscope (Hitachi, Tokyo, Japan).

Preparation of Ceramic Bovine Bone (CBB) and Chemically Conditioned Root Dentin (CCRD)

Blocks of CBB (Research and Development Center for Tissue Engineering, Fourth Military Medical University, Xi'an, China) [23] were produced from fresh bovine rib bones (Shaanxi Kingbull Slaughterhouse, Xi'an, China) and shaped to a hollow tubule. CCRD specimens were prepared from collected human teeth and remodeled into slices (thickness, 1.0 mm; length, 2.0 mm), then they were treated by a series of chemical procedures as previously described [24].

Regeneration Effects of HPDLSC and PPDLSC Sheets Combined with CBB and CCRD in Immunodeficient Mice

HPDLSC and PPDLSC cell sheets were prepared and placed on the surfaces of CCRD scaffolds and wrapped from one side to the other. Then, the constructs containing HPDLSC/PPDLSC sheets and CCRD were inserted into CBB tubules to mimic a natural root for heterotopic transplantation into immunodeficient mice. All animal procedures were approved by the Animal Care

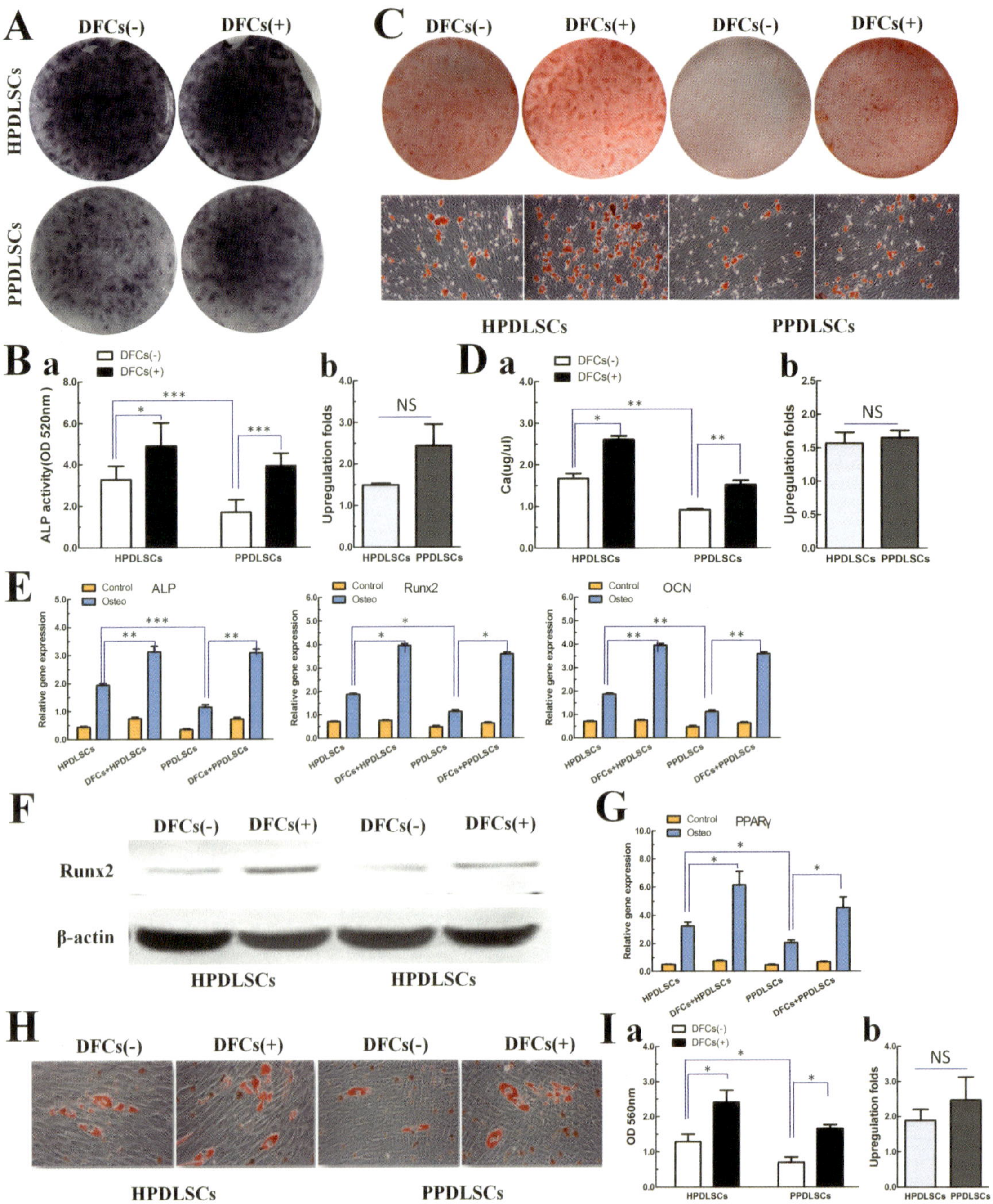

Figure 4. Effects of DFCs on the osteogenic and adipogenic differentiation of HPDLSCs and PPDLSCs in vitro. ALP activity was detected by (**A**) ALP staining and (**Ba**) ALP activity assay at day 7; **Bb:** Upregulation folds of ALP activity in HPDLSCs and PPDLSCs by cocultured with DFCs. **C:** Osteogenic differentiation was determined by Alizarin Red S staining after 28 days of culture with osteogenic supplements. **Da:** Calcium concentration was examined by calcium level analysis after 28 days of culture with osteogenic supplements; **Db**: Upregulation folds of calcium concentration in HPDLSCs and PPDLSCs by cocultured with DFCs. **E:** The expression levels of the osteogenic genes ALP, Runx2, and OCN were measured by real time PCR after 7 days of culture with osteogenic supplements. **F:** Runx2 protein expression was determined by western blot analysis after 7 days of culture with osteogenic supplements. **G:** The expression levels of the adipogenic genes PPARγwas measured by real time RT-PCR after 7 days of culture with adipogenic supplements. **H:** Adipogenic differentiation was evaluated by Oil Red O staining after 21 days of culture with adipogenic supplements. **Ia:** Quantitative data for Oil Red O staining; **Ib:** Upregulation folds of the quantitative data in HPDLSCs and PPDLSCs by cocultured with DFCs. Notes: DFCs (–), monocultured PDLSCs that were cultured with transwell containing no DFCs; DFCs (+), co-cultured PDLSCs that were cultured with transwell seeded with a specific number of DFCs. Bars represent the mean ± S.D. (n = 3). *$p<0.05$, **$p<0.01$, ***$p<0.001$.

Committee of the Fourth Military Medical University (Permit Number: 12046), and was conducted according to the Guidelines for Animal Experimentation of the Fourth Military Medical University (Xi'an, China). Six 6-week-old male mice (BALB/c-nu; FMMU Medical Laboratory Animal Center, Xi'an, China) with severe combined immunodeficiency were used as hosts. Each mouse received four samples. Composites of HPDLSC/PPDLSC sheets plus CBB and CCRD scaffolds were transplanted into

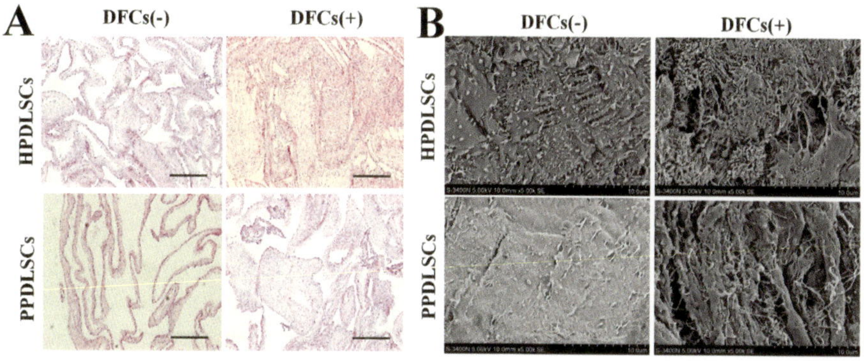

Figure 5. Effects of DFCs on cell sheet formation by HPDLSCs and PPDLSCs in vitro. A: H&E staining of cell sheets. HPDLSCs formed more cell layers and ECM than PPDLSCs. In the co-cultured systems, both HPDLSCs and PPDLSCs formed more cell layers and ECM than in the monocultured systems (hematoxylin-eosin staining, magnification: 400×, scale bar = 50 mm). **B:** SEM of cell sheets; HPDLSCs secreted richer ECM than PPDLSCs, and co-culture with DFCs enhanced the ECM secretion by both HPDLSCs and PPDLSCs. Notes: DFCs (–), monocultured PDLSCs that were cultured with transwell containing no DFCs; DFCs (+), co-cultured PDLSCs that were cultured with transwells seeded with a specific number of DFCs.

subcutaneous pockets on the left side; composites of HPDLSCs/ PPDLSCs from the monoculture system plus CBB and CCRD scaffolds were implanted on the right side as controls. General anesthesia was administered by intramuscular injection of pentobarbital sodium (0.1 mL/100 g) for all surgical procedures. The mice were checked carefully to prevent infection of the wound, and the health status of animals were observed every day post-transplantation. Eight weeks after implantation, the mice were euthanized by cervical dislocation after general anesthesia, and the implants were removed for H&E and Masson's trichrome staining.

Statistical analysis

All experiments were performed in triplicate with three different groups of co-culture systems. All data are expressed as the mean ± standard deviation (S.D.). Statistical significance was assessed with a χ^2 test and an independent-samples t test using SPSS13.0 software (SPSS, San Rafael, CA, USA). Statistical significance was defined as $p<0.05$. All data acquisition and analyses were performed in a blinded manner.

Results

Culture and Identification of HPDLSCs, PPDLSCs and DFCs

HPDLSCs and PPDLSCs were successfully isolated from PDL tissues derived from healthy donors and patients diagnosed with periodontitis, respectively. Putative stem cells were isolated using a limiting dilution technique and cultured to the third passage. Additionally, DFCs were harvested from dental follicle tissue and cultured to the third passage. Using a microscope, HPDLSCs, PPDLSCs, and DFCs were observed growing in an adherent manner with a long spindle shape. Although no obvious difference was observed between HPDLSCs and PPDLSCs, PPDLSCs appeared slightly irregular (Figure 1A). All three cell populations expressed the mesenchymal stem cell markers Stro-1, CD146, CD105, CD90, and CD29 and were negative for the hematopoi-

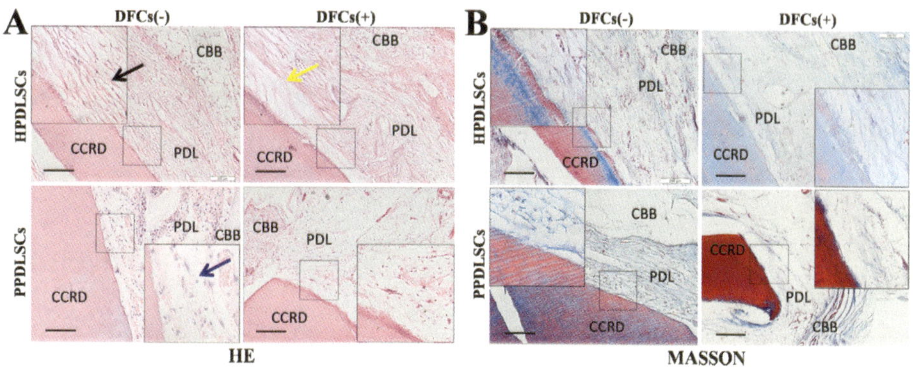

Figure 6. Transplantation of HPDLSC and PPDLSC cell sheets in immunodeficient mice. A: H&E staining of cell sheets. Monocultured HPDLSCs formed PDL-like fibers parallel to the CCRD and CBB (black arrow). Co-cultured HPDLSCs formed perpendicular Sharpey-like fibers (yellow arrow) and also generated a root/periodontal ligament-like complex in the CCRD side and periodontal ligament/bone-like complex in the CBB side. In the monocultured PPDLSC group, the fibers did not adhere very well to the CCRD and CBB, and many inflammatory cells were observed in the tissue (blue arrow). In the co-cultured PPDLSC group, no inflammatory cells were observed, and more fibers were formed (hematoxylin-eosin staining, magnification: 400×, scale bar = 50 mm). **B:** Masson's trichrome staining consistently confirmed the results of the H&E staining for each group (Masson's trichrome staining: 400×, scale bar = 50 mm). Notes: DFCs (–), monocultured PDLSCs that were cultured with transwell containing no DFCs; DFCs (+), co-cultured PDLSCs that were cultured with transwell seeded with a specific number of DFCs; CBB: ceramic bovine bone; CCRD: chemically conditioned root dentin; PDL: periodontal ligament-like tissue.

etic marker CD45 (Figure 1B). In addition, the experiments described below confirmed the osteogenic and adipogenic potential of the HPDLSCs and PPDLSCs.

Effect of DFCs on the stemness of HPDLSCs and PPDLSCs

To evaluate the influence of DFCs on the stemness of HPDLSCs and PPDLSCs, real-time PCR was used to evaluate the expression of the stemness-related genes Oct4, Sox2, and Klf4, which are associated with self-renewal and multi-lineage differentiation. PPDLSCs exhibited lower Oct4, Sox2, and Klf4 mRNA expression than HPDLSCs in the monoculture systems; however, in the co-culture systems, DFCs increased the expression of these three genes in both HPDLSCs and PPDLSCs ($p<0.05$; Figure 2Aa, Ba, Ca). The DFC-mediated upregulation folds of Oct4, Sox2, and Klf4 were higher in PPDLSCs than those in HPDLSCs, especially for Sox2 with statistical significance ($p<0.05$; Figure 2Ab, Bb, Cb).

Effect of DFCs on Proliferation of HPDLSCs and PPDLSCs

HPDLSCs and PPDLSCs were cultured in monoculture and co-culture systems, and their proliferation abilities were determined using the colony-forming assay at day 10 and cell cycle analysis at day 5. PPDLSCs had a higher proliferation capacity than HPDLSCs based on their colony-forming rate ($p<0.05$; Figure 3A, B) and the percentages of cells in G_2 and S phases (PI) ($p<0.05$; Figure 3C, D). In addition, co-cultured HPDLSCs/PPDLSCs showed an increased proliferation ability compared to monocultured cells, as indicated by their higher colony-forming rate ($p<0.05$; Figure 3A, B) and PI ($p<0.05$; Figure 3C, D). Interestingly, HPDLSCs and PPDLSCs had different sensitivities to DFCs in terms of the observed increase in proliferation. Specifically, DFCs more strongly promoted the proliferation of PPDLSCs than that of HPDLSCs, especially in the cell cycle assay ($p<0.05$; Figure 3B, D).

Effects of DFCs on the osteogenic and adipogenic differentiation of HPDLSCs and PPDLSCs in vitro

At day 7, osteogenic differentiation was analyzed by ALP staining and the ALP activity assay. Additionally, mRNA expression of the osteogenic genes ALP, Runx2, and OCN was determined by real time PCR, and Runx2 protein expression was assessed by western blot analysis. Furthermore, mineralized nodule formation and calcium concentration were examined by Alizarin Red S staining and calcium level analysis at day 28, respectively. HPDLSCs had a better osteogenic capacity than PPDLSCs, with the evidence of higher ALP activity ($p<0.05$; Figure 4A, Ba), gene expression of ALP, Runx2, and OCN ($p<0.05$; Figure 4E), protein expression of Runx2 (Figure 4F), as well as more mineralized nodules (Figure 4C) and higher calcium levels ($p<0.05$; Figure 4Da). These results indicate that the periodontitic microenvironment decreased the osteogenic capacity of PPDLSCs. When we investigated the effect of DFCs on the osteogenic differentiation potential of HPDLSCs and PPDLSCs, we found that DFCs significantly enhanced the osteogenic potential of both HPDLSCs and PPDLSCs in the assays described above ($p<0.05$; Figure 4A, Ba, C, Da, E, F). Furthermore, co-culture with DFCs appeared to increase the osteogenic potential of PPDLSCs to a greater extent than that of HPDLSCs, based on the quantitative analyses of the upregulation folds of ALP activity (Figure 4Bb) and calcium concentration (Figure 4Db). However, the differences were not statistically significant.

We also evaluated the effects of DFCs on the adipogenic ability of HPDLSCs and PPDLSCs by real time PCR at day 7 and Oil Red O staining at day 21. HPDLSCs showed a higher level of PPARγ gene expression (Figure 4G) and a higher number of lipid droplets than PPDLSCs ($p<0.05$; Figure 4H, Ia), and co-culture with DFCs increased the adipogenic ability of both HPDLSCs and PPDLSCs ($p<0.05$; Figure 4H, Ia). Co-culture improved the formation of lipid droplets similarly for PPDLSCs and HPDLSCs ($p>0.05$; Figure 4Ib).

Effect of DFCs on cell sheet formation by HPDLSCs and PPDLSCs in vitro

H&E staining showed that HPDLSCs formed more cell layers and extracellular matrix (ECM) than PPDLSCs in the monoculture groups. Co-culture with DFCs improved cell sheet formation for both HPDLSCs and PPDLSCs. Cell aggregates formed and no necrosis was observed, especially in the co-cultured HPDLSCs (Figure 5A).

SEM showed that in the monoculture groups, HPDLSCs secreted only a limited amount of extracellular matrix (ECM), whereas PPDLSCs only produced a small granule of ECM on the surface of the cell sheets. In the co-culture groups, thick and interwoven ECM was present in both HPDLSC and PPDLSC cell sheets, with more ECM secretion being observed in HPDLSCs (Figure 5B).

Effect of implantation of cell sheets of HPDLSCs and PPDLSCs in immunodeficient mice

After implantation of the cell sheets into the subcutaneous space of immunodeficient mice for 8 weeks, the regenerated tissue specimens were harvested and their morphology was examined by light microscopy after H&E and Masson's trichrome staining. In the HPDLSC group, several PDL-like fibers were observed in the monocultured HPDLSC sheet, which presented a parallel orientation between the CCRD and CBB. However, in the co-cultured HPDLSC sheet, a typical arranged tissue with Sharpey-like perpendicular fibers was regenerated between the CCRD and CBB. Additionally, a root/periodontal ligament-like complex and a periodontal ligament/bone-like complex were observed on the CCRD and CBB sides, respectively. The collagen fiber bundles between the CCRD and CBB closely resembled the physiological structure of the periodontium. However, in the PPDLSC group, the fibers and bone did not adhere well, and many inflammatory cells were present in the regenerated tissue. In the co-cultured PPDLSC sheet, some Sharpey fiber-like tissue formed between the CCRD and CBB without inflammatory cells (Figure 6A). Masson's trichrome staining further confirmed the deposition of collagen and the regeneration of mineralized matrix in each group (Figure 6B).

Discussion

PDLSCs are promising stem cells for periodontal regeneration, as they have been shown to form PDL/cementum and bone-like tissues in vivo [8–11]. However, the extracellular microenvironment has a direct effect on PDLSC function [15,16]. In our study, PDLSCs from two distinct microenvironments were evaluated, i.e. a healthy periodontal environment and an inflammatory periodontal environment. We found that PPDLSCs exhibit high proliferation ability, as they had significantly more colony-forming units and a higher proliferation index. However, pluripotency and differentiation capacity are more vital for tissue regeneration, and both of these capacities were decreased in PPDLSCs, which expressed stemness-associated genes at lower levels and showed reduced osteogenic and adipogenic differentiation. These results are consistent with a previous report [18] demonstrating that the periodontitic microenvironment can have adverse effects on the characteristics of PPDLSCs and lead to impaired periodontal regeneration.

The purpose of our study was to optimize the function of HPDLSCs and PPDLSCs by modulating their extracellular microenvironment. A previous report showed that a young microenvironment supplied by young PDLSCs can improve the proliferation and differentiation ability of aged PDLSCs [19]. DFCs are young precursor cells existing in the periodontium. Thus, we speculated that DFCs could enhance the function of both HPDLSCs and PPDLSCs by providing a beneficial young microenvironment. Because conventional in vitro culture cannot mimic the complicated environment present during cell growth and development, it is common to use special culture techniques to imitate the in vivo microenvironment and guide cells to a specific differentiation fate [25,26]. Co-culture methods have thus been developed to promote an optimal cell phenotype by mimicking the natural environment in vivo. Co-culture can also be used to observe interactions between different cell types and explore the mechanisms underlying diseases [27–29].

In the present study, we established co-culture systems of DFCs/HPDLSCs and DFCs/PPDLSCs. Oct4, Sox2, and Klf4 are transcription factors associated with self-renewal and pluripotency, and we demonstrated that both HPDLSCs and PPDLSCs showed higher expression of these genes after co-culture with DFCs, indicating that DFCs can improve the comprehensive potency of HPDLSCs and PPDLSCs. In addition, colony-formation and cell cycle analyses further demonstrated that DFCs can provide a favorable microenvironment to optimize the proliferation capacity of HPDLSCs and PPDLSCs.

Soleymaninejadian et al. [30] reported that MSCs secrete a variety of cytokines and factors, including transforming growth factor-β (TGF-β), hepatic growth factor (HGF), prostaglandin E2 (PGE2), IL-10, nitric oxide (NO), indolamine2, 3-dioxygenase (IDO), heme oxygenase-1 (HO-1), and human leukocyte antigen-G (HLA-G). Many of these soluble factors have been shown to maintain the stemness of MSCs and also increase their proliferation ability [31]. DFCs are a type of MSCs present in periodontal tissue. In our co-culture system, DFCs and HPDLSCs or PPDLSCs were separated by a 0.4 μm polycarbonate membrane, allowing the transport of molecular but not cellular components [32]. Therefore, soluble factors secreted by the DFCs likely diffused into the medium to affect the HPDLSCs and PPDLSCs.

In some studies, opposite effects on proliferation and differentiation have been observed, i.e., when stemness was enhanced, proliferation was enhanced but differentiation was inhibited [33]. Such a phenomenon is beneficial for maintaining the pluripotency of MSCs in vitro but is not ideal for directing tissue regeneration. In our study, in addition to improving the proliferation, co-culture also had advantageous effects on differentiation. We found that DFCs improved the in vitro osteogenic capacity, as osteogenic gene and protein activity, ALP activity and mineralized nodule formation were enhanced. The adipogenic capacity was also improved based on the increased PPARγ expression and the formation of lipid droplets. Transplantation of cells into tissues is considered to be an appropriate method for evaluating the function of the cells [34]. The omentum is usually chosen as the implantation site because it provides sufficient space for the transplantation of immunoprotective tissue as well as an adequate blood supply [35]. Upon transplantation, HPDLSCs co-cultured with DFCs grew well and produced root/periodontal ligament-like and periodontal ligament/bone-like tissues. Several studies [36,37] have shown that after engraftment, MSCs contribute to tissue repair secretion of trophic molecules, including soluble extracellular matrix glycoproteins, cytokines, and growth factors, and through direct cell-to-cell contact. Moreover, as a type of MSC, DFCs are also young precursor cells. Cells with a young phenotype have been confirmed to enhance the proliferation and differentiation ability of PDLSCs by providing a young microenvironment [19]. However, the environment supplied by DFCs is complicated, which suggests that a combination of multiple factors from DFCs may influence the proliferation and differentiation of HPDLSCs and PPDLSCs, subsequently providing better periodontal regeneration in vivo.

In our study, co-culture with DFCs had a greater effect on PPDLSCs than HPDLSCs. Specifically, the stemness-associated gene expression, number of colony-forming units, proliferation index, ALP activity and osteogenic gene expression were all enhanced to a greater degree. Several studies have indicated that, in addition to secreting trophic factors as mentioned above, MSCs also have immunomodulatory and anti-inflammatory properties [36]. MSCs have been shown to modulate the microenvironment of injured tissues and protect damaged tissues by releasing anti-inflammatory molecules [38,39]. These molecules may not only reduce inflammation, apoptosis and fibrosis in damaged tissues but also enhance tissue regeneration. The PPDLSCs in this study were derived from an inflammatory microenvironment. Epigenetics studies have shown that PPDLSCs may constitutively secrete inflammatory factors, such as TNF-α and IL-1β, in vitro [40]. Thus, PPDLSCs are distinct from HPDLSCs with regard to both the cell source and the microenvironment. For example, inflammatory factors secreted by PPDLSCs may stimulate the immunomodulatory effects of DFCs, causing the DFCs to produce more anti-inflammatory cytokines and trophic factors, thereby enhancing the biological properties of the PPDLSCs. Future studies should further explore the specific mechanism.

Conclusion

In summary, our data from in vitro and in vivo assays demonstrated a positive role for DFCs, as a type of MSCs and precursor cells from periodontal tissues, in providing a favorable microenvironment for optimizing the self-renewal and multi-differentiation capacity of HPDLSCs. Furthermore, DFCs helped to ameliorate the biological impairment of PPDLSCs caused by inflammation and may ultimately be useful in enhancing periodontal regeneration using PDLSCs.

Author Contributions

Conceived and designed the experiments: YJ ZJ JL LW WL. Performed the experiments: JL LW. Analyzed the data: JL WL QL. Contributed to the writing of the manuscript: JL. Interpreted the findings: WL ZJ YJ.

References

1. Pihlstrom BL, Michalowicz BS, Johnson NW (2005) Periodontal diseases. Lancet 366: 1809–1820.
2. Nanci A, Bosshardt DD (2000) Structure of periodontal tissues in health and disease. Periodontol 2000 40: 11–28.
3. Chen FM, Zhang J, Zhang M, An Y, Chen F, et al. (2010) A review on endogenous regenerative technology in periodontal regenerative medicine. Biomaterials 31: 7892–7927.
4. Douglass GL (2005) Periodontics–tissue engineering and the future. J Calif Dent Assoc 33: 203–204.
5. Chen FM, Jin Y (2010) Periodontal tissue engineering and regeneration: current approaches and expanding opportunities. Tissue Eng Part B Rev16: 219–255.
6. Zhang W, Abukawa H, Troulis MJ, Kaban LB, Vacanti JP, et al. (2009) Tissue engineered hybrid tooth-bone constructs. Methods 47: 122–128.

7. Peng L, Ye L, Zhou XD (2009) Mesenchymal stem cells and tooth engineering. Int J Oral Sci 1: 6–12.
8. Ma Z, Li S, Song Y, Tang L, Ma D, et al. (2008) The biological effect of dentin noncollagenous proteins (DNCPs) on the human periodontal ligament stem cells (HPDLSCs) invitro and invivo. Tissue Eng Part A 14: 2059–2068.
9. Grzesik WJ, Narayanan AS (2002) Cementum and periodontal wound healing and regeneration. Crit Rev Oral Biol Med 13: 474–484.
10. Chen FM, Zhao YM, Wu H, Deng ZH, Wang QT, et al. (2006) Enhancement of periodontal tissue regeneration by locally controlled delivery of insulin-like growth factor-I from dextran-co-gelatin microspheres. J Control Release 114: 209–222.
11. Ramseier CA, Abramson ZR, Jin Q, Giannobile WV (2006) Gene therapeutics for periodontal regenerative medicine. Dent Clin North Am 50: 245–263.
12. Lin NH, Gronthos S, Bartold PM (2009) Stem cells and future periodontal regeneration. Periodontol 2000 51: 239–251.
13. Rios HF, Lin Z, Oh B, Park CH, Giannobile WV (2011) Cell- and gene-based therapeutic strategies for periodontal regenerative medicine. J Periodontol 82: 1223–1237.
14. Chen FM, Sun HH, Lu H, Yu Q (2012). Stem cell-delivery therapeutics for periodontal tissue regeneration. Biomaterials 33: 6320–6344.
15. Monje ML, Toda H, Palmer TD (2003) Inflammatory blockade restores adult hippocampal neurogenesis. Science 302: 1760–1765.
16. Pluchino S, Muzio L, Imitola J, Deleidi M, Alfaro-Cervello C, et al. (2008) Persistent inflammation alters the function of the endogenous brain stem cell compartment. Brain 31: 2564–2578.
17. Zhang J, An Y, Gao LN, Zhang YJ, Jin Y, et al. (2012) The effect of aging on the pluripotential capacity and regenerative potential of human periodontal ligament stem cells. Biomaterials 33: 6974–6986.
18. Liu N, Shi S, Deng M, Tang L, Zhang G, et al. (2011) High levels of beta-catenin signaling reduce osteogenic differentiation of stem cells in inflammatory microenvironments through inhibition of the noncanonical Wnt pathway. J Bone Miner Res 26: 2082–2095.
19. Zheng W, Wang S, Ma D, Tang L, Duan Y, et al. (2009) Loss of proliferation and differentiation capacity of aged human periodontal ligament stem cells and rejuvenation by exposure to the young extrinsic environment. Tissue Eng Part A 15: 2363–2371.
20. Morsczeck C, Schmalz GJ (2010) Transcriptomes and proteomes of dental follicle cells. J Dent Res 89: 445–456.
21. Seo BM, Miura M, Gronthos S, Bartold PM, Batouli S, et al. (2004) Investigation of multipotent postnatal stem cells from human periodontal ligament. Lancet 364: 149–155.
22. Yang Z, Jin F, Zhang X, Ma D, Han C, et al. (2009) Tissue engineering of cementum/periodontal-ligament complex using a novel three-dimensional pellet cultivation system for human periodontal ligament stem cells. Tissue Eng Part C Methods 15: 571–581.
23. Liu W, Liu Y, Guo T, Hu C, Luo H, et al. (2013) TCF3, a novel positive regulator of osteogenesis, plays a crucial role in miR-17 modulating the diverse effect of canonical Wnt signaling in different microenvironments. Cell Death Dis 4, e539; doi:10.1038/cddis.2013.65.
24. Guo W, He Y, Zhang X, Lu W, Wang C, et al. (2009) The use of dentin matrix scaffold and dental follicle cells for dentin regeneration. Biomaterials 30: 6708–6723.
25. Trottier V, Marceau-Fortier G, Germain L, Vincent C, Fradette J (2008) IFATS collection: using human adipose-derived stem/stromal cells for the production of new skin substitutes. Stem Cells 26: 2713–2723.
26. Rajnicek AM, Foubister LE, McCaig CD (2008) Alignment of corneal and lens epithelial cells by co-operative effects of substratum topography and DC electric fields. Biomaterials 29: 2082–2095.
27. Prgeeth Pandula PK, Samaranayake LP, Jin LJ, Zhang CF (2014) Human umbilical vein endothelial cells synergize osteo/odontogenic differentiation of periodontal ligament stem cells in 3D cell sheets. J Periodontal Res 49: 299–306 doi:10.1111/jre.12107.
28. Wu Y, Cao H, Yang Y, Zhou Y, Gu Y, et al. (2013) Effects of vascular endothelial cells on osteogenic differentiation of noncontact co-cultured periodontal ligament stem cells under hypoxia. J Periodontal Res 48: 52–65.
29. Bai Y, Bai Y, Matsuzaka K, Hashimoto S, Fukuyama T, et al. (2011) Cementum- and periodontal ligament-like tissue formation by dental follicle cell sheets co-cultured with Hertwig's epithelial root sheath cells. Bone 48: 1417–1426.
30. Soleymaninejadian E, Pramanik K, Samadian E (2012) Immunomodulatory properties of mesenchymal stem cells: cytokines and factors. Am J Reprod Immunol 67: 1–8.
31. Wu J, Huang GT, He W, Wang P, Tong Z, et al. (2012) Basic fibroblast growth factor enhances stemness of human stem cells from the apical papilla. J Endod 38: 614–622.
32. Mizuno N, Ozeki Y, Shiba H, Kajiya M, Nagahara T, et al. (2008) Humoral factors released from human periodontal ligament cells influence calcification and proliferation in human bone marrow mesenchymal stem cells. J Periodontol 79: 2361–2370.
33. Pricola KL, Kuhn NZ, Haleem-Smith H, Song Y, Tuan RS (2009) Interleukin-6 maintains bone marrow-derived mesenchymal stem cell stemness by an ERK1/2-dependent mechanism. J Cell Biochem 108: 577–588.
34. Song AM, Shu R, Xie YF, Song ZC, Li HY, et al. (2007) A study of enamel matrix proteins on differentiation of porcine bone marrow stromal cells into cementoblasts. Cell Prolif 40: 381–396.
35. Kin T, Korbutt GS, Rajotte RV (2003) Survival and metabolic function of syngeneic rat islet grafts transplanted in the omental pouch. Am J Transplant 3: 281–285.
36. Ankrum J, Karp JM (2010) Mesenchymal stem cell therapy: two steps forward, one step back. Trends Mol Med 16: 203–209.
37. Plotnikov MB, Aliev OI, Vasil'ev AS, Andreeva VY, Krasnov EA, et al. (2008) Effect of Rhaponticumcarthamoides extract on structural and metabolic parameters of erythrocytes in rats with cerebral ischemia. Bull Exp Biol Med 146: 45–48.
38. von Bahr L, Sundberg B, Lönnies L, Sander B, Karbach H, et al. (2012) Long-term complications, immunologic effects, and role of passage for outcome in mesenchymal stromal cell therapy. Biol Blood Marrow Transplant 18: 557–564.
39. Meirelles Lda S, Fontes AM, Covas DT, Caplan AI (2009) Mechanisms involved in the therapeutic properties of mesenchymal stem cells. Cytokine Growth Factor Rev 20: 419–427.
40. Palacios D, Mozzetta C, Consalvi S, Caretti G, Saccone V, et al. (2010) TNF/p38α/polycomb signaling to Pax7 locus in satellite cells links inflammation to the epigenetic control of muscle regeneration. Cell Stem Cell 7: 455–469.

Leukotoxic Activity of *Aggregatibacter actinomycetemcomitans* and Periodontal Attachment Loss

Carola Höglund Åberg[1], Dorte Haubek[2], Francis Kwamin[3], Anders Johansson[1], Rolf Claesson[4]*

1 Division of Molecular Periodontology, Department of Odontology, Faculty of Medicine, Umeå University, Umeå, Sweden, 2 Section for Pediatric Dentistry, Department of Dentistry, Health, Aarhus University, Aarhus, Denmark, 3 Dental School University of Ghana, Accra, Ghana, 4 Oral Microbiology, Department of Odontology, Faculty of Medicine, Umeå University, Umeå, Sweden

Abstract

Aggregatibacter actinomycetemcomitans is a Gram-negative periodontitis-associated bacterium that expresses a toxin that selectively affects leukocytes. This leukotoxin is encoded by an operon belonging to the core genome of this bacterial species. Variations in the expression of the leukotoxin have been reported, and a well-characterized specific clonal type (JP2) of this bacterium with enhanced leukotoxin expression has been isolated. In particular, the presence of the JP2 genotype significantly increases the risk for the progression of periodontal attachment loss (AL). Based on these findings we hypothesized that variations in the leukotoxicity are linked to disease progression in infected individuals. In the present study, the leukotoxicity of 239 clinical isolates of *A. actinomycetemcomitans* was analysed with different bioassays, and the genetic peculiarities of the isolates were related to their leukotoxicity based on examination with molecular techniques. The periodontal status of the individuals sampled for the presence of *A. actinomycetemcomitans* was examined longitudinally, and the importance of the observed variations in leukotoxicity was evaluated in relation to disease progression. Our data show that high leukotoxicity correlates with an enhanced risk for the progression of AL. The JP2 genotype isolates were all highly leukotoxic, while the isolates with an intact leukotoxin promoter (non-JP2 genotypes) showed substantial variation in leukotoxicity. Genetic characterization of the non-JP2 genotype isolates indicated the presence of highly leukotoxic genotypes of serotype b with similarities to the JP2 genotype. Based on these results, we conclude that *A. actinomycetemcomitans* harbours other highly virulent genotypes besides the previously described JP2 genotype. In addition, the results from the present study further highlight the importance of the leukotoxin as a key virulence factor in aggressive forms of periodontitis.

Editor: Michael Glogauer, University of Toronto, Canada

Funding: This study was supported by the Swedish National Graduate School in Odontological Science, the Research Fund (TUA), County of Västerbotten, Sweden, the Swedish Dental Association, Sweden, Ingeborg and Leo Dannins Foundation, Aarhus University Research Foundation (F-2009-SUN-1-57), funds from the Danish Dental Association. The funders had no role in the study design, data collection and analysis, decision to publish, or preparation of the manuscript.

Competing Interests: The authors have declared that no competing interests exist.

* Email: rolf.claesson@odont.umu.se

Introduction

Periodontitis is an inflammatory disease, initiated by a bacterial biofilm on the teeth and characterized by the degradation of the tooth-supporting tissues [1]. The disease usually progresses slowly among adults, whilst in young individuals rapidly progressing forms of the disease are usually seen. The bacterium, *Aggregatibacter actinomycetemcomitans*, is strongly associated with the aggressive forms of the disease [2]. Based on longitudinal studies, the presence of *A. actinomycetemcomitans* is considered a risk marker for the progression of periodontal attachment loss (AL), i.e. degradation of the periodontal tissues around the teeth [3,4,5]. While a cytolethal distending toxin (CDT) produced by this bacterial species seems to have limited effect on disease progression, the opposite has been reported for the leukotoxin, another toxin produced by the bacterium [6]. A specific genotype of *A. actinomycetemcomitans*, JP2, with the capacity to produce substantial amounts of the leukotoxin, has been shown to be highly associated with aggressive forms of periodontitis [5,7].

The leukotoxin exerts its effect on the immune defense cells in different ways [8]. It binds to the lymphocyte function-associated antigen-1 (LFA-1) molecule of haematopoetic cells and induces an activation and secretion of lysosomal proteases from neutrophils and IL-1β from macrophages [9,10,11]. This leukotoxin-induced cellular activation subsequently causes death of the target cells. It has also been shown that leukotoxin induces β-haemolysis in erythrocytes, although these cells lack the LFA-1 molecule on the cell surface [12,13].

The leukotoxin operon consists of the *ltxC*, *ltxA*, *ltxB*, and *ltxD* genes and a promoter region [14,15]. The *ltxA* codes for the protein, while the *ltxC* encodes components responsible for the posttranslational acylation. The two other genes, the *ltxB* and the *ltxD*, are involved in the transport of the leukotoxin to the bacterial surface [14,15,16].

The leukotoxicity varies among different strains of *A. actinomycetemcomitans*. The presence of specific sequences within the promoter region and the binding of regulation proteins to these sequences are thought to control the expression of the leukotoxin

[17,18,19]. Environmental factors, such as levels of oxygen or fermentable sugars, have also been shown to regulate the leukotoxicity [20,21,22]. High levels of leukotoxin production have been detected in *A. actinomycetemcomitans* strains with a 530-base pair (bp) deletion within the leukotoxin promoter region [23,24]. Strains with such truncated promoter regions are described as JP2-like or JP2 clonal strains [24].

The JP2 genotype is thought to have originated in North Africa, spread to West Africa and then spread among individuals of African descent living in South America, North America and Europe [7,25,26,27]. Reports on the carriage of the JP2 genotype of *A. actinomycetemcomitans* in Caucasians are scarce, but a few exist [28,29].

Individuals carrying the JP2 genotype of *A. actinomycetemcomitans* have a significantly higher risk for progression of AL than carriers of the non-JP2 genotypes [5]. It has been suggested that this enhanced risk for disease progression is due to the higher leukotoxicity of the JP2 genotype compared with the non-JP2 genotypes [24,30]. In other words, the prevailing opinion is that the JP2 genotype is highly leukotoxic, while non-JP2 genotypes, strains with a complete leukotoxin promoter, are minimally leukotoxic. However, since the majority of individuals developing rapid bone loss at a young age are colonized with non-JP2 genotypes, it seems that the usage of methods which only distinguish between JP2 and non-JP2 genotypes provides too little information on the actual virulence capacity of the various clones of the bacterium.

Therefore, in the present study we focus on the *de facto* variations in leukotoxicity in different genotypes of *A. actinomycetemcomitans*. We hypothesize that the leukotoxic activity of this bacterial species is of importance for the progression of periodontitis of the infected individuals, and that the leukotoxicity can be used as a virulence marker.

Results

Leukotoxicity of different *A. actinomycetemcomitans* isolates

For studying the leukotoxicity of clinical isolates of *A. actinomycetemcomitans*, we used two established methods, one based on cell lysis and the other based on cell death. We also tested if haemolysis that is induced when *A. actinomycetemcomitans* is grown on blood agar can be used as a leukotoxin assay [12].

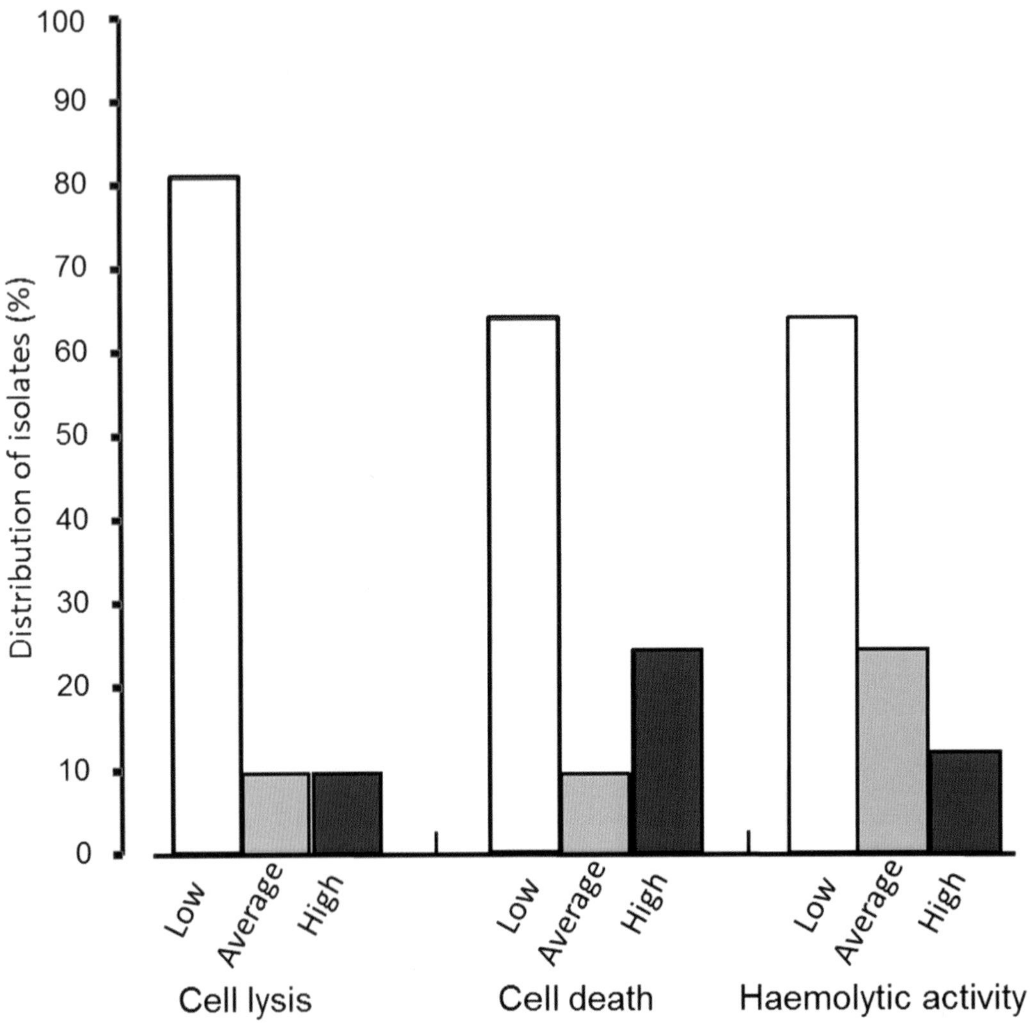

Figure 1. Distribution of *A. actinomycetemcomitans* isolates into three categories according to their leukotoxicity (n = 239). Cell lysis (LDH) and cell death (NRU) assay: 1 = minimal leukotoxicity (0–30%), 2 = average leukotoxicity (31–60%), 3 = high leukotoxicity (≥61%). Haemolysis-based assay: 1 = minimal leukotoxicity (no or small zone), 2 = average leukotoxicity (average zone), 3 = high leukotoxicity (large zone).

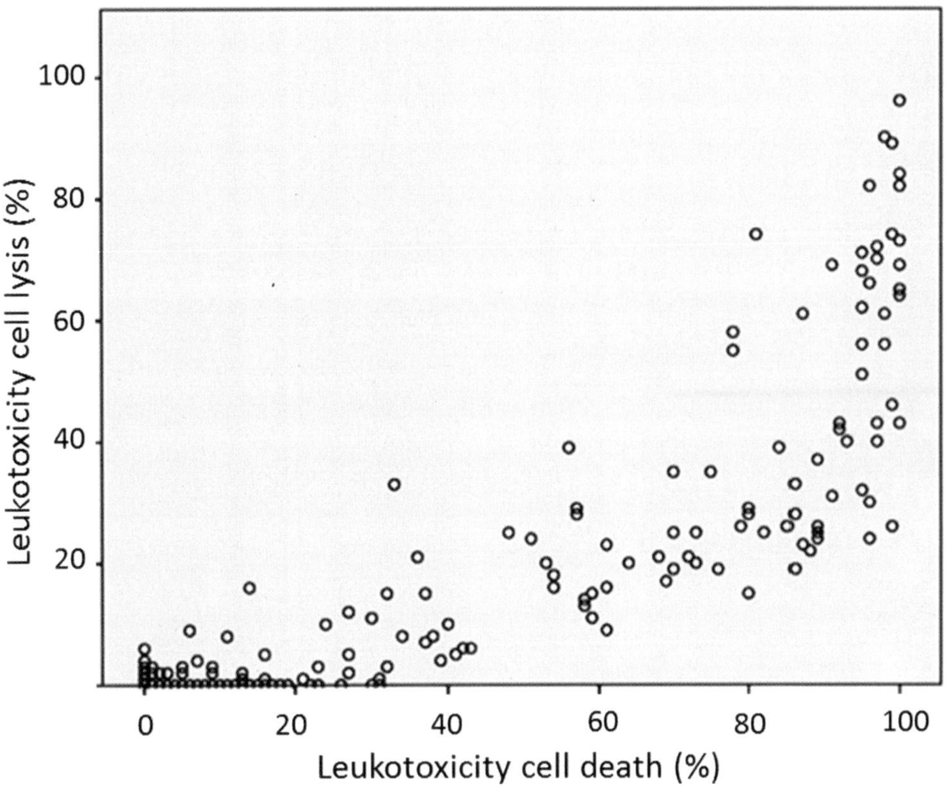

Figure 2. Correlation between the cell lysis (LDH) method and the cell death (NRU) method according to leukotoxicity in isolates (n = 239).

We found that the majority of the isolates (n = 239) showed low leukotoxicity (Fig. 1). Using the cell lysis method (LDH release), a smaller proportion of the isolates were placed in the highly leukotoxic category than when the cell death method (NRU) was used (Fig. 1). This discrepancy between the two methods is further illustrated in a scatter plot diagram (Fig. 2). This figure indicates that the majority of the isolates that show average leukotoxicity (31–60%) with the cell lysis method (LDH), show a high level of leukotoxicity (>61%) with the cell death (NRU) method. This figure shows that the majority of the isolates that show average leukotoxicity (31–60%) with the cell lysis method (LDH) roughly correspond to the isolates that show high leukotoxicity (≥61%) with the cell death (NRU) method. The results were correlated from the three different tests (leukotoxin assay based on haemolytic activity, cell lysis assay (LDH), and cell death (NRU) assay) (Fig. 2 and Fig. 3A, B).

When focusing on the leukotoxicity of the serotypes a to f, we found diversity both between and within the different serotypes. Most striking was that serotype b isolates were represented by both highly leukotoxic and low leukotoxic isolates. These results were determined by the cell lysis (LDH) methd and the cell death (NRU) method (Fig. 4A, B). The results of the haemolysis-based leukotoxicity assay were consistent with this (Table 1).

As determined by the cell lysis (LDH) method, fifteen (36.6%) out of the 41 non-JP2 genotype isolates, serotype b were classified as highly leukotoxic and expressed leukotoxicity similar to that of the 10 JP2 genotype isolates examined (Fig. 5).

Sequencing of the leukotoxin promoter

The differences in the leukotoxicity of *A. actinomycetemcomitans* strains have been suggested to be due to variations in the leukotoxin promoter sequence [17]. When we sequenced the promoter region of the 41 non-JP2 genotype serotype b isolates, only three sequence types (ST) were identified: ST 1 (n = 39), ST 2 (n = 1), and ST 3 (n = 1). The polymorphic sites which define the sequence types are shown in Table 2.

Isolates of ST2 and ST3 were found to have average and minimal leukotoxicity, respectively. These findings indicate that the differences in the leukotoxicity between these Ghanaian isolates are not due to the genetic organization of the promoter of the leukotoxin operon.

The sequence of the undeleted part of the promoter of the five JP2 strains isolated at baseline was identical to the corresponding part of the promoter of ST 1 and ST 3-isolates and of Y4, i.e., all differences within the promoter sequence of 40 (ST 1 and ST 3) of the Ghanaian isolates were located in the part of the promoter that is deleted in the JP2 genotype of *A. actinomycetemcomitans*.

Sequencing of the *hbpA-2* gene

Among the identified nucleotide mutations within *hbpA*-2, one has been suggested to distinguish JP2 isolates of North African and West African origin [25]. When we sequenced this particular gene in the 10 JP2 genotype isolates included in the present study, we found the previously reported point G to A SNP (position 525285 in the HK 1651 genome) which indicates a West-African origin of the Ghanaian JP2 genotype isolates.

Characterization of non-JP2 and JP2 genotypes by Arbitrarily primed (AP) PCR

When we used the AP PCR technique to study our *A. actinomycetemcomitans* isolates of serotype b, it revealed >10 different banding patterns (Fig. 6A–D). The patterns produced by

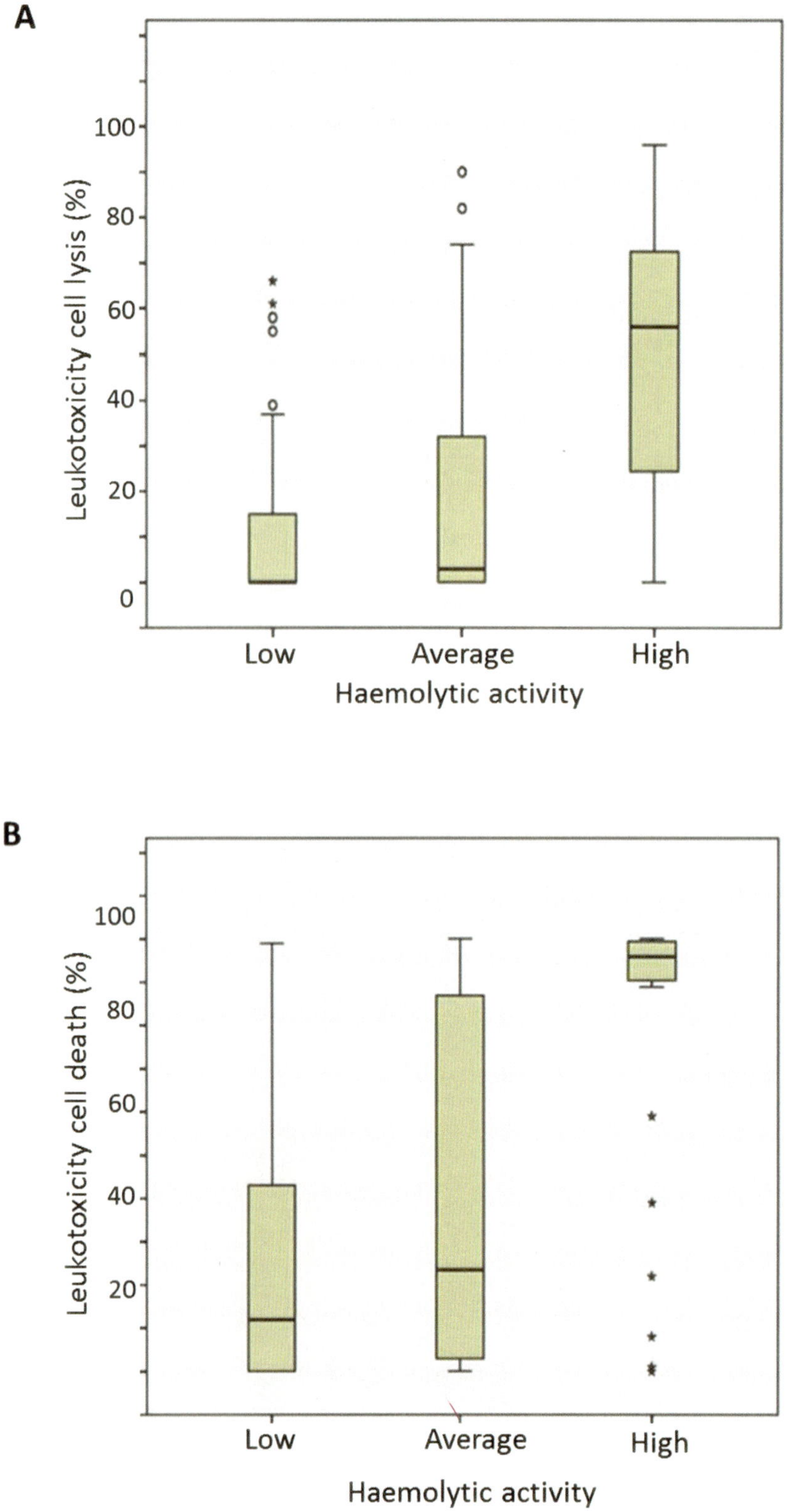

Figure 3. Distribution of *A. actinomycetemcomitans* isolates into three categories (minimal, average, high) according to leukotoxicity (n = 239). A. Correlation between the cell lysis (LDH) method and the haemolysis method. **B.** Correlation between the cell death (NRU) method and the haemolysis method.

the 10 JP2 genotype isolates were identical (Fig. 6A). Interestingly, most of the non-JP2 genotype isolates distributed from the highly leukotoxic cell lysis (LDH) category exhibited a pattern identical to that of the JP2 genotype isolates (Fig. 6, Table 3). The banding pattern was more diverse among the isolates of the average and minimal leukotoxicity cell lysis (LDH) groups (Fig. 6, Table 3).

Table 1. Haemolytic activity of various serotypes (n = 239) of *A. actinomycetem-comitans* determined by the haemolysis method.

	minimal	average	high	total
serotypes	*n (%)*	*n (%)*	*n (%)*	*n*
a	43 (75.4)	14 (24.6)		57
b	1 (2.2)	18 (39.1)	27 (58.7)	46
c	83 (83.0)	17 (17.0)		100
d	10 (83.3)	2 (16.7)		12
e	5 (83.3)	1 (16.7)		6
f	10 (55.5)	7 (38.9)	1 (5.6)	18

Leukotoxicity and increased risk for progression of AL

The leukotoxicity of *A. actinomycetemcomitans* isolates obtained from a subgroup of the study population, consisting of 146 adolescents living in Ghana, was studied (Table 4). We also evaluated the risk for a progression of AL≥3 mm in 146 of these individuals in relation to the carriage of the different genotypes of *A. actinomycetemcomitans* with varying leukotoxicity. The isolates examined were grouped into categories of minimal, average and high leukotoxicity when the cell lysis (LDH) and the cell death (NRU) methods were used. In the analysis of the risk (OR) for the progression of AL at the individual level (Table 4), the results from the cell lysis (LDH)- and the cell death (NRU)-methods were combined into two categories. In order to represent individuals that were carriers of strains with high leukotoxicity, the average category for the cell lysis (LDH) method was combined with the high leukotoxicity category, and the average category was combined with the minimal leukotoxicity category when the more sensitive cell death (NRU) method was used (Table 4).

A significantly increased risk of progression of AL≥3 mm was found among individuals who carried *A. actinomycetemcomitans* in relation to the reference group (the *A. actinomycetemcomitans*-negative individuals) (Table 4). Those individuals with a notably increased risk (OR>10) of developing progression of AL were colonized with average to highly leukotoxic *A. actinomycetemcomitans* (Table 4). Consequently, highly leukotoxic *A. actinomycetemcomitans* correlated most strongly with the progression of AL. Corresponding results were obtained when the semi-quantitative haemolysis-based leukotoxin assay was used, i.e. the carriage of highly haemolytic genotypes (category 3) was strongly associated with the progression of AL≥3 mm (Table 4).

After exclusion of the carriers harbouring the JP2 genotype, the remaining carriers of the highly leukotoxic *A. actinomycetemcomitans* were still at a significantly enhanced risk for disease progression. An exclusion of the JP2 genotype-positive individuals in the "minimal LDH" category resulted in an OR of 3.9 (95% CI [2.1–7.0], $p<0.001$), and in the "average–high (LDH)" category the OR was 6.9 (95% CI [2.9–16.2], $p<0.001$). In the "minimal–average" category according to the cell death (NRU) method, the exclusion resulted in an OR of 4.1 (95% CI [2.2–7.6], $p<0.001$), and in the "high (NRU)" category the OR was 5.1 (95%CI [2.4–10.9], $p<0.001$). Exclusion of the carriers with the JP2 genotype in the "minimal haemolysis" category, resulted in an OR of 4.2 (95% CI [2.3–7.8], $p<0.001$), in the "average haemolysis" category the OR was 3.5 (95% CI [1.5–8.0], $p=0.004$), and in the "high haemolysis" category the OR was 11.1 (95% CI [3.3–36.6], $p<0.001$). For the cell lysis (LDH) method, we consider isolates that cause ≥31% cell lysis (LDH) as having an enhanced leukotoxic activity, and these were all classified as highly leukotoxic when examined by the cell death (NRU) method (Fig. 2).

In the present study population (n = 146), 32 out of 41 carriers of the non-JP2 genotypes of *A. actinomycetemcomitans* of serotype b were clinically examined at the follow-up two years later. Among 20 of these examined individuals having a progression of AL> 3 mm, 14 (70%) carried *A. actinomycetemcomitans* with a leukotoxicity ≥31%. In contrast, among 12 of the examined individuals with a progression of AL<3 mm, only 5 (40%) were colonized with *A. actinomycetemcomitans* belonging to the category with high leukotoxicity.

Discussion

In the present study we have shown that individuals harbouring highly leukotoxic *A. actinomycetemcomitans*, independently of carrying a complete or truncated (JP2-genotype) leukotoxin promoter, had a significantly increased risk of progression of AL. We observed that the non-JP2 genotype isolates with high leukotoxicity comprised a subgroup of serotype b, and we found that the sequence of the leukotoxin promoter region in the non-JP2 genotype isolates of serotype b was similar, independent of leukotoxicity of the isolates. Taken together, these findings provide new insights into the leukotoxin as a virulence factor. As other genotypes than the JP2 genotype are shown to be highly leukotoxic, the association of *A. actinomycetemcomitans* to disease should be considered in a broader perspective than previously.

Based on our findings, we suggest that the generally accepted concept that *A. actinomycetemcomitans* can be divided into two categories based on leukotoxicity and organization of the leukotoxin promoter region should be further developed. In our point of view, the JP2 genotype of *A. actinomycetemcomitans*, characterized by a leukotoxin promoter region missing a 530-bp fragment, is highly leukotoxic [24]. This is further supported by reports that individuals carrying the JP2 genotype of *A. actinomycetemcomitans* are at increased risk for the development of AL [5,31].

However, in the present study, we have shown that there is more extensive variation in leukotoxicity among genotypes with a complete leukotoxin promoter than earlier assumed. Our results also show that the progression of AL in infected individuals is associated with the leukotoxicity (minimal, average or high) of *A. actinomycetemcomitans*, as determined *in vitro*. This indicates that analysis of virulence characteristics of *A. actinomycetemcomitans* should not be limited to leukotoxin promoter typing but should also include the determination of leukotoxic activity.

A. actinomycetemcomitans of serotype b has been reported to be associated with an increased risk for the development of

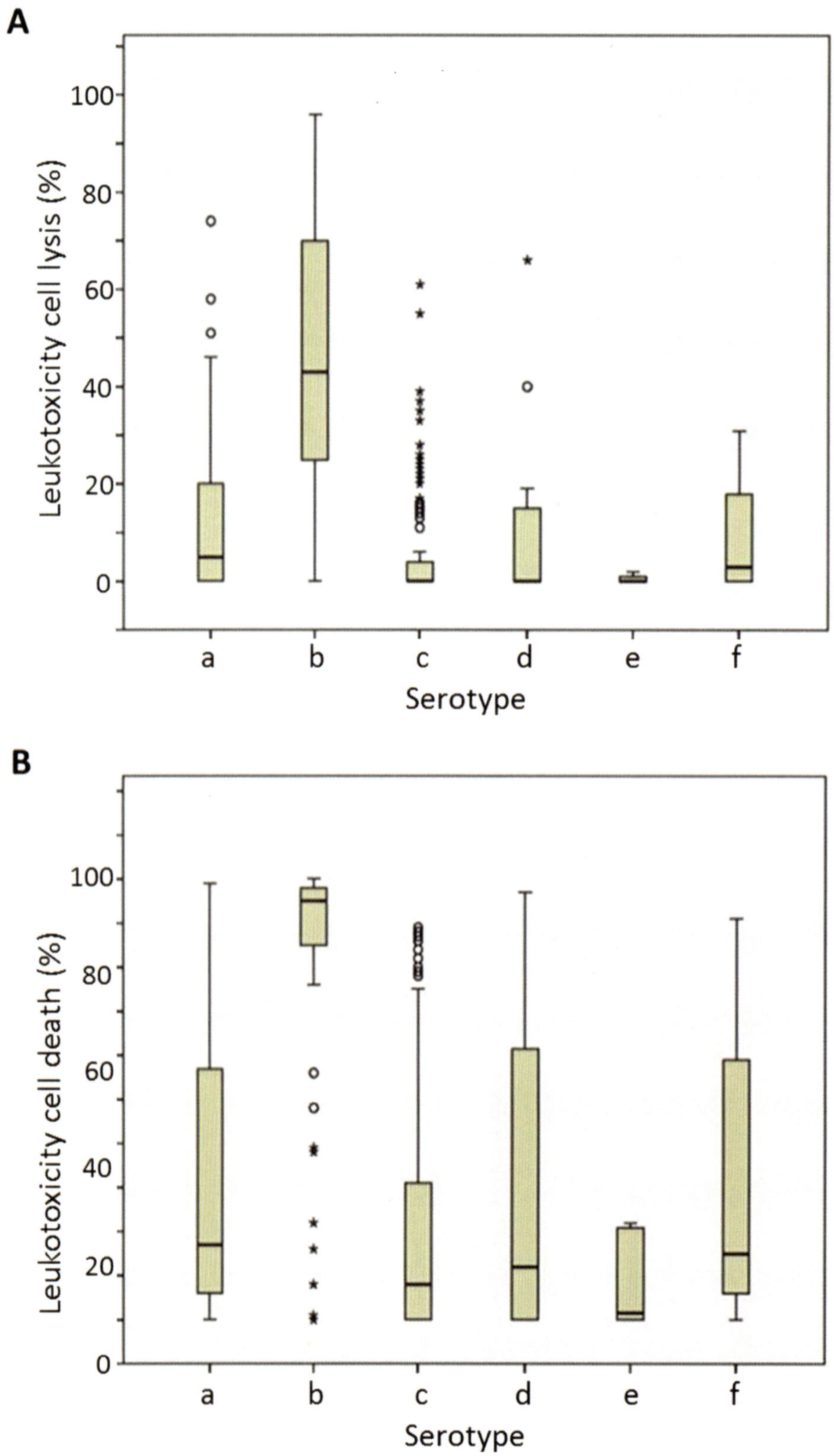

Figure 4. Leukotoxicity of various serotypes of *A. actinomycetemcomitans* (n = 239) determined by **A.** The cell lysis (LDH) method. **B.** The cell death (NRU) method.

periodontitis for decades [32,33]. Higher leukotoxicity within serotype b, as compared with the other serotypes, has been suggested to be one reason [30]. The present study shows that there is a substantial variation in leukotoxicity among serotype-b strains. We identified isolates of serotype b that exert high leukotoxicity as well as some that showed no leukotoxic activity at

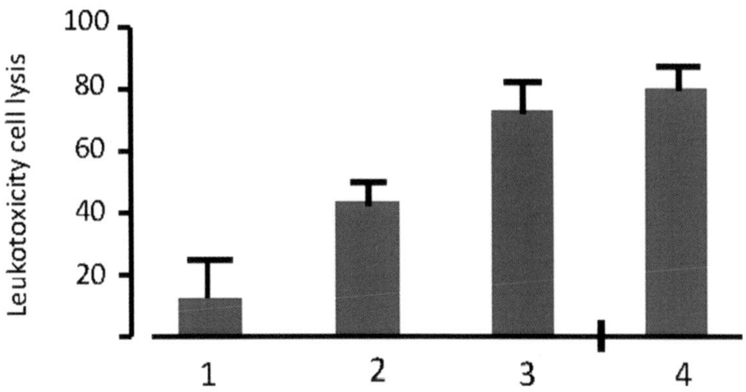

Figure 5. Distribution of serotype b isolates (n = 51) in various leukotoxicity categories based on data obtained by the cell lysis (LDH) method. 1. Minimal leukotoxicity, serotype b, non-JP2 genotype isolates (n = 15), **2.** Average leukotoxicity, serotype b, non-JP2 genotype isolates (n = 11) **3.** High leukotoxicity, serotype b, non-JP2 genotype isolates (n = 15), **4.** JP2 genotype isolates (n = 10). Mean LDH-release ± SD.

all. The most striking observation was that the highly leukotoxic group of serotype b comprised both JP2 and non-JP2 genotype isolates. This means that more than one highly leukotoxic genotype can be found within the b serotypes. Based on this novel finding it would be valuable if focus were moved from distinguishing between JP2 and non-JP2 genotypes, to also include determination of the actual leukotoxicity of *A. actinomycetemcomitans*, serotype b.

In order to further study the variation in the leukotoxicity among *A. actinomycetemcomitans* isolates of serotype b, the leukotoxin promoter region of the serotype b isolates was sequenced. However, almost no differences in the organization of the promoter region among the isolates were observed. This indicates that the organization of the promoter region was not responsible for the observed variations in leukotoxicity. However, the AP PCR-based characterization of the isolates revealed different banding patterns. As expected, the JP2 genotype isolates had an identical banding pattern. Interestingly, the majority of the isolates with high leukotoxicity showed a 'JP2-like' pattern. The AP PCR banding pattern of the remaining isolates was more diverse. The AP PCR method has previously been used for the characterization of *A. actinomycetemcomitans* strains isolated from healthy and diseased individuals [34,35,36]. For the identification of putative virulence genes, the AP PCR technique provides limited information. However, our observations indicate that screening for highly leukotoxic non-JP2 genotypes of *A. actinomycetemcomitans* of serotype b might be successful if extended gene level comparisons between different *A. actinomycetemcomitans* isolates of serotype b are performed.

For the determination of leukotoxicity, we used three different assays. Based on the results from the cell lysis (LDH) and the cell death (NRU) methods, the isolates were categorized into groups with high, average, or minimal leukotoxicity. Although the two methods gave similar results, fewer isolates were identified as highly leukotoxic by the cell lysis (LDH) method than with the cell death (NRU) method. Taken together, we concluded that the cell lysis (LDH) method seemed to identify the "true" highly leukotoxic isolates with greater accuracy than the cell death (NRU) method. However, this latter method identified low leukotoxic producers which otherwise could have been overlooked by the cell lysis (LDH) method.

The JP2 genotype of *A. actinomycetemcomitans* induces β-haemolysis on blood agar plates [12,37]. As far as we know, this is the first study in which haemolytic activity has been used for the determination of the leukotoxicity of clinical *A. actinomycetmcomitans* isolates. The results were in accordance with those achieved by the cell lysis (LDH) and cell death (NRU) methods. However, further studies of the relevance of the method are required before it can be recommended as a screening method for highly leukotoxic *A. actinomycetemcomitans* genotypes.

In the present study, we provide new information about the diversity of the *de facto* leukotoxicity within the species *A. actinomycetemcomitans*. The importance of these data was substantially improved since we were able to evaluate the progression of AL in relation to the leukotoxicity of *A. actinomycetemcomitans* isolates collected from healthy or diseased individuals. Previous reports showing the virulence mechanisms of the leukotoxin and the enhanced risk of the progression of AL for individuals carrying the highly leukotoxic genotype (JP2) of this bacterium further strengthen the relevance of the present study [5,7,8,31].

In conclusion, our data provide evidence for a substantial variation in the leukotoxicity among the non-JP2 genotype strains of *A. actinomycetemcomitans* that were often previously grouped into the category of minimally leukotoxic strains. These data clearly support leukotoxicity of *A. actinomycetemcomitans* as an important virulence factor and a causative agent implicated in the progression of periodontitis.

Materials and Methods

Ethics statement

Ethical clearance for the study was obtained from the Noguchi Memorial Institute for Medical Research, University of Ghana (IRB 000 1276), and from the local Ethical committee of Umeå University, Sweden (Dnr 2010-188-31M). Signed consents were received from the parents or the guardians of the children before they entered the study.

Study collection

This study is based on a characterization of 239 *A. actinomycetemcomitans* isolates (234 non-JP2 and 5 JP2 genotypes) obtained from 199 Ghanaian adolescents [38]. This collection is a part of a collection previously described [6].

In addition, based on a subpopulation of 146 individuals we evaluated the potential risk for progression of AL for the carriers of the different genotypes of *A. actinomycetemcomitans* [6].

Table 2. Polymorphic sites in the leukotoxin promoter region of serotype b isolates (n = 41).

ST	n	-1	-79	-219	-220	-221	-436	-646	-1109
1	39	T	A	A	T	A	C	C	T
2	1	T	A	A	T	A	C	T	T
3	1	T	A	*	*	*	T	C	T

The leukotoxin promoter sequence of the isolates was compared with the corresponding sequence of the reference strain Y4 (accession number HAU51861). Y4 sequence was identical to ST 3.
ST (sequence types). Position -1 corresponds to the first nucleotide upstream of the start codon for *lkt*. Position – 1109 corresponds to the first nucleotide after the terminal codon of *glyA*.
*Deletion of a single nucleotide at this position.

Determination of leukotoxic activity

Three different methods were used for analyzing the leukotoxicity of the 239 different isolates: 1) Cell lysis, 2) Cell death, and 3) Haemolytic activity.

Cell lysis (LDH). Leukotoxicity analysis with the cell lysis (LDH) assay reveals loss of membrane integrity determined by the activity of lactate dehydrogenase that is released from damaged THP-1 cells (human acute monocytic leukemia cell line, ATCC 16) after 60-min exposure to the leukotoxic extract [8]. Briefly, each of the 239 isolates was re-cultivated on blood agar until conversion to a smooth phenotype was obtained. The isolates were then cultured in polyethylene glucose broth (PYG, peptone 20 g/l, glucose 5 g/l, Baptist yeast powder 10 g/l, NaCl 0.08 g/l cysteine hydrochloride 0.5 g/l, $CaCl_2$ 0.008 g/l, $MgSO_4$ 0.008 g/l, KH_2HPO_4 0.04 g/l, K_2HPO_4 0.04 g/l, $NaHCO_3$ 0.4 g/l, pH 7.1–7.3) for 72 hours at 37°C, and the optical density ($OD_{600\ nm}$) was measured. The bacterial suspensions were centrifuged for 5000×g for 20 min at 4°C, and the pellet was re-suspended in 300 mM NaCl in PBS to a final concentration corresponding to $OD_{600\ nm} = 20$. The THP-1 cells were seeded in 96-well plates with 10^5 cells/well in the presence of RPMI with 10% fetal calf serum and 50 nM PMA. After 24 h incubation at 37°C in 5% CO_2, the medium was replaced with 100 µl RPMI with 10% FBS and 5% leukotoxic extract. Extracts from each isolate were analyzed in triplicate, and the mixtures were incubated for 60 min at 37°C in 5% CO_2. The LDH activity in the supernatants was analyzed through the decreased absorbance at 340 nm as a result of NADH oxidation catalyzed by the release of cytosolic LDH. The release of LDH was expressed as % of the maximal release (100%) caused by incubation with 0.1% Triton x-100. The leukotoxicity of the isolates was classified in relation to their capacity to induce LDH-release: minimal leukotoxicity ≤30%, average leukotoxicity ≥31–60% or high leukotoxicity ≥61% release of cytosolic LDH.

Cell death (NRU). The cell viability assay (NRU) quantifies viability in relation to the capacity to accumulate neutral red in the lysosomes of leukotoxin-exposed THP-1 cells. The accumulation of neutral red in the lysosomes requires cells with an intact proton potential in the lysosomal membrane [39]. THP-1 cells and the leukotoxic extracts were processed as described for the cell lysis (LDH) assay. After a 60-min incubation period with the leukotoxic extracts, the culture medium was replaced with 100 µl fresh culture medium containing neutral red. After a 2-h staining period at 37°C in 5% CO_2, the staining medium was discarded and the cell monolayer was rinsed with 150 µl PBS. The cells were dissolved in 150 µl lysis solution (50% ethanol with 1% acetic acid), and the absorbance from the stain was measured at 550 nm. Cell viability (%) was calculated in relation to the absorbance of a sample incubated without leukotoxic extract. The leukotoxicity of the isolates was classified according to their capacity to induce cell death: minimal leukotoxicity ≤30%, average leukotoxicity ≥31–60% or high leukotoxicity ≥61% reduction of viable cells.

Haemolytic activity. The haemolytic activity has been suggested to reflect the effect of leukotoxin on erythrocytes. It has not previously been used for quantification of leukotoxicity. The haemolytic activity of the bacterial isolates was measured according to the following protocol. The bacterial isolates were cultivated on blood agar plates (as above) for 3–5 days. Subsequently, 5 µl OD 2-suspensions in 0.9% NaCl (approximately 4×10^9 cells/ml) of the isolates were added to blood agar plates (Columbia blood agar base, Acumedia, Neogen, Lansing, Michigan, USA) containing 5% horse blood and 10 µM deferoxamine (Sigma Aldrich; St. Louise, MO, USA.). Suspensions from six different isolates and three reference strains (JP2, D7s and a leukotoxin mutant of the D7s strain ([D7S*ΔltxA*]) were applied to

Table 3. AP PCR types with serotype b isolates (n = 51) divided into leukotoxicity categories based on results of the cell lysis (LDH) method.

	AP PCR types	
Genotypes of A.a*	**JP2/JP2-like, n (%)**	**Other, n (%)**
JP2	10 (100)	0 (0)
non-JP2 high leukotoxicity	10 (67)	5 (33)
non-JP2 average leukotoxicity	2 (18)	9 (82)
non-JP2 minimal leukotoxicity	2 (13)	13 (87)

**A.a; A. actinomycetemcomitans.*
(%): proportion of isolates within each leukotoxicity group.

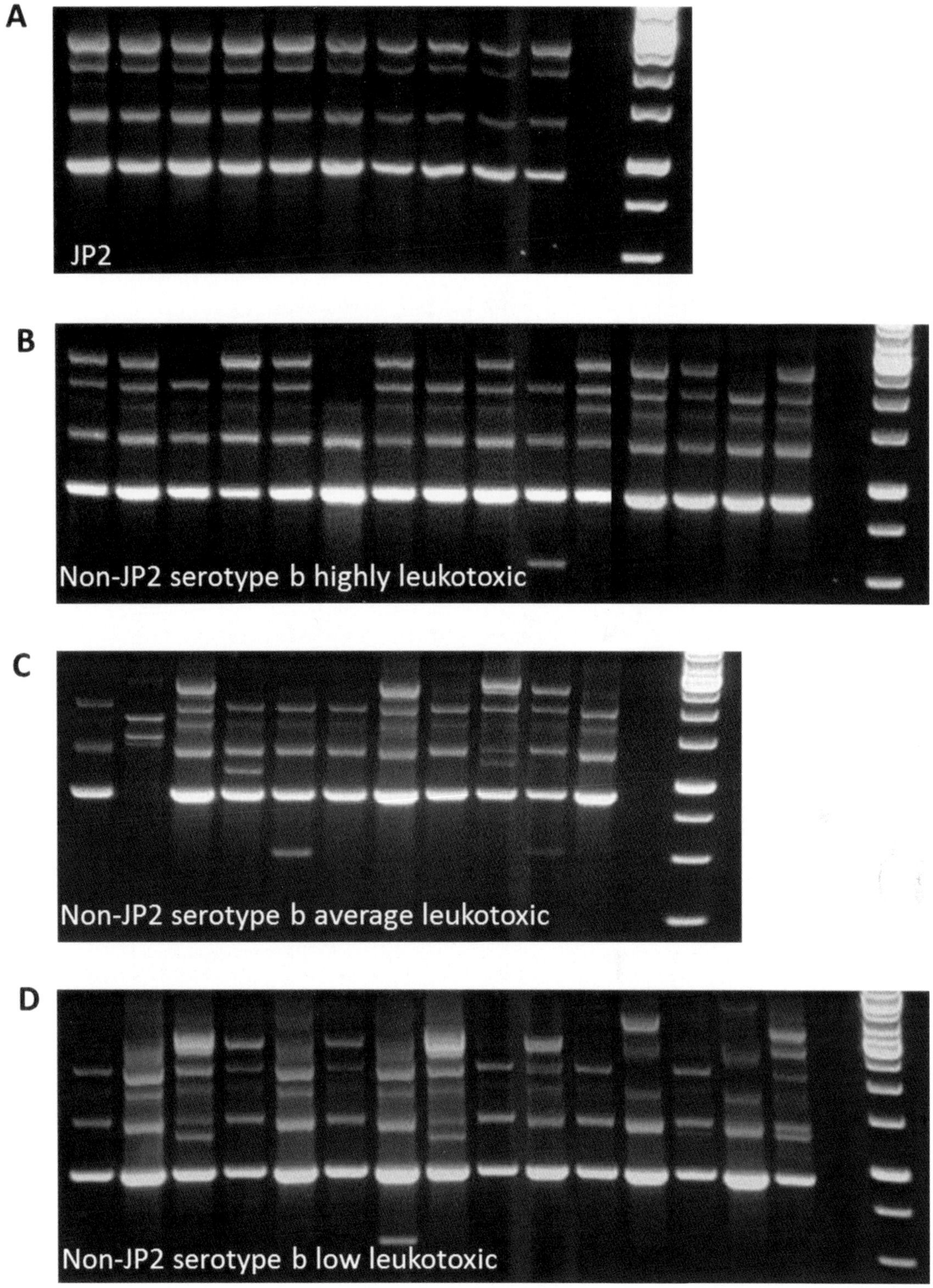

Figure 6. AP PCR banding pattern of **A.** JP2 genotype isolates (n = 10), **B.** High leukotoxicity non-JP2 genotype isolates of serotype b (n = 15), **C.** Average leukotoxicity non-JP2 genotype isolates of serotype b (n = 11), **D.** Minimal leukotoxicity non-JP2 genotype isolates of serotype b (n = 15). The classification of the non-JP2 genotype serotype-b isolates is based on results from the cell lysis (LDH) method.

each plate. The plates were incubated 5–7 days at 37°C in 5% CO_2 before examination. The haemolytic activity was scored as high (zone similar in size to that produced by JP2), average (zone similar to that produced by D7s), or low (minimal zone as produced by D7S*ΔltxA*).

Estimated risk (OR) of progression of AL in relation to leukotoxicity. To assess the estimated risk (OR) of the progression of AL within individuals harbouring strains from the three leukotoxicity categories (minimal, average or high), with the LDH and NRU-methods, the definition was as follows: The isolate

Table 4. Odds ratio (OR) for the progression of attachment loss (AL) according to leukotoxicity.

Variable	OR	95% CI	*p*-values	Individuals, total number (n)	Individuals, with progression of AL≥3 mm, n (%)
Cell lysis					
minimal	4.1	2.3–7.3	<0.001	110	41 (37.3)
Average + high	10.9	4.9–24.1	<0.001	36	22 (61.1)
Cell death					
Minimal + average	4.3	2.4–7.7	<0.001	97	37 (38.1)
high	7.8	3.9–15.8	<0.001	49	26 (53.1)
Haemolysis					
minimal	4.8	2.6–8.8	<0.001	90	37 (41.1)
average	3.9	1.8–8.5	<0.001	39	14 (35.9)
high	16.6	5.4–51.3	<0.001	17	12 (70.9)
A.a negative*	1.0	reference		190	24 (12.6)

Cell lysis (minimal = 0–30%, *average + high* = ≥31% release of cytosolic LDH), Cell death (*minimal + average* = 0–60%, *high* = ≥61% reduction of viable cells), Haemolysis (1 = minimal, none or small zone, 2 = *average*, average size zone, 3 = *high*, large size zone). Subgroup of individuals (n = 146) positive for *A. actinomycetemcomitans*. The reference group consisted of individuals (n = 190) who were negative for *A. actinomycetemcomitans*. OR, odds ratio; confidence interval; AL, attachment loss. Significance ($p<0.05$).
**A.a; A. actinomycetemcomitans.*

of *A. actinomycetemcomitans*, with the highest leukotoxicity score was determined to be representative for the individual studied. Therefore, if more than one serotype of *A. actinomycetemcomitans* was detected in an individual, the isolate/serotype with the highest score of leukotoxicity was chosen to be representative for that individual.

PCR-based characterization

Before the PCR-based analyses were performed, DNA was purified with GenElute Bacterial DNA kit (Sigma-Aldrich, St. Louise, MO, USA). For preparation of the PCR mixtures, PureTaq Ready-To-Go PCR (GE Healthcare; Buckinghamshire, UK) was used. For the sequencing procedure, DNA of amplified genes was sent to Eurofins MWG Operon (Ebersberg, Germany).

AP PCR. Arbitrarily-primed (AP) PCR, which can be carried out without previous knowledge of specific DNA sequence, was used for the characterization of the serotype b isolates. For amplification, the random sequence oligonucleotide OPB-3 (AGTCAGCCAC) (Invitrogen, Carlsbad, CA, USA) (0.4 µM) was used. The concentration of $MgCl_2$ in the PCR mixture was increased to 2.5 µM. The amplification was carried out as described by Dogan and co-workers [40].

Sequencing of the house-keeping gene hbpA-2. By sequencing *hbpA-2*, the origin of the JP2 genotype isolates used in this study could be determined. For amplification the primers TATTTTGACGCAATTGCTGTTC and TAGGGCACTTAT-CATTTCCATC (0.4 µM each) were used. The amplification was carried out as described by Eriksen and co-workers [41].

Sequencing of the leukotoxin promoter region. Sequencing the promoter region of the leukotoxin operon was carried out to determine sequence differences among the serotype b isolates. For amplification primer ltx3 (GCCGA-CACCAAAGACAAAGTCT') and primer ltx4 (GCCCATAAC-CAAGCCACATAC) (0.4 µM each) were used. The amplification was carried out as described by Poulsen and co-workers [42].

Statistical analysis. Data analyses were performed using SPSS 21.0 (SPSS Inc., Chicago, IL, USA). In the statistical analyses, the primary outcome was the progression of AL≥3 mm in one or more sites at individual level, based on the collection of data performed at the baseline examination (in 2009) and at the follow-up examination (in 2011). The estimated risk associated with the progression of AL≥3 mm during a two-year follow-up period according to leukotoxicity determined by the three methods (cell lysis, cell death and haemolysis) was evaluated by calculation of odds ratios (OR). A value of $p<0.05$ was considered statistically significant.

Acknowledgments

The authors would like to express their profound thanks for valuable support in the data collection of this study to the staff at the Dental School, University of Ghana, Accra, Ghana. We also want to thank all the school children who participated and made this study possible.

Author Contributions

Conceived and designed the experiments: RC AJ CHÅ DH. Performed the experiments: RC CHÅ AJ. Analyzed the data: CHÅ AJ RC DH. Contributed reagents/materials/analysis tools: RC AJ. Wrote the paper: RC CHÅ AJ FK DH.

References

1. Pihlstrom BL, Michalowicz BS, Johnson NW (2005) Periodontal diseases. Lancet 366: 1809–1820.
2. Henderson B, Ward JM, Ready D (2010) *Aggregatibacter (Actinobacillus) actinomycetemcomitans*: a triple A* periodontopathogen? Periodontol 2000 54: 78–105.
3. Van der Velden U, Abbas F, Armand S, Loos BG, Timmerman MF, et al. (2006) Java project on periodontal diseases. The natural development of periodontitis: risk factors, risk predictors and risk determinants. J Clin Periodontol 33: 540–548.
4. Fine DH, Markowitz K, Furgang D, Fairlie K, Ferrandiz J, et al. (2007) *Aggregatibacter actinomycetemcomitans* and its relationship to initiation of localized aggressive periodontitis: longitudinal cohort study of initially healthy adolescents. J Clin Microbiol 45: 3859–3869.

5. Haubek D, Ennibi OK, Poulsen K, Vaeth M, Poulsen S, et al. (2008) Risk of aggressive periodontitis in adolescent carriers of the JP2 clone of *Aggregatibacter (Actinobacillus) actinomycetemcomitans* in Morocco: a prospective longitudinal cohort study. Lancet 371: 237–242.
6. Höglund Åberg C, Antonoglou G, Haubek D, Kwamin F, Claesson R, Johansson A (2013) Cytolethal distending toxin in isolates of *Aggregatibacter actinomycetemcomitans* from Ghanaian adolescents and association with serotype and disease progression. PLOSONE 8(6): e65781.
7. Haubek D (2010) The highly leukotoxic JP2 clone of *Aggregatibacter actinomycetemcomitans*: evolutionary aspects, epidemiology and etiological role in aggressive periodontitis. APMIS 118 (S 130): 1–53.
8. Johansson A (2011) *Aggregatibacter actinomycetemcomitans* leukotoxin: a powerful tool with capacity to cause imbalance in the host inflammatory response. Toxins 3: 242–259.
9. Johansson A, Claesson R, Hänström L, Sandström G, Kalfas S (2000) Polymorphonuclear leukocyte degranulation induced by leukotoxin from *Actinobacillus actinomycetemcomitans*. J Periodontal Res 35: 85–92.
10. Claesson R, Johansson A, Belibasakis G, Hänström L, Kalfas S (2002) Release and activation of matrix metalloproteinase 8 from human neutrophils triggered by the leukotoxin of *Actinobacillus actinomycetemcomitans*. J Periodontal Res 37: 353–359.
11. Kelk P, Johansson A, Claesson R, Hänström L, Kalfas S (2003) Caspase 1 involvement in human monocyte lysis induced by *Actinobacillus actinomycetemcomitans* leukotoxin. Infect Immun 71: 4448–4455.
12. Balashova NV, Crosby JA, Al Ghofaily L, Kachlany SC (2006) Leukotoxin confers beta-hemolytic activity to *Actinobacillus actinomycetemcomitans*. Infect Immun 74: 2015–2021.
13. Reinholdt J, Poulsen K, Brinkmann CR, Hoffmann SV, Stapulionis R, et al. (2013) Monodisperse and LPS-free *Aggregatibacter actinomycetemcomitans* leukotoxin: interactions with human β_2 integrins and erythrocytes. Biochim Biophys Acta 1834: 546–558.
14. Lally ET, Kieba IR, Demuth DR, Rosenbloom J, Golub EE, et al. (1989) Identification and expression of the *Actinobacillus actinomycetemcomitans* leukotoxin gene. Biochem Biophys Res Commun 159: 256–262.
15. Kraig E, Dailey T, Kolodrubetz D (1990) Nucleotide sequence of the leukotoxin gene from *Actinobacillus actinomycetemcomitans*: homology to the alpha-hemolysin/leukotoxin gene family. Infect Immun 58: 920–929.
16. Kolodrubetz D, Dailey T, Ebersole J, Kraig E (1989) Cloning and expression of the leukotoxin gene from *Actinobacillus actinomycetemcomitans*. Infect Immun 57: 1465–1469.
17. Kolodrubetz D, Spitznagel J Jr, Wang B, Phillips LH, Jacobs C, et al. (1996) cis Elements and trans factors are both important in strain-specific regulation of the leukotoxin gene in *Actinobacillus actinomycetemcomitans*. Infect Immun 64: 3451–3460.
18. Mitchell C, Gao L, Demuth DR (2003) Positive and negative cis-acting regulatory sequences control expression of leukotoxin in *Actinobacillus actinomycetemcomitans* 652. Infect Immun 71: 5640–5649.
19. He T, Nishihara T, Demuth DR, Ishikawa I (1999) A novel insertion sequence increases the expression of leukotoxicity in *Actinobacillus actinomycetemcomitans* clinical isolates. J Periodontol 70: 1261–1268.
20. Inoue T, Tanimoto I, Tada T, Ohashi T, Fukui K, et al. (2001) Fermentable-sugar-level-dependent regulation of leukotoxin synthesis in a variably toxic strain of *Actinobacillus actinomycetemcomitans*. Microbiology 147: 2749–2756.
21. Kolodrubetz D, Phillips L, Jacobs C, Burgum A, Kraig E (2003) Anaerobic regulation of *Actinobacillus actinomycetemcomitans* leukotoxin transcription is ArcA/FnrA-independent and requires a novel promoter element. Res Microbiol 154: 645–653.
22. Feuerbacher LA, Burgum A, Kolodrubetz D (2011) The cyclic-AMP receptor protein (CRP) regulon in *Aggregatibacter actinomycetemcomitans* includes leukotoxin. Microb Pathog 51: 133–141.
23. Spitznagel J Jr, Kraig E, Kolodrubetz D (1991) Regulation of leukotoxin in leukotoxic and nonleukotoxic strains of *Actinobacillus actinomycetemcomitans*. Infect Immun 59: 1394–1401.
24. Brogan JM, Lally ET, Poulsen K, Kilian M, Demuth DR (1994) Regulation of *Actinobacillus actinomycetemcomitans* leukotoxin expression: analysis of the promoter regions of leukotoxic and minimally leukotoxic strains. Infect Immun 62: 501–508.
25. Haubek D, Poulsen K, Kilian M (2007) Microevolution and patterns of dissemination of the JP2 clone of *Aggregatibacter (Actinobacillus) actinomycetemcomitans*. Infect Immun 75: 3080–3088.
26. Macheleidt A, Muller HP, Eger T, Putzker M (1999). Absence of an especially toxic clone among isolates of Actinobacillus actinomycetemcomitans recovered from army recruits. Clin Oral Invest 3: 161–167.
27. Jentsch H, Cachovan G, Guentsch A, Eickholz P, Pfister W, Eick S (2012). Characterization of *Aggregatibacter actinomycetemcomitans* strains in periodontitis patients in Germay. Clin Oral Invest 16: 1589–1597.
28. Guthmiller JM, Lally ET, Korostoff J (2001) Beyond the specific plaque hypothesis: are highly leukotoxic strains of *Actinobacillus actinomycetemcomitans* a paradigm for periodontal pathogenesis? Crit Rev Oral Biol Med 12: 116–124.
29. Claesson R, Lagervall M, Höglund Åberg C, Johansson A, Haubek D (2011) Detection of the highly leucotoxic JP2 clone of *Aggregatibacter actinomycetemcomitans* in members of a Caucasian family living in Sweden. J Clin Periodontol 38: 115–121.
30. Kelk P, Claesson R, Chen C, Sjöstedt A, Johansson A (2008) IL-1β secretion induced by *Aggregatibacter (Actinobacillus) actinomycetemcomitans* is mainly caused by the leukotoxin. Int J Med Microbiol 298: 529–541.
31. Höglund Åberg C, Kwamin F, Claesson R, Dahlén G, Johansson A, et al. (2014) Progression of attachment loss is strongly associated with presence of the JP2 genotype of *Aggregatibacter actinomycetemcomitans*: a prospective cohort study of a young adolescent population. J Clin Periodontol 41: 232–241.
32. Zambon JJ, Slots J, Genco RJ (1983) Serology of oral *Actinobacillus actinomycetemcomitans* and serotype distribution in human periodontal disease. Infect Immun 41: 19–27.
33. Yang HW, Asikainen S, Dogan B, Suda R, Lai CH (2004) Relationship of *Actinobacillus actinomycetemcomitans* serotype b to aggressive periodontitis: frequency in pure cultured isolates. J Periodontol 75: 592–599.
34. He T, Hayashi J, Yamamoto M, Ishikawa I (1998) Genotypic characterization of *Actinobacillus actinomycetemcomitans* isolated from periodontitis patients by arbitrarily primed polymerase chain reaction. J Periodontol 69: 69–75.
35. Paju S, Saarela M, Alaluusua S, Fives-Taylor P, Asikainen S (1998) Characterization of serologically nontypeable *Actinobacillus actinomycetemcomitans* isolates. J Clin Microbiol 36: 2019–2022.
36. Paju S, Carlson P, Jousimies-Somer H, Asikainen S (2000) Heterogeneity of *Actinobacillus actinomycetemcomitans* strains in various human infections and relationships between serotype, genotype, and antimicrobial susceptibility. J Clin Microbiol 38: 79–84.
37. Haubek D, Dirienzo JM, Tinoco EM, Westergaard J, Lopez NJ, et al. (1997) Racial tropism of a highly toxic clone of *Actinobacillus actinomycetemcomitans* associated with juvenile periodontitis. J Clin Microbiol 35: 3037–3042.
38. Höglund Åberg C, Kwamin F, Claesson R, Johansson A, Haubek D (2012) Presence of JP2 and non-JP2 genotypes of *Aggregatibacter actinomycetemcomitans* and attachment loss in adolescents in Ghana. J Periodontol 83: 1520–1528.
39. Repetto G, del Peso A, Zurita JL (2008) Neutral red uptake assay for the estimation of cell viability/cytotoxicity. Nat Protoc 3: 1125–1131.
40. Dogan B, Saarela MH, Jousimies-Somer H, Alaluusua S, Asikainen S (1999) *Actinobacillus actinomycetemcomitans* serotype e–biotypes, genetic diversity and distribution in relation to periodontal status. Oral Microbiol Immunol 14: 98–103.
41. Eriksen KT, Haubek D, Poulsen K (2005) Intragenomic recombination in the highly leukotoxic JP2 clone of *Actinobacillus actinomycetemcomitans*. Microbiology 151: 3371–3379.
42. Poulsen K, Ennibi OK, Haubek D (2003) Improved PCR for detection of the highly leukotoxic JP2 clone of *Actinobacillus actinomycetemcomitans* in subgingival plaque samples. J Clin Microbiol 41: 4829–4832.

23

The Pro-Apoptotic and Pro-Inflammatory Effects of Calprotectin on Human Periodontal Ligament Cells

Yunfei Zheng[1,2¶], Jianxia Hou[2¶], Lei Peng[3], Xin Zhang[4], Lingfei Jia[1,5], Xian'e Wang[2], Shicheng Wei[1], Huanxin Meng[2*]

1 Department of Oral and Maxillofacial Surgery, Peking University School and Hospital of Stomatology, Beijing, P.R. China, **2** Department of Periodontology, Peking University School and Hospital of Stomatology, Beijing, P.R. China, **3** Department of Stomatology, Beijing Friendship Hospital, Capital Medical University, Beijing, P.R. China, **4** Department of Stomatology, Peking Union Medical College Hospital, Chinese Academy of Medical Science, Beijing, P.R. China, **5** Laboratory of Molecular Biology, Peking University School and Hospital of Stomatology, Beijing, China

Abstract

Calprotectin, a heterodimer of S100A8 and S100A9 subunits, is associated with inflammatory disorders such as rheumatoid arthritis and cystic fibrosis. Although calprotectin levels are increased significantly in the gingival crevicular fluid (GCF) of periodontitis patients, its effects on periodontal ligament cells (PDLCs) remain largely unknown. The aim of this study was to evaluate calprotectin levels in the GCF of generalized aggressive periodontitis (AgP) patients and to investigate the effects of recombinant human calprotectin (rhS100A8/A9) and its subunits (rhS100A8 and rhS100A9) in PDLCs. Both the concentration and amount of crevicular calprotectin were significantly higher in the AgP group compared with healthy controls. In addition, the GCF calprotectin levels were correlated positively with clinical periodontal parameters including bleeding index, probing depth, and clinical attachment loss. rhS100A8/A9 promoted cell apoptosis, whereas rhS100A8 and rhS100A9 individually exerted little effect on apoptosis in PDLCs. rhS100A9 and rhS100A8/A9 increased the activation of nuclear factor-κB (NF-κB) by promoting the nuclear translocation of p65 in PDLCs, subsequently inducing expression of the pro-inflammatory cytokines IL-6, IL-8, TNFα, and COX2. Treatment with an NF-κB inhibitor partially reversed the rhS100A9- and rhS100A8/A9-induced upregulation of the pro-inflammatory cytokines. rhS100A9, and not rhS100A8, was mainly responsible for the pro-inflammatory role of calprotectin. Collectively, our results suggest that calprotectin promotes apoptosis and the inflammatory response in PDLCs via rhS100A9. These findings might help identify novel treatments for periodontitis.

Editor: Michael Glogauer, University of Toronto, Canada

Funding: This work was supported by the National Natural Science Foundation of China (30271411, 30471882, 30973319), and HX Meng received the funding for this work. The funders had no role in study design, data collection and analysis, decision to publish, or preparation of the manuscript.

Competing Interests: The authors have declared that no competing interests exist.

* Email: kqhxmeng@bjmu.edu.cn

¶ These authors contributed equally to this work.

Introduction

Periodontitis is an infectious disease that affects the tissues supporting the teeth and leads to eventual tooth loss [1]. Apart from the type associated with systemic conditions, periodontitis can be divided into two broad categories; chronic periodontitis, which occurs primarily in adults and progresses relatively slowly, and aggressive periodontitis, a more aggressive form that may occur in adolescents. Current knowledge regarding the pathogenesis of periodontal disease suggests that its central cause is an imbalance in the host-parasite relationship. The host inflammatory response also plays a role. A large number of cytokines and other effector molecules released by resident and migrating cells contribute to the destruction of soft and hard tissues seen in periodontitis [2].

Calprotectin is a heterodimeric calcium-binding protein consisting of S100A8 and S100A9 subunits [3]. It is expressed constitutively in neutrophils [4], monocytes [4], keratinocytes [5]. It also plays role in epithelial cells [6] and several different cancer cells [3,7,8]. Calprotectin is estimated to constitute ~40% of the total cytosolic proteins in polymorphonuclear neutrophil [4,7]. It is released during inflammatory events, either after cell death or via an active secretary mechanism [9]. Calprotectin exerts antiproliferative and antitumoral effects [10,11]. In addition, it acts not only as a chemoattractant [12], but also as a pro-inflammatory factor that exerts cytokine-like activities. For example, it can bind to Toll-like receptor 4 (TLR-4) or the advanced glycation end product receptor to activate the intracellular signaling pathways including the mitogen-activated protein kinase and nuclear factor-κB (NF-κB) pathways [13,14]. Increased levels of calprotectin in extracellular fluid were reported in numerous inflammation-associated pathological conditions, such as rheumatoid arthritis, Sjögren's syndrome, Crohn's Diseas, colorectal cancer and periodontitis [7]. The levels of calprotectin in the gingival crevicular fluid (GCF) of patients with gingivitis and periodontitis were reported, and its concentration was correlated with clinical factors such as probing depth (PD), bleeding on probing (BOP), and gingival index [15,16]. Conversely, non-surgical therapy using antibiotics decreased local calprotectin levels [17].

Interestingly, human S100A8 is a potent and specific autocrine chemotactic factor in periodontal ligament cells (PDLCs); therefore, it might be an attractive therapeutic candidate for the treatment of periodontal disease [18,19]. However, the concentration of S100A8 that stimulates the chemotactic activity of PDLCs is far lower than the concentration *in vivo*. PDLCs reside in the periodontal ligament space and play a key role in forming the periodontal ligament and its fibers by secreting extracellular matrix components such as collagen and mineralized tissue [20]. PDLCs also play a role in the production of various pro-inflammatory cytokines, thereby participating in the development of periodontal inflammation.

In recent years the regenerative potential of PDLCs in tissue repair has received increasing attention [21]. Given the importance of PDLCs in maintaining of the integrity of periodontal tissue, the effects of calprotectin and its subunits in PDLCs, other than their chemotactic activity, is worthy of investigation. To determine a potential correlation between calprotectin levels and periodontitis and to examine the mechanism of calprotectin's influence on the behavior of PDLCs, calprotectin levels in the GCF of patients with generalized aggressive periodontitis (AgP) were evaluated and the pro-apoptotic and pro-inflammatory effects of recombinant S100A8, S100A9, and S100A8/A9 in PDLCs were investigated.

Materials and Methods

Ethics statement

The Ethics Committee of Peking University School of Stomatology approved the study protocol, and all clinical specimens were obtained from patients who provided written informed consent to use their tissues for research purposes (approval number PKUSSIRB-2011007).

Study population

A total of 40 participants were included in the study. Of these, 20 patients <36 years old with generalized aggressive periodontitis were recruited from the Department of Periodontology, Peking University Hospital of Stomatology, China. The diagnostic criteria for generalized aggressive periodontitis were defined according to the classification proposed at the International Workshop for the Classification of Periodontal Diseases and Conditions in 1999 [22]. The details of inclusion criteria were as follows: (1) patients are affected at <35 years of age; (2) at least eight teeth had a probing depth (PD) >6 mm, three or more of which were not first molars or incisors; and (3) radiographs showed alveolar bone loss. In addition, 20 periodontally healthy controls were selected from the staff and students at the School of Stomatology; they were included if they meet the following criteria as previously described [22]: (1) PD ≤3 mm; (2) bleeding on probing (BOP) was <10%; (3) no attachment loss (AL); and (4) no bone loss visible on radiographs. All participants were non-smokers and no participants had a concomitant systemic disease or received antibiotics within the 4 months prior to the study. Patients who had received periodontal therapy within the previous year and females who were post-menopausal, pregnant, in lactation or taking oral contraceptive drugs were excluded from the study. The purpose of the study and the procedures involved were explained to all participants in advance and written informed consent was obtained.

Clinical examination

All subjects underwent a clinical periodontal examination including PD, BI, and CAL using a Williams periodontal probe at six sites of each tooth to determine their clinical periodontal status [22]. A set of full-mouth periapical radiographs was also taken from each subject.

Collection of GCF samples

Two sites of each subject were selected for GCF sampling, one from the mesial buccal site of the right maxillary central incisor and the other from the mesial buccal site of the left mandibular first molar. GCF samples were collected using a paper strip (Whatman, Maidstone, U.K.) from healthy gingival crevices (PD ≤2 mm, BI = 0, CAL = 0 mm) for periodontally healthy controls and from periodontal pockets (PD ≥4 mm, BI ≥1, CAL ≥1 mm) in patients with generalized aggressive periodontitis. Supragingival plaques were removed from the interproximal surfaces using a sterile curette prior to the sampling. Paper strips were then inserted carefully into the crevice until mild resistance was felt and left there for 30 seconds.

Measuring calprotectin levels

GCF samples were eluted from the strips by placing them in 300 μl of phosphate buffered saline (PBS). The calprotectin levels were then assayed using commercially available ELISA kits according to the manufacturer's instructions (Phicaltest; Calpro AS, Oslo, Norway). The amount of calprotectin in each sample was calculated based on the dilutions as described previously [23].

Production of recombinant human S100A8 (rhS100A8) and S100A9 (rhS100A9)

The methods used to produce and purify the recombinant proteins were described previously [24]. Briefly, the hS100A8 and hS100A9 plasmids (kind gifts from Dr. Tessier, Infectious Diseases Research Center, Laval University Hospital Center, Québec, Canada) [24] were transformed into *Escherichia coli* BAL21 (DE3) and their expression was induced using isopropyl β-D-thiogalactosidein (Sigma-Aldrich, St. Louis, MO, USA). Next, a nickel column and a polymyxin B-agarose column (Pierce, Rockford, IL, USA) were used to purify the recombinant His-tagged proteins. The endotoxins contamination was <1 pg/μg protein, as measured using a Limulus amebocyte assay (Sigma-Aldrich). Recombinant proteins were analyzed on SDS-PAGE gels and stained using Coomassie brilliant blue. As shown in Figure S1, rhS100A8 and rhS100A9 migrated to their expected molecular masses and were free of contaminating bacteria-derived proteins after purification. Equimolar amounts of rhS100A8 and rhS100A9 were mixed to generate rhS100A8/A9 in the presence of 1.3 mM Ca^{2+} according to Vandal et al [25].

Cell culture

Primary normal human periodontal ligament cells were obtained from explant cultures using methods described previously [26]. Briefly, periodontal ligament explants were obtained from the middle third of premolar roots extracted for orthodontic treatment and were minced into smaller portions. The cells were maintained in Dulbecco's modified Eagle medium (DMEM; Gibco, Gaithersburg, MD, USA) supplemented with 10% heat-inactivated fetal bovine serum (Hyclone, Logan, UT, USA) in tissue culture flasks (Corning, NY, USA). Cells from passages four to eight were used all experiments.

Apoptosis analysis

To detect cell apoptosis, an annexin V-fluorescein isothiocyanate (FITC) kit (Roche, Mannheim, Germany) was used according to the manufacturer's protocol. Briefly, PDLCs were treated with rhS100A8, rhS100A9 or rhS100A8/A9, incubated for 48 h, trypsinized, and then re-suspended in the binding buffer containing 5 μL of annexin V-FITC and 4 μg/mL of propidium iodide after incubation in the dark at room temperature for 10 min. Apoptosis were then analyzed using fluorescence-activated cell sorting (Beckman Coulter, Fullerton, CA, USA). At least 10,000 cells per sample were analyzed and annexin-V-FITC-positive cells were regarded to be apoptotic.

The morphology of PDLCs treated with calprotectin were evaluated using fluorescence microscopy after staining with 4′,6-diamidino-2-phenylindole (DAPI). Approximately 5×10^4 PDLCs per well of a 24-well plate were incubated with rhS100A8, rhS100A9 or rhS100A8/A9 at a final concentration of 10^{-6} M for 48 h. They were then fixed with 4% paraformaldehyde (Sigma-Aldrich), stained with DAPI and visualized using a fluorescence microscope as described previously [27].

RNA extraction and real-time PCR analysis

Subconfluent cell monolayers were serum-depleted overnight in DMEM and were then treated with rhS100A8, rhS100A9 or rhS100A8/A9 alone or in combination with the NF-κB specific inhibitor pyrrolidine dithiocarbamate (PDTC; Sigma-Aldrich) for 12 h. Total RNA was isolated using RNA isolation reagent TRIzol (Invitrogen, Carlsbad, CA, USA) according to the manufacturer's instructions, and the concentration was determined spectrophotometrically. First-strand cDNA was synthesized using a first-strand cDNA synthesis kit (MBI Fermentas, Inc., Burlington, ON, Canada) using oligo dT primers. The primers used were as follows: human IL-1β forward 5′-ATG GCT TAT TAC AGT GGC A-3′ and reverse 5′-GTA GTG GTG GTC GGA GAT T-3′, human IL-6 forward 5′-GTG AGG AAC AAG CCA GAG C-3′ and reverse 5′-TAC ATT TGC CGA AGA GCC-3′, human IL-8 forward 5′-TTT TGC CAA GGA GTG CTA AAG A-3′ and reverse 5′-AAC CCT CTG CAC CCA GTT TTC-3′, human TNFα forward 5′-CGA GTG ACA AGC CTG TAG CC-3′ and reverse 5′-TGA AGA GGA CCT GGG AGT AGA T-3′, human COX2 forward 5′-CTG GCG CTC AGC CAT ACA G-3′ and reverse 5′-ACA CTC ATA CAT ACA CCT CGG T-3′, human GAPDH forward 5′-ATG GGG AAG GTG AAG GTC G-3′ and reverse 5′-GGG GTC ATT GAT GGC AAC AAT A-3′. Real-time PCR was performed using a 7500 Fast Real-time RT-PCR System (Applied Biosystems, Foster City, CA) according to the manufacturer's instructions. The relative expression of the targed gene was then normalized to GAPDH expression using $2^{-\Delta\Delta Ct}$ method.

ELISA

The concentrations of IL-6 and IL-8 in cell culture supernatants were determined using ELISA (Gersion, Beijing, China) according to the manufacturer's instructions. Briefly, the supernatants of PDLCs treated with 10^{-6} M rhS100A8, rhS100A9 and rhS100A8/A9 were added to the ELISA plates incubated with antibodies, aspirated and then washed with washing buffer. The optical density at 450 nm was then measured.

Immunofluorescent analysis of p65

PDLCs were seeded on glass slides at a density of 5×10^4 cells/mL, and treated with rhS100A8, rhS100A9 or rhS100A8/A9 for 6 h. Immunofluorescent analysis of the p65 was then performed as described previously [28]. Briefly, cultures were fixed in 4% paraformaldehyde, permeabilized with 0.1% Triton X-100 and blocked with 10% goat serum. After incubation overnight at 4°C in a humid chamber with antibodies against the 65 kDa subunit of NF-κB (1:100) (Beyotime, Jiangsu, China), slides were incubated with tetramethyl rhodamine isothiocyanate-conjugated goat anti-rabbit secondary antibodies (1:200) (Chemicon, Hofheim, Germany) for 30 min at room temperature; 5 μg/mL DAPI was used for conterstaining. Finally, the slides were embedded in mounting medium and the fluorescence signals were measured using a Zeiss laser scanning microscope (LSM 510; Carl Zeiss, Jena, Germany).

EMSA

Nuclear PDLC extracts were prepared and EMSAs were performed as described previously [28]. 3′-Biotin-labeled and unlabeled probes containing the NF-κB consensus binding site (5′-AGT TGA GGG GAC TTT CCC AGG C-3′) were synthesized, and the binding reaction was performed using a Light Shift Chemiluminescent EMSA Kit (Pierce, Rockford, IL, USA).

Statistical analysis

Statistical analyses were performed using SPSS PASW version 18. Distribution of the variables was tested using the Shapiro-Wilk test. Continuous normally distributed variables were presented as means ± standard deviations (SD). The median (lower to upper quartile) was used to describe non-normally distributed data. Differences for age and calprotectin levels in the GCF between groups were analyzed using Student's t-test, whereas differences for clinical parameters between groups were analyzed using Mann-Whitney U-test. Gender was analyzed using chi-square test. Spearman's correlation tests were used to identify the associations between local clinical variables and the calprotectin levels. Pearson's correlation coefficient is used to identify the association between the age and GCF calprotectin level. Cell culture experiments were performed at least in triplicate, and the differences among groups were analyzed using one-way ANOVA. A two-tailed p value <0.05 was considered to indicate statistical significance.

Results

Increased GCF calprotecin levels in the AgP group

The demographic characteristics of the 40 study participants are summarized in Table 1. There were no significant differences in age or gender between the two groups. Generally, patients in the AgP group had more severe clinical indices with respect to BI, PD and CAL. Both the concentration and amount of GCF calprotectin were significantly higher in the AgP group compared with the control group (2,332±383.200 μg/mL *vs.* 471±51.120 μg/mL, and 4,378±741.4 ng *vs.* 87.82±12.38 ng, respectively; $p<0.05$). The calprotectin levels in the GCF were moderately positively correlated with clinical periodontal parameters including BI, PD and CAL ($p<0.05$, Table 2). There was no association with age or gender.

Pro-apoptotic activity of rhS100A8, rhS100A9 and rhS100A8/A9

Flow cytometry revealed that the number of annexin V-positive PDLCs increased significantly upon exposure to rhS100A8/A9 for 48 h, whereas only ~5% of cells were annexin V-positive in the vehicle group. Fewer apoptotic cells were detected in the presence of rhS100A8 or rhS100A9 compared with rhS100A8/A9 (Figure 1).

Table 1. Demographic and clinical variables.

variables	Healthy group (n = 20)	AgP group (n = 20)	*p* value
Age(years)[a]	24.40±0.3434	26.80±1.615	0.1543
Gender (n; male/female)[b]	10/10	6/14	0.197
BI[c]	2 (1–3)	4 (3–4)	**<0.01**
PD(mm)[c]	2.5 (2.0–3.0)	7.0 (5.3–7.0)	**<0.01**
CAL(mm)[c]	0	6.0 (5.0–7.75)	**<0.01**
CPT Conc. in GCF(μg/mL)[a]	471±51.120	2332±383.200	**<0.01**
CPT amount in GCF(ng)[a]	87.82±12.38	4378±741.4	**<0.01**

Data are given as Mean ± SD or number of subjects, or median (lower-upper quartile).
Between-group comparisons were performed using the [a]t-test, [b]chi-square test, or [c]Mann-Whitney U-test.
Values in bold indicate a statistically significant difference ($p<0.01$).
AgP, generalized aggressive periodontitis; BI, bleeding index; PD, probing depth; CAL, clinical attachment loss; CPT Conc., calprotectin concentration; CPT amount, the amount of calprotectin; GCF, gingival crevicular fluid.

Morphological changes in PDLCs treated with rhS100A8, rhS100A9 and rhS100A8/A9 were analyzed using fluorescence microscopy following DAPI staining (Figure 2). Viable cells exhibit a normal-sized nucleus and blue fluorescence, whereas apoptotic cells contain condensed chromatin and fragmented nuclei. After treatment with rhS100A8/A9 for 48 h, the number of apoptotic cells increased significantly (24.5%±5.1% *vs.* 6.7%±3.1%, $p<0.05$). Fewer apoptotic cells were observed in rhS100A8-treated cultures compared with rhS100A9-treated cultures. Because the recombinant S100A proteins used in these studies were derived from *E. coli* extracts, it is possible that the response was due to trace contamination with bacterial LPS. To exclude this possibility, an aliquot of the recombinant protein was heated at 100°C for 10 min to inactivate the protein; this abrogated its pro-apoptotic activity.

rhS100A8, rhS100A9 and rhS100A8/A9 induce pro-inflammatory cytokines

The mRNA levels of IL-6, IL-8, TNFα and COX2 were increased significantly in cells treated with rhS100A9 and rhS100A8/A9 compared with the vehicle and heat-inactivated groups (Figure 3A). IL-6 and IL-8 were the most responsive genes, both upregulated several hundred-fold. Although these genes were also upregulated by rhS100A8, the levels were lower than those induced by rhS100A9 or rhS100A8/A9. Heat-inactivated rhS100A9 and rhS100A8/A9 failed to upregulation IL-6, IL-8, TNFα or COX2, which excluded the possibility of trace LPS contamination. rhS100A9 also increased the protein expression of IL-6 and IL-8 significantly ($p<0.05$; Figure 3B).

rhS100A9 and rhS100A8/A9 activate NF-κB

To determine the mechanism for the pro-inflammatory effects of rhS100A9 and rhS100A8/A9, indirect immunohistofluorescence was performed to detect the nuclear translocation of NF-κB-p65. The presence of red fluorescence in the nucleus, which is suggestive of NF-κB translocation, typically indicates its functional activation because it is otherwise retained in the cytoplasm as inactive complexes with IκB proteins. In untreated PDLCs, p65 was localized almost exclusively in the cytoplasm. In contrast, rhS100A9 and rhS100A8/A9 induced the nuclear translocation of p65, as indicated by the pink nuclear signal in the merged images

Table 2. Correlations between crevicular calprotecin levels and the variables evaluated in the study cohort (n = 40).

Variables	crevicular calprotectin conc.		crevicular calprotectin amount	
	r	*p*-value	r	*p*-value
Demographic parameters				
age	0.03373	0.8363[a]	0.2539	0.1138[a]
gender	−0.07515	0.6449[b]	0.2520	0.1167[b]
Clinical parameters				
Mean BI	0.5503	**<0.01[b]**	0.6271	**<0.01[b]**
Mean PD	0.5010	**<0.01[b]**	0.7246	**<0.01[b]**
Mean CAL	0.5350	**<0.01[b]**	0.7659	**<0.01[b]**
CPT conc. in GCF	—	—	0.7626	**<0.01[a]**
CPT amount in GCF	0.7626	**<0.01[a]**	—	—

Correlation analysis was performed using [a]Pearson's rank correlation analyses or [b]Spearman's rank correlation analyses.
Bold numbers indicate a statistically significant difference ($p<0.01$).
BI, bleeding index; PD, probing depth; CAL, clinical attachment loss; CPT Conc., calprotectin concentration; CPT amount, the amount of calprotectin; GCF, gingival crevicular fluid.

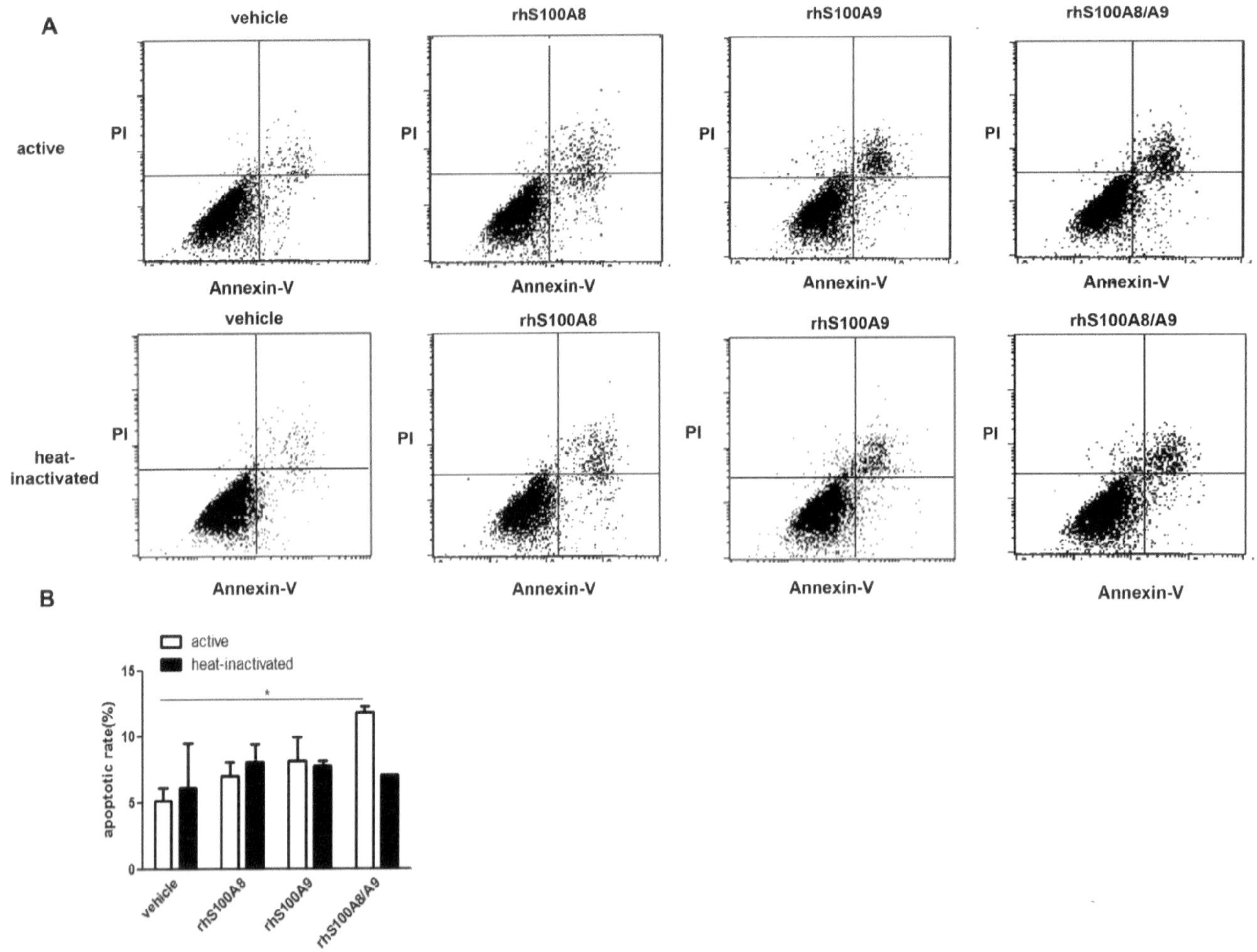

Figure 1. Analysis of PDLC apoptosis using annexin V/PI staining. PDLCs were treated with 10^{-6} M rhS100A8, rhS100A9, rhS100A8/A9 or heat-inactivated rhS100A8, rhS100A9, rhS100A8/A9 for 48 h. Apoptosis was then assessed using flow cytometry after annexin V/PI staining. The fluorescence intensity of 10,000 cells was measured and the number of annexin-V-FITC-positive cells was calculated. Statistical analysis revealed that there were significantly more apoptotic cells in the rhS100A8/A9-treated group (10.2475%±2.019%, $p<0.05$) compared with the control group (5.653%±2.914%). There were no differences between the rhS100A8- and rhS100A9-treated groups. * $p<0.05$ *vs.* the control group.

caused by the overlapping blue (DAPI staining) and red fluorescence signals (NF-κB-p65 subunit) in the nucleus (Figure 4A). rhS100A8 did not stimulate significant translocation of NF-κB-p65, although some small patches of positive NF-κB staining were present in the nuclei.

To further assess the effects of rhS100A8, rhS100A9 and rhS100A8/A9 on NF-κB signaling, oligonucleotides containing the NF-κB-binding sequences were reacted with nuclear extracts. As shown in Figure 4B, a DNA-protein complex was visible in the samples incubated with the nuclear extracts (lanes 2, 3 and 4) compared with the oligonucleotides without the nuclear extracts (lanes 1). A competition assay was then used to verify the binding specificity. The DNA-binding activity of NF-κB in the rhS100A9-treated group was increased compared with the rhS100A8- and rhS100A8/A9-treated groups. The activation of NF-κB signaling was confirmed by the addition of PDTC, an NF-κB inhibitor, which attenuated the rhS100A9- and rhS100A8/A9-induced cytokines upregulation (Figure 4C).

Discussion

The present study revealed that calprotectin levels were significantly higher in the GCF of AgP patients compared with the control group, which is consistent with the previous studies [15,29,30]. Therefore, local calprotectin levels have the potential to be used as a diagnostic marker of periodontitis. However, the biological function of calprotectin in PDLCs and the mechanism by which calprotectin contributes to the pathogenesis of periodontitis remain unclear. Therefore, the biological effect of rhS100A8, rhS100A9 and rhS100A8/A9 in PDLCs was measured in the current study.

S100A8/A9 was reported to have broad apoptosis-inducing activity in various cells including cancer cells such as AGS [31], HaCaT keratinocytes [32], EL-4 lymphoma cells [33], colon carcinoma cells [34], and normal cells like HMEC-1 cells [10]. The apoptosis-inducing effects of rhS100A8, rhS100A9 and rhS100A8/A9 were examined in PDLCs *in vitro* and data revealed that rhS100A8/A9 had greater apoptosis-inducing effects than did rhS100A8 or rhS100A9 alone. Consistent with this, cytotoxic effects of rhS100A8/A9 in EL-4 cells were detected with

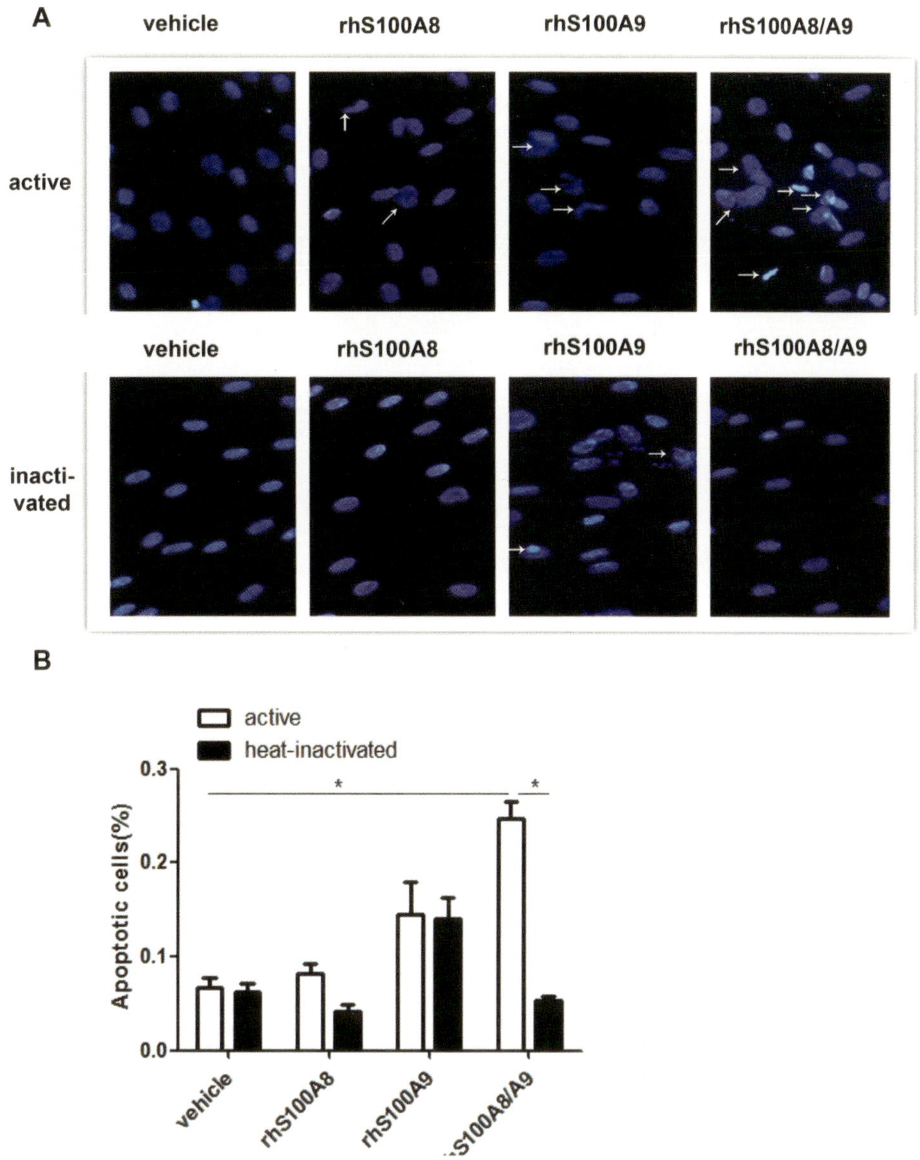

Figure 2. Morphology of PDLCs after DAPI staining. The morphological changes of PDLCs treated with rhS100A8, rhS100A9, rhS100A8/A9, or heat-inactivated rhS100A8, rhS100A9, or rhS100A8/A9 were evaluated by fluorescence microscopy after DAPI staining. Viable cells displayed a normal-sized nucleus and blue fluorescence, whereas apoptotic cells exhibited condensed chromatin and fragmented nuclei. Treatment with rhS100A8/A9 increased the percentage of apoptotic cells significantly compared with the control (24.5%±5.1% *vs.* 6.7%±3.1%, $p<0.05$) and heat-inactivated rhS100A8/A9 (24.5%±5.1% *vs.* 5.273%±1.14%, $p<0.05$). Fewer apoptotic cells were observed in rhS100A8-treated cultures whereas more apoptotic cells were present in rhS100A9-treated cells. * $p<0.05$ *vs.* the control or heat-inactivated groups.

relatively low concentrations in a standard medium, whereas rhS100A8 and S100A9 caused only marginal cytotoxicity at even higher concentrations [33]. To verify whether the observed pro-apoptotic effects of calprotectin were specific, the cytotoxic activity of heat-inactivated calprotectin was also examined to exclude the possible effects of trace LPS contamination. Heat-inactivating calprotecin abrogated its pro-apoptotic effects in PDLCs. However, fewer PDLCs underwent apoptosis after treatment with rhS100A8/A9 in the current study compared with the previous study in tumor cells. Because cells exhibit variable sensitivity to S100A8/A9 [34], this discrepancy might be because tumor cells are more sensitive to calprotectin, or because of the eukaryotic origin of the protein used in previous studies. Clinically, the pro-apoptotic activity of S100 proteins toward tumor cells raises the possibility that they could be used to treat tumors. However, the apoptosis-inducing activities of calprotectin in normal PDLCs might contribute to periodontal tissue destruction and delayed tissue repair.

Anatomically, periodontal ligament cells are in close proximity to infiltrating inflammatory cells [35]; therefore they are readily accessible to the promoters of inflammation. To determine whether S100 proteins also exacerbate inflammation, the effects of rhS100A8, rhS100A9 and rhS100A8/9 on the expression of several pro-inflammatory cytokines in PDLCs were investigated. Data revealed that treatment with rhS100A9, and rhS100A8/A9 upregulated the expression of IL-6, IL-8, TNFα and COX2 in PDLCs. Importantly, treatment with rhS100A9 and rhS100A8/A9 resulted in the robust expression of IL-6 and IL-8. IL-6 induces

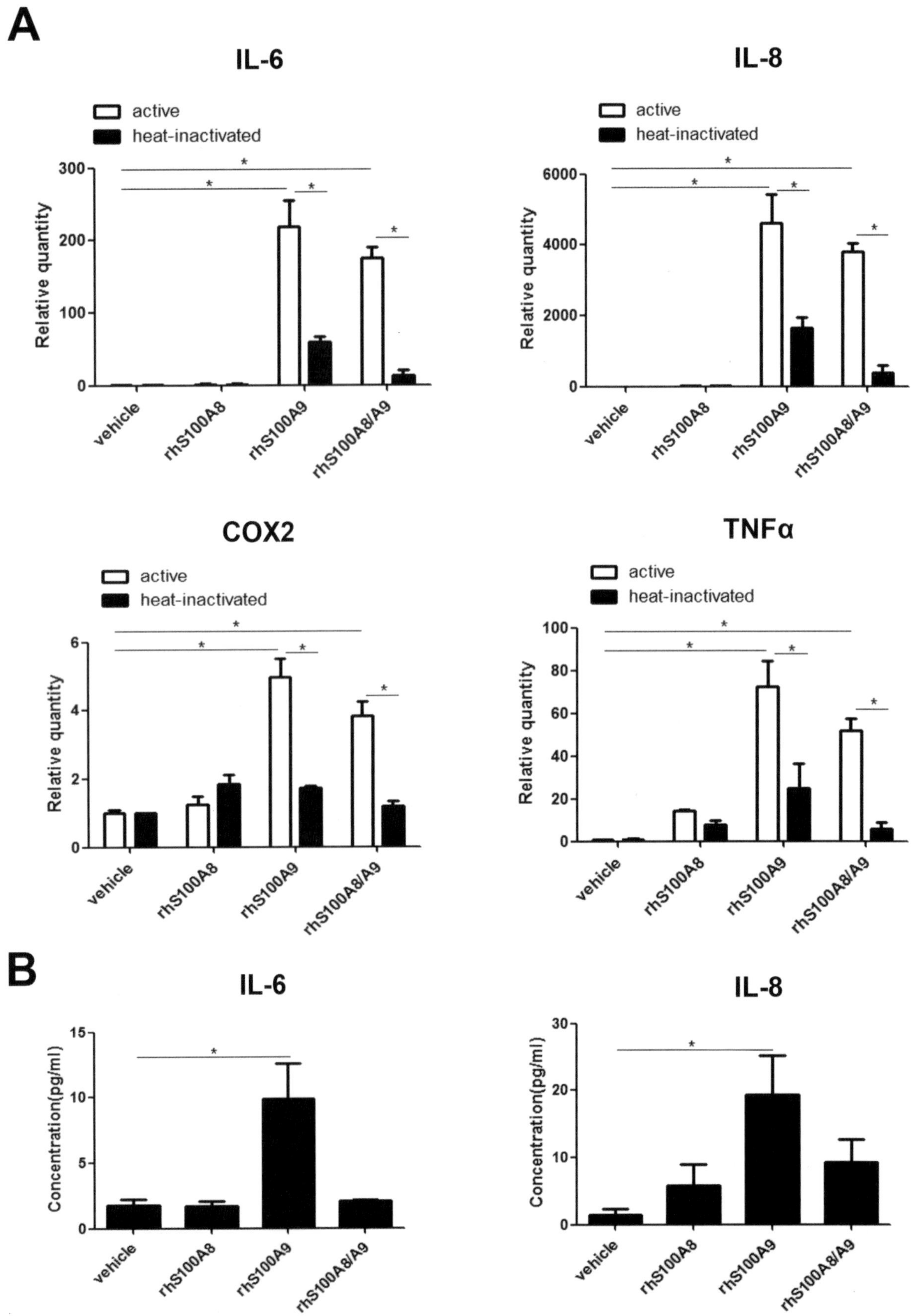
A
IL-6
active
heat-inactivated
Relative quantity
300
200
100
0
vehicle
rhS100A8
rhS100A9
rhS100A8/A9
IL-8
active
heat-inactivated
Relative quantity
6000
4000
2000
0
COX2
active
heat-inactivated
Relative quantity
6
4
2
0
TNFα
active
heat-inactivated
Relative quantity
100
80
60
40
20
0
B
IL-6
Concentration(pg/ml)
15
10
5
0
IL-8
Concentration(pg/ml)
30
20
10
0
vehicle
rhS100A8
rhS100A9
rhS100A8/A9

Figure 3. rhS100A8, rhS100A9 and rhS100A8/9 upregulate pro-inflammatory cytokines in PDLCs. (A). PDLCs were treated with rhS100A8, rhS100A9 or rhS100A8/A9 for 12 h, and the mRNA levels of cytokines were analyzed. rhS100A9 and rhS100A8/A9 upregulated the expression of IL-6, IL-8, TNFα, and COX2 significantly compared with rhS100A8 and the control group ($p<0.05$). (B). PDLCs were treated with rhS100A8, rhS100A9 or rhS100A8/A9 for 12 h, and the protein levels of IL-6 and IL-8 in PDLCs culture supernatants were detected using ELISA. rhS100A9 promoted the protein expression of IL-6 and IL-8 significantly ($p<0.05$). * $p<0.05$ *vs.* the control or heat-inactivated groups.

osteoclastogenesis [36] and IL-8 functions as a chemoattractant for neutrophils [37]; therefore, their induction leads to further bone destruction and neutrophils infiltration. Furthermore, rhS100A9 and rhS100A8/A9 promoted the activation of NF-κB signaling significantly in the current study, which might explain the upregulation of pro-inflammatory cytokines. Consistent with this,

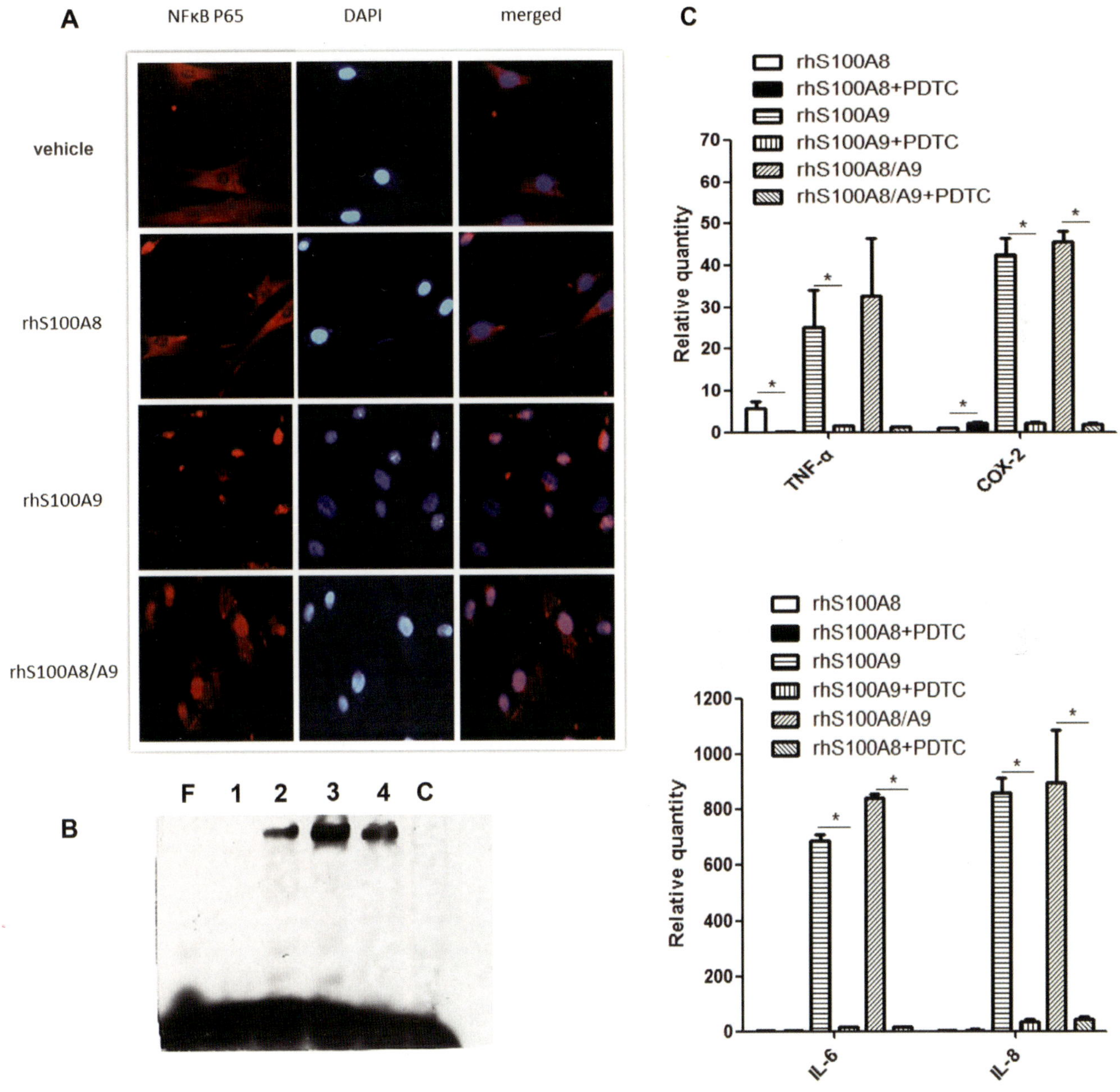

Figure 4. rhS100A8, rhS100A9 and rhS100A8/9 increase NF-κB signaling in PDLCs. (A). PDLCs were treated with rhS100A8, rhS100A9 or rhS100A8/A9 for 6 h, fixed, and then incubated with NF-κB p65 antibodies. The translocation of p65 was observed in cells treated with rhS100A9 and rhS100A8/A9, whereas p65 remained mainly in the cytoplasm of cells treated with rhS100A8. (B). NF-κB activation was assessed using EMSA 12 h after treatment with rhS100A8, rhS100A9, or rhS100A8/A9. Compared with lane F, which contains oligonucleotides without nuclear extracts, a band representing binding was visible after the addition of PDLCs nuclear extracts from cells treated with rhS100A8 (lanes 2), rhS100A9 (lane 3), or rhS100A8/A9 (lane 4). A competition assay was then used to confirm the binding specificity (lane C). The addition of rhS100A8 attenuated the rhS100A9-induced DNA-binding activity of NF-κB. (C). PDTC reversed rhS100A9- and rhS100A8/A9-induced cytokines upregulation. * $p<0.05$ *vs.* the control or heat-inactivated groups.

a previous study revealed that S100A8/A9 enhanced the activation of NF-κB by binding to advanced glycation end product receptors and Toll-like receptors [38]. Although both S100A8 and S100A9 induced the NF-κB-dependent transcriptional activity [39,40], S100A8 induced only mild activation of NF-κB signaling in the current study.

The pro-inflammatory effects of rhS100A9 and rhS100A8/A9 in the current study were significantly greater than those of rhS100A8. Although there is a general consensus that the function of S100A8 or S100A9 is dependent on heterodimer formation, increasing evidence suggests that each subunit alone might exert specific effects. The present study revealed that treatment with rhS100A9 induced more apoptotic cells and a more significant upregulation of pro-inflammatory cytokines compared with rhS100A8. This suggests that S100A9 plays a more important role in the pro-apoptotic and pro-inflammatory actions of rhS100A8/A9 than does S100A8. Consistent with this, S100A9 exerts pro-inflammatory effects by triggering NF-κB activation in human THP1 cells, which is dependent on TLR-4 [13]. Because the effect of rhS100A9 was reversed partly by rhS100A8 as observed in the rhS100A8/A9 group, it is possible that the effects of S100A9 are neutralized in part by S100A8. Other studies support this hypothesis. For example, the S100A9-mediated enhanced integrin-mediated adhesion was inhibited by S100A8 [41], and the addition of S100A8 abrogated the candidastatic effects of S100A9 [42]. Recently, Tessier et al demonstrated that treatment with anti-S100A9 antibodies inhibited the amplified immune response and helped to preserve tissue integrity in a murine arthritis model [43]. Therefore, the protective role of anti-S100A9 might facilitate the treatment of periodontitis; ongoing *in vivo* trials using anti-S100A9 might support this.

In conclusion, rhS100A8/A9 exerted PDLCs apoptosis, whereas rhS100A8 or rhS100A9 were less effective. In addition, rhS100A9 and rhS100A8/A9 amplified the pro-inflammatory cytokine response by activating NF-κB signaling in PDLCs; rhS100A8 was less potent. These results suggest that reducing local S100A9 or S100A8/A9 levels might have therapeutic potential for periodontitis.

Supporting Information

Figure S1 SDS-PAGE analysis of recombinant S100A8 and S100A9 stained with Coomassie brilliant blue. Recombinant human S100A8 (lane 3) and S100A9 (lane 5) were expressed after induction with β-D-thiogalactoside but were absent in uninduced lysate (lane 2). Purified rhS100A8 and rhS100A9 were free from other contaminants (lanes 4 and 6).

Author Contributions

Conceived and designed the experiments: HXM YFZ JXH. Performed the experiments: YFZ LP XZ XW. Analyzed the data: YFZ LP. Contributed reagents/materials/analysis tools: XZ XW LFJ. Wrote the paper: YFZ JXH HXM SCW LFJ.

References

1. Reynolds JJ, Meikle MC (1997) Mechanisms of connective tissue matrix destruction in periodontitis. Periodontol 2000 14: 144–157.
2. Amano A (2010) Host-parasite interactions in periodontitis: microbial pathogenicity and innate immunity. Periodontol 2000 54: 9–14.
3. Kerkhoff C, Klempt M, Sorg C (1998) Novel insights into structure and function of MRP8 (S100A8) and MRP14 (S100A9). Biochim Biophys Acta 1448: 200–211.
4. Hessian PA, Edgeworth J, Hogg N (1993) MRP-8 and MRP-14, two abundant Ca(2+)-binding proteins of neutrophils and monocytes. J Leukoc Biol 53: 197–204.
5. Abtin A, Eckhart L, Glaser R, Gmeiner R, Mildner M, et al. (2010) The antimicrobial heterodimer S100A8/S100A9 (calprotectin) is upregulated by bacterial flagellin in human epidermal keratinocytes. J Invest Dermatol 130: 2423–2430.
6. Nishii K, Usui M, Yamamoto G, Yajima S, Tsukamoto Y, et al. (2013) The distribution and expression of S100A8 and S100A9 in gingival epithelium of mice. J Periodontal Res 48: 235–242.
7. Yui S, Nakatani Y, Mikami M (2003) Calprotectin (S100A8/S100A9), an inflammatory protein complex from neutrophils with a broad apoptosis-inducing activity. Biol Pharm Bull 26: 753–760.
8. Driemel O, Escher N, Ernst G, Melle C, von Eggeling F (2010) S100A8 cellular distribution in normal epithelium, hyperplasia, dysplasia and squamous cell carcinoma and its concentration in serum. Anal Quant Cytol Histol 32: 219–224.
9. Rammes A, Roth J, Goebeler M, Klempt M, Hartmann M, et al. (1997) Myeloid-related protein (MRP) 8 and MRP14, calcium-binding proteins of the S100 family, are secreted by activated monocytes via a novel, tubulin-dependent pathway. J Biol Chem 272: 9496–9502.
10. Viemann D, Barczyk K, Vogl T, Fischer U, Sunderkotter C, et al. (2007) MRP8/MRP14 impairs endothelial integrity and induces a caspase-dependent and -independent cell death program. Blood 109: 2453–2460.
11. Gebhardt C, Nemeth J, Angel P, Hess J (2006) S100A8 and S100A9 in inflammation and cancer. Biochem Pharmacol 72: 1622–1631.
12. Hiratsuka S, Watanabe A, Aburatani H, Maru Y (2006) Tumour-mediated upregulation of chemoattractants and recruitment of myeloid cells predetermines lung metastasis. Nat Cell Biol 8: 1369–1375.
13. Riva M, Kallberg E, Bjork P, Hancz D, Vogl T, et al. (2012) Induction of nuclear factor-kappaB responses by the S100A9 protein is Toll-like receptor-4-dependent. Immunology 137: 172–182.
14. Ghavami S, Rashedi I, Dattilo BM, Eshraghi M, Chazin WJ, et al. (2008) S100A8/A9 at low concentration promotes tumor cell growth via RAGE ligation and MAP kinase-dependent pathway. J Leukoc Biol 83: 1484–1492.
15. Kido J, Nakamura T, Kido R, Ohishi K, Yamauchi N, et al. (1999) Calprotectin in gingival crevicular fluid correlates with clinical and biochemical markers of periodontal disease. J Clin Periodontol 26: 653–657.
16. Nakamura T, Kido J, Kido R, Ohishi K, Yamauchi N, et al. (2000) The association of calprotectin level in gingival crevicular fluid with gingival index and the activities of collagenase and aspartate aminotransferase in adult periodontitis patients. J Periodontol 71: 361–367.
17. Kaner D, Bernimoulin JP, Kleber BM, Heizmann WR, Friedmann A (2006) Gingival crevicular fluid levels of calprotectin and myeloperoxidase during therapy for generalized aggressive periodontitis. J Periodontal Res 41: 132–139.
18. Nishimura F, Terranova V P., Sawa T, Y M (1999) Migration inhibitory factor related protein-8 (MRP-8) is an autocrine chemotactic factor for periodontal ligament cells. J Dent Res 78: 1251–1255.
19. Nishimura F, Takahashi K, Kurihara M, Takashiba S, Murayama Y (1998) Periodontal disease as a complication of diabetes mellitus. Ann Periodontol 3: 10.
20. Jonsson D, Nebel D, Bratthall G, Nilsson BO (2011) The human periodontal ligament cell: a fibroblast-like cell acting as an immune cell. J Periodontal Res 46: 153–157.
21. Ikeda H, Sumita Y, Ikeda M, Okumura T, Sakai E, et al. (2011) Engineering bone formation from human dental pulp- and periodontal ligament-derived cells. Ann Biomed Eng 39: 26–34.
22. Zhang X, Meng H, Sun X, Xu L, Zhang L, et al. (2013) Elevation of vitamin D-binding protein levels in the plasma of patients with generalized aggressive periodontitis. J Periodontal Res 48: 74–79.
23. Liu K, Meng H, Lu R, Xu L, Zhang L, et al. (2010) Initial periodontal therapy reduced systemic and local 25-hydroxy vitamin D(3) and interleukin-1beta in patients with aggressive periodontitis. J Periodontol 81: 260–266.
24. Ryckman C, Vandal K, Rouleau P, Talbot M, Tessier PA (2003) Proinflammatory activities of S100: proteins S100A8, S100A9, and S100A8/A9 induce neutrophil chemotaxis and adhesion. J Immunol 170: 3233–3242.
25. Vandal K, Rouleau P, Boivin A., Ryckman C, McColl SR, et al. (2003) Blockade of S100A8 and S100A9 Suppresses Neutrophil Migration in Response to Lipopolysaccharide. J Immunol: 2602–2609.
26. Liu K, Meng H, Hou J (2012) Characterization of the autocrine/paracrine function of vitamin D in human gingival fibroblasts and periodontal ligament cells. PLoS One 7: e39878.
27. Yin H, Guo C, Wang Y, Liu D, Lv Y, et al. (2013) Fengycin inhibits the growth of the human lung cancer cell line 95D through reactive oxygen species production and mitochondria-dependent apoptosis. Anticancer Drugs 24: 587–598.
28. Kou XX, Wu YW, Ding Y, Hao T, Bi RY, et al. (2011) 17 beta-estradiol aggravates temporomandibular joint inflammation through the NF-kappaB pathway in ovariectomized rats. Arthritis Rheum 63: 1888–1897.
29. Sun X, Meng H, Shi D, Xu L, Zhang L, et al. (2011) Analysis of plasma calprotectin and polymorphisms of S100A8 in patients with aggressive periodontitis. J Periodontal Res 46: 354–360.

30. Kaner D, Bernimoulin JP, Dietrich T, Kleber BM, Friedmann A (2011) Calprotectin levels in gingival crevicular fluid predict disease activity in patients treated for generalized aggressive periodontitis. J Periodontal Res 46: 417–426.
31. Zali H, Rezaei-Tavirani M, Kariminia A, Yousefi R, Shokrgozar MA (2008) Evaluation of growth inhibitory and apoptosis inducing activity of human calprotectin on the human gastric cell line (AGS). Iran Biomed J 12: 7–14.
32. Voss A, Bode G, Sopalla C, Benedyk M, Varga G, et al. (2011) Expression of S100A8/A9 in HaCaT keratinocytes alters the rate of cell proliferation and differentiation. FEBS Lett 585: 440–446.
33. Yui S, Nakatani Y, Hunter MJ, Chazin WJ, Yamazaki M (2002) Implication of extracellular zinc exclusion by recombinant human calprotectin (MRP8 and MRP14) from target cells in its apoptosis-inducing activity. Mediators Inflamm 11: 165–172.
34. Ghavami S, Kerkhoff C, Los M, Hashemi M, Sorg C, et al. (2004) Mechanism of apoptosis induced by S100A8/A9 in colon cancer cell lines: the role of ROS and the effect of metal ions. J Leukoc Biol 76: 169–175.
35. Moskow BS, Polson AM (1991) Histologic studies on the extension of the inflammatory infiltrate in human periodontitis. J Clin Periodontol 18: 534–542.
36. Cheung WY, Simmons CA, You L (2012) Osteocyte apoptosis regulates osteoclast precursor adhesion via osteocytic IL-6 secretion and endothelial ICAM-1 expression. Bone 50: 104–110.
37. Mitsuyama K, Toyonaga A, Sasaki E, Watanabe K, Tateishi H, et al. (1994) IL-8 as an important chemoattractant for neutrophils in ulcerative colitis and Crohn's disease. Clin Exp Immunol 96: 432–436.
38. Volz HC, Laohachewin D, Seidel C, Lasitschka F, Keilbach K, et al. (2012) S100A8/A9 aggravates post-ischemic heart failure through activation of RAGE-dependent NF-kappaB signaling. Basic Res Cardiol 107: 250.
39. Vogl T, Tenbrock K, Ludwig S, Leukert N, Ehrhardt C, et al. (2007) Mrp8 and Mrp14 are endogenous activators of Toll-like receptor 4, promoting lethal, endotoxin-induced shock. Nat Med 13: 1042–1049.
40. Boyd JH, Kan B, Roberts H, Wang Y, Walley KR (2008) S100A8 and S100A9 mediate endotoxin-induced cardiomyocyte dysfunction via the receptor for advanced glycation end products. Circ Res 102: 1239–1246.
41. Newton RA, Hogg N (1998) The human S100 protein MRP-14 is a novel activator of the beta 2 integrin Mac-1 on neutrophils. J Immunol 160: 1427–1435.
42. Murthy AR, Lehrer RI, Harwig SS, Miyasaki KT (1993) In vitro candidastatic properties of the human neutrophil calprotectin complex. J Immunol 151: 6291–6301.
43. Cesaro A, Anceriz N, Plante A, Page N, Tardif MR, et al. (2012) An inflammation loop orchestrated by S100A9 and calprotectin is critical for development of arthritis. PLoS One 7: e45478.

24

Pro-inflammatory, Th1, Th2, Th17 Cytokines and Dendritic Cells

Giovanna Ribeiro Souto[1]*, Celso Martins Queiroz-Junior[1], Mauro Henrique Nogueira Guimarães de Abreu[2], Fernando Oliveira Costa[1], Ricardo Alves Mesquita[1]

1 Department of Oral Surgery and Pathology, School of Dentistry, Universidade Federal de Minas Gerais, Belo Horizonte, Minas Gerais, Brazil, 2 Department of Social and Preventive Dentistry, School of Dentistry, Universidade Federal de Minas Gerais, Belo Horizonte, Minas Gerais, Brazil

Abstract

There are a limited number of studies correlating the different stages of dendritic cells (DC) maturation with cytokines in individuals presented chronic periodontitis (CP). The aim of the study was to evaluate the correlation among the expression of IL-2, IL-10, IL-4, IL-6, IFN-Ɣ, TNF-α, and IL-17A with the presence of DC and mild-moderate or advanced CP. Gingival samples were obtained from 24 individuals with CP and six samples of normal mucosa (NM) overlapping third molar for controls of the levels of cytokines. Periodontal examination was performed. Immunohistochemical staining was carried out, revealing CD1a+ immature, Fator XIIIa+ immature, and CD83+ mature DCs. The inflammatory infiltrate was counted, and the cytokines were measured by flow cytometry. Densities of DCs and inflammatory infiltrate, cytokines, subtypes of CP, and clinical periodontal parameters were correlated and compared. IL-6 expression was correlated positively with the increased numbers of CD1a+ immature DCs. Levels of IL-2, TNF-α, IFN-Ɣ, IL-10, and IL-17A were increased when compared with NM. The percentage of sites with clinical attachment level (CAL)>3 were positively correlated with densities of inflammatory infiltrate and negatively correlated with densities of immature DCs. IL-6 can contribute to the increase of the immature DCs in the CP. Higher levels of IL-2, TNF-α, IFN-Ɣ, IL-10, and IL-17A cytokines were observed in CP. Higher densities of inflammatory infiltrate as well as lower densities of immature DCs can result in a more severe degree of human CP.

Editor: Paul Proost, University of Leuven, Rega Institute, Belgium

Funding: The authors wish to thank the National Council for Scientific and Technological Development (CNPq) (309209/2010-2; 472045/2011-3). RA Mesquita, MH de Abreu and FO Costa are researchers funded by CNPq. The funders had no role in study design, data collection and analysis, decision to publish, or preparation of the manuscript

Competing Interests: The authors have declared that no competing interests exist.

* E-mail: grsouto@hotmail.com

Introduction

Chronic periodontitis (CP) [1] is the most frequent form of periodontitis [2,3]. The bacterial biofilm is required, but not sufficient, for disease initiation. Major periodontal tissue destruction results from persistent host inflammatory immune reaction in response to bacteria [4–6]. The host inflammatory immune reaction begins when the recognition of the bacterial pathogens occurs by means of antigen-presenting cells, such as dendritic cells (DCs) [7].

Myeloid DCs, also known as conventional DCs, present a strong capability of capturing antigens, which enables them to stimulate T cells [8]. In this context, in CP, DC activation occurs after coming into contact with lipopolysaccharide (LPS) [9,10] or immune complexes [11] produced by periodontal pathogens [12,13]. After activation, these DCs become mature, express co-stimulatory molecules, and produce distinct cytokine patterns, such a INF-Ɣ and IL-17, which will determine the selective migration of CD4 T-helper subsets and the subsequent production of characteristic cytokines [7,11].

CD4 T-cells can be subdivided into Th1, Th2, Th17, and Treg subsets on the basis of their pattern of cytokine production [14,15]. Protective Th1-related cytokines (Interleukin (IL)-2 and interferon (IFN)-Ɣ) are involved in cellular immune responses [16-20]. Th2-related cytokines (IL-4 and IL-10) are associated with humoral immunity and anti-inflammatory properties [16–20]. Th2-related cytokinees (IL-4 and IL-10) are associated with humoral immunity and anti-inflammatory properties. However, these arise in a later period of periodontitis and are involved in the chronic progression of the disease[14,17–19]. Th17 was identified as cells that recruited neutrophils and macrophages to participate and amplify the inflammatory reaction [4,13,21].

The role of T-helper cells and DCs in the pathogenesis of CP has not yet been fully clarified. There are a limited number of studies correlating the different stages of DC maturation with pro-inflammatory (IL-6 and tumor necrosis factor (TNF)-α), Th1 (IL-2 and interferon (IFN)-Ɣ), Th2 (IL-4 and IL-10), and Th17 (IL-17A) cytokines in individuals with different stages of CP. In this light, the present study aimed to investigate the correlation among the expression of pro-inflammatory, Th1, Th2, and Th17 cytokines with the presence of DCs in gingival samples of mild-moderate and advanced CP.

Materials and Methods

Patients and periodontal samples

This study was approved by the Committee of Ethics in Research from Universidade Federal de Minas Gerais (UFMG), Brazil (423/11). Thirty patients provided written informed consent to participate in this study. All individuals received a full-mouth periodontal examination in which probing depth (PD), clinical attachment level (CAL), bleeding on probing, and oral hygiene index were determined [2,22]. Individuals presenting four or more teeth with one or more sites containing PD≥4 and CAL≥3 within the same site were diagnosed as CP. Individuals presenting four or more teeth with one or more sites containing CAL≥5 were diagnosed as advanced CP; otherwise, participants were diagnosed as mild-moderate CP [2]. The patients evaluated in this study reported no presence of systemic diseases or immunologic abnormalities. Individuals with smoking habit were excluded [23]. All subjects included in the study had untreated CP at the moment of the sample collection. After diagnostic of mild-moderate or advanced CP, two samples of gingival tissues were collected from each individual during extractions for prosthetic or endodontic reasons in tooth with CP and CAL≥5. The first sample was stored in a buffer (0.4 mM NaCl, 10 mM $NaPO_4$, pH 7.4) containing inhibitors of proteases (0.1 mM PMSF – phenylmethylsulfonyl fluoride – 0.1 mM benzethonium chloride, 10 mM EDTA, and 0.01 mg/mL aprotinin A) and Tween 20 (0.05%), pH 7.4, at a ratio of 1 ml of solution per 100 mg of tissue to perform the cytometric bead array (CBA). The second sample was set in 10% buffered formalin, histologically processed, sectioned, and stained with hematoxylin and eosin or subjected to immunohistochemistry. Due to losses during processing of samples, 24 samples were examined by means of Cytometric Bead Array (CBA), and 22 samples by means of hematoxylin and eosin and immunohistochemistry.

Six samples were collected from the mucosa overlapping the third molar that had been recommended for extraction. These samples were used to control the cytokine levels.

Detection of tissue cytokines

Multiple gingival tissue cytokines (IL-2, IL-10, IL-4, IL-6, IFN-γ, TNF-α, and IL-17A) were simultaneously measured by flow cytometry by means of CBA. The human Th1/Th2/Th17 kit (BD Biosciences, San Jose, CA, USA) was applied following manufacturer instructions. The limit of detection of each cytokine is 0.1 pg/ml (IL-2), 0.03 pg/ml (IL-4), 1.4 pg/ml (IL-6), 0.5 pg/ml (IFN-γ), 0.9 pg/ml (TNF-α), 0.8 pg/ml (IL-17A), 16.8 pg/ml (IL-10). Acquisition was performed with a FACSCanto II flow cytometer (BD Biosciences, San Jose, CA, USA). The instrument was checked for sensitivity and overall performance using Cytometer Setup & Tracking beads (BD Biosciences, San Jose, CA, USA) prior to data acquisition. Quantitative results were generated using FCAP Array v1.0.1 software (Soft Flow Inc., Pecs, Hungary).

Inflammatory assessment

The inflammatory infiltrate in gingival tissue was measured using hematoxylin and eosin stained sections (Figure 1A). These sections were digitized using a microscope (Axio Scoup A1, Zeiss, Göttingen, Germany) at 400x magnification and interfaced to a computer. Cell counts were taken during the sectioning by a blinded examiner (GRS). The mean of inflammatory infiltrate was determined by counting the number of inflammatory cells on the lamina propria (LP) in consecutive fields of all gingival samples (field area: 0.04652 mm^2) using the Image Tool software (version 3.0, University of Texas Health Science Center, San Antonio, TX). The mean number of cells per unit area (cell number per square millimeters) was obtained. Inflammatory infiltrate density was correlated with periodontal indexes, densities of DCs, and cytokine levels. Furthermore, data were dichotomized by medians: mild and intense inflammatory infiltrate [23]. The periodontal indexes, densities of DCs, and cytokine levels were compared between mild and intense inflammatory infiltrate groups.

Immunohistochemistry

An immunohistochemical reaction was performed using the streptavidin-biotin standard protocol. Anti-CD1a and anti-Factor XIIIa are considered markers for immature DCs. Anti-CD1a is typical epidermal Langerhans cells (LC) characterized by the expression of Birbeck granules, while Factor XIIIa is described as dermal dendritic cells [24-26] Anti-CD83 is considered a marker for mature DCs [27]. Serial sections of 3μm from paraffin-embedded blocks were deparaffinized and dehydrated. Antigen retrieval was carried out using the Dewaxing & Antigen Retrieval Buffer 4 (pH 9.0, Spring bioscience, Pleasanton, CA, USA) for 12 minutes at 98°C for anti-CD1a and anti-CD83. Antigen retrieval was carried out using a 10-mM citrate buffer (Laboratory Synth, Diadema, SP, Brazil), pH = 6.0, for 20 minutes at 98°C for anti-Factor XIIIa. Endogenous peroxidase activity was blocked using 0.3% hydrogen peroxide. Primary antibodies were incubated at room temperature for 1 hour. The following monoclonal antibodies were used: anti-CD1a (clone MTB1; BioSB, Santa Barbara, CA, USA), at a dilution of 1:20; anti-Factor XIIIa (clone AC-1A1; BioSB, Santa Barbara, CA, USA), at a dilution of 1:500; and anti-CD83 (clone 1H4b; Abcam, Cambridge, UK), at a dilution of 1:10. Detection was performed using the Advance HRP system (Dako, Carpinteria, CA, EUA) for CD1a, the LSAB system (Dako, Carpinteria, CA, EUA) for Fator XIIIa, and the Reveal system (Spring bioscience, Pleasanton, CA, USA) for CD83. Counter-staining was performed using 3.3′-diaminobenzidine tetrahydrochloride chromogen (DAB, Sigma-Aldrich, St. Louis, MO) and Mayer hematoxylin.

Immunoexpression analysis and cell counts

Densities of immunolabeled cells (cell number per square millimeters) were calculated for CD1a, Factor XIIIa, and CD83. Positive cell counts were restricted to immunolabeled cells that exhibited well-defined nuclei. The slices were digitized with a microscope (Axio Scoup A1, Zeiss, Göttingen, Germany) at 400x magnification and interfaced to a computer. Cell counts were performed throughout the sections by a blinded examiner (GRS). Areas were delineated using a mouse and measured using the software AxioVision (version 4.8, Zeiss).

Statistical analyses

SPSS statistic software (SPSS Inc., version 17.0, Chicago, IL, USA) was used for statistical analyses. Normal distribution was tested using the Shapiro-Wilks procedure. In samples with a normal distribution, the Student t test was applied and P values were <0.05. Kruskal–Wallis and Mann-Whitney U tests were used to analyze the samples with abnormal distributions. After Bonferroni correction, the statistical significance was achieved when P values were <0.016. For correlation tests, all samples demonstrated abnormal distribution, and Spearman correlation was applied; the α level was set to 0.05. The correlation was graded according to the Cohen classification as weak (<0.30), moderate (0.30 to 0.50), or strong (>0.50) [28].

Sample calculation considered both type I and II errors. For this, we assumed a 95% confidence interval, 80% power of test,

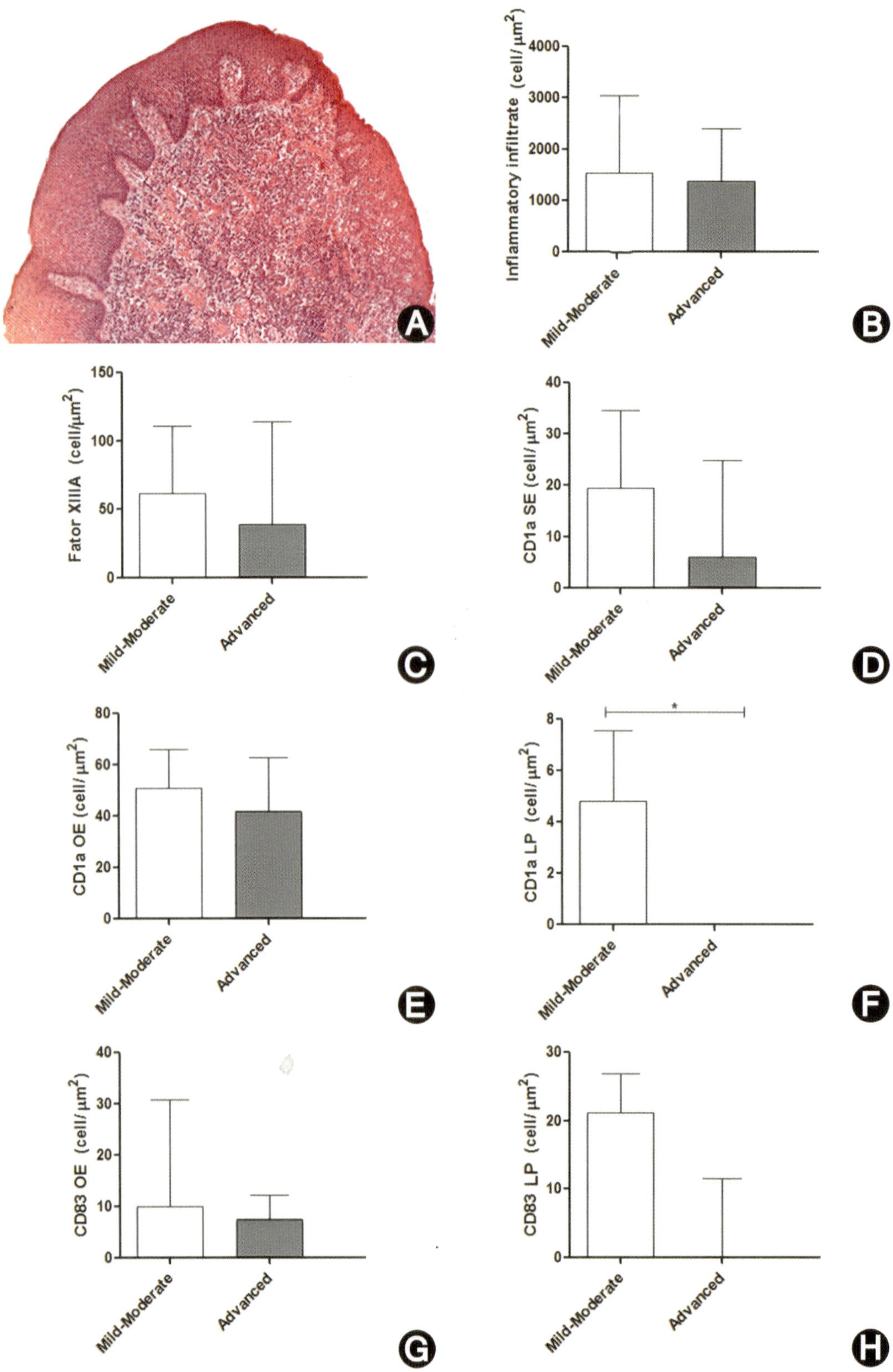

Figure 1. Inflammatory infiltrate cells and dendritic cells (DCs) in individuals with mild-moderate or advanced chronic periodontitis. A) Gingival tissue with intense inflammatory infiltrate on the lamina propria (LP) (haematoxilin-eosin, 50x original magnification). Distribution of the inflammatory infiltrate cells and DCs in groups of individuals with mild-moderate or advanced chronic periodontitis. B) Density of inflammatory infiltrate cells (cells/mm^2). C) Density of Factor XIIIa+ immature DCs (cells/mm^2). Density of CD1a+ immature DCs (cells/mm^2) in the sulcular epithelium (D), oral epithelium (E), and LP (F). Density of CD83+ mature DCs (cells/mm^2) in the oral epithelium (G) and LP (H). *Mann-Whitney U test, statistically significant difference at $P<0.05$.

and parameters of values of levels of IL17A obtained in study of periodontal disease of Behfarnia et al. [29].

Results

Clinical date

The studied population presented a mean age of 44.50±12.19 years (12 males, mean age: 45.70; and 12 females, mean age: 43.30). Periodontal clinical parameters of the samples are presented in Table 1. In accordance with periodontal parameters for cytokine analysis and DC evaluation, individuals were classified as presenting either mild-moderate CP (n = 10) or advanced CP (n = 14 for cytokines; n = 12 for DCs).

Inflammatory infiltrate cells, dendritic cells and CP

All regions of the gingival tissue were evaluated for each antibody. Factor XIIIa+ immature DCs could be observed only in the LP (Figure 2A and 2D); CD1a+ immature DCs could only be observed in the oral epithelium (OE), sulcular epithelium (SE), and LP (Figure. 2B, 2E and 2F); while CD83+ mature DCs could be observed in the OE and LP regions (Figure 2C, 2G, 2H). CD1a+ immature DCs showed cytoplasmic processes in the OE and SE (Figure 2E and 2F, respectively), CD1a+ immature DCs in the LP (Figure 2F), Factor XIIIa+ immature DCs in the LP (Figure 2D), and CD83+ mature DCs in the OE and LP (Figure 2G and 2H, respectively), all of which presented a rounded or oval shape. The density of inflammatory cells and DCs was compared between mild-moderate CP and advanced CP (Figure 1B, 1C, 1D, 1E, 1F, 1G, and 1H). Despite the lack of statistical significance, the group of individuals with advanced CP presented slightly less inflammatory infiltrate cells and DCs than did individuals with mild-moderate CP. A statistically significant difference could be observed for the CD1a+ immature DCs of the LP (Figure 1F).

Regarding possible altered phenotypes between the female and male genders, when comparing the density of inflammatory infiltrate cells and the density of immature and mature DCs, no significant differences between genders could be observed.

Intensity of inflammatory infiltrate and DC densities

The present study evaluated whether or not the density of inflammatory infiltrate cells influenced the quantity of DCs. Eleven samples were grouped in mild inflammatory infiltrate and eleven in intense inflammatory infiltrate. The density of Factor XIIIa+ immature DCs was higher in individuals presenting an intense, as compared to mild, inflammatory infiltrate density ($P<0.05$) (table 2). For this reason, correlations between inflammatory infiltrate cells and DCs also were performed. In this regard, there was a positive correlation ($P<0.05$) between the density of Factor XIIIa+ immature DCs and inflammatory infiltrate cells. Furthermore, positive correlations ($P<0.05$) could be observed between the density of CD1a+ immature DCs in the OE and CD1a+ immature DCs in the LP with inflammatory infiltrate cells. By contrast, negative correlations ($P<0.05$) were observed between the density of CD83+ mature DCs in the OE and inflammatory infiltrate cells.

Pro-inflammatory, Th1, Th2, and Th17 cytokine profiles correlated with CP

Pro-inflammatory (IL-6 and TNF-α), Th1 (IL-2 and INF-Y), Th2 (IL-4 and IL-10), and Th17 (IL-17A) cytokine profiles were compared among the groups with mild-moderate CP (n = 10), advanced CP (n = 14), and NM (n = 6) (Figure 3). IL-2, INF-Y, IL-10, and IL-17A levels were higher ($P<0.016$) in the individuals presenting mild-moderate and advanced CP, when compared to NM (Figure 3C, 3D, 3F and 3G, respectively). By contrast, TNF-α levels were higher ($p<0.016$) in the individuals presenting advanced CP, as compared to NM (Figure 3A). In addition, cytokines correlations was performed and presented in the table 3. Pro-inflammatory, Th1, Th2, and Th17 profiles of cytokines were correlated among themselves. Then, the samples were grouped according to the classification of CP and cytokines were correlated (table 3). No differences between females and males could be observed when comparing cytokines.

Correlations among cytokine levels, dendritic cells, inflammatory infiltrate cells, and clinical periodontal parameters of CP

Positive correlation ($P<0.05$) could be observed between IL-6 and the density of CD1a+ immature DCs, as well as the density of inflammatory infiltrate cells, in both the SE and LP. A positive correlation ($P<0.05$) could also be observed between IL-6 and the percentage of sites with PD>4. By contrast, a negative correlation ($P<0.05$) could be identified between IL-2 and the percentage of sites with CAL>3.

Positive correlations ($p<0.05$) could be observed between the percentage of sites with PD>4 and the density of inflammatory infiltrate cells, CD1a+ immature DCs in the SE, and Factor XIIIa+ immature DCs. Moreover, a positive correlation ($p<0.05$) could also be identified between the percentage of sites with CAL>3 and the density of inflammatory infiltrate cells. However, negative correlations ($p<0.05$) could be observed between the number of teeth with CAL>3 and CD1a+ immature DCs in the SE, as well as between the number of teeth with CAL>5 and CD1a+ immature DCs in the SE and LP.

Table 1. Periodontal clinical parameters of samples (n = 24).

Clinical Parameters	Median (minimum-maximum)
Number of teeth	16 (4–28)
Number of teeth PD>4 mm	6 (4–21)
Number of teeth CAL>3 mm	12 (4–27)
Number of teeth CAL>5 mm	5 (1–18)
% sites PD>4 mm	19.0 (4.0–100.0)
% sites CAL>3 mm	80.0 (22.0–100.0)
% sites BOP	54.5 (18.0–100.0)

PD - probing depths; CAL - clinical attachment levels; BOP – bleeding on probing.

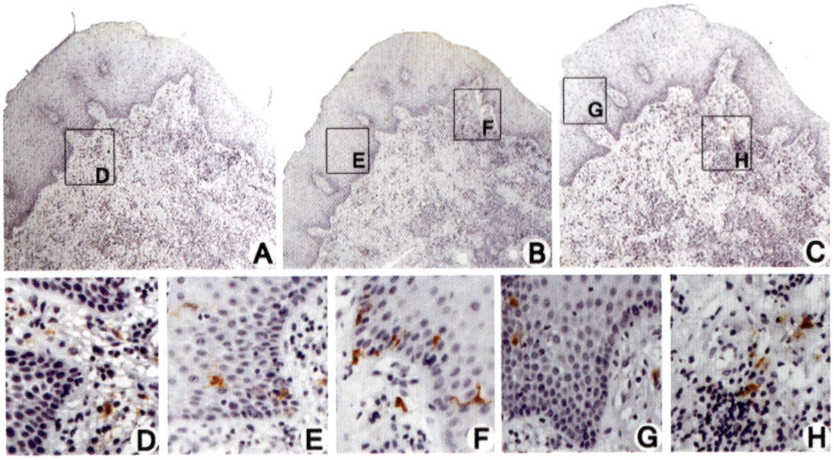

Figure 2. Regions of the gingival tissue evaluated for immature and mature DCs. Immunohistochemical staining of Factor XIIIa+ immature DCs (A), CD1a+ immature DCs (B), and CD83+ mature DCs (C) (streptavidin-biotin, 50x original magnification). Factor XIIIa+ immature DCs could be observed in the lamina propria (LP) region (D). CD1a+ immature DCs could be observed in the oral epithelium (E), sulcular epithelium and LP regions (F). CD83+ mature DCs could be observed in the oral epithelium (G) and LP regions (H) (streptavidin-biotin, 400x original magnification).

Discussion

DCs are the most potent antigen-presenting cells (APCs), whose function is to initiate an adaptive immune response. Activation and maturation of DCs are induced by infectious agents and inflammatory products [7,30], as well as by host cytokines [31,32]. Cytokines affect DC differentiation and are important in controlling states of perpetual inflammation, as can be seen in CP, when DCs are continuously exposed to antigens [33]. Prior reports have shown that, in regions such as the lymph nodes, spleen, and liver, where DCs are continually exposed to potential antigens, IL-6 avoids a state of perpetual inflammation and protects central immune organs from overstimulation [34,35]. In this regard, *in vitro* studies have shown that IL-6 plays a major role in maintaining immature DCs and in blocking DC maturation. IL-6-mediated negative feedback may well contribute to the down-regulation of the immune response initiated by pathogens or in persistent infections [36]. In fact, in the present study, the IL-6 expression in gingival tissues was positively correlated with the increased number of immature DCs in patients presenting CP. It is therefore possible to conclude that IL-6 may well contribute to the inhibition of DC maturation in human CP.

In addition, it is known that macrophages are important APCs. It was demonstrate that these cells can contribute to innate immunity employing various cytokines and chemokines [13,37]. However, it was not possible to evaluate macrophages in the present study. It was demonstrated that responses of the macrophages and DCs in the production of cytokines and chemokines were similar for the various microbial challenges [37]. Huang et al. [37] demonstrated that only response of immature DC to polymicrobial challenge could contribute to production of IL-6 [37]. Furthermore, others studies are necessary to understand mechanisms that affect the relation between immature DCs and IL-6.

IL-6 levels showed no increase when compared with NM, whereas the levels of IL-2, TNF-α, INF-Y, IL-10, and IL-17A did present a significant increase. It is well-known that, when there is an absence of cytokines, such as TNF-α, IL-12, or IFN-Y, the IL-6 cytokine can favor immune tolerance, in turn contributing to homeostasis [34]. By contrast, as can be witnessed with other pro-inflammatory cytokines and in inflammatory conditions, IL-6 can aggravate the inflammatory disease pattern [34]. Therefore, it can be proposed that the increased expression of IL-2, TNF-α, INF-Y, IL-10, and IL-17A cytokines can influence the role of IL-6, in turn causing alterations in host immune responses, thus contributing to the pathogenesis of CP.

In line with these results, the IL-6 expression proved to be positively correlated with PD. Guillot et al. [38] and Baker, et al [39] reported on the role of IL-6 in the resorption of the alveolar bone in periodontal disease. IL-6 also induces bone resorption,

Table 2. Densities of dendritic cells (DCs) in gingival samples of individuals presenting mild and intense inflammatory infiltrate.

DC (cells/mm^2)	mild inflammatory infiltrate (n = 11)	intense inflammatory infiltrate (n = 11)
Fator XIIIA*	38.64 (± 23.84)	99.60 (± 63.81)
CD1a SE	15.47 (± 14.88)	18.91 (± 23.42)
CD1a OE	50.91 (± 28.21)	48.87 (± 22.05)
CD1a LP	1.81 (± 2.62)	5.52 (± 7.08)
CD83 OE	11.18 (± 13.86)	17.02 (± 15.95)
CD83 LP	15.40 (± 21.72)	7.67 (± 11.11)

SE – sulcular epithelium; OE – oral epithelium; LP – lamina própria.
* $p<0.05$, Student t test.

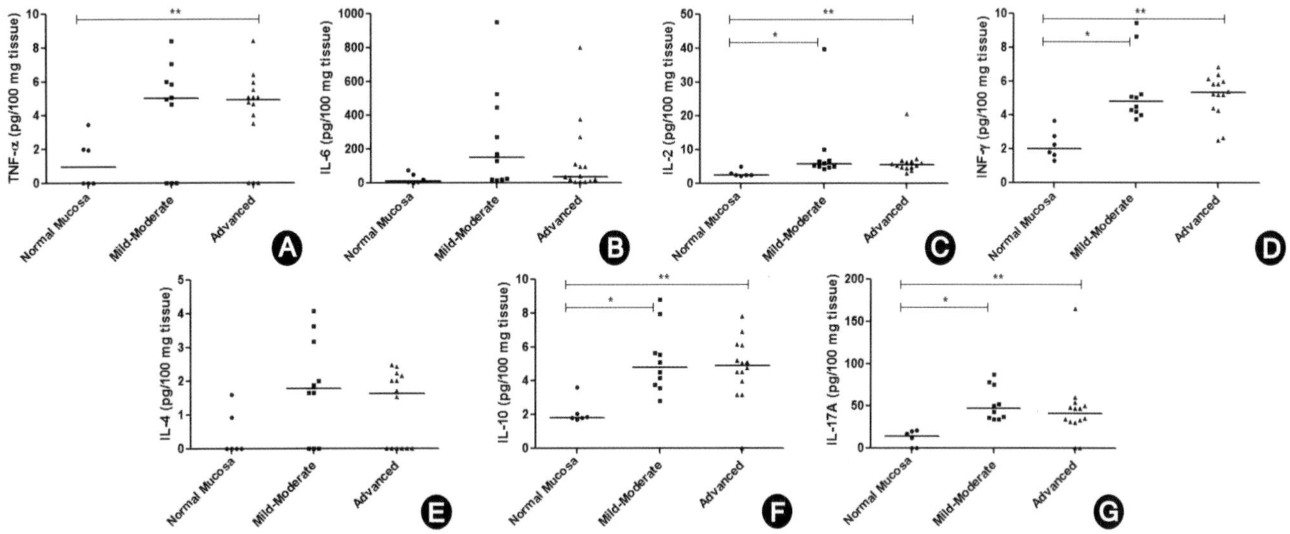

Figure 3. Cytokine levels in individuals with mild-moderate or advanced chronic periodontitis and normal mucosa. Levels of TNF-α (A), IL-6 (B), IL-2 (C), INF-γ (D), IL-4 (E), IL-10 (F), and IL-17A (G). *Statistically significant difference at P<0.016 in normal mucosa *versus* mild-moderate chronic periodontitis. **Statistically significant difference at P<0.016, in normal mucosa *versus* advanced chronic periodontitis.

both alone and together with other bone-resorption agents [40]. However, Moutsopoulos et al., [10] demonstrated that only IL-17 was positively correlated with bone loss in CP, suggesting that the Th17 subset may well drive or contribute to bone destruction. It could also be observed that female mice without an IL-17 receptor proved to be much more susceptible to bone loss in periodontal disease than in males, demonstrating a gender-dependent effect of IL-17 signaling [41]. In addition, estrogen loss resulted in an IL-6-mediated stimulation of osteoclastogenesis, which suggests a mechanism for the increased bone resorption in postmenopausal osteoporosis [42]. Nevertheless, although the present study's results demonstrated that IL-17A, IL-2, TNF-α, INF-γ, and IL-10 levels were higher in CP when compared to NM, it was impossible to demonstrate any form of altered phenotypes between genders when comparing cytokine levels, the density of inflammatory infiltrate cells, or the densities of immature and mature DCs.

Th1-related cytokines are related to the early process of periodontal disease [19,43], while Th2-related cytokines were related to the later stages of the periodontal disease [14,19]. In addition, Th17 cells amplified the inflammatory destruction through the recruitment of inflammatory cells to the target site [4,13,21]. In the present study, IL-2 was negatively related to CAL, which is related to advanced CP, resulting in a greater severity of the disease [2]. Accordingly, our data showed that, in individuals presenting mild-moderate CP, the Th17 cytokine (IL-17) proved to be positively correlated with the Th1 (IL-2 and INF-γ) cytokine profile, while in individuals presenting advanced CP these correlations were not observed. This result suggests that the balance of Th17/Th1 cytokines is involved in the amplification of inflammatory reaction, especially in the early stages of periodontal disease.

Differences in cytokines levels can be observed in accordance with the applied methodology. Analysis of the IL-6 levels in gingival crevicular fluid (GCF) of patients with CP showed a decrease in disease sites, as compared to non-diseased sites [37,44]. However, an increase in IL-6 levels could be identified in the gingival connective tissue adjacent to the intra-bony pocket [38] and the GCF of sites with CP [45–47]. The present study's data showed no significant differences in IL-4 and IL-6 but did register a significant increase in TNF-α, IL-2, INF-γ, IL-10, and IL-17 levels in tissues with CP when compared to the NM. By contrast, IL-4 [29] and IFN-γ [29,47] levels showed a significant reduction in patients with CP, as compared to those of healthy gingival samples, while other studies demonstrated an increase in IL-4 [4] and IL-6 [44] after treatment, suggesting a protective role for these cytokines.

In most studies evaluating DCs in periodontal disease, an increase in these cells can be observed in diseased tissues, as compared to healthy samples, although a decrease in the later processes of the disease can also be seen [48–55]. In the present study, positive correlations could be identified between immature DCs and probing depth. Likewise, fewer immature DCs could be found in the group of individuals with advanced CP. Although no comparisons were performed between diseased tissue and NM, these data indicate that increased numbers of immature DCs are associated with the initial stage of periodontal disease. In addition, negative correlations could be observed between immature DCs and CAL>3, as well as between immature DCs and CAL>5, thus suggesting that these cells decrease with the severity of CP.

The present study found an increase in the percentage of sites with PD>4 and CAL >3, and IL-6 levels and immature DCs with higher inflammatory infiltrate. In a previous study by our research group, an increase in immature DCs with inflammatory infiltrate was identified, while mature DCs proved to be positively correlated with mild inflammatory infiltrate in samples presenting chronic gingivitis [23]. In this study, a decrease in mature DCs, with higher inflammatory infiltrate, could be observed. This observation was also associated with the absence of these cells in the SE, a region characterized by intense inflammatory infiltrate in the adjacent LP. Therefore, the inverse relation of mature DCs with inflammatory infiltrate may well explain their absence in the SE.

In conclusion, the IL-6 can contribute to the increase of the immature DCs in the CP, in turn impacting the inflammatory response. Higher levels of IL-2, TNF-α, INF-γ, IL-10, and IL-17A cytokines in the gingival tissue are related to human CP, while higher densities of inflammatory infiltrate and lower densities of

Table 3. Correlations between pro-inflammatory, Th1, Th2 and Th7 profiles of cytokines in all individuals with chronic periodontitis (CP), or in individuals with mild-moderate CP and individuals with advanced CP.

	Pro-inflammatory cytokines		Th1 cytokines		Th2 cytokines		Th17 cytokines
Individuals with CP (n = 24)	TNF-α	IL-6	IFN- γ	IL-2	IL-4	IL-10	IL-17
TNF-α	1	−0.20	0.42*	0.65*	0.75*	0.70*	0.60*
IL-6		1	0.07	−0.09	0.03	−0.03	0.04
IFN-γ			1	0.59*	0.59*	0.56*	0.50*
IL-2				1	0.58*	0.73*	0.52*
IL-4					1	0.55*	0.63*
IL-10						1	0.50*
Mild-moderate CP group (n = 10)	TNF-α	IL-6	IFN-γ	IL-2	IL-4	IL-10	IL-17
TNF-α	1	−0.05	0.47	0.76*	0.61	0.86*	0.65*
IL-6		1	0.51	0.00	0.23	0.20	0.34
IFN-ɣ			1	0.43	0.78*	0.67*	0.72*
IL-2				1	0.51	0.75*	0.75*
IL-4					1	0.61	0.58
IL-10						1	0.87*
Advanced CP group (n = 14)	TNF-α	IL-6	IFN-γ	IL-2	IL-4	IL-10	IL-17
TNF-α	1	−0.24	0.27	0.52	0.86*	0.54*	0.64*
IL-6		1	−0.17	−0.11	−0.16	−0.21	10.15
IFN-ɣ			1	0.65*	0.37	0.38	0.44
IL-2				1	0.55*	0.60*	0.43
IL-4					1	0.42	0.66*
IL-10						1	0.40

* $p < 0.05$, Spearman correlation coefficient.

immature and mature DCs may well result in much more severe degree of human CP.

Author Contributions

Conceived and designed the experiments: FOC RAM. Performed the experiments: GRS CMQJ. Analyzed the data: GRS MHNGA. Contributed reagents/materials/analysis tools: RAM. Wrote the paper: GRS RAM.

References

1. Wykes M, Pombo A, Jenkins C, MacPherson GG (1998) Dendritic cells interact directly with naive B lymphocytes to transfer antigen and initiate class switching in a primary T-dependent response. J Immunol 161:1313–1319.
2. Armitage GC (2004) Periodontal diagnoses and classification of periodontal diseases. Periodontol 2000 34:9–21.
3. Tonetti MS, Claffey N (2005) Advances in the progression of periodontitis and proposal of definitions of a periodontitis case and disease progression for use in risk factor research. Group C consensus report of the 5th European Workshop in Periodontology. J Clin Periodontol 32 Suppl 6:210–213.
4. Zhao L, Zhou Y, Xu Y, Sun Y, Li L, et al. (2011) Effect of non-surgical periodontal therapy on the levels of Th17/Th1/Th2 cytokines and their transcription factors in Chinese chronic periodontitis patients. J Clin Periodontol 38:509–516.
5. Graves D (2008) Cytokines that promote periodontal tissue destruction. J Periodontol 79:1585–1591.
6. Liu YC, Lerner UH, Teng YT (2010) Cytokine responses against periodontal infection: protective and destructive roles. Periodontol 2000 52:163–206.
7. Cutler CW, Jotwani R (2004) Antigen-presentation and the role of dendritic cells in periodontitis. Periodontol 2000 35:135–157.
8. Schmidt SV, Nino-Castro AC, Schultze JL (2012) Regulatory dendritic cells: there is more than just immune activation. Front Immunol 3:274.
9. Jotwani R, Moonga BS, Gupta S, Cutler CW (2010) Nuclear factor-kappaB p50 subunits in chronic periodontitis and Porphyromonas gingivalis lipopolysaccharide-pulsed dendritic cells. Ann N Y Acad Sci 1192:278–285.
10. Moutsopoulos NM, Kling HM, Angelov N, Jin W, Palmer RJ, et al. (2012) Porphyromonas gingivalis promotes Th17 inducing pathways in chronic periodontitis. J Autoimmun 39:294–303.
11. Tew JG, El Shikh ME, El Sayed RM, Schenkein HA (2012) Dendritic cells, antibodies reactive with oxLDL, and inflammation. J Dent Res 91:8–16.
12. Jotwani R, Palucka AK, Al-Quotub M, Nouri-Shirazi M, Bell D, et al. (2001) Mature dendritic cells infiltrate the T cell-rich region of oral mucosa in chronic periodontitis: in situ, in vivo, and in vitro studies. J Immunol 167:4693–4700.
13. Allam JP, Duan Y, Heinemann F, Winter J, Götz W, et al. (2011) IL-23-producing CD68(+) macrophage-like cells predominate within an IL-17-polarized infiltrate in chronic periodontitis lesions. J Clin Periodontol 38:879–886.
14. Murphy KM, Reiner SL (2002) The lineage decisions of helper T cells. Nat Rev Immunol 2:933–944.
15. Sallusto F, Lanzavecchia A (2009) Heterogeneity of CD4+ memory T cells: functional modules for tailored immunity. Eur J Immunol 39:2076–2082.
16. Kawashima N, Stashenko P (1999) Expression of bone-resorptive and regulatory cytokines in murine periapical inflammation. Arch Oral Biol 44:55–66.
17. Jankovic D, Liu Z, Gause WC (2001) Th1- and Th2-cell commitment during infectious disease: asymmetry in divergent pathways. Trends Immunol 22:450–457.
18. Lappin DF, MacLeod CP, Kerr A, Mitchell T, Kinane DF (2001) Anti-inflammatory cytokine IL-10 and T cell cytokine profile in periodontitis granulation tissue. Clin Exp Immunol 123:294–300.
19. Gemmell E, Yamazaki K, Seymour GJ (2007) The role of T cells in periodontal disease: homeostasis and autoimmunity. Periodontol 2000 43:14–40.
20. Garlet GP, Cardoso CR, Campanelli AP, Garlet TP, Ávila-Campos MJ, et al. (2008) The essential role of IFN-gamma in the control of lethal Aggregatibacter actinomycetemcomitans infection in mice. Microbes Infect 10:489–496. \
21. Laurence A, O'Shea JJ (2007) T(H)-17 differentiation: of mice and men. Nat Immunol 8:903–905.
22. Lopez NJ, Da Silva I, Ipinza J, Gutierrez J (2005) Periodontal therapy reduces the rate of preterm low birth weight in women with pregnancy-associated gingivitis. J Periodontol 76:2144–2153.
23. Souto GR, Segundo TK, Costa FO, Aguiar MC, Mesquita RA (2011) Effect of smoking on Langerhans and dendritic cells in patients with chronic gingivitis. J Periodontol 82:619–625.
24. Caux C, Vanbervliet B, Massacrier C, Dezutter-Dambuyant C, Saint-Vis B, et al. (1996) CD34+ hematopoietic progenitors from human cord blood differentiate along two independent dendritic cell pathways in response to GM-CSF+TNF alpha. J Exp Med 184:695–706.
25. Caux C, Massacrier C, Vanbervliet B, Dubois B, Dubois I, et al. (1997) CD34+ hematopoietic progenitors from human cord blood differentiate along two independent dendritic cell pathways in response to granulocyte-macrophage colony-stimulating factor plus tumor necrosis factor alpha: II. Functional analysis. Blood 90:1458–1470.
26. Dereka XE, Tosios KI, Chrysomali E, Angelopoulou E (2004) Factor XIIIa+ dendritic cells and S-100 protein+ Langerhans' cells in adult periodontitis. J Periodontal Res 39:447–452.
27. Lechmann M, Berchtold S, Hauber J, Steinkasserer A (2002) CD83 on dendritic cells: more than just a marker for maturation. Trends Immunol 23:273–275.
28. Cohen J (1988) Statistical Power Analysis for the Behavioral Sciences, 2nd ed. Hillsdale, NJ: Lawrence Erlbaum Associates. 140–151p.
29. Behfarnia P, Birang R, Andalib AR, Asadi S (2010) Comparative Evaluation of IFNgamma, IL4 and IL17 Cytokines in Healthy Gingiva and Moderate to Advanced Chronic Periodontitis. Dent Res J (Isfahan) 7:45–50.
30. Cella M, Sallusto F, Lanzavecchia A (1997) Origin, maturation and antigen presenting function of dendritic cells. Curr Opin Immunol 9:10–16.
31. Reis e Sousa C (2001) Dendritic cells as sensors of infection. Immunity 14:495–498.
32. Lannes N, Summerfield A (2013) Regulation of Porcine Plasmacytoid Dendritic Cells by Cytokines. PLoS ONE 8(4): e60893. doi:10.1371/journal.pone.0060893
33. Bridges RB, Kraal JH, Huang LJ, Chancellor MB (1977) Effects of cigarette smoke components on in vitro chemotaxis of human polymorphonuclear leukocytes. Infect Immun 16:240–248.
34. Frick JS, Grunebach F, Autenrieth IB (2010) Immunomodulation by semi-mature dendritic cells: a novel role of Toll-like receptors and interleukin-6. Int J Med Microbiol 300:19–24.
35. Lunz JG 3rd, Specht SM, Murase N, Isse K, Demetris AJ (2007) Gut-derived commensal bacterial products inhibit liver dendritic cell maturation by stimulating hepatic interleukin-6/signal transducer and activator of transcription 3 activity. Hepatology 46:1946–1959.
36. Hegde S, Pahne J, Smola-Hess S (2004) Novel immunosuppressive properties of interleukin-6 in dendritic cells: inhibition of NF-kappaB binding activity and CCR7 expression. FASEB J 18:1439–1441.
37. Huang CB, Altimova Y, Strange S, Ebersole JL (2011) Polybacterial challenge effects on cytokine/chemokine production by macrophages and dendritic cells. Inflamm Res. 60(2):119–25.
38. Guillot JL, Pollock SM, Johnson RB (1995) Gingival interleukin-6 concentration following phase I therapy. J Periodontol 66:667–672.
39. Baker PJ, Dixon M, Evans RT, Dufour L, Johnson E, et al. (1999) CD4(+) T cells and the proinflammatory cytokines gamma interferon and interleukin-6 contribute to alveolar bone loss in mice. Infect Immun 67:2804–2809.
40. Ishimi Y, Miyaura C, Jin CH, Akatsu T, Abe E, et al. (1990) IL-6 is produced by osteoblasts and induces bone resorption. J Immunol 145:3297–3303.
41. Yu JJ, Ruddy MJ, Conti HR, Boonanantanasarn K, Gaffen SL (2008) The interleukin-17 receptor plays a gender-dependent role in host protection against Porphyromonas gingivalis-induced periodontal bone loss. Infect Immun 76:4206–4213.
42. Jilka RL, Hangoc G, Girasole G, Passeri G, William DC, et al. (1992) Increased osteoclast development after estrogen loss: mediation by interleukin-6. Science 257:88–91.
43. Trombone AP, Claudino M, Colavite P, de Assis GF, Àvila-Campos MJ, et al. (2010) Periodontitis and arthritis interaction in mice involves a shared hyper-inflammatory genotype and functional immunological interferences. Genes Immun 11:479–489.
44. Goutoudi P, Diza E, Arvanitidou M (2012) Effect of periodontal therapy on crevicular fluid interleukin-6 and interleukin-8 levels in chronic periodontitis. Int J Dent 362905.
45. Cardoso CR, Garlet GP, Crippa GE, Rosa AL, Júnior WM, et al. (2009) Evidence of the presence of T helper type 17 cells in chronic lesions of human periodontal disease. Oral Microbiol Immunol 24:1–6.
46. Tymkiw KD, Thunell DH, Johnson GK, Joly S, Burnell KK, et al. (2011) Influence of smoking on gingival crevicular fluid cytokines in severe chronic periodontitis. J Clin Periodontol 38:219–228.
47. Thunell DH, Tymkiw KD, Johnson GK, Joly S, Burnell KK, et al. (2010) A multiplex immunoassay demonstrates reductions in gingival crevicular fluid cytokines following initial periodontal therapy. J Periodontal Res 2010;45:148–152.
48. Seguier S, Godeau G, Brousse N (2000) Immunohistological and morphometric analysis of intra-epithelial lymphocytes and Langerhans cells in healthy and diseased human gingival tissues. Arch Oral Biol 45:441–452.
49. Cury PR, Furuse C, Rodrigues AE, Barbuto JA, Araujo VC, et al. (2008) Interstitial and Langerhans' dendritic cells in chronic periodontitis and gingivitis. Braz Oral Res 22:258–263.
50. Anjana R, Joseph L, Suresh R (2012) Immunohistochemical localization of CD1a and S100 in gingival tissues of healthy and chronic periodontitis subjects. Oral Dis 18:778–785.
51. Vassallo R, Kroening PR, Parambil J, Kita H (2008) Nicotine and oxidative cigarette smoke constituents induce immune-modulatory and pro-inflammatory dendritic cell responses. Mol Immunol 45:3321–3329.

52. Bratke K, Klug M, Bier A, Julius P, Kuepper M, et al. (2008) Function-associated surface molecules on airway dendritic cells in cigarette smokers. Am J Respir Cell Mol Biol 38:655–660.
53. Newcomb GM, Seymour GJ, Powell RN (1982) Association between plaque accumulation and Langerhans cell numbers in the oral epithelium of attached gingiva. J Clin Periodontol 9:297–304.
54. Smyth LJ, Starkey C, Gordon FS, Vestbo J, Singh D (2008) CD8 chemokine receptors in chronic obstructive pulmonary disease. Clin Exp Immunol 154:56–63.
55. Rezavandi K, Palmer RM, Odell EW, Scott DA, Wilson RF (2002) Expression of ICAM-1 and E-selectin in gingival tissues of smokers and non-smokers with periodontitis. J Oral Pathol Med 31:59–64.

Permissions

All chapters in this book were first published in PLOS ONE, by The Public Library of Science; hereby published with permission under the Creative Commons Attribution License or equivalent. Every chapter published in this book has been scrutinized by our experts. Their significance has been extensively debated. The topics covered herein carry significant findings which will fuel the growth of the discipline. They may even be implemented as practical applications or may be referred to as a beginning point for another development.

The contributors of this book come from diverse backgrounds, making this book a truly international effort. This book will bring forth new frontiers with its revolutionizing research information and detailed analysis of the nascent developments around the world.

We would like to thank all the contributing authors for lending their expertise to make the book truly unique. They have played a crucial role in the development of this book. Without their invaluable contributions this book wouldn't have been possible. They have made vital efforts to compile up to date information on the varied aspects of this subject to make this book a valuable addition to the collection of many professionals and students.

This book was conceptualized with the vision of imparting up-to-date information and advanced data in this field. To ensure the same, a matchless editorial board was set up. Every individual on the board went through rigorous rounds of assessment to prove their worth. After which they invested a large part of their time researching and compiling the most relevant data for our readers.

The editorial board has been involved in producing this book since its inception. They have spent rigorous hours researching and exploring the diverse topics which have resulted in the successful publishing of this book. They have passed on their knowledge of decades through this book. To expedite this challenging task, the publisher supported the team at every step. A small team of assistant editors was also appointed to further simplify the editing procedure and attain best results for the readers.

Apart from the editorial board, the designing team has also invested a significant amount of their time in understanding the subject and creating the most relevant covers. They scrutinized every image to scout for the most suitable representation of the subject and create an appropriate cover for the book.

The publishing team has been an ardent support to the editorial, designing and production team. Their endless efforts to recruit the best for this project, has resulted in the accomplishment of this book. They are a veteran in the field of academics and their pool of knowledge is as vast as their experience in printing. Their expertise and guidance has proved useful at every step. Their uncompromising quality standards have made this book an exceptional effort. Their encouragement from time to time has been an inspiration for everyone.

The publisher and the editorial board hope that this book will prove to be a valuable piece of knowledge for researchers, students, practitioners and scholars across the globe.

List of Contributors

Teresa Lorenzi, Maria Lorenzi, Francesca Paolinelli, Giorgio Barbatelli and Mario Castellucci
Department of Experimental and Clinical Medicine, Universita` Politecnica delle Marche, Ancona, Italy

Elena Annabel Nițulescu, Monica Baniță and Ștefania Crăițoiu
Department of Histology, University of Medicine and Pharmacy of Craiova, Craiova, Romania

Antonio Zizzi, Gaia Goteri and Corrado Rubini
Pathological Anatomy, Department of Medical Sciences and Public Health, Universita` Politecnica delle Marche, United Hospitals, Ancona, Italy

Simone Domenico Aspriello
Department of Clinical Specialistic and Dental Sciences, Periodontology, Universita` Politecnica delle Marche, Ancona, Italy

Tommaso Lombardi
Laboratory of Oral and Maxillofacial Pathology, Division of Stomatology and Oral Surgery, University of Geneva, Geneva, Switzerland

Roberto Di Felice
Private Dental Practice, San Benedetto del Tronto, Ascoli Piceno, Italy

Matteo Serino, Elodie Riant, Jean-François Arnal, , Pierre Gourdy and Rémy Burcelin
Institut National de la Santé et de la Recherche Me´dicale (INSERM), Toulouse, France
Université Paul Sabatier, Unité Mixte de Recherche (UMR) 1048, Institut de Maladies Métaboliques et Cardiovasculaires (I2MC), Toulouse, France

Vincent Blasco-Baque and Pascale Loubieres
Institut National de la Santé et de la Recherche Me´dicale (INSERM), Toulouse, France
Université Paul Sabatier, Unité Mixte de Recherche (UMR) 1048, Institut de Maladies Métaboliques et Cardiovasculaires (I2MC), Toulouse, France
L.U. 51, Parodontites et Maladies G énérales, Université Paul Sabatier, Faculté de Chirurgie Dentaire, 3, Chemin des Maraîchers, Toulouse, France

Jean-Noël Vergnes, Michel Sixou and Philippe Kemoun
L.U. 51, Parodontites et Maladies G énérales, Université Paul Sabatier, Faculté de Chirurgie Dentaire, 3, Chemin des Maraîchers, Toulouse, France

Juhi Bagaitkar and Carlo A. Daep
Department of Microbiology and Immunology, University of Louisville, Louisville, Kentucky, United States of America

Donald R. Demuth and David A. Scott
Department of Microbiology and Immunology, University of Louisville, Louisville, Kentucky, United States of America
Center of Oral Health and Systemic Disease, University of Louisville, Louisville, Kentucky, United States of America

Carol K. Patel and Diane E. Renaud
Center of Oral Health and Systemic Disease, University of Louisville, Louisville, Kentucky, United States of America

Akiko Kukita, Yuka Ichigi, Ippei Takigawa and Hiroshi Miyamoto
Department of Microbiology, Faculty of Medicine, Saga University, Saga, Japan

Toshiyuki Watanabe and Toshio Kukita
Molecular Cell Biology and Oral Anatomy, Faculty of Dental Science, Kyushu University, Fukuoka, Japan

Tamaki Takahashi, Shigeo Muro, Naoya Tanabe, Kunihiko Terada, Hirofumi Kiyokawa, Susumu Sato, Yuma Hoshino and Michiaki Mishima
Department of Respiratory Medicine, Kyoto University, Kyoto, Japan

Emiko Ogawa
Health Administration Center, Shiga University of Medical Science, Shiga, Japan

Kazuko Uno
Louis Pasteur Center for Medical Research, Kyoto, Japan

Koji Naruishi
Division of Endodontology, Iwate Medical University, Department of Conservative Dentistry and Oral Rehabilitation, Iwate, Japan

Shogo Takashiba
Department of Pathophysiology–Periodontal Science, Okayama University Graduate School of Medicine, Dentistry and Pharmaceutical Sciences, Okayama, Japan

Daniel H. Fine, Kenneth Markowitz, Karen Fairlie, Debbie Tischio-Bereski, Javier Ferrandiz, Dipti Godboley and David Furgang
Department of Oral Biology, School of Dental Medicine, Rutgers University, Newark, New Jersey, United States of America

John Gunsolley and Al Best
Department of Periodontics, School of Dentistry, Virginia Commonwealth of Virginia, Richmond, Virginia, United States of America

Jieun Shin, Yun S. Choi, Yong C. Kim and Youngnim Choi
Department of Immunology and Molecular Microbiology, BK21 CLS, School of Dentistry and Dental Research Institute, Seoul National University, Seoul, Korea

Sang-A Kho and In-Chul Rhyu
Department of Periodontology, BK21 CLS, School of Dentistry and Dental Research Institute, Seoul National University, Seoul, Korea

Kaining Liu, Huanxin Meng and Jianxia Hou
Department of Periodontology, Peking University School and Hospital of Stomatology, Beijing, China

Alisha G. Campbell
Genome Science and Technology Program, University of Tennessee, Knoxville, Tennessee, United States of America
Biosciences Division, Oak Ridge National Laboratories, Oak Ridge, Tennessee, United States of America

Mircea Podar
Genome Science and Technology Program, University of Tennessee, Knoxville, Tennessee, United States of America
Biosciences Division, Oak Ridge National Laboratories, Oak Ridge, Tennessee, United States of America
Department of Microbiology, University of Tennessee, Knoxville, Tennessee, United States of America

James H. Campbell and Steve Allman
Biosciences Division, Oak Ridge National Laboratories, Oak Ridge, Tennessee, United States of America

Patrick Schwientek, Tanja Woyke and Alexander Sczyrba
DOE Joint Genome Institute, Walnut Creek, California, United States of America

Clifford J. Beall, Ann Griffen and Eugene Leys
College of Dentistry, Ohio State University, Columbus, Ohio, United States of America

Dominik Kraus
Department of Prosthodontics, Preclinical Education, and Material Sciences, University of Bonn, Bonn, Germany
Clinical Research Unit 208, University of Bonn, Bonn, Germany

Jochen Winter and Søren Jepsen
Clinical Research Unit 208, University of Bonn, Bonn, Germany
Department of Periodontology, Operative and Preventive Dentistry, University of Bonn, Bonn, Germany

Andreas Jäger
Clinical Research Unit 208, University of Bonn, Bonn, Germany
Department of Orthodontics, University of Bonn, Bonn, Germany

James Deschner
Clinical Research Unit 208, University of Bonn, Bonn, Germany
Experimental Dento-Maxillo-Facial Medicine, University of Bonn, Bonn, Germany

Rainer Meyer
Institute of Physiology II, University of Bonn, Bonn, Germany

Anna Carolina Ratto Tempestini Horliana, Leandro Chambrone, Adriana Moura Foz, Hilana Paula Carillo Artese, Mariana de Sousa Rabelo, Cláudio Mendes Pannuti and Giuseppe Alexandre Romito
Department of Stomatology, School of Dentistry, University of São Paulo, São Paulo, Brazil

Yi Liu
Pediatric Research Institute, Qilu Children's Hospital of Shandong University, Ji'nan, Shandong, China

Yujie Zhang, Yang Guo and Shuiqing Xiao
Department of Orthodontic, Jinan Stomatological Hospital, Jinan, Shandong, China

Lili Wang
Clinical Laboratory, Jinan Central Hospital of Shandong University, Jinan, Shandong, China

Toshiyuki Nagasawa, Reiko Yashiro, Yukiko Bando and Hiroaki Kobayashi
Department of Periodontology, Tokyo Medical and Dental University, Tokyo, Japan

Hiromi Nanbara and Yuichi Izumi
Department of Periodontology, Tokyo Medical and Dental University, Tokyo, Japan

Global Center of Excellence Program, International Research Center for Molecular Science in Tooth and Bone Diseases, Tokyo Medical and Dental University, Tokyo, Japan

Nawarat Wara-aswapati, Janjura Khongcharoensuk and Doosadee Hormdee
Department of Periodontology, Faculty of Dentistry, Khon Kaen University, Khon Kaen, Thailand

Yasuhiro Yoshida
Department of Immunology, School of Medicine, University of Occupational and Environmental Health, Fukuoka, Japan

Waranuch Pitiphat
Department of Community Dentistry, Faculty of Dentistry, Khon Kaen University, Khon Kaen, Thailand

Jason A. Boch
Department of Oral Medicine, Infection and Immunity, Harvard School of Dental Medicine, Boston, Massachusetts, United States of America

Koichi Tabeta
Center for Transdisciplinary Research, Niigata University, Niigata, Japan

Tomoki Maekawa, Naoki Takahashi, Yukari Aoki, Hirotaka Miyashita, Sayuri Miyauchi, Haruna Miyazawa and Kazuhisa Yamazaki
Center for Transdisciplinary Research, Niigata University, Niigata, Japan
Laboratory of Periodontology and Immunology, Division of Oral Science for Health Promotion, Niigata University Graduate School of Medical and Dental Sciences, Niigata, Japan

Takako Nakajima
Center for Transdisciplinary Research, Niigata University, Niigata, Japan
General Dentistry and Clinical Education Unit, Niigata University Medical and Dental Hospital, Niigata, Japan

Karola Prior, Rafael Szczepanowski, Inga Harks, Benjamin Ehmke and Dag Harmsen
Department for Periodontology, University of Münster, Münster, Germany

Sebastian Jünemann
Department for Periodontology, University of Münster, Münster, Germany
Institute for Bioinformatics, Center for Biotechnology, Bielefeld University, Bielefeld, Germany

Alexander Goesmann
Institute for Bioinformatics, Center for Biotechnology, Bielefeld University, Bielefeld, Germany
Bioinformatics Resource Facility, Center for Biotechnology, Bielefeld University, Bielefeld, Germany

Jens Stoye
Institute for Bioinformatics, Center for Biotechnology, Bielefeld University, Bielefeld, Germany
Genome Informatics Group, Faculty of Technology, Bielefeld University, Bielefeld, Germany

Adrien Boillot, Bechara El Halabi, Hélène Rangé and Philippe Bouchard
Department of Periodontology, Service of Odontology, Rothschild Hospital, AP-HP, Paris 7 - Denis Diderot University, U.F.R. of Odontology, Paris, France
Department of Nutrition, Ambroise Pare´ Hospital, University Versailles St-Quentin, Boulogne-Billancourt, France

Sébastien Czernichow
Department of Nutrition, Ambroise Pare´ Hospital, University Versailles St-Quentin, Boulogne-Billancourt, France
INSERM, U1018, Centre for Research in Epidemiology and Population Health, Villejuif, France

George David Batty
Department of Epidemiology and Public Health, University College London, London, United Kingdom

Mi Zhou and Chunxia Zhu
State Key Laboratory Breeding Base of Basic Science of Stomatology, Key Laboratory of Oral Biomedicine Ministry of Education, School and Hospital of Stomatology, Wuhan University, Wuhan, Hubei, China

Qi Zhang
State Key Laboratory Breeding Base of Basic Science of Stomatology, Key Laboratory of Oral Biomedicine Ministry of Education, School and Hospital of Stomatology, Wuhan University, Wuhan, Hubei, China
Department of Endodontics, School of Stomatology, Tongji University, Shanghai, China

Ruichen Rong, Daniel Munro and Xiang Gao
Department of Biological Sciences, University of North Texas, Denton, Texas, United States of America

Qunfeng Dong
Department of Biological Sciences, University of North Texas, Denton, Texas, United States of America

Department of Computer Science and Engineering, University of North Texas, Denton, Texas, United States of America

Rajendra P. Settem, Kiyonobu Honma and Ashu Sharma
Department of Oral Biology, School of Dental Medicine, University at Buffalo, State University of New York, Buffalo, New York, United States of America

Georgios Papantonopoulos
Center for Research and Applications of Nonlinear Systems, Department of Mathematics, University of Patras, Patras, Greece

Keiso Takahashi
Department of Conservative Dentistry, School of Dentistry, Ohu University, Fukushima, Japan

Tasos Bountis
Laboratory of Nonlinear Systems and Applied Analysis, Department of Mathematics, University of Patras, Patras, Greece

Bruno G. Loos
Department of Periodontology, Academic Center for Dentistry Amsterdam (ACTA), University of Amsterdam and VU University, Amsterdam, The Netherlands

Adrian Markus Ramseier and Tuomas Waltimo
Department of Preventive Dentistry and Oral Microbiology, School of Dental Medicine, University of Basel, Basel, Switzerland

Matti Mauramo
Department of Preventive Dentistry and Oral Microbiology, School of Dental Medicine, University of Basel, Basel, Switzerland
Institute of Dentistry, University of Helsinki, Helsinki, Finland

Andreas Buser
The Blood Transfusion Service SRC Basel, Basel, Switzerland

Jean-Marie Tiercy
National Reference Laboratory for Histocompatibility, Geneva University Hospital and University of Geneva, Geneva, Switzerland

Roland Weiger
Clinic for Periodontology, Endodontology and Cariology, School of Dental Medicine, University of Basel, Basel, Switzerland

Virginia M. Barnes, Fotinos Panagakos, William Devizio and Harsh M. Trivedi
Colgate Palmolive Technology Center, Piscataway, NJ, United States of America

Shannon Cervi and Frank A. Scannapieco
Metabolon, Durham, NC, United States of America

Adam D. Kennedy, Thomas Jönsson and Lining Guo
Department of Oral Biology, School of Dental Medicine, University at Buffalo, State University of New York, Buffalo, NY, United States of America

Yung-Kai Huang
School of Oral Hygiene, College of Oral Medicine, Taipei Medical University, Taipei, Taiwan,

Wei-Fang Lee
School of Dental Technology, College of Oral Medicine, Taipei Medical University, Taipei, Taiwan

Meng-Jiy Wang
Department of Chemical Engineering, National Taiwan University of Science and Technology, Taipei, Taiwan

Yus-Han Sophie Chang and Wen-Shiun Tchaou
Division of Oral Rehabilitation and Center of Pediatric Dentistry, Department of Dentistry, Taipei Medical University Hospital, Taipei, Taiwan

Nai-Chia Teng
Division of Oral Rehabilitation and Center of Pediatric Dentistry, Department of Dentistry, Taipei Medical University Hospital, Taipei, Taiwan
School of Dentistry, College of Oral Medicine, Taipei Medical University, Taipei, Taiwan

Wei- Jen Chang
School of Dentistry, College of Oral Medicine, Taipei Medical University, Taipei, Taiwan

Sheng-Yang Lee
School of Dentistry, College of Oral Medicine, Taipei Medical University, Taipei, Taiwan
Dental Department of Wan-Fang Hospital, Taipei Medical University, Taipei, Taiwan

Joen-Rong Sheu
Department of Pharmacology, School of Medicine, College of Medicine, Taipei Medical University, Taipei, Taiwan
Graduate Institute of Medical Sciences, College of Medicine, Taipei Medical University, Taipei, Taiwan

Zuolin Jin
State Key Laboratory of Military Stomatology, Department of Orthodontics, School of Stomatology, The Fourth Military Medical University, Xi'an, Shaanxi, China

Jia Liu and Liying Wang
State Key Laboratory of Military Stomatology, Department of Orthodontics, School of Stomatology, The Fourth Military Medical University, Xi'an, Shaanxi, China
State Key Laboratory of Military Stomatology, Center for Tissue Engineering, School of Stomatology, The Fourth Military Medical University, Xi'an, Shaanxi, China

Wenjia Liu and Yan Jin
State Key Laboratory of Military Stomatology, Center for Tissue Engineering, School of Stomatology, The Fourth Military Medical University, Xi'an, Shaanxi, China
Research and Development Center for Tissue Engineering, Fourth Military Medical University, Xi'an, Shaanxi, China

Qiang Li
State Key Laboratory of Military Stomatology, Department of General Dentistry and Emergency, School of Stomatology, The Fourth Military Medical University, Xi'an, Shaanxi, China

Carola Höglund Åberg and Anders Johansson
Division of Molecular Periodontology, Department of Odontology, Faculty of Medicine, Umea° University, Umeå, Sweden

Dorte Haubek
Section for Pediatric Dentistry, Department of Dentistry, Health, Aarhus University, Aarhus, Denmark

Francis Kwamin
Dental School University of Ghana, Accra, Ghana

Rolf Claesson
Oral Microbiology, Department of Odontology, Faculty of Medicine, Umeå University, Umeå, Sweden

Yunfei Zheng
Department of Oral and Maxillofacial Surgery, Peking University School and Hospital of Stomatology, Beijing, P.R. China
Department of Periodontology, Peking University School and Hospital of Stomatology, Beijing, P.R. China

Lingfei Jia
Department of Oral and Maxillofacial Surgery, Peking University School and Hospital of Stomatology, Beijing, P.R. China
Laboratory of Molecular Biology, Peking University School and Hospital of Stomatology, Beijing, China

Jianxia Hou, Xian'e Wang and Huanxin Meng
Department of Periodontology, Peking University School and Hospital of Stomatology, Beijing, P.R. China

Lei Peng
Department of Stomatology, Beijing Friendship Hospital, Capital Medical University, Beijing, P.R. China

Xin Zhang
Department of Stomatology, Peking Union Medical College Hospital, Chinese Academy of Medical Science, Beijing, P.R. China

Alisha G. Campbell and Mircea Podar
Biosciences Division, Oak Ridge National Laboratory, Oak Ridge, Tennessee, United States of America
Genome Science and Technology Program, University of Tennessee, Knoxville, Tennessee, United States of America

Ann L. Griffen
Division of Pediatric Dentistry and Community Oral Health, College of Dentistry, The Ohio State University, Columbus, Ohio, United States of America

Juan Wu, Yu Liu and Weibin Sun
Department of Periodontology, Hospital of Stomatology, Medical School, Nanjing University, Nanjing, Jiangsu Province, China

Jie Yang
Department of Periodontology, Hospital of Stomatology, Medical School, Nanjing University, Nanjing, Jiangsu Province, China
Central Laboratory of Stomatology, Hospital of Stomatology, Medical School, Nanjing University, Nanjing, Jiangsu Province, China

Jin Huang and Zhipin Lu
Department of Cardiology, Nanjing Chest Hospital, Nanjing, Jiangsu Province, China

Liping Xie and Yong Ji
Key Laboratory of Cardiovascular Disease and Molecular Intervention, Atherosclerosis Research Centre, Nanjing Medical University, Nanjing, Jiangsu Province, China

Mutsumi Miyauchi, Toshihiro Inubushi, Hisako Furusho, Toshinori Ando, Nurina Febriyanti Ayuningtyas, Atsuhiro Nagasaki and Takashi Takata
Department of Oral and Maxillofacial Pathobiology, Institute of Biomedical and Health Sciences, Hiroshima University, Hiroshima, Japan

Min Ao.
Department of Oral and Maxillofacial Pathobiology, Institute of Biomedical and Health Sciences, Hiroshima University, Hiroshima, Japan
Department of Pediatric Dentistry, Institute of Biomedical and Health Sciences, Hiroshima University, Hiroshima, Japan

Katsuyuki Kozai
Department of Pediatric Dentistry, Institute of Biomedical and Health Sciences, Hiroshima University, Hiroshima, Japan

Masae Kitagawa
Center of Oral Clinical Examination, Hiroshima University Hospital, Hiroshima University, Hiroshima, Japan

Kazuyuki Ishihara
Department of Microbiology, Tokyo Dental College, Tokyo, Japan

Hidetoshi Tahara
Department of Cellular and Molecular Biology, Institute of Biomedical and Health Sciences, Hiroshima University, Hiroshima, Japan

Aurigena Antunes de Araú jo
Post Graduation Program Public Health/Post Graduation Program in Pharmaceutical Science/ Department of Biophysics and Pharmacology, UFRN, Natal, Rio Grande do Norte, Brazil

Hugo Varela
Post Graduation Program Public Health/Department of Dentistry, UFRN, Natal, Rio Grande do Norte, Brazil

Gerly Anne de Castro Brito
Post Graduation Program in Pharmacology/ Department of Morphology, UFC, Fortaleza, Ceará, Brazil

Caroline Addison Carvalho Xavier de Medeiros
Department of Biophysics and Pharmacology, UFRN, Post Graduation Program in Health and Society, UERN, Natal, Rio Grande do Norte, Brazil

Lorena de Souza Araú jo
Department of Dentistry, UFRN, Natal, Rio Grande do Norte, Brazil

José Heriberto Oliveira do Nascimento
Department of Textile Engineered, UFRN, Natal, Rio Grande do Norte, Brazil,

Raimundo Fernandes de Araú jo Júnior
Post Graduation Program in Functional and Structural Biology/Post Graduation Program Health Science/ Department of Morphology, UFRN, Natal, Rio Grande do Norte, Brazil

Clifford J. Beall, Daniel M. Dayeh and Eugene J. Leys
Division of Oral Biology, College of Dentistry, The Ohio State University, Columbus, Ohio, United States of America

Giovanna Ribeiro Souto, Celso Martins Queiroz-Junior, Fernando Oliveira Costa and Ricardo Alves Mesquita
Department of Oral Surgery and Pathology, School of Dentistry, Universidade Federal de Minas Gerais, Belo Horizonte, Minas Gerais, Brazil

Mauro Henrique Nogueira Guimarães de Abreu
Department of Social and Preventive Dentistry, School of Dentistry, Universidade Federal de Minas Gerais, Belo Horizonte, Minas Gerais, Brazil

Index